LIFE AND HEALTH

CONTRIBUTING CONSULTANTS

S. Howard Bartley, Ph.D., *Michigan State University*

Abraham I. Braude, M.D., Ph.D., *School of Medicine, University of California, San Diego*

George M. Briggs, Ph.D., *University of California, Berkeley*

G. A. DeLaria, M.D., Ph.D. candidate, *University of California, San Diego*

J. Anthony Deutsch, Ph.D., *University of California, San Diego*

Joyce A. F. Diener, Ph.D., *Del Mar, California*

Fitzhugh Dodson, Ph.D., *La Primera Preschool, Redondo Beach, California*

Joel Fort, M.D., *Fort Help, San Francisco, California*

Paul H. Gebhard, Ph.D., *Institute for Sex Research, Indiana University*

Luigi Giacometti, Ph.D., *Oregon Zoology Research Center*

Jeoffry B. Gordon, M.D., *School of Medicine, University of California, San Diego*

Ralph M. Grawunder, Ed.D., *San Diego State College*

Clifford Grobstein, Ph.D., *School of Medicine, University of California, San Diego*

Ruth H. Grobstein, Ph.D., *School of Medicine, University of California, San Diego*

Barbara E. Gunning, Ph.D., *San Diego State College*

Seymour L. Halleck, M.D., Ph.D., Sc.D., *University of Wisconsin*

Daniel Horn, Ph.D., *National Clearinghouse for Smoking and Health*

Michael C. Hosokawa, Ed.D., *University of Oregon*

Morton Hunt, B.A., *New York*

J. Willis Hurst, M.D., *School of Medicine, Emory University*

Warren R. Johnson, Ed.D., *University of Maryland, College Park*

Francis C. Kenel, Ed.D., *University of Maryland*

Lois P. Kessler, M.A., *San Diego State College*

Robert W. Kistner, M.D., *Harvard Medical School, Boston Hospital for Women*

Dennis Krebs, Ph.D., *Harvard University*

Fred Leavitt, Ph.D., *California State College at Hayward*

Charles E. Lewis, M.D., D.Sc., *University of California, Los Angeles*

Purvis L. Martin, M.D., *School of Medicine, University of California, San Diego*

Jean Mayer, Ph.D., D.Sc., *Harvard University*

David C. McClelland, Ph.D., *Harvard University*

Aubrey C. McTaggart, Ph.D., *San Diego State College*

William Montagna, Ph.D., D.Sc., D. Biol. Sci., *Oregon Regional Primate Research Center*

William D. Ross, Ph.D., *Simon Fraser University*

Marvin J. Schissel, D.D.S., *Triboro Hospital, New York*

Eugene Schoenfeld, M.D., *San Francisco*

Michael B. Shimkin, M.D., *School of Medicine, University of California, San Diego*

William C. Sloan, Ph.D., *San Diego State College*

David E. Smith, M.D., *Haight-Ashbury Medical Clinic, San Francisco General Hospital, San Francisco Medical Center*

Walter D. Sorochan, Ph.D., *San Diego State College*

Curt Stern, Ph.D., D.Sc., *University of California, Berkeley*

Robert Straus, Ph.D., *College of Medicine, University of Kentucky, Lexington*

Jared R. Tinklenberg, M.D., *Stanford University*

Silvio S. Varon, M.D., Engin.D., *University of California, San Diego*

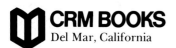

CRM BOOKS
Del Mar, California

LIFE AND HEALTH

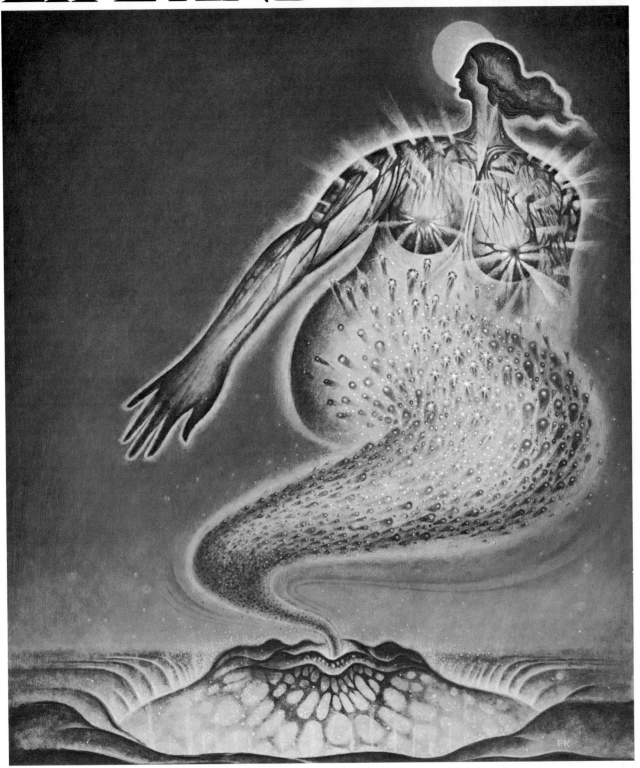

PREFACE

Imagine yourself as a cave dweller whose energies are confined to collecting firewood and stalking wild animals whose bodies provide food and clothing. Your life, if you are successful in your daily tasks, allows you approximately twenty years filled with the burden of mere survival. ¶ As a resident of fourteenth-century England, while your daily existence is less fraught with the endless search for food and fuel, you hear the village bell toll again and again, marking yet another victim of the dreaded Black Death. Your life will probably end before you are fifty. ¶ As an American in the 1970s, you no longer face the daily need for time-consuming food gathering or dread the devastating plague; the satisfaction of your basic needs is taken for granted. Through the centuries man's foes have slowly evolved from being obvious external ones to predominantly self-inflicted ones: degenerative diseases such as atherosclerosis and emphysema; aggravating, sometimes fatal pollutants; ignorant abuse of dangerous drugs; and tremendous psychological pressures that arise out of societal and personal demands. ¶ In a setting that overflows with phenomenal scientific advances, each man's life (and most of us can expect to live to at least seventy) is no longer a conscious quest for sheer physical survival but is focused on achieving increasingly higher degrees of well-being. But all the knowledge science has to offer is of little value in and of itself—it must be comprehended, evaluated, and applied. It is therefore the goal of this book, *Life and Health*, to help you determine your personal needs and values in the light of current thought in the areas of mental and emotional health, the potentials and limitations of drugs, the functioning of the human body, disease facts and theories, nutrition, ecology, and trends and techniques in current medical practice. ¶ *Life and Health* is not just a book for the classroom (an endless list of dos and don'ts); it is current thought and information to be applied to individual daily lives. The purpose of this book, then, is not to suggest a list of *solutions* to health problems but to isolate some of the most perplexing *questions* and provide opinions, data, and facts that help in investigating those questions. If you want to rise above the level of the barely subsisting caveman or the disease-fearing medieval Englishman, if you are to thrive, to achieve your own personal goals, you must see yourself as having a life that you, rather than external forces, can direct and control.

John H. Painter Jr.
Publisher

I Foundations of Health Science 3

1 Introduction to Health Science 5
MEANS TO HEALTH 6
Health Research 7
Health Education 7
Health Implementation 8
OBSTACLES TO HEALTH 9
THE PERSONAL STAKE IN HEALTH 11

2 The Body in Action 15
THE SKELETAL SYSTEM 20
THE MUSCULAR SYSTEM 21
THE CIRCULATORY SYSTEM 23
THE RESPIRATORY SYSTEM 27
THE DIGESTIVE SYSTEM 29
THE EXCRETORY SYSTEM 35
THE ENDOCRINE SYSTEM 37
The Thyroid and Pituitary Glands 37
The Adrenal Glands 38
THE NERVOUS SYSTEM 38
THE REPRODUCTIVE SYSTEM 43
A SYSTEM OF CELLS 45
MORE THAN THE SUM OF ITS PARTS 47

II Mental and Emotional Functioning 51

3 Physiological Basis of Behavior 53
THE PHYSIOLOGY OF THE NERVOUS SYSTEM 54
The Neuron 54
Transmission of Signals Between Neurons 57
Interaction Among Neurons 58
Topical Insert: "Autonomic Control" 55
THE NERVOUS SYSTEM AND BEHAVIOR 59
BRAIN FUNCTION 61
Visual Abstraction 61
Studies on Epilepsy 63
Brain Injury 64
The Neuron and Memory 66
EMOTIVE BEHAVIOR 66
Fight or Flight 66
Switches for Stereotyped Behavior 68
The Role of Chemical Transmitters in Emotions 70
THE DYNAMICS OF INVESTIGATION 73

4 Psychological Development 75
EMOTIONS 75
The Nature of Emotions 76
Unconscious Behavior 76
Emotional Development 78
THE ROLE OF HEREDITY 78
Ethological Theory 79

Freud's Psychoanalytic Theory 81
Erikson's Psychosocial Theory 81
The Competence Theory of Robert White 82
THE ROLE OF ENVIRONMENT 84
Learning Theory 85
Social Learning Theory 86
Cognitive-Developmental Theory 86
Enriched Environments 88
THE MATURE PERSONALITY 88
Rogerian Theory 88
Maslow's Humanistic Theory 89
CRITERIA FOR EMOTIONAL HEALTH 91

5 Mental Health and Mental Illness 93
THE PROBLEM OF DEFINITION 93
PROBLEMS IN EVERYDAY LIVING 95
Stress 96
Dealing with Stress 101
WHEN PROBLEMS GET OUT OF HAND 103
Neuroses 103
Depression 104
Psychoses 105
Personality Disorders 106
Psychophysiological Reactions 109
Topical Insert: "Schizophrenia" 107
HELP FOR PROBLEMS 109
Community Psychiatry 109
Symptomatic Treatment 110
Psychotherapy 111
Therapists and Their Training 115
Involuntary Commitment 115

III Chemical Alteration of Behavior 117

6 The Role of Drugs in the Good Life 119
PSYCHOACTIVE DRUGS 120
THE HISTORICAL PERSPECTIVE 120
DRUG ABUSE 122
HAZARDS AND COSTS OF DRUG USE 124
Habituation 124
Tolerance 124
Addiction 124
CAUSES OF DRUG USE AND ABUSE 126
Psychological Factors 126
Sociological Factors 127
Pharmacological Factors 130
Interaction of Factors 130
BEYOND DRUGS 131

7 Common Drugs of Misuse and Abuse 133
DEPRESSANTS 138
Sedative-Hypnotics 138
Opiates (Narcotics) 139
STIMULANTS 142
Caffeine 142
Amphetamines 143
Cocaine 145
PSYCHEDELIC-HALLUCINOGENS 145
LSD Effects 146
Other Hallucinogen-Psychedelics 148

Contents

CANNABIS (MARIJUANA) 148
Short-Term Effects 148
Long-Term Effects 150
TRANQUILIZERS 150
OTHER PSYCHOACTIVE AGENTS 151
AN ENDLESS LIST 151

8 Alcohol Abuse 153
SOURCES AND TYPES OF ALCOHOL 153
THE PHYSIOLOGICAL EFFECTS OF ALCOHOL 154
Alcohol Absorbtion and Blood Alcohol Level 155
Other Biochemical Factors 158
PSYCHOLOGICAL EFFECTS OF ALCOHOL 159
Motivation 160
Role of Experience 160
Drinking and the Family 161
Drinking Customs 161
DRINKING IN AMERICAN SOCIETY 162
Drinking Among Youth 162
Intoxication and Society 164
ALCOHOLISM 165
What Causes Alcoholism? 165
Treatment 169
FACING THE PROBLEM 169

9 Smoking and Health 171
THE MAN-MADE EPIDEMIC 172
COMPONENTS OF CIGARETTE SMOKE 173
SMOKE AS A DISEASE AGENT 174
Lung Cancer 174
Coronary Artery Disease 175
Bronchitis and Emphysema 175
Other Related Problems 175
PROFILE OF THE SMOKER 176
WHY PEOPLE SMOKE 177
SOLUTIONS TO THE SMOKING PROBLEM 178
For Those Who Smoke 180
The Bigger Picture 180

10 Controlling Drug Use and Abuse 183
PATTERNS OF DRUG USE AND ABUSE 184
Heroin 184
Pills 186
Alcohol and Nicotine 186
LSD-type Drugs 186
Marijuana 189

Topical Insert: "The Marijuana To Heroin Controversy" 187
DRUG TRAFFIC 189
Alcohol and Cigarettes 189
The Pill Traffic 189
LSD-type Drugs 189
Marijuana 190
Narcotics 191
DRUGS AND THE LAW 191
The Trend Changes 193
TREATMENT 195
Methadone Maintenance Treatment 198
Cyclazocine and Naloxone 199
TOWARD A SOLUTION 199

11 Drugs in Perspective 203
DRUGS AND SOCIETY 203
THE DRUG CREDIBILITY GAP 204
Sensationalism 204
LSD and Chromosomal Breakage 204
TOWARD ELIMINATING DRUG HYPOCRISY 206
THE FUTURE OF DRUG USE 207

IV Family Health 211

12 Human Sexuality 213
PSYCHOSOCIAL ASPECTS OF SEXUAL BEHAVIOR 213
PATTERNS OF SEXUAL ACTIVITY 214
Masturbation 214
Petting 214
Coitus 217
Homosexuality 218
Prostitution 220
PHYSIOLOGY OF COITUS 221
Female Cycle 222
Male Cycle 227
Sex Differences 229
Sexual Techniques 229
THE SEXUAL REVOLUTION 230

13 Reproduction and Birth Control 233

THE MALE CONTRIBUTION 233
THE FEMALE SYSTEM 234
The Uterus 234
The Fallopian Tubes 236
The Ovaries 237
Problems of Menstruation 239
Feminine Hygiene 240
PRENATAL DEVELOPMENT 241
PREGNANCY 243
Early Changes in Pregnancy 243
Visits to the Doctor 243
Blood Examinations 244
Discomforts of Pregnancy 245
Miscarriage 246
LABOR AND BIRTH 246
INFERTILITY 249
Male Infertility 249
Female Infertility 250
THE MENOPAUSE 250
Topical Insert: "You Can Choose Your Baby's Sex" 253
BIRTH CONTROL 252
Condoms 252
Coitus Interruptus 253
Rhythm Method 253
Spermicides and Diaphragms 253
Intrauterine Devices 258
Oral Contraceptives 259
Surgical Sterilization 259
Abortion 260
Future Methods of Contraception 262

14 Heredity and Health 265

THE TOOLS OF INHERITANCE 266
DNA and the Genetic Code 267
Genetic Machinery of the Cell 271
MECHANISMS OF INHERITANCE 273
HEREDITY VERSUS ENVIRONMENT 276
Schizophrenia 276
Intelligence 277
GENE ABNORMALITIES 278
Sickle Cell Anemia 278
Phenylketonuria (PKU) 279
Sphingolipidoses 280
Drug Abnormalities 280
Sex-Linked Gene Mutations 281

CHROMOSOME ABNORMALITIES 283
CONGENITAL DEFECTS 285
GENETIC COUNSELING 287

15 Marriage in American Society 291

CHANGING PERSPECTIVES 292
DIVORCE 295
INFIDELITY 296
COMARITAL SEX 297
NONLEGAL MARRIAGES 299
GROUP MARRIAGE 300
THE FUTURE OF MARRIAGE 302
THE WOMAN'S ROLE 304

16 Parenthood 309

TO HAVE OR NOT TO HAVE 309
Unwed Mothers 310
Effects of Children on Marriage 310
THE PARENTS' ROLE 311
Role in Emotional Development 312
Role in Social Development 313
Role in Intellectual Development 314
PARENT-CHILD INTERACTION 315
Discipline 316
No-Lose Method 317
Adolescence 318
SOCIAL-CLASS DIFFERENCES 319
A CHANGING SOCIETY 320
Topical Insert: "Wanted: A Dr. Spock for Black Mothers" 321
WHAT MAKES A GOOD PARENT? 323

V Personal Health Care 327

17 Nutrition 329
NUTRITION AND SOCIETY 329
COMPONENTS OF NUTRITION 330
Carbohydrates 332
Fats 333
Proteins 333
Vitamins 334
Minerals 336
THE WELL-BALANCED DIET 336
WEIGHT CONTROL 338
Obesity 338
Dieting 339
DIET AND HEART DISEASE 340
NUTRITION DURING PREGNANCY 342
Topical Insert: "The Health Food Myth" 343
THE NUTRITION GAP 342
World Food Needs 345
The Green Revolution 345
MISCONCEPTIONS ABOUT NUTRITION 349

18 Physical Fitness 351
ROLE OF FITNESS 351
ELEMENTS OF FITNESS 353
EXERCISE AND HEALTH 354
Role of Exercise in Hypokinetic Disorders 355
HOW FIT IS "FIT ENOUGH"? 356
WHAT EXERCISE AND HOW MUCH? 359
TOO MUCH OR TOO LITTLE 361
A LIFETIME NEED 362
FATIGUE 362
Physical Fatigue 364
Mental Fatigue 364
Causes of Fatigue 365
Overcoming Fatigue 365
SLEEP 366
Topical Insert: "Biological Clocks" 367

19 The Eyes and Ears 371
THE EYES 371
Structure and Function 371
Problems in Vision 374
Contact Lenses 377
THE EARS 378
Structure and Function 378
Hearing Losses 381
Hearing Aids and Tests 383

20 The Teeth, Skin, and Hair 385
THE TEETH AND SUPPORTING STRUCTURES 385
Structure and Function 386
Major Dental Diseases 389
Restorative Dental Procedures 391
Dental Prosthetics 392
Prevention 395
Topical Insert: "The Dr. Poorwork Affair" 393
THE SKIN AND HAIR 396
The Epidermis 397
The Dermis 397
The Pigment System 400
Nerve Endings 400
Common Skin Disorders 400
Plastic Surgery 401

VI Health and Disease 403

21 The Conquest of Disease 405
EPIDEMIOLOGY 406
Topical Insert: "Prescription Drugs" 409
CHANGING PATTERNS OF DISEASE 411
CAUSES OF DISEASE 413
Heredity 413
Diet 414
Infection 415
Environment 416
Stress 417
Degenerative Processes 418
CHEMOTHERAPY 419
CONQUEST – OR PARTIAL TRUCE? 421

22 Infectious Diseases 423

AGENTS OF INFECTION 424

Topical Insert: "Life on Man" 425

HOW INFECTION SPREADS 427

THE COURSE OF AN INFECTION 428

BODY DEFENSES 429

IMMUNITY 431

PREVENTION AND TREATMENT 432

COMMON INFECTIOUS DISEASES 434

The Common Cold 434

Influenza 435

Tuberculosis 436

Pneumonia 436

Mononucleosis 437

VENEREAL DISEASE 437

Syphilis 438

Gonorrhea 440

Prevention and Control of Infectious Disease 442

THE ROLE OF INFECTIOUS DISEASE 443

23 Cancer 445

UNCONTROLLED GROWTH 446

TYPES OF CANCER 448

DISTRIBUTION OF CANCER 448

HEREDITY AND ENVIRONMENT 448

CAUSES OF CANCER 450

Chemical Agents 450

Radiation 450

Viruses 451

Defective Immune Mechanism 453

PREVENTION OF CANCER 453

DETECTION AND DIAGNOSIS 454

CANCER TREATMENT 456

CANCER QUACKERY 457

24 Cardiovascular Diseases 459

ATHEROSCLEROSIS 460

Diet 462

Blood Pressure 462

Cigarette Smoking 462

Exercise 464

Multiplying the Risks 464

HEART ATTACKS 464

A Faltering Heartbeat 465

Heart Block 466

OTHER HEART PROBLEMS 466

Heart Failure 466

Cardiac Arrest and Emergency Treatment 466

Congenital Heart Disease 467

Rheumatic Heart Disease 468

HIGH BLOOD PRESSURE 468

STROKES 469

HEART TRANSPLANTATION AND ARTIFICIAL HEARTS 470

25 Systemic Diseases 473

DISORDERS OF THE IMMUNE SYSTEM 473

Allergy 474

Autoimmune Disease 475

DISORDERS OF THE RESPIRATORY SYSTEM 475

Chronic Bronchitis 475

Emphysema 477

KIDNEY DISORDERS 477

DISEASES OF THE DIGESTIVE TRACT 479

Inflammations 479

Gastric (Peptic) Ulcer 479

The Liver 480

The Pancreas 480

DISEASES OF THE ENDOCRINE SYSTEM 481

The Pituitary 481

Adrenals 481

Thyroid 483

Islet Cells of the Pancreas 483

DISEASES OF THE NERVOUS SYSTEM 484

26 Pollution and Health 487

POLLUTION AND POPULATION 488

ECOLOGY AS A SCIENCE 489

Topical Insert: "Survival Is Not Enough" 493

AIR POLLUTION 498

WATER POLLUTION 500

FOOD POLLUTION 501

NOISE POLLUTION 502

DIRECTIONS FOR THE FUTURE 505

27 Accidents and Safety 507

SCOPE OF THE ACCIDENT PROBLEM 508

THE CONCEPT OF ACCIDENT 508

ACCIDENTS AND THEIR VICTIMS 510

CAUSATION OF ACCIDENTS 513

The Individual 513

The Agent 515

The Environment 517

SAFETY AND CONSUMER PROTECTION 518

The Food and Drug Administration 519

State and Local Protection 523

Private Organizations 523

What Can Consumers Do? 524

Topical Insert: "The Safety-Happy FDA" 521

FOR A FUTURE WITH SAFETY 525

VII Health Care in America 527

28 Health Providers 529

CHANGING VIEWS OF COMMUNITY HEALTH 529

1900 to 1945 530

1945 to 1970 531

HEALTH ORGANIZATIONS 531

International Health Efforts 532

Government Agencies 533

Corporate Organizations 536

Volunteer Groups and Private Foundations 536

Professional Organizations 537

HEALTH PRACTITIONERS 538

Physicians 539

Selected Medical Practitioners 545

Medical Allied Manpower 545

Doctor of Dental Surgery (D.D.S.) 546

Dental Allied Manpower 546

Registered Nurses 547

Nursing Allied Manpower 547

Topical Insert: "Can Doctors Cause Disease?" 543

QUACKERY 548

Why Quacks Succeed 548

Health Advertising 550

Recognizing Quackery 551

29 Health Care Delivery 553

PROBLEM AREAS 554

Health Manpower 554

The Cost of Health Care 555

IMPROVING THE SYSTEM 558

Personnel Reforms 558

Health Coverage Reforms 560

The Delivery System 563

THE ROLE OF COMMUNITIES 566

Early Attempts at Community Involvement 566

Community-Generated Action 567

Prospective Roles of the Community 568

HEALTH CARE AND MEDICAL CARE 569

30 Health and the Individual 571

BASIC CONCEPTS OF HEALTH 571

CHALLENGES FOR THE FUTURE 573

INDIVIDUAL ACTION 576

Appendix A
Common Diseases of Man 578

Appendix B
A Survey of Drug Laws in the United States 587

Further Readings 600

Contributing Consultants 610

Glossary 618

Index 632

Credits and Acknowledgments 640

LIFE AND HEALTH

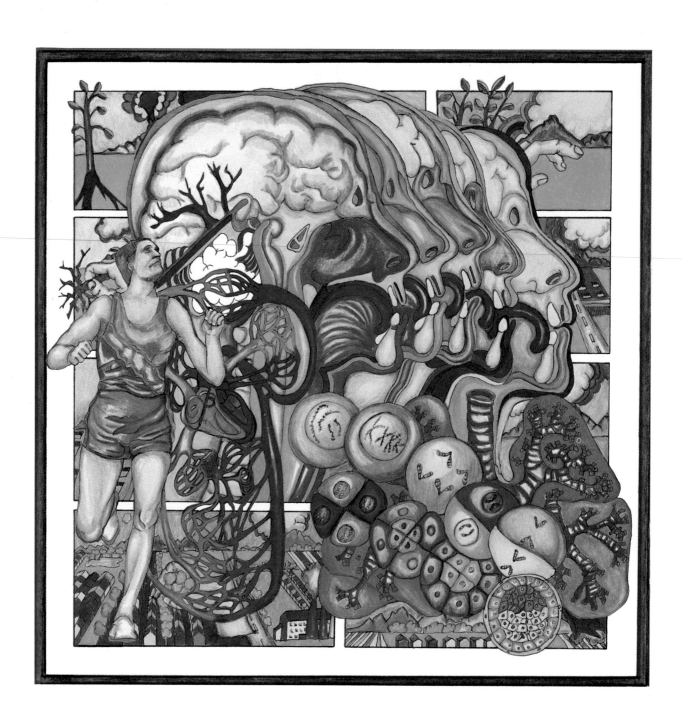

I FOUNDATIONS OF HEALTH SCIENCE

Whatever people do or fail to do regarding their health ultimately comes from one motive: to help one feel better. That is why people do or do not go to doctors, eat pizza, take dope, exercise, use deodorants, or buy insurance. But although the motive is always the same, the results differ widely. This difference is in part due to the individual's priorities—he may prefer the short-term "feeling better" of a banana split over the long-term benefits he would gain by maintaining a trim build. Another main reason is that many people simply do not know how to make health decisions or do not have the information with which to do so. ¶ Health is intricately involved in every aspect of human life, and to be a health expert an individual would need to be well versed not only in medicine but in psychology, sociology, political science, child development, economics, law, biology, sexology, pharmacology, urban engineering, genetics, ecology, and uncountable other fields. It is the purpose of health science to draw material from all these diverse fields, integrate it, and pass it along to individuals who can use the knowledge to make intelligent health-related decisions in their daily lives that will lead them to *feel* better because they will *be* better. ¶ What, then, are healthy people like? They are *not* fearful or neurotically driven people who compulsively observe the rules of health behavior, smugly, not only for their own sake but for "what people will think of them." They *are* people who do what they "ought to do" because such actions facilitate a full, abundant, get-every-thing-out-of-life existence. And they are people who make health decisions on the best possible knowledge available to them, including a fundamental understanding of the workings of the human body. Health is not a static condition, existing only in the absence of disease, but is an ongoing process of learning, decision making, and action for optimizing one's well-being.

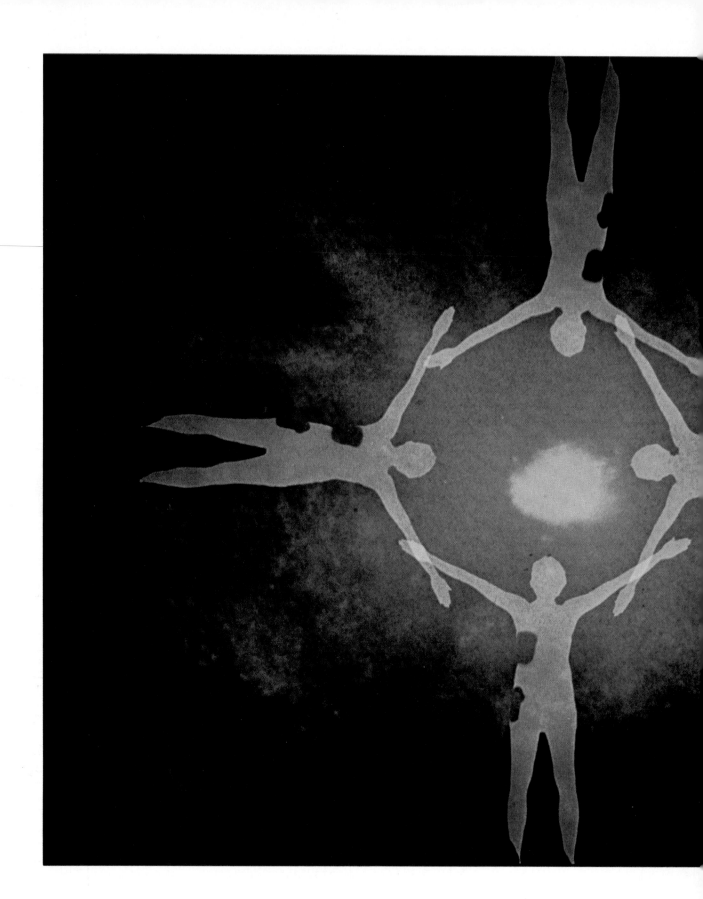

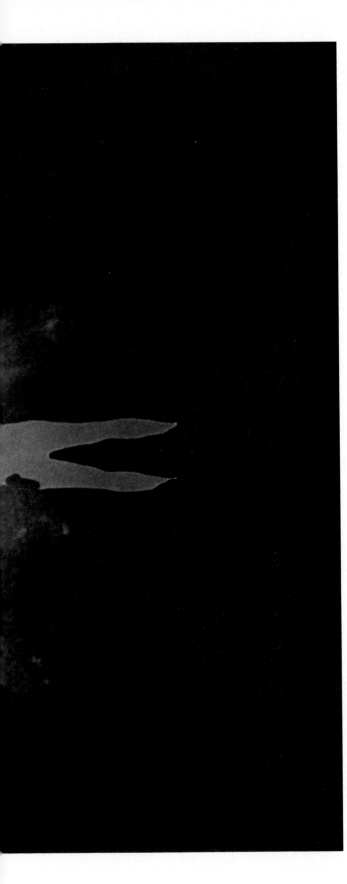

1 *Life and Health* is a book about health *science*, which means that it treats health from a foundation of reliable knowledge. It approaches problems with the assumption that accumulation of relevant facts and logical interpretation of them are the best methods of finding adequate solutions. Not all the facts about health are known, nor has everything presented in this book been established beyond the shadow of a doubt. One must recognize, however, that even the most rigorous sciences cannot be accepted as fixed and final and that reassessment of past conclusions plays a critical role in the progress of knowledge. What a health science book can do, then, is to put together available facts with respect to a number of health problems and point out the ways in which people can live in a more healthful manner. Many health questions are too important to too many people to be left totally unanswered until the complete analysis and evidence required for scientific certainty have been accumulated. For example, many people decided to stop smoking cigarettes—and recommended that others do so—before it was fully certain that cigarette smoking causes lung cancer. Even today, physicians cannot say for sure who will and who will not contract the disease, even if a person is a heavy smoker. Nevertheless, the facts are judged sufficient by competent analysts to warrant labeling cigarette smoking a health hazard—and one of a magnitude that requires public attention and regulation.

Scientists have less assurance in predicting that regular exercise will reduce incidence of heart dis-

Introduction to Health Science

ease. On the other hand, they can predict consequences much more confidently when people are exposed, for instance, to measles or to gonorrhea. In all these instances, the recommendations are made in the light of the most recent knowledge available, and they represent the best possible interpretation of all the facts involved. Thus they still follow a health science approach, in that the attempt is made to be as factual as possible. In contrast, there are certain other approaches to health—such as faith healing or witchcraft—that proceed from the premise that preconceptions or ritual can counteract disease, leading sometimes to recommendations that are in total defiance of the scientific facts. Ignorance and wishful thinking also at times are the bases for recommendations vitally affecting health. It is hoped that this book will provide the reader with some capacity to recognize the basis on which a given health recommendation is made and thus to make intelligent decisions.

MEANS TO HEALTH

Health represents effective function both within the individual and by the individual in his environment. Effective function is not an absolute but rather is dependent upon circumstance and values. One can be more or less healthy both as an individual system and as a part of a larger system. Some factors tend to promote health, and others tend to decrease it. The scientific approach to health calls for identification of the significant health-influencing factors, both within the individual and in his environment.

Health science, however, is concerned not only with the acquisition of knowledge about health and the identification of health-influencing factors, but also seeks to improve health, and in this respect is a *social* science as well as a *natural* science. The social approach to health calls for measures to promote the health-favoring factors and to overcome the health-threatening ones.

Animals and babies may be healthy "automatically"—that is, without knowledge or deliberate effort. But an understanding of the problems of health is required to *consciously* improve health—whether the improvement be over disease or over an otherwise unsatisfactory level of health. *Understanding* rests upon *knowledge* and becomes effective through *implementation*.

Basically, knowledge is acquired through experience. During the course of human history, man has learned to deliberately control experience so as to maximize the knowledge it yields. When he controls his experience to solve a new problem, he calls the process *research*. When he controls experience to pass on or to acquire existing knowledge, he calls the process *education*. When he applies his new or transmitted knowledge to promote health, he deals with health *implementation*. All three components involve both individuals and communities.

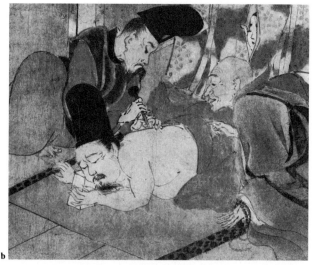

b

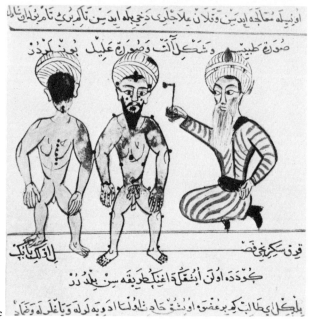

c

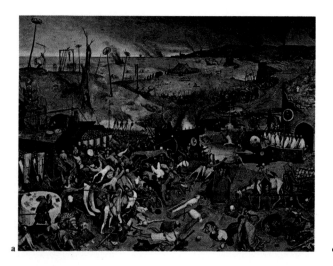

a

Health Research

Health research (the acquisition of health knowledge) must have begun before recorded history. Certainly the earliest known societies had rules for living — religious dietary rules for example — that are explainable on the basis of health experience. Whether prohibition of undercooked foods that are prone to parasitic infection stemmed from observation or from deliberate experimentation, the conclusion was an early result of health "research." True health research, in the sense of deliberate experimentation, must have preceded such ancient practices as trephining the skull, acupuncture, and blood-letting. *Scientific* health research, however, awaited the development of a new, rigorous intellectual approach and did not really begin to flower until the Renaissance.

Despite all that went before, there has been more health research in the past century — and particularly in the past two decades — than in all of previous history. In fact, a good case can be made for the possibility that future historians will date the beginning of true health knowledge in the twentieth century. Why did this spurt in research happen?

Explanation of such sociohistorical questions is never easy or simple. For one thing, scientific research in general had grown and prospered in the preceding period. Health research critically depends upon reliable knowledge in physics, chemistry, and biology, and these fields all had progressed substantially in the nineteenth and early twentieth centuries. Not only had they progressed, they had supplied specific tools that health research and treatment of health problems could use for their own development. For example, physical studies of the fundamental nature of matter led to an understanding of radioactivity, which led to the x-ray machine, which, in turn, has been applied in ever more effective ways to solving and treating health problems.

Besides contributing *directly* to health science and health research, advances in the basic sciences also created a favorable *climate* for such research. Impressed by the power of science when applied to physical problems, such as in the case of the atomic bomb, people were willing and even anxious to turn this power to more rewarding objectives. Health-related research accelerated astonishingly after World War II and continued to grow for two decades. Today, the issues are not whether to conduct health research, but rather how much, in what direction, and how best to support it.

Health Education

In past times, accumulated experience became the property of the priesthood and other ruling groups, who hoarded it and used it as a source of power. Today, the power of knowledge is protected as the public domain. Knowledge is stored — in

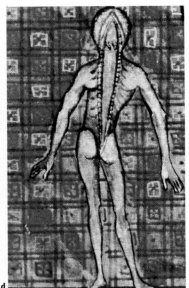
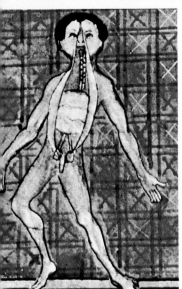
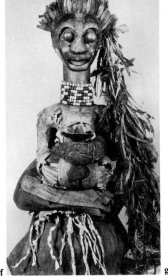

Figure 1.1 Concepts of medicine in history. Each society had its own ideas of what disease is and how it can be cured. (a) Pieter Breugel's painting depicts the ravages of the Black Death in fourteenth-century Europe. (b) "The Scroll of the Sickness" from twelfth-century Japan shows acupuncture being applied. (c) An illustration from a fourteenth-century Persian manuscript shows a doctor about to apply a hot iron to the sores of a leper. Fire was the standard remedy for all kinds of ailments for several centuries and still remains in the form of cauterization. (d, e, f) The fourteenth-century physician Henri de Mondeville used these drawings as teaching aids in anatomy. They show (d) a skeleton, (e) the internal organs as seen from the back, (f) the viscera as seen from the front. (g) An African medicine man's "fetish figure." The orifices in the stomach hold the "medicine."

people's minds, in libraries, in computers—but it also is disseminated, through the process of health education.

One aim of health education is *professional* preparation and training. Competent physicians, dentists, nurses, and other health professionals are needed to carry out the implementation of knowledge. Also needed are capable and talented health scientists, with a thorough grounding in both basic and medical disciplines, to continue the research effort necessary to expand health knowledge. And dedicated and inspiring teachers are needed to help younger people develop their talents in pursuing a health-related career.

The rapid accumulation of health science knowledge has increased the number of professionals needed, the extent of their initial training, and the importance of a continuing, up-dating process; it thus has posed an enormous educational problem. America's present educational system is creaking and straining in its efforts to achieve new ways to cope adequately with this problem.

An important consideration that is slowly being recognized is that the life style of individuals and the character of social structures are increasingly involved in determining the health problems one has to deal with and how they can or will be handled. Because cultural values or prejudices, economic pressures, technological impositions, legal considerations, and political activities are inextricably interwoven into the basic issues of health, health knowledge can no longer be relinquished or limited to the professional categories.

Every individual needs to be aware of the main health issues, so that he can make more informed and rational choices—whether directed to a better handling of his own health problems or to an effective influencing of the decision-making processes whose consequences ultimately will dictate the individual's problems and options. Therefore, health education has a second, equally important, aim: the encouragement of health understanding at the *individual*, nonprofessional level. Here, too, educational processes have yet to be revised so as to release the vast flood of health science knowledge to a general public—this book is but one step in this general direction.

Health Implementation

The whole history of knowledge accumulation emphasizes that there is a close relationship between learning and implementation. People learn best when they have an objective, apply what they learn to this original objective, and use it as a platform to look beyond, toward new objectives. Science always has grown this way, and health science is no exception. Conversely, the way one takes care of his health problems is molded by the knowledge he has about them and the new knowledge acquired in the process of implementing it. The nature of the changes affecting his *health care* is expressed in the increasing use of another term, the *health-care system*.

The concept of "system" emphasizes that it is no longer possible to think of health care as a simple relationship between a patient and a doctor. The fact is that the traditional one-to-one relationship between a single person and a single doctor is no longer the *total* process in health care. No single doctor can possibly know and command all the resources now available to deal with a single seriously ill patient, even with an easily recognizable disease. No patient can ensure his health by passive adherence to a doctor's instructions, without his own understanding of and personal commitment to his health problems. And neither doctor nor patient can singly control the social and physical environments upon which depend the health of both individuals and communities. When one considers the variety of diseases and the complexity of the known health-relevant variables in human populations, it

Figure 1.2 (a) "The Stones of Folly" by Hieronymous Bosch, painted in the sixteenth century, shows a surgeon plucking "stones of folly" from a fool's head. The funnel represents fraud, and the jug is a symbol for Satan. Such charlatans deluded people into thinking that stones in the brain were the cause of madness. (b) A medieval presentation of what must have been one of the first hospitals. (c) Leonardo da Vinci's drawing of the artery tree, one of the sketches he did on the basis of his dissection of human bodies.

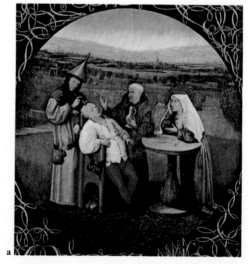

is no wonder that modern health care requires a *system* of people and operations to succeed.

The first and foremost component of the health-care system is, of course, *personnel*. The image of the doctor as the knowledgeable and caring person with respect to illness has multiplied and diversified. The image now has a number of components. First, there is the primary physician, sometimes called the family physician, who provides personal contact with the unwell. However, even the family physician has become many doctors—a general practitioner, a pediatrician, an internist, and so on. Specialization of training is the consequence of expanding and diversifying knowledge. In some ways the specialist is more effective than a generalist (and more expensive) because he focuses greater experience on a defined and localized medical problem. Thus there are otolaryngologists, ophthalmologists, neurosurgeons, endocrinologists, psychiatrists, gynecologists, and a host of others. If for no other reason, a *system* is needed to relate properly the patient and the several physicians who frequently must be involved in all but the simplest health-care problems.

Health-care personnel are not, of course, all physicians. The nurse has long been a familiar participant in health care, but today even the nurse has differentiated into many nursing specialties, each with a particular role. Beyond the nurse there is the optometrist, the dentist, the optician, the psychologist, the physiotherapist, the radiologist, and many others. Whereas in 1900 there were only two nonphysicians for every physician involved in health care, today there are about ten and the number is climbing steadily. Within the United States there are about 300,000 physicians but there are more than 3 million health-care personnel.

The second major component of the health-care system is *technology*. Compare the facilities and equipment of a modern community hospital with the early twentieth-century physician's office, with its bookshelves, mounted skeleton, examining table, and microscope. Compare the modern electrocardiograph with the stethoscope, the electron microscope with the microscope, the ultracentrifuge with the blood sedimentation tube. This massive, elaborate, and expensive array of facilities and equipment reflects the advance of biomedical knowledge, concentrated and focused by technology on human health problems.

The third major component of the health-care system is *organization*, that is, the ways in which the various aspects and processes of health care are related to each other. A physician may be in solo practice, with his own office, his own assistants whom he pays, and receive a fee from the patient for his services. A group of physicians may share an office (and staff) where they individually see patients, or where they collectively assume responsibility. The group may operate a clinic, with or without beds, for overnight care. They may operate a hospital for critical illness or for chronic care. A governmental agency may provide health care, employing physicians in suitable numbers to care for a particular population. All of these setups are different organizations for health care and each, with its personnel, technology, and particular set of relationships, makes up a health-care system. Today more and more thought is going into designing and innovating new systems of health care to meet the needs presented by particular problems.

OBSTACLES TO HEALTH

In the areas of both health research and health education directed to the training of health-related professionals, the United States has gained for itself a well-deserved reputation of excellence. Yet, infant mortality and average life expectancy lag behind those prevailing in many other countries, and a large fraction of the American population—per-

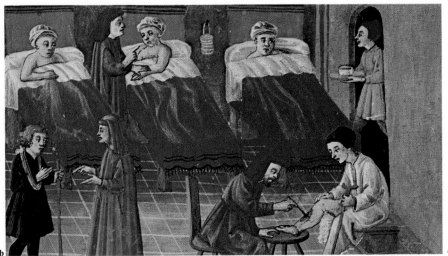

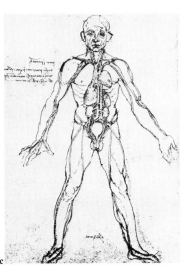

haps as large as 10 percent—is still not getting any health-care service at all. In addition, all American people are increasingly subject to new health hazards that are gradually replacing infectious diseases as the primary obstacles to health. It is increasingly clear that the whole process of ensuring health for the nation needs a critical reassessment.

The cost and the financing of health-care systems have become a central concern in recent years. As the United States entered the 1970s it was spending more than 60 billion dollars a year on health-care services, a figure second only to manufacturing in the national budget. So great a financial investment, and the effort it represents, cannot fail to be a major concern. The question raised is whether expenditures could be cut without sacrifice of essential services, while at the same time expanding the availability of health services to all people in need of them.

Three major factors contribute to the high cost of health care: (1) health manpower shortage, (2) high-cost technology, and (3) inefficiency of organization. Because these factors relate to the three major components of the health-care system, it is clear that the whole system itself is under criticism and analysis. Essentially, the critics seem to be saying that knowledge and understanding of health is not being matched by implementation procedures and that implementation must be improved in the interest of more effective health services for all.

Who is responsible for improvement of the health-care system? Some feel that the answer has been: "Everyone, hence no one." Increasingly, however, it appears that government will be more heavily involved. The United States government has been concerned with health since its inception, and state and local governments have followed suit. The major research effort of the National Institutes of Health, the impact of the long-established federal programs for veterans and recent new programs for the aged and the needy, and the rising health

expectations of almost everyone seem to assure increasing governmental participation. On the other hand, rising insistence on personal involvement and resentment of "establishment" dominance emphasize that the cared-for should have at least as large a say as the health provider. It is perhaps in the health-care arena that one may find the best opportunity to solve some of the immediate problems of the individual forced to confront a massive system that simultaneously affords benefits and imposes constraints.

There is another critical factor involved in the cost of health care—the *demand.* Just as doctors are beginning to stress the importance of prevention in the fight against defined diseases—and reorganization of health services will increasingly be concerned with preventive treatments—a society aiming at being healthy must address itself to fostering conditions where its members are in less and less

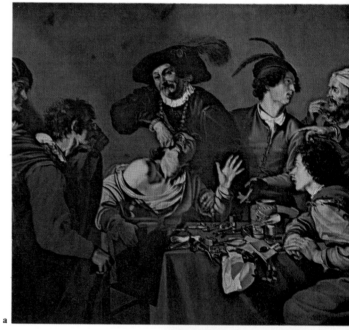

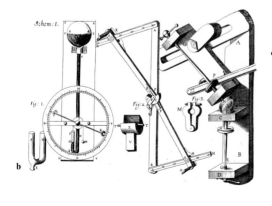

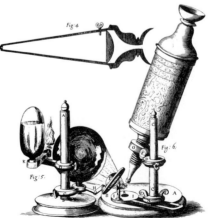

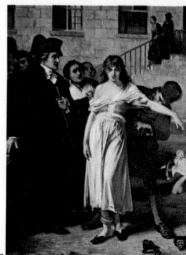

need of health care because the opportunities for ill or insufficient health have been effectively minimized. No social problem—poverty, racial tension, technological stress, environmental deterioration, and so on—is without a powerful influence on the health of society as a whole and on that of its individual members.

THE PERSONAL STAKE IN HEALTH

Although health may be the subject of research, education, and governmental concern, ultimately each individual personalizes it in terms of his own experience with illness and his hopes for his life.

Health was defined earlier in this chapter in terms of effective function, both within the individual and by the individual in his environment. It is not hard to turn this definition into one for personal health: *Health is a sense of well-being, of vigor and effectiveness, of purpose and fulfillment, of* maximum utilization and expression of oneself in interaction with others and one's environment.

There are three keys to achieving this way of living. The first lies in man's "inner working," in the multifarious components and processes that make up the extraordinarily complex human body. It takes experts to understand this inner functioning, and even they have only partial comprehension. Each person however, must understand his body well enough to know when to turn to experts, to understand what they are doing, and to evaluate their competence to some degree. Few people can fix an automobile but they try to know enough about one so that they are not at the mercy of an unscrupulous mechanic. Each person must thus recognize that one aspect of "self" is affected by structural and functional components and is best dealt with at the functional level. Drugs, for example, whether for better or for worse, interact with chemical components of the body and affect the self through these interactions. Knowledge of and attention to inner working is therefore essential to health.

The second key to a healthy way of life is one's sense of self. Whatever may be the intricacies that underlie this identification, the most overwhelming fact of each person's conscious life is—*I exist.* The objective of health science—and any given individual's study of it—is a *healthy I.* In this sense there is no more personal science than health science. Everyone, as an expression of his sense of individual self, can resolve to live in a given way, can make decisions to support his resolution, and can persist until the task is accomplished. The capacity to do so belongs only to human beings and is fully actualized only by healthy ones. Indeed, the realization of this capacity is another way to define health.

The third key stems from the growing understanding that man is a *social being.* As John Donne wrote, "No man is an island." If anything were still needed to convince man of this idea, the discovery

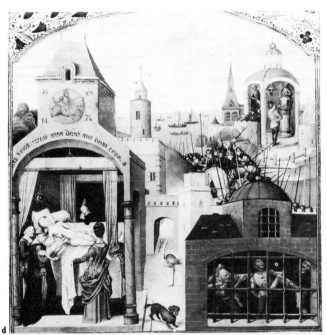

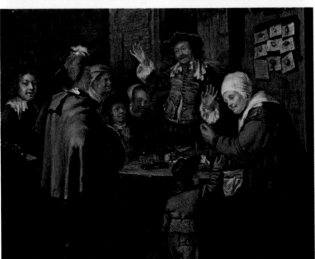

Figure 1.3   (a) A seventeenth-century Italian painter's representation of a tooth extraction. (b) Robert Hooke's refined version of the microscope, through which he saw and identified the cell. Present-day microscopes are based on the same principles he established in the seventeenth century. (c) The great French physician of the eighteenth century Phillippe Pinel is immortalized in this painting. Pinel, while chief physician at the Bicetre mental hospital, took the unprecedented step of removing the chains from his patients. He advocated humane treatment of the mentally ill. (d) A fifteenth-century French representation of a Caesarean section. (e) A quack deluding people in seventeenth-century Italy.

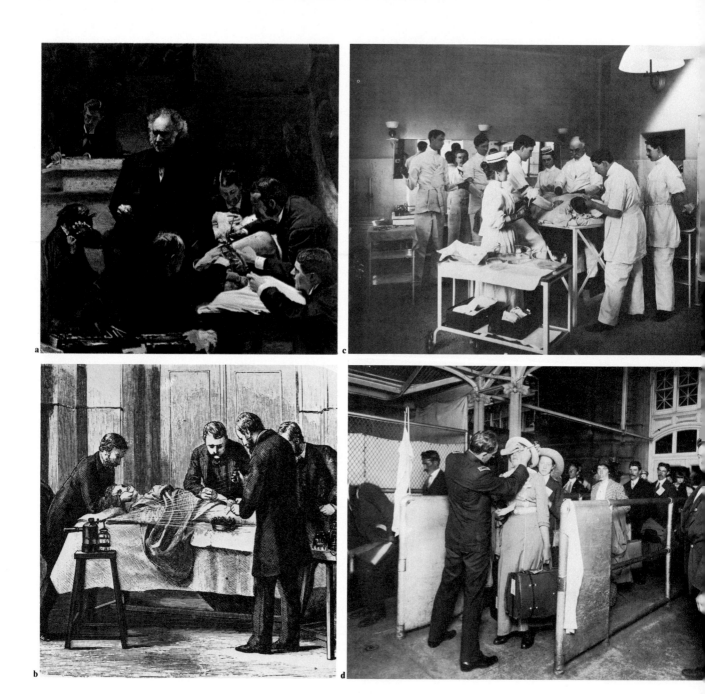

Figure 1.4   Advances in medicine in the late nineteenth century and early twentieth century. (a) "The Gross Clinic," done by Thomas Eakins in 1875, depicts the demonstration of a surgical operation to a group of students. (b) This engraving shows surgeons operating in 1882 with the use of a sprayer that emits a germicidal mist. The spray was the idea of Joseph Lister, who wanted to provide a germ-free atmosphere for operations. (c) Roosevelt Hospital operating room, 1900. (d) Early in this century, all immigrants arriving at Ellis Island had to undergo an eye examination. Those with infections and other eye problems were sent back to their country of origin for treatment.

of infectious disease should have done it. "Love thy neighbor" was a religious teaching probably stemming from the desire to reduce discord. If, however, one's neighbor is a source of infectious disease, one either shuns him or loves him well enough to help make him well. Public health and personal health are ever more closely linked as population density grows. Moreover, it is not only infectious disease that increases as a threat. Nutritional insufficiency becomes a spectre, and the waste products of living accumulate and press not only upon man but upon other species and the entire balance of the environment. Pollution and its ecological consequences alter man's way of life, threatening his health, and force him to recognize that if man is not an island, earth is, and that it is rapidly being exhausted as a suitable habitat for healthy living.

Of the three keys to health, only the second is one's own. The first is shared with the experts on whom one must partly rely. The third is shared with all humanity, and it poses what is certainly one of the most fateful questions in human history. Even if one properly uses the first and second keys, his personal health is threatened by improper use of the third. Even if one personally resolves and together with doctors properly controls his "inner workings," his health is not guaranteed. Whether it be high levels of radiation resulting from nuclear weapons tests (as was feared in the 1950s and 1960s) or the overproliferation of the human species, he is threatened by events he cannot control.

Whether the decisions that cause these problems are economic, political, or social, the fact is that the most threatening conditions for future health stem from human activities. These conditions include the accelerating growth of human populations, the occurrence of war or the preparation for it, and the impact of the replacement of human labor by chemical and physical energy sources. The question is whether these directions of human social development are or can be made compatible with health. If they are not compatible and are not changed, then all that is known about health science indicates that human health will decline and the continuance of mankind may be threatened. It is the task of health scientists to provide the information on which wise choices facilitating survival can be made. But it is the task of each individual to become informed enough and concerned enough to bring about the right decisions and behavior necessary for survival and health.

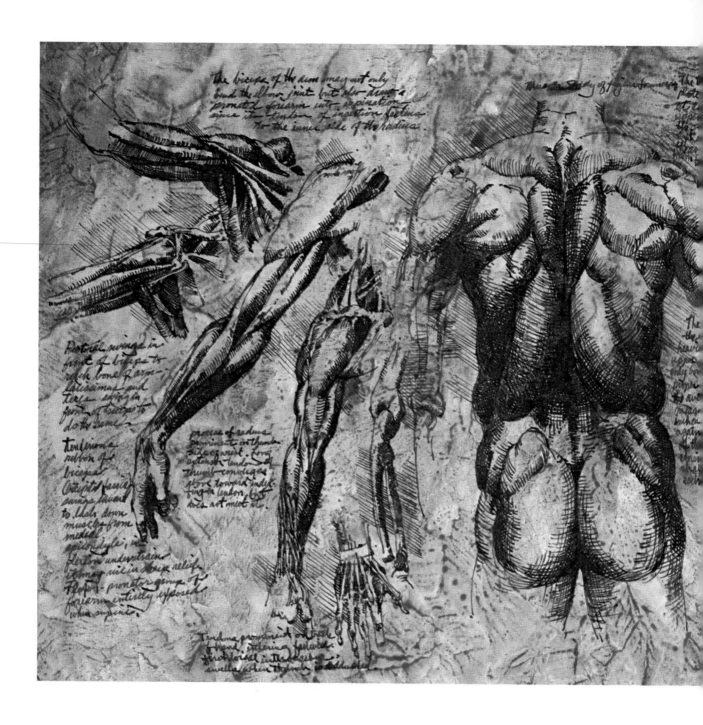

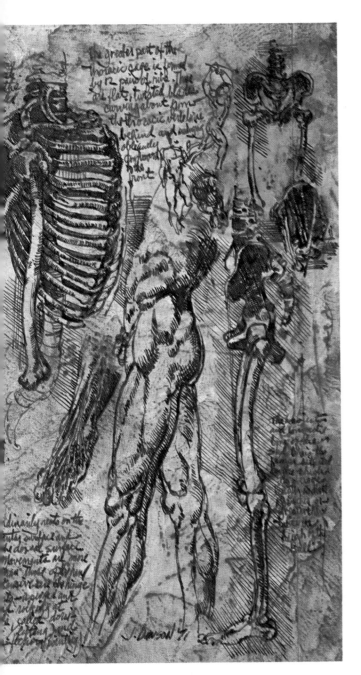

2The human body is a marvel of engineering and construction. It is made up of materials that man has not been able to improve upon artificially, and it contains machinery that man can only duplicate in a more clumsy, bulky, and less efficient form. In addition, it is so well designed that it can usually stand up under needless wear and tear, decade after decade.

The body performs myriad functions, most of them not under conscious control. It provides protection—the ribs are like barrel staves around the heart and lungs, and the skull's sturdy dome caps the brain. It produces motion with wide flexibility—the same hand that softly caresses a baby may chop down a tree.

The body experiences the world through the senses. The eyes respond to certain forms of radiation and the brain "sees" it as color. The other senses—touch, smell, hearing, taste—also add their input to the brain. What each individual believes the world to be like is determined in part by the senses, which vary considerably from individual to individual. Thus the capabilities and inadequacies of the body not only determine how each person functions as an individual, they determine his entire outlook on the world he lives in. And, through the actions of the human body, the world is changed.

Even before men could understand many of the accomplishments of the human body, they recognized its inherent beauty. Throughout history, artists have depicted the body in paintings, sculpture,

The Body in Action

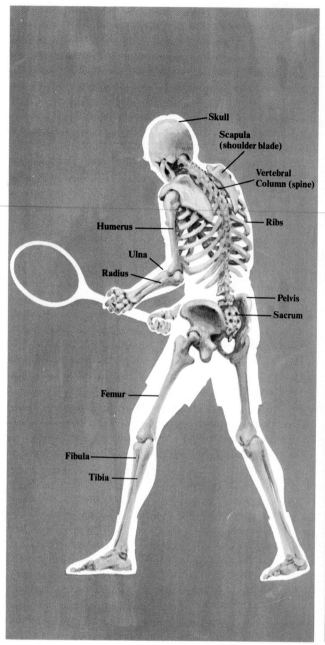

Figure 2.1   The skeletal system.

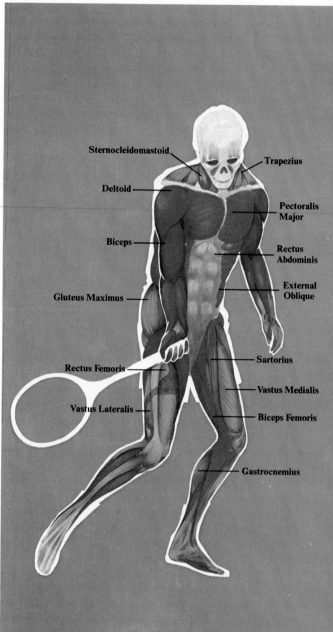

Figure 2.2   The muscular system.

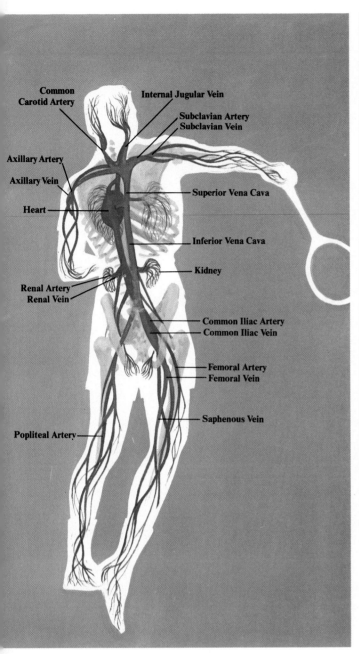

Figure 2.3   The cardiovascular system.

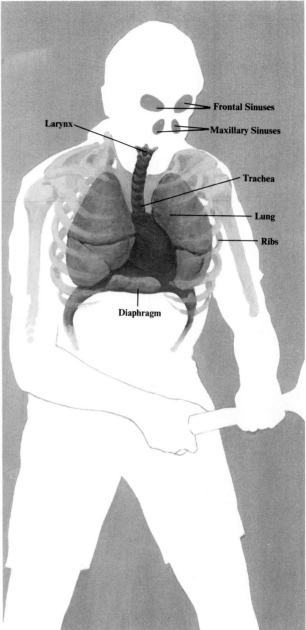

Figure 2.4   The respiratory system.

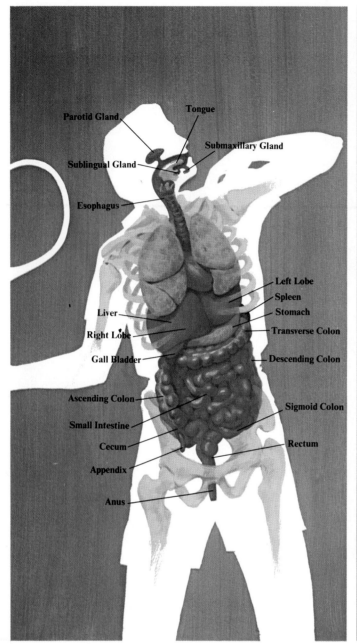

Figure 2.5   The digestive system.

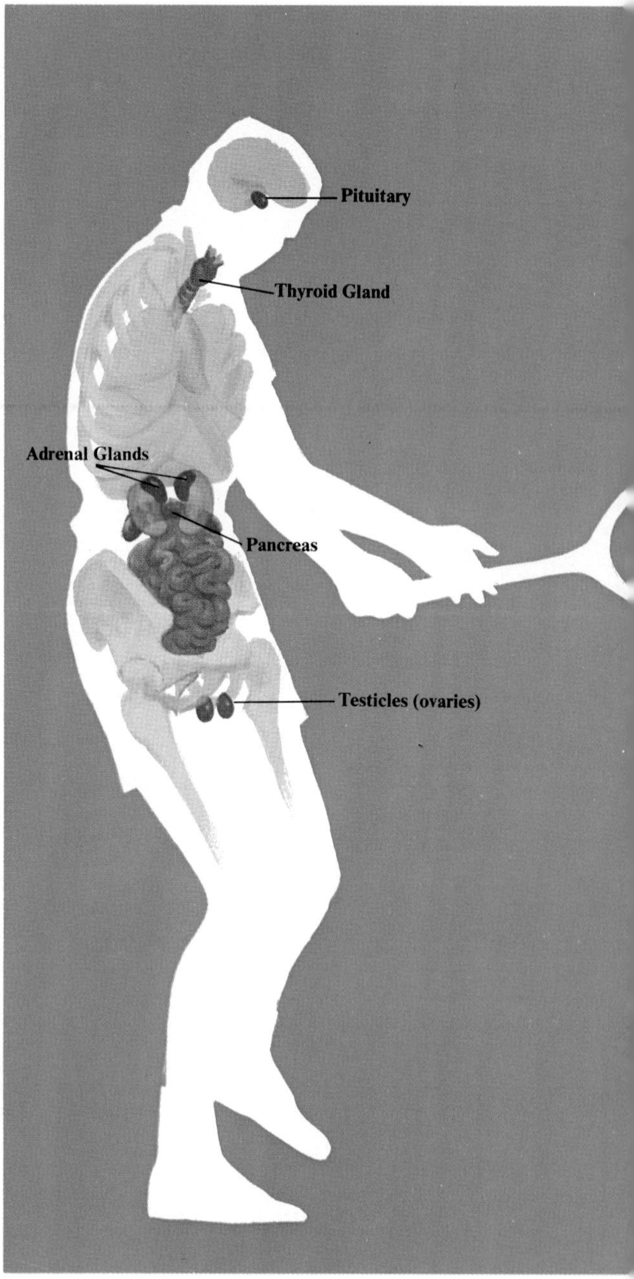

Figure 2.6   The endocrine system.

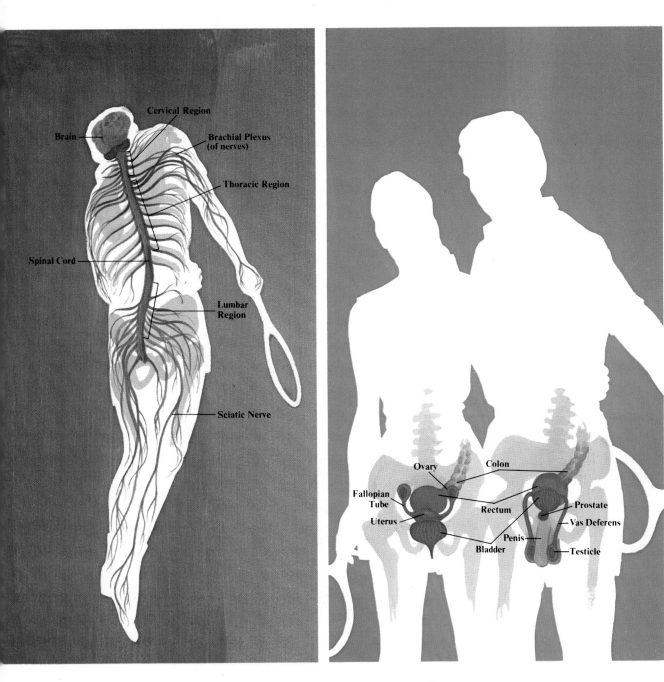

Figure 2.7   The nervous system.

Figure 2.8   The reproductive systems.

and photography. Today, however, scientific understanding can be added to aesthetic appreciation.

The human body is enormously complex. But it also is a system, functioning as a balanced unit despite its overwhelming complexity, because its parts are disposed in a regular pattern and interact in accord with a definable set of rules. Most complex systems can be separated into subsystems, and the human body is no exception. Defining and comprehending bodily subsystems are the great achievements of human anatomy and physiology—a process that has only recently approached completion. One cannot fully appreciate the human body, either in health or in disease, unless he understands its major subsystems, its lesser subsystems, and its components. The building blocks of all the systems and subsystems of the body are the *cells;* and yet, they, too, at their own microscopic level, are systems made up of subsystems and components within components.

The function of this chapter will be to examine the marvelous human organism system by system, from its major organs down to its cells and back up

to a broader view once again. The chapters that follow will be heavily dependent on the material presented here—to study disease, for example, one must understand the nature of the body part that a particular disease attacks. Throughout the book, therefore, constant reference will be made to this chapter, for understanding of the remarkable human body is the foundation to any understanding of health.

THE SKELETAL SYSTEM
Each individual has a characteristic bodily shape that identifies him both as human and as a particular person. Because of earth's strong gravitational field, this shape could not be maintained without mechanical support. The chief supporting structure is the skeletal system, composed of more than 200 bones arranged in characteristic configurations that determine not only the shape of the body but the patterns of its potential movement.

The main skeletal axis includes the skull, with its hinged lower jaw, and the vertebral or spinal column. Articulating with the spinal column are the

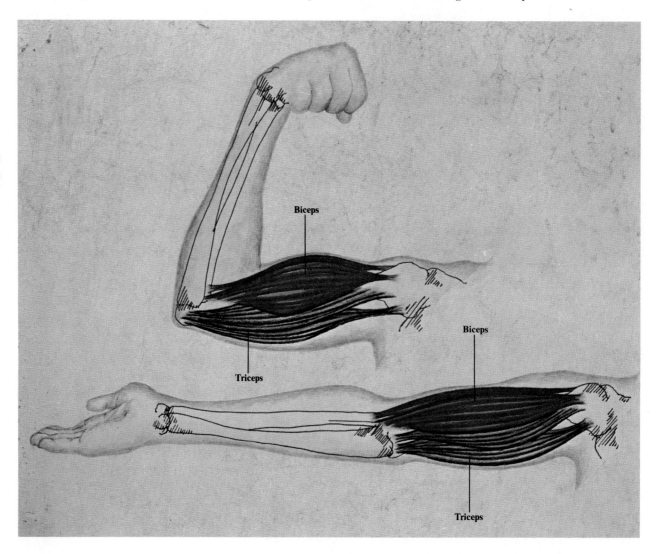

ribs and sternum, which make up the thoracic basket (chest). Also attached to the spinal column—indirectly via connecting girdle elements—are the skeletal elements of the arms and legs, each in turn involving long bones and smaller ones that are connected to them.

If everything but bones were to be dissolved away, almost all of the skeleton would collapse in a disorderly heap, because most of the bones are separate units that are held together by nonbony material. This arrangement is essential if body movement is to be possible. The bones fit together to form the *joints*, which are usually held together by tough, fibrous *ligaments*. Frequently the joint is surrounded by a special fluid-filled capsule. Joints are easily damaged and are the special sites of such diseases as arthritis and gout.

THE MUSCULAR SYSTEM

A skeleton cannot stand alone. With its joints intact it would still collapse of its own weight, not into a disorderly heap but into a limp and flaccid one. The bones are held in position as well as moved by the *muscles*. Individual muscles are long, fibrous bundles. Each bundle is strong enough to resist the pull from a large load without breaking or tearing. But the muscle's most important property is its capacity to contract or shorten, thereby reducing the distance between its two ends. When the two ends are attached to movable objects (usually by means of tough, fibrous *tendons*), one or both objects will be moved.

For example, a simple leverlike movement results when the biceps muscle contracts across the hinged joint of the elbow. Bending or flexion of the lower arm results from shortening the distance between the muscle's connection on the *radius* and its origin on the head of the *humerus*. Alternatively, rotational movement of the lower arm is produced by muscles that run partly around the axis of the

long bones. Still more complicated movements are produced by more elaborate arrangements of muscles and bones. The tongue can perform many complex and subtle movements in the processes of eating and talking, all of which derive from the simple property of muscle contraction.

A muscle seldom acts alone. Usually one muscle or a muscle group is paired against one or more other muscles. This pairing is called *antagonism*, illustrated in Figure 2.9. For example, contraction of the biceps flexes the forearm but contraction of the triceps extends the forearm; when one contracts, the other must relax or the arm will not move. Antagonism of the biceps and triceps gives a person greater control of the forearm because it can be moved back and forth in either direction. Wielding

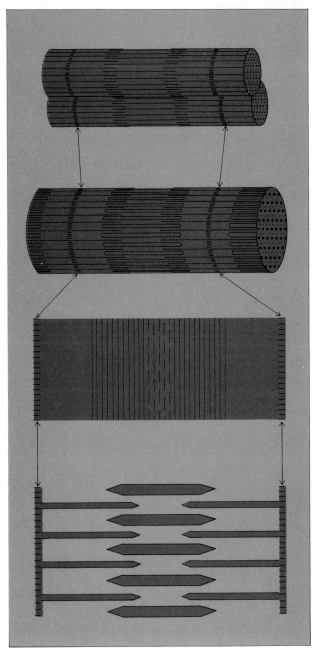

Figure 2.9   (*left*) An example of muscle antagonism. This pairing of two muscles also is found in such areas of the body as the sphincter muscles of the stomach, the muscles that move the eye from side to side, and the muscles of the penis that close off the ureters during sexual excitement and ejaculation.

Figure 2.10   (*right*) Muscle fibers. Within every fiber are many smaller units called myofibrils that are made of interlocking strands. Thick filaments are found between thinner strands. As the muscle contracts the thinner strands slide in and out while the thicker strands remain stationary.

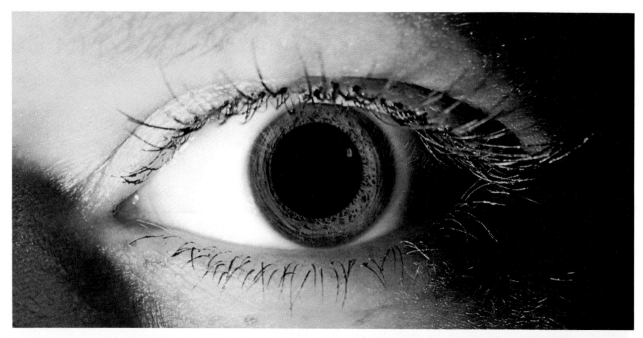

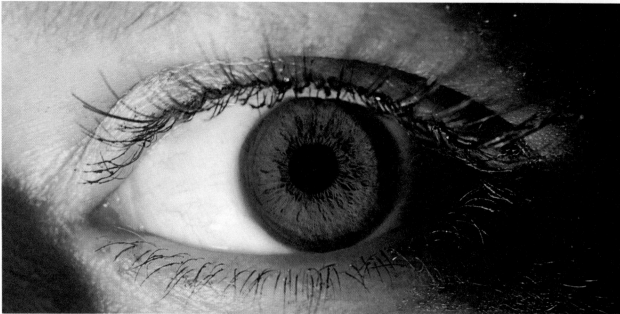

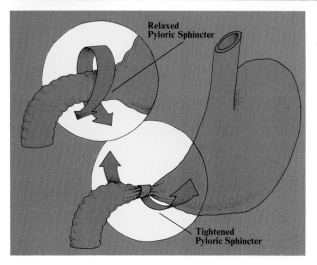

Relaxed Pyloric Sphincter

Tightened Pyloric Sphincter

Figure 2.11 The sphincter muscle of the eye, like all sphincter muscles, is a smooth circular muscle band. The sphincter of the eye allows the colored iris to open and close in response to light and distance from object.

Figure 2.12 The stomach sphincters open and close as if a knot were being tightened or loosened.

a tennis racket or rowing a boat obviously would be difficult or impossible without an antagonistic system of muscles. In fact, just standing up against gravity would not be feasible without such pairing of muscles.

The body also has many muscles that work independently of the skeleton. Many parts of the body are in the form of a tube or have circular openings. An example of the latter is the pupil of the eye, which changes diameter depending on the amount of light available or on the viewer's interest in what he sees. Here muscle fibers are arranged in a circle around the opening. When the fibers shorten, they reduce the circumference and hence the diameter of the opening (see Figure 2.11). Such circular muscle systems are called *sphincters*, and they are widely distributed throughout the body. Many of them control the flow of contents through such tubular structures as the gut (see Figure 2.12).

The muscles associated with the gut and other internal organs are somewhat different from those that move the skeleton. An individual can move his arms or legs at will, and muscles that make this movement possible are voluntary muscles. Those muscles of the internal organs contract much more slowly and often rhythmically; they are largely beyond voluntary control. The muscles of the heart are different from the other two sorts of muscle

and have their own distinct properties and structure. Thus, muscles are arranged in subsystems primarily related to their function.

In general, muscles do mechanical work; that is, they exert force and move the bodily parts or their contents, which means that they require energy—no work occurs without expenditure of energy. Muscles are energy converters, for they convert the chemical energy derived from foods into mechanical energy and heat. The mechanical energy is apparent when one lifts something, the heat energy when one flushes and perspires during hard work.

THE CIRCULATORY SYSTEM

The skeletal system would collapse without muscles, but muscles would not function long without blood circulation. Both bone and muscle—like practically all other tissues of the body—are thoroughly permeated by the circulatory system. In the case of muscle, circulation is essential in bringing new sources of chemical energy and removing the heat and other by-products of contraction. The circulatory structures that permeate the tissues are the capillaries, tiny thin-walled vessels finer than hairs, that form networks intimately related to all the tissue components. Through these networks the blood is brought into close contact with all elements of the body (see Figure 2.15). Nutrients and oxygen pass through the capillary walls to reach nearby cells, and waste products from the cells pass the other way into the blood to be transported elsewhere in the body (to the lungs and kidneys, in particular).

The *blood* is itself a tissue of the body, in the sense that like any other tissue it comprises a society of cells with characteristic cell composition and properties. But it differs from all other body tissues in two particular aspects. Although the bulk of it, about five quarts in the average person, is within the circulatory system, its boundaries blend with

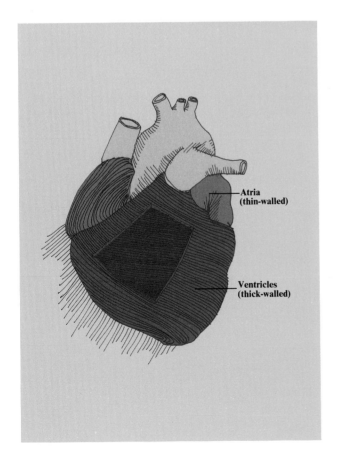

Atria
(thin-walled)

Ventricles
(thick-walled)

Figure 2.13 The heart is one large muscle with layered muscle tissue, which varies in thickness. The atria are relatively thin-walled compared to the thick-walled ventricles.

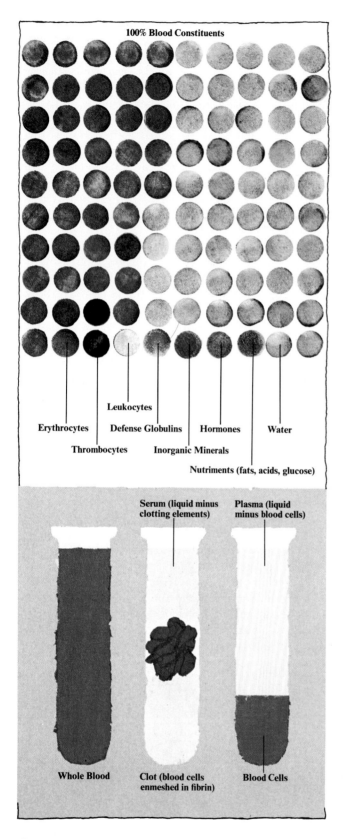

100% Blood Constituents

Erythrocytes

Thrombocytes

Leukocytes

Defense Globulins

Inorganic Minerals

Hormones

Nutriments (fats, acids, glucose)

Water

Serum (liquid minus clotting elements)

Plasma (liquid minus blood cells)

Whole Blood

Clot (blood cells enmeshed in fibrin)

Blood Cells

Figure 2.14 (*top*) Blood constituents and their proportions. (*bottom*) When normal blood is drawn from the body and allowed to sit at room temperature for several minutes, the fibrin-associated clotting phenomenon occurs. The plasma, which separates from the cells when centrifuged (spun at high velocity), makes up 55 percent of the blood.

the rest of the body, with which it exchanges fluid, fluid constituents, and cells. Also, 55 percent of the blood "tissue" is made up of fluid and only 45 percent of it is cells. The blood fluid is known as *plasma* and contains minerals, proteins, hormones, and various other soluble substances. One of its proteins, fibrinogen, confers to it the ability to coagulate or *clot*, that is, to form a fibrous jelly that plays a critical role in sealing broken or cut blood vessels and preserving the integrity of the circulatory system; the fluid that can be collected from the plasma, after it has clotted, is called *serum* (see Figure 2.14).

The blood cells comprise three major categories. First, there are the *red blood cells*, some 30 billion of them, which are constantly replaced with new cells mainly produced in the *bone marrow*, the pulpy inside of the bones. Red cells are devoted essentially to one function, the carrying of oxygen and carbon dioxide between tissues and lungs; this function is executed by a special protein, *hemoglobin*, which is the primary constituent of these cells. A second major category is made up by the *white blood*

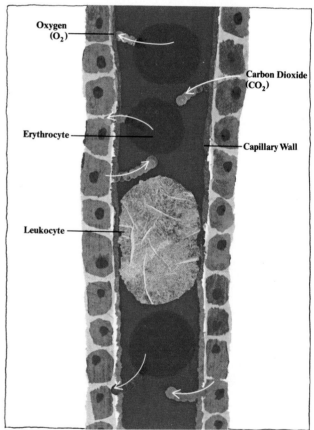

Oxygen (O_2)

Carbon Dioxide (CO_2)

Erythrocyte

Capillary Wall

Leukocyte

Figure 2.15 Exchange of oxygen and carbon dioxide in the capillaries. The red blood cells file through one at a time, and the larger leukocytes must elongate in order to squeeze through.

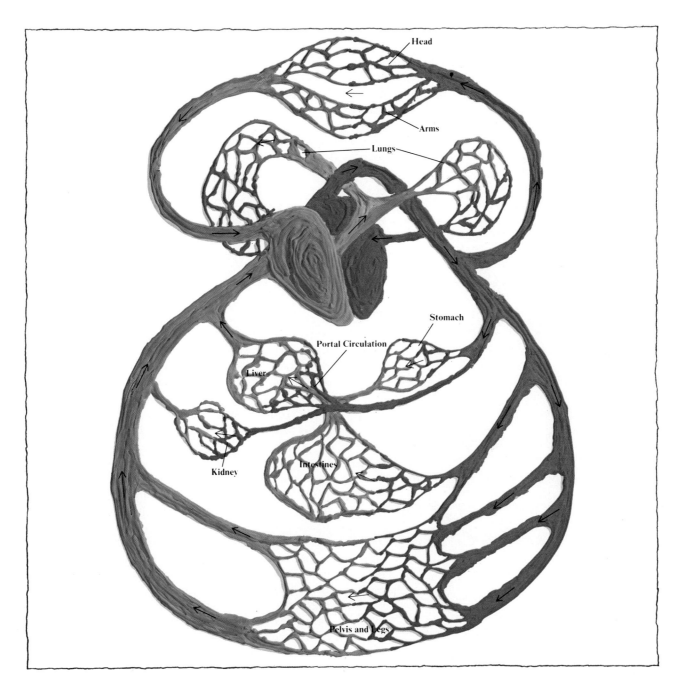

Figure 2.16   The circulatory system. This schematic diagram shows the basic manner in which blood circulates, first going to the lungs for aeration and then being pumped to the rest of the body.

cells, which comprise three main varieties: granulocytes, lymphocytes, and monocytes. All three varieties are involved in specific ways in the defense of the body against invasion by foreign substances or organisms as, for example, occurs in infectious disease (see Chapter 22). White blood cells are a thousand times fewer than the red cells. They, too, are rapidly replaced all the time from the bone marrow, except for lymphocytes, whose main source is the *lymphoid tissue* of the thymus, spleen, and lymph nodes. *Platelets* constitute the third category of blood

cells. They are smaller than red cells and fifty times less numerous, and they also come from the bone marrow. They serve a variety of functions, mainly connected with the repair of damaged vessels and the blood-clotting process.

The blood makes a complete circuit through the body (see Figure 2.16). It is pumped by the heart into the relatively thick-walled and muscular *arteries*. The arteries branch into smaller and smaller *arterioles* before reaching the *capillaries*. *Venules* leaving the capillaries converge to form larger and larger *veins*. The largest veins empty into the heart. Altogether these various components constitute what is called the *cardiovascular* (heart-vessels) system.

The heart consists of two pumps side by side, each equipped with two chambers. The pump on the left side of the heart is more powerful, for it must push blood the full length of the body—upward to the brain, downward to the toes, and outward to the fingertips. The right side of the heart has less physical work to do, but its task is no less important. It forces blood toward the capillaries in the lungs, where waste carbon dioxide is released and life-giving oxygen is absorbed into the blood. Blood returns from the lungs to the left side of the heart ready for distribution to the body.

Blood enters the heart at the top in two paired chambers called *atria*. The blood from the lungs pours into the left atrium, and the blood from the rest of the body, into the right atrium. Below the atria are two muscular pumping chambers, the *ventricles*. Blood from the left atrium moves into the left ventricle, that from the right atrium into the right ventricle. The left and right sides are separated by a solid wall, the *septum*. Valves let blood flow from each atrium into the proper ventricle, but will not permit it to return. Similar outlet valves for the ventricles keep blood from flowing back into the heart after its pumping action is completed (see Figure 2.17).

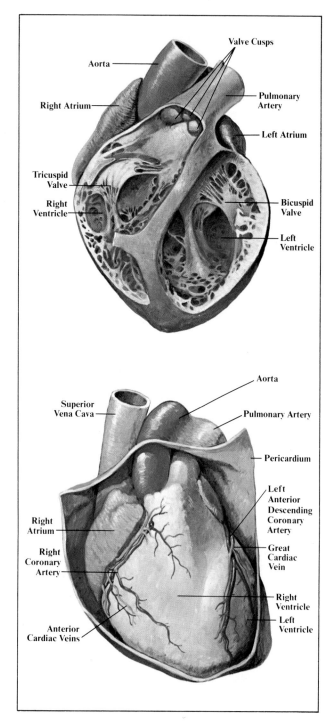

Figure 2.17 The heart is a tireless organ, roughly the size of a clenched fist and weighing between eight and twelve ounces in the normal adult. (*top*) Note the fibrous interior of the heart. It is made up of chambers, which contract with regular rhythmic motions, and of valves, which, as in other muscle systems, work in coordinated pairs—as one valve opens to admit blood, its antagonistic counterpart snaps closed. (*bottom*) Note that the heart is enclosed in a membranous sac, called the pericardium, and that the exterior muscle wall is fed by an intricate system of veins and arteries.

During a heart cycle, the atria, filled with blood, contract first. Blood is forced into the relaxed ventricles, which contract shortly afterward. This second contraction sends blood pulsing from the left side through the body's largest artery, the *aorta*, and then to the countless branches leading from it—arteries, arterioles, and capillaries. At the same time, the right ventricle pushes its load of blood into the *pulmonary artery* leading to the lungs. Then, as the heart relaxes, blood is sucked into the atria again to begin the cycle once more. Outside the heart, blood flow is helped along by the contraction or relaxation of the thin, smooth muscles and elastic fibers embedded within the walls of the arteries; returning of blood to the heart is facilitated by valves in the veins that prevent backward flow (see Figure 2.18).

THE RESPIRATORY SYSTEM

All the cells of the body require oxygen to release the energy stored in the nutrients they use. The circulatory system delivers oxygen and nutrients to the bones, muscles, and other tissues and carries away their waste products. The respiratory system's function is to enable the body to bring in its needed oxygen and to dispose of the waste gas, carbon dioxide.

The major organs of this system are the *lungs*. They are provided with an extensive capillary network in extremely close contact with a similar network of air passages. Exchange of gases occurs across thin membranes separating the air and blood. Because the pressure of oxygen on the air side of the membrane is greater than in the blood arriving in the capillaries, oxygen moves from the air into the blood. Because the reverse is true of carbon dioxide, it moves from the blood into the air and is thus eliminated.

Thus blood moves through the lung capillaries, gives up the carbon dioxide it picked up in the body tissues, and acquires a fresh load of oxygen to distribute to the tissues on its next cycle. Because the air in the lungs would soon become too rich with carbon dioxide and short of oxygen if it were unchanged, air must be moved in and out of the lungs regularly in exchange with the atmosphere outside the body.

Just as the blood vessels in the lungs divide over and over again until the minute capillaries bring blood only two thin membranes away from the air, so the airways leading from the nose and mouth through the throat and into the lungs branch over and over again. The upper duct, the windpipe, is called the *trachea;* its first two main branches, each leading to one lung, are called *bronchi;* and the smaller and smaller branches from them are the *bronchioli.* The tiny air sacs of the lungs in which the exchange of gases finally occurs are known as *alveoli* (see Figure 2.19). The walls of the alveoli and the smallest bronchioli reaching them are elastic, so that the total air space in the lungs can change. Thus, if air under pressure is introduced through the trachea, the lungs increase in volume, which is what happens during artificial resuscitation.

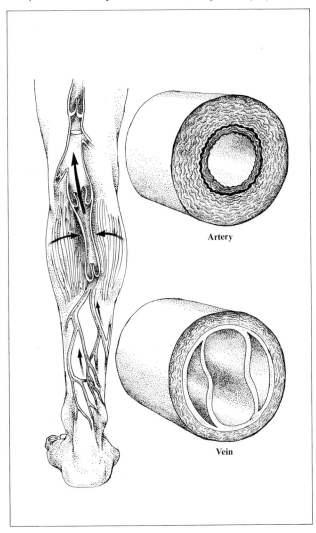

Artery

Vein

Figure 2.18   How blood returns to the heart through the veins. Valves prevent the blood from flowing in the wrong direction, while muscular action serves to push the blood along. (*right*) Cutaways of an artery and a vein. Note that arteries have thicker walls than do veins because they must expand and contract with greater force to direct blood flow to tissues and organs.

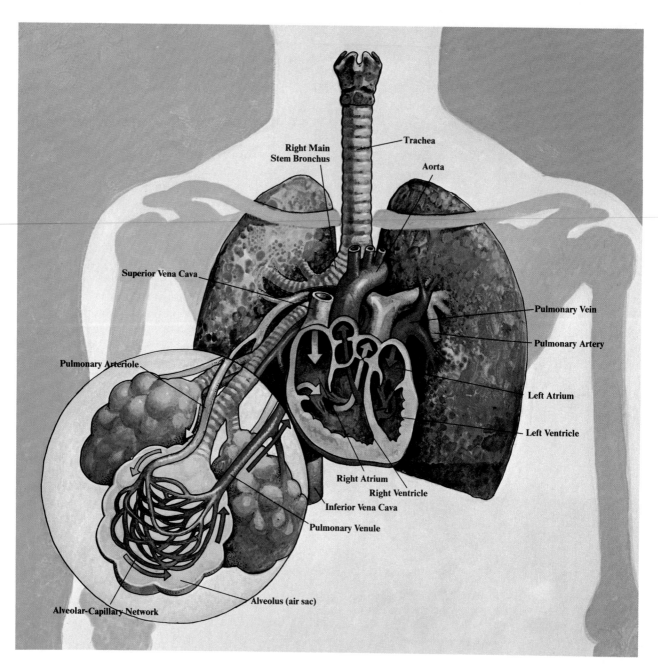

Right Main
Stem Bronchus

Trachea

Aorta

Superior Vena Cava

Pulmonary Vein

Pulmonary Artery

Pulmonary Arteriole

Left Atrium

Left Ventricle

Right Atrium

Right Ventricle

Inferior Vena Cava

Pulmonary Venule

Alveolar-Capillary Network

Alveolus (air sac)

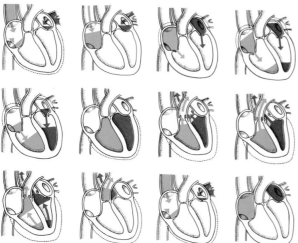

Figure 2.19 (*above*) Exchange of gases in the lungs occurs in the tiny alveoli, the smallest units of the respiratory system. (*below*) Diagrammatic representation of blood flow and action of valves in the heart during a heart cycle. Note the changes in the size of the heart at each stage. Arrows indicate direction of flow.

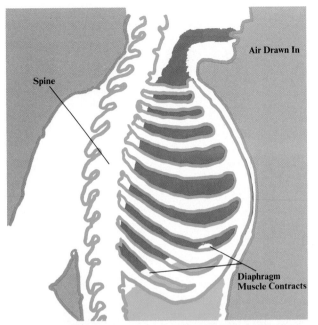

Spine

Air Drawn In

Diaphragm Muscle Contracts

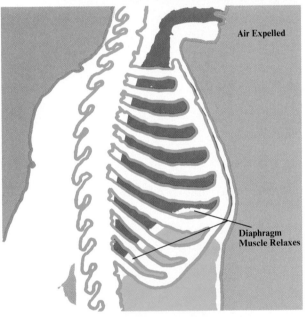

Air Expelled

Diaphragm Muscle Relaxes

Figure 2.20   The process of respiration. When the rib cage expands and the diaphragm drops, air is sucked into the lungs. Contraction of the ribs and raising of the diaphragm cause air to be expired.

During normal breathing, however, something different happens. Inspiration, or intake of breath, occurs because the volume of the lungs is increased mechanically so that air is sucked in through the nose and windpipe. Subsequently, the volume of the lungs is made to decrease, and air is forced out as expiration. The regular respiratory cycle, some twelve times a minute in a normal resting man, maintains oxygen and carbon dioxide levels in the alveolar air that are intermediate between those in the atmosphere and those in the tissues. Therefore, gas exchange continues in a favorable direction.

Muscles have the main responsibility for changing lung volume so that air is drawn in and expelled. The muscles involved are chiefly those between the ribs and the muscle called the *diaphragm*, which forms a dome between the abdomen and the chest. When it contracts, the diaphragm flattens downward, pressing on the abdominal contents and tending to expand the chest volume. Similarly, contraction of one of the sets of muscles between the ribs raises them so they are slightly more horizontal, which also tends to increase chest volume. Because the elastic lungs almost entirely fill the closed space within the chest, except for a thin film of relatively inelastic fluid, the lungs expand following an increase in chest volume (see Figure 2.20). When the lung volume increases, pressure within each lung drops below the atmospheric pressure and air flows inward. Relaxation of the diaphragm and rib muscles allows the lungs to contract due to their own elasticity, thus raising pressure within the lung and pushing air out.

THE DIGESTIVE SYSTEM

Just as there is a special capillary network in the lungs for exchange between the blood and the gaseous environment, there are special capillary networks for exchange of materials between the blood and the tissues. One of these networks is responsi-

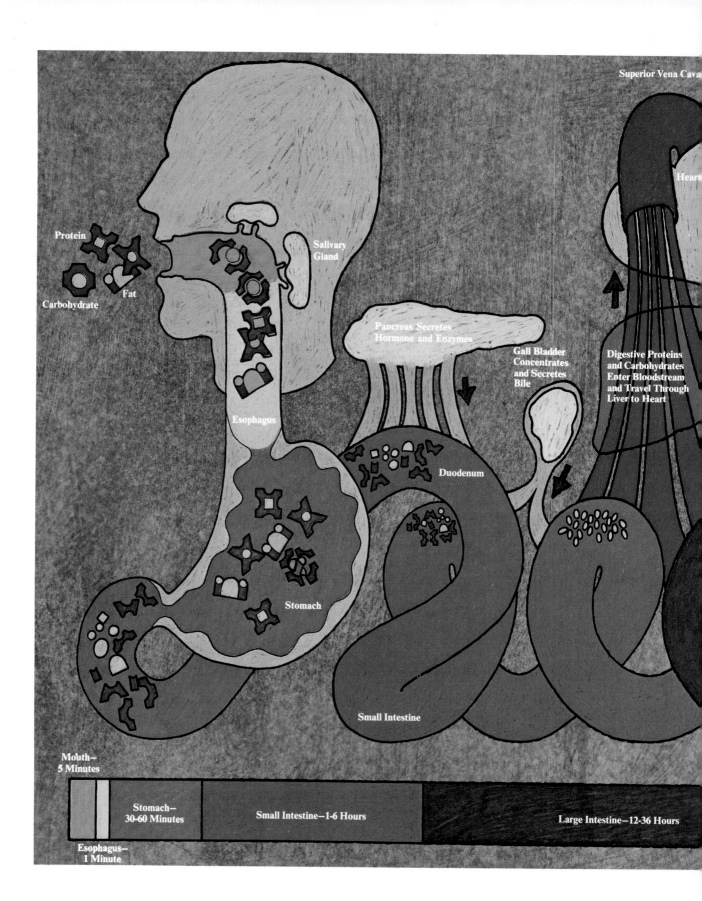

Superior Vena Cava

Heart

Protein

Carbohydrate

Fat

Salivary Gland

Pancreas Secretes Hormone and Enzymes

Gall Bladder Concentrates and Secretes Bile

Digestive Proteins and Carbohydrates Enter Bloodstream and Travel Through Liver to Heart

Esophagus

Duodenum

Stomach

Small Intestine

Mouth-- 5 Minutes

Stomach-- 30-60 Minutes

Small Intestine—1-6 Hours

Large Intestine—12-36 Hours

Esophagus-- 1 Minute

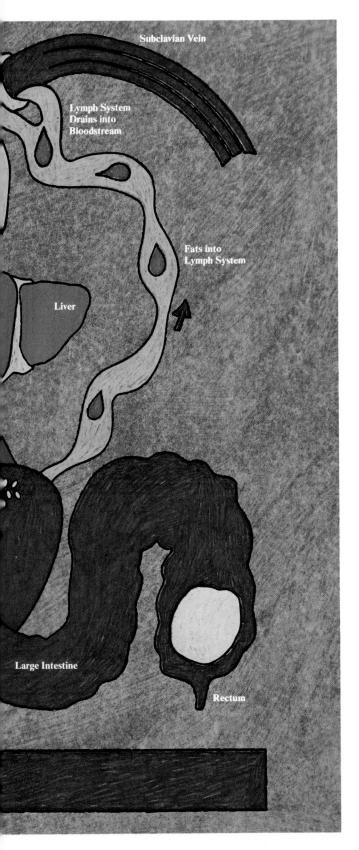

ble for the uptake of nutrients derived from food. *Nutrients* are substances that can be used by the body to supply energy or building blocks for growth or activity. The body obtains these nutrients from the food an individual takes in, or *ingests*. Ingested nutrients frequently must be broken down, or *digested*, before they can be absorbed into the blood by a capillary network. Material from the food that is not digested and absorbed is eliminated as a part of the feces. Ingestion, digestion, absorption, and elimination are functions of the *digestive tract*, a continuous tube leading from mouth to anus (see Figure 2.21). Different portions of this continuous tube are known by different names, depending on their location and specific functions.

The first step in food processing is *mastication*, or chewing, during which the food is partially broken down physically. Subsequent breakdown steps are largely chemical, meaning that large chemical molecules are split down to smaller molecules until they reach a size at which they can be transported across membranes into the capillary blood. Both chemical breakdown and membrane transport occur best in water solution. Chewing is therefore accompanied by the mixing in of watery *saliva*, secreted by the salivary glands to assist in bringing nutrients into solution. Saliva also contains an enzyme that helps break down large sugar molecules into simple sugars the body can later absorb. *Enzymes* are proteins that accelerate specific chemical reactions.

The mechanically dispersed food, still in the early stages of digestion, is swallowed into the esophagus by movements of the muscular canal at the back of the mouth, the pharynx. The food mass is pushed along the esophagus by muscular movements of its wall. These movements are known as *peristalsis*—periodic waves of squeezing contractions that progress along the length of a tube. These waves normally push the food on into the stomach.

Figure 2.21 The digestive system. Basically, food is taken in in the form of protein, carbohydrates, and fats, which are broken down and eventually absorbed into the bloodstream. Carbohydrates and proteins are broken down more readily than fats. The time food spends in each part of the gastrointestinal tract is extremely variable—the "normal" amount of time from mouth to anus can vary from eight to seventy-two hours. The figures presented here are reasonable averages.

In vomiting, however, when partially digested food is moved in the opposite direction, the peristaltic wave is reversed.

The *stomach* is an enlargement of the digestive tube with walls whose contractions are less regular than those of the esophagus but just as powerful—they produce a generalized churning rather than a motion that moves the food onward. The stomach (gastric) wall further aids in digestion by secreting hydrochloric acid and certain digestive enzymes. Food entering the stomach not only is further broken up and liquified but undergoes several chemical changes. As it accumulates during a meal it is thoroughly churned and mixed before moving on to the next section of the gut. It is kept from moving on by a sphincter between the stomach and the small intestine. Only food in semifluid form is allowed to pass this sphincter.

The *small intestine* is a long, coiled tube whose wall is thrown into folds, and the surface of these folds is increased by fingerlike projections, called *villi.* In the small intestine food is thoroughly broken down both mechanically and chemically and the nutrients are released and absorbed into the circulation. Chemical breakdown is completed by a number of additional enzymes, some from the intestinal wall and some from the *pancreas,* a major digestive gland that lies outside the main digestive tube. The digestive secretion produced by this gland is transported through a tube or duct that joins another duct leading from the *gall bladder.* The gall bladder stores the bile produced by the *liver;* bile helps break fats and oils into small droplets. Thus bile and pancreatic juice are secreted together into the small intestine.

Nutrients are actually absorbed in the villi, each of which contains elements of two extensive circulatory networks (see Figure 2.23). The first of these networks is closer to the surface of the villi and is made up of typical capillaries, with arterioles leading into the capillary network and venules collecting the blood back into veins. Nutrients are so highly concentrated in the intestine that they move across the capillary wall into the bloodstream. The nutrient-rich blood collected from the intestinal capillary networks flows through veins to the liver. The liver processes many nutrients before they are utilized by the body. Nutrients processed in the liver are transferred back to the capillary blood, which now enters veins to be transported to the right atrium for aeration in the lungs before distribution through the circulatory system to the body generally.

The secondary circulatory network in the intestine is present in each villus at its central core, which contains a single vessel larger than the capillaries and with more penetrable walls. Larger molecules, particularly fats, that are not quickly absorbed into the capillaries end up in this central *lymphatic vessel.* Lymphatics from the intestinal villi flow together with other lymphatics that drain off excess fluid from most body tissues and form larger and larger lymphatic vessels that eventually empty into the large veins just before they enter the heart.

The lymphatic system provides an auxiliary system for returning fluids from the tissues to the heart (see Figure 2.22). The *lymph* flowing through it can carry somewhat larger molecules and particles than the ordinary venous blood. Therefore, fat droplets picked up in the intestinal villi bypass the liver, allowing fat to go directly to fat storage depots. The lymph also carries a number of white blood cells, particularly granulocytes and lymphocytes, that it collects from all the various tissues. While some of these cells are returned to the large veins and therefore to the bloodstream, others are delayed or replaced at various way stations along the lymphatic system, known as *lymph nodes.* Lymph nodes are small lumps of lymphoid tissue (one of the body

Figure 2.22   (*top*) The lymphatic system. Fluid and other substances seep out of the blood capillaries into the tissue spaces and are returned to the bloodstream by the lymph capillaries and larger lymphatic vessels. (*bottom*) Present theory of fluid exchange. Large molecules, such as proteins and lipids (white dots) leave the blood capillaries along with fluid and salts. Some of the fluid and salts are reabsorbed; the excess, along with large molecules that cannot reenter the blood capillaries, is returned via the lymphatic system.

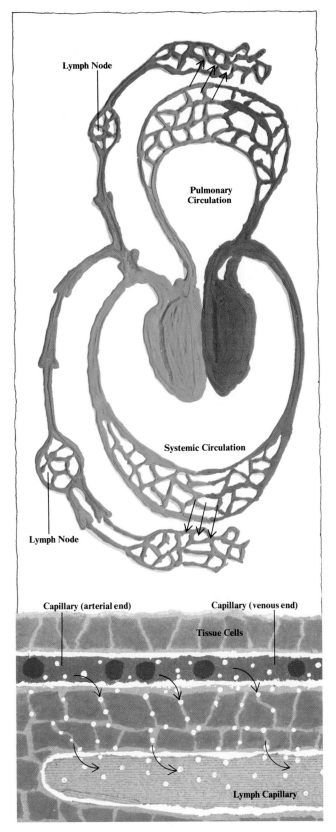

Lymph Node

Pulmonary Circulation

Systemic Circulation

Lymph Node

Capillary (arterial end)

Capillary (venous end)

Tissue Cells

Lymph Capillary

sources of lymphocytes) criss-crossed by distended lymph spaces.

Undigested, unabsorbed material in the small intestine is carried to the *large intestine*, where some water and salts are reabsorbed and some other soluble and insoluble waste products are added. The residue moves on into the rectum where it is stored as feces prior to elimination.

The time required for a meal to complete this course through the digestive tract varies with the nature of the food. Proper digestion and absorption, however, usually requires many hours. Nearly all of the activity occurs involuntarily via delicate, unlearned controls. The digestive process is easily upset, not only by disease but by emotional disturbances, because the controls for digestion operate via pathways that are shared with controls for some other forms of physiological behavior. Before discussing these control pathways, however, the passage of food through the rest of the body will be followed to see how unused and potentially harmful by-products are removed.

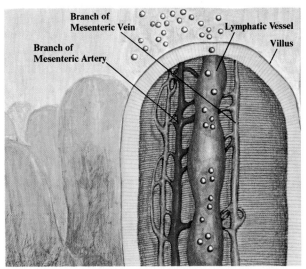

Branch of Mesenteric Vein

Lymphatic Vessel

Villus

Branch of Mesenteric Artery

Figure 2.23   Intestinal villi. Large molecules, particularly fats, enter the lymphatic system through these villi. Lymph vessels carry these large particles to tissues that require them and transport the fat molecules to storage depots.

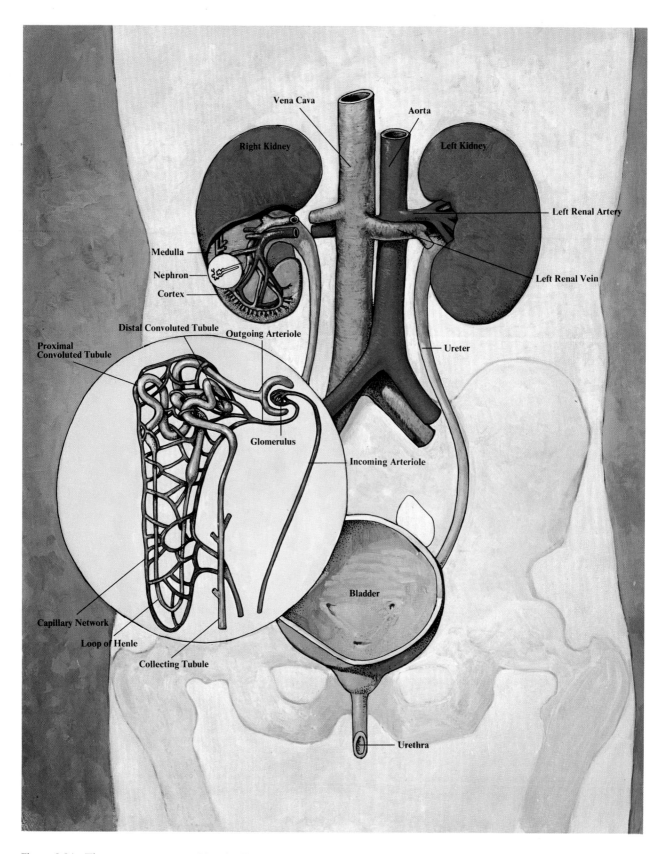

Figure 2.24   The excretory system, with a detail of a nephron.

THE EXCRETORY SYSTEM

If a specialist in nutrition were asked to define an ideal food—to be used, for example, most efficiently on a space voyage—he might suggest that it consist entirely of nutrients that could be converted to body substance or that would provide energy for activity without leaving any residue. There are, however, no such ideal foods. Even simple energy-yielding nutrients such as sugars produce water and carbon dioxide when they are combined with oxygen to yield energy. Carbon dioxide is expelled by the lungs. Water is lost through several channels, one of which is the kidneys. Few foods, moreover, are totally digestible, and the undigested residue is eliminated as a component of feces. Finally, a number of other components of food are utilized by the body but eventually produce residues that would be toxic (poisonous) if accumulated within the body. Particularly important are the breakdown products of amino acids, the building blocks of proteins. In most instances these amino acids break down to yield, among other products, ammonia, a simple compound of nitrogen and hydrogen.

Ammonia cannot be further decomposed by the body and is extremely toxic if it accumulates. It normally does not accumulate, however, because it is converted to *urea*, which is nontoxic at normal concentrations. Urea, in turn, is excreted—expelled out of the body—largely through the *kidneys*. Thus, water, carbon dioxide, and urea are among the by-products of the chemical reactions by which less-than-ideal foods are converted and decomposed within the body. Many other by-products of the chemical reactions by which nutrients are converted to energy and body substance are excreted by the kidneys. The kidneys not only remove potentially poisonous substances left over from the build-up and breakdown of nutrients, they also maintain a delicate chemical balance of many materials circulating in the bloodstream.

The kidneys, like the lungs and liver, depend upon an elaborate capillary network. The arterioles in the kidneys give rise to tufts of capillaries, or *glomeruli*, each of which fits inside the cup-shaped end of a kidney tubule. Each individual tubule and its glomerulus constitute one unit, or *nephron* (see Figure 2.24). There are about 1 million nephrons within each kidney, joined into larger collecting ducts that enter a common space within the kidney from which the *ureter* emerges. The ureter conveys the fluid gathered from the tubules—urine—to a reservoir, the *bladder*, from which the *urethra* will carry it outside the body during urination.

The blood in each capillary tuft is separated from the fluid-filled space of the tubule by two thin membranes (those of the capillary and of the tubule). Because the blood is under pressure produced by the heart pump, and because the membranes are permeable to moderate-sized molecules, water and a number of molecules can pass across the membranes and move into the tubular space while larger molecules are held back in the blood. Urea is among the small molecules that are filtered out of the blood (just as carbon dioxide leaves the blood and moves into the alveolar space in the lung).

As the filtrate from the blood moves along the tubule, other substances are exchanged between the filtrate and the blood, especially where the blood vessels emerging from the tuft form more capillaries located close to twists and turns of the tubule. At these points some substances are reabsorbed from the tubule and others are added. What finally emerges from the tubules is not the simple filtrate that is found in the space around the tuft, but a modified version of it. Because the composition of the urine varies depending upon activity, diet, and other factors, it is a useful clinical indicator of many processes going on in the body.

The complex regulatory mechanism of the healthy kidney maintains the chemical contents of

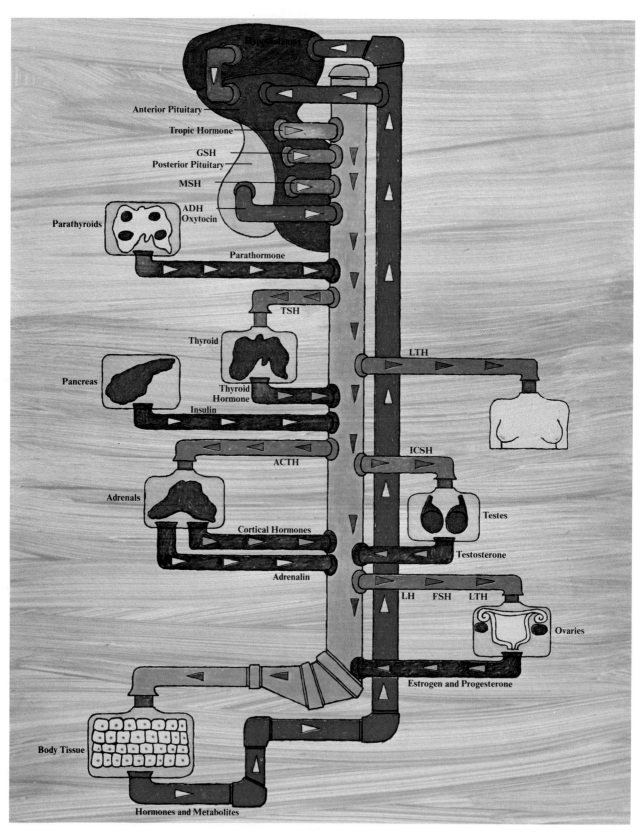

GSH = growth-stimulating hormone

TSH = thyroid-stimulating hormone

ICSH = interstitial-cell-stimulating hormone

MSH = melanocyte-stimulating hormone

ACTH = adrenocorticotropic hormone

LH = luteinizing hormone

ADH = antidiuretic hormone

LTH = luteotropic hormone

FSH = follicle-stimulating hormone

the blood within normal limits by removing some substances and allowing others to be retained. All tissues of the body directly or indirectly exchange substances with the blood in their own capillary networks. By preserving the composition of the blood, therefore, the kidneys make an important contribution to the constancy of the internal environment of the whole body. Much can go wrong when the internal environment is altered. Conversely, when something goes wrong anywhere in the body, it is much more difficult for the kidneys to maintain proper balance. Disease and injury are likely to throw a greater load on the kidneys. A kidney weakened by disease in turn makes the body less able to withstand disease or injury. Kidney disorders are further discussed in Chapter 25.

THE ENDOCRINE SYSTEM

Changes in one part of the body may drastically affect the activities of another part. For instance, when food enters the small intestine from the stomach, bile and pancreatic juice are released into the small intestine. How do the pancreas and gall bladder "know" that food has reached the intestine?

To discover the answer to this question, scientists treated pieces of the intestinal wall with acid and then filtered the residue. When the clear extract was injected into the bloodstream, it caused bile and pancreatic juice to flow. The extract can be purified to yield an active component that is a short chain of amino acids known as *secretin*. Secretin, found at the beginning of the twentieth century, was the first *hormone* to be discovered. Hormones are chemical messengers that are produced in one part of the body and influence activities elsewhere. Some hormones, like secretin, are produced in tissues that primarily are involved in other functions. Others are manufactured in tissues and organs specialized for hormone production. Either way, the tissues discharge the hormones directly into the

circulation, unlike such glands as the salivary glands that discharge their secretions through a duct. For this reason these hormone-producing glands are called ductless, or *endocrine* (inward-secreting), glands. Extensive study has shown that they make up a system whose parts interact with one another and influence other tissues through the circulation. Some of these parts are discussed here; others appear in Figure 2.25.

The Thyroid and Pituitary Glands

The thyroid gland illustrates how the endocrine system works. It is an H-shaped tissue mass, lying astride the trachea, that produces the hormone *thyroxin*. Thyroxin affects all tissues of the body because it promotes certain key chemical reactions. If the body has too little thyroxin, one feels lazy and lethargic; if it has too much, one is overactive. Disease or removal of the thyroid causes the former effect; injection of thyroid extract or excess hormone itself causes the latter effect. Similar effects are produced, however, by removing the *pituitary gland* at the base of the brain or by injecting suitable extracts of this gland into the body. In other words, the pituitary influences the thyroid with a chemical messenger.

The pituitary produces a substance known as thyroid-stimulating hormone (TSH), which is necessary for the thyroid to make and discharge thyroxin. Moreover, high levels of thyroxin in the blood reduce the output of TSH, whereas insufficient thyroxin leads to greater output of TSH. Pituitary and thyroid therefore regulate each other, and the combination regulates general tissue activity. The pituitary is involved in several similar relationships with other endocrine glands. In fact, the pituitary sometimes is referred to as the "master gland" because most of the hormones it produces act indirectly by controlling the hormonal output of other endocrine glands.

Figure 2.25   The endocrine system. The control of the endocrine system is complex and delicately balanced so as to provide sufficient hormones to meet the body's needs. These controls are of three types. The first interrelates endocrine glands to the hypothalamus and anterior pituitary through feedback. The thyroid, for example, releases its hormone (blue arrow), the amount of which (white arrow) is fed back to the hypothalamus. If the level is low, a hypothalamic releasing factor instructs the anterior pituitary to secrete TSH, a tropic hormone (green arrow). This secretion in turn stimulates thyroid production, and the circle is completed. When hormone level is sufficient, stimulation and production decrease. Similarly, cortical hormone-ACTH, testosterone-ICSH, estrogen-FSH, and progesterone-LH are controlled through feedback. In the second type of control, substances other than hormones control gland output, and the hypothalamus is bypassed. The pancreas and parathyroids secrete insulin and parathormone (yellow arrows) according to the levels of glucose and calcium, rather than tropic hormones. In the third type of control, the stimulation for secretion may by physiological and not chemical, as when the adrenal medulla responds to stress with adrenalin or the posterior pituitary makes ADH after the hypothalamus senses excessive plasma concentration. With the remaining hormones, LTH, GSH, MSH, and oxytocin, the controls are not defined, although they may well fit into the above schemes.

The Adrenal Glands

No hormone is more spectacular in its effects than the one called *adrenalin* (also known as epinephrine). It is produced by the *adrenal glands* that lie just above the kidneys. This hormone is carried by the blood, as is true for all hormones, and also acts in part by controlling the circulation itself.

From what has been said so far, one might have the impression that the many blood vessels in the body always have the same diameter and the same rate of blood flow. In fact, the flow of blood through any given capillary bed is constantly changing, depending on the activity of the particular organ involved. After a heavy meal there is increased blood flow to the digestive tract and decreased flow to the brain, often producing drowsiness. During exercise, on the other hand, more blood flows to the skeletal muscles and less to the digestive tract. These changes in blood flow occur because of changes in the number of capillaries utilized and changes in the diameter of the smallest vessels leading to them, the arterioles. When the circular muscles in these vessels contract, the vessels become constricted and less blood moves through them. When the muscles relax, on the other hand, more blood gets through.

Adrenalin acts, among other ways, in contracting and relaxing these muscles, but does not affect all arterioles in the same way. Its effect is oppositely directed in different capillary beds. For example, adrenalin dilates vessels and thus increases blood flow to the skeletal muscles, liver, and heart while constricting vessels and thus decreasing blood flow to the skin and kidneys.

The role of adrenalin is, however, far from limited to circulatory regulation. At the same time as it directs the appropriate redistribution of blood supply, adrenalin intensifies the heartbeat and accelerates and deepens breathing. It reduces the activity of the digestive tract and tends to contract all sphincter muscles of the gut while dilating the pupil of the eye. Because such changes all function to increase the body's capacity to react to external threat, whether in defense or aggression, the effect of adrenalin is often referred to as preparing the body for "fight or flight." It is a neatly coordinated response, directed by the discharge of adrenalin into the common carrier afforded by the circulation. In times of danger or excitement the adrenal glands pour adrenalin into the bloodstream and quickly prepare many parts of the body for action—an excellent example of chemical coordination. (The fight-flight response is further discussed in Chapter 3.)

THE NERVOUS SYSTEM

The endocrine system is one way by which the body controls the functioning of many of its internal organs. The *nervous system* is another. It is a network of nerve cells controlled by the brain and spinal cord and served by nerves reaching throughout the body. The nerve cells, or *neurons*, of the body number in the billions. They each send out one or more *nerve fibers* of variable length and extent of branching, through which they extensively communicate with one another. Many of the longer fibers bundle together to form the *nerves* that link portions of the nervous system with other body organs and tissues. Neurons send signals, or impulses, down the length of their fibers; these signals, while confined within the neuron, are electrical. They must, however, be converted into chemical signals at the end of the fiber in order to jump across the narrow gap—or *synapse*—that separates it from the next nerve cell or from the muscle or gland to which they are directed (see Figure 2.26). This leap is accomplished by the release of special chemicals, called *neurotransmitters*, which diffuse across the synaptic gap and trigger into activity the cell on the other side.

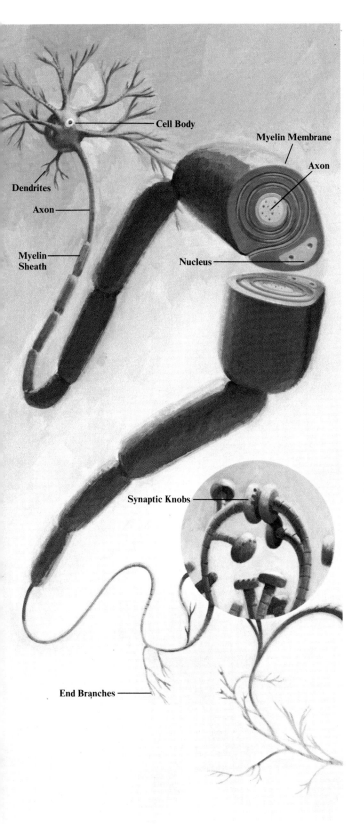

Cell Body

Myelin Membrane

Axon

Dendrites

Axon

Myelin
Sheath

Nucleus

Synaptic Knobs

End Branches

The great majority of the nerve cells are massed together in what is known as the *central nervous system*, the main subdivisions of which are the brain and the spinal cord, surrounded by protective membrane sheaths and encased in the bony structures of the skull and the vertebral canal inside the spinal column. The *peripheral nervous system* comprises the major nerves emerging from the central portion and the remaining, relatively few neurons gathered in small clusters or in patchy networks in various locations of the body. Through its *sensory* branch, the nervous system gathers information from the outside world and from all parts of the body and carries it to the processing and coordinating centers.

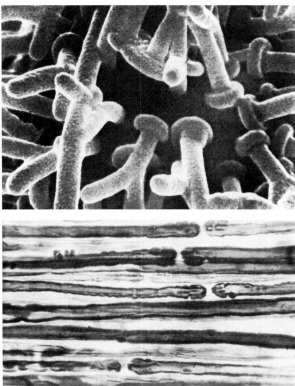

Figure 2.26   Basic components of the nervous system. (*left*) The structure of a neuron. (*above top*) Photomicrograph of synaptic knobs. (*above bottom*) Photomicrograph of nerve fibers.

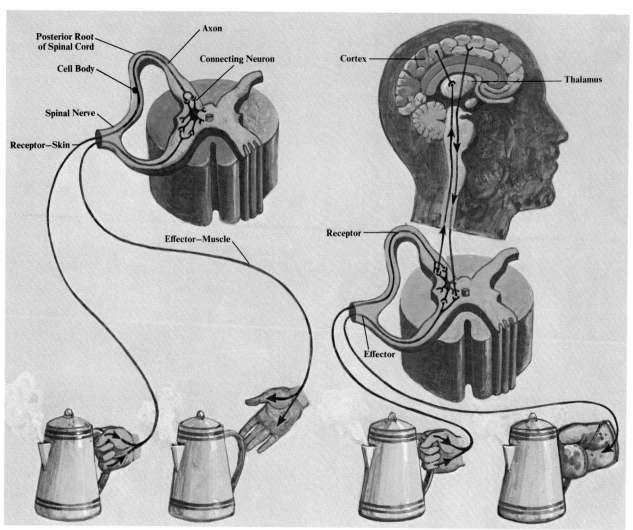

Figure 2.27 (*above*) Human behavior can be divided into those activities that are voluntary, and are therefore mediated by the brain (*right*), and those that are "automatic"—either reflexes (knee jerk) or learned (walking, eating), as is shown on the left. Both types involve reflex arcs that include a sensor, input path, control center, output path, and effector.

Fig. 2.28 (*right*) Regulatory influences on the heart. The heart has its own pacemaker, a patch of tissue that emits electrical signals that control the heartbeat. The heart rate also can be controlled via the vagus nerve by the brain, which is constantly monitoring heart activity through feedback, and by hormones such as adrenalin.

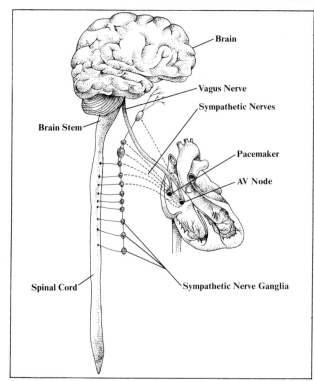

Through its *motor* branch, it sends out the directions necessary to control all the various body activities. Essentially, there are two broad motor subsystems. One is self-governing, involuntary, autonomous; it is known as the *autonomic nervous system.* The other can be consciously directed in its activity; it is the *voluntary nervous system.*

The autonomic system resembles the adrenalin-message system in some of its effects and in fact duplicates some of adrenalin's effects. The autonomic system alters the circulation, both in terms of heart action and capillary flow. Its influence is exerted by antagonistic directions that are balanced one against the other. The heart has two sets of nerves reaching it from the brain and spinal cord. One of these sets acts to increase the force and rate of heart contraction, the other to decrease them. Because both sets of nerves are normally active, heart performance will result from the balance of the two. An increase in heart rate may occur either because the stimulating nerve becomes more active or because the inhibitory nerve becomes less active. Both nerves carry messages from the centers of nervous control in the spinal cord and brain, and these centers in turn respond to information from the periphery. The typical sequence of nervous control in the autonomic systemic is called a *reflex arc,* which consists of a sensor, input path, control center, output path, and effector.

The autonomic division of the nervous system, with its antagonistic nerve circuitry, serves primarily the viscera (lungs, heart, gut, kidneys, reproductive organs), where continuous regulation is required, where actions and reactions are relatively slow, and where the resulting behavior is largely involuntary. Control of skeletal muscles, which is under the voluntary nervous system, is fundamentally similar to that exercised on other organs by the autonomic system, but it differs in a number of details. For example, skeletal-muscle action is rela-

tively quick compared to visceral activity. Also, no antagonistic directions ever reach an individual skeletal muscle: arriving impulses always stimulate it, causing it to contract. The interplay between stimulatory and inhibitory signals is settled at the level of interconnected central neurons, and the only possible outcome is an order to contract or no order at all.

The voluntary nervous system may be used to deliberately control skeletal muscles of the body, such as when one wants to pick up a book or take a walk. Much of the skeletal-muscle activity, however, occurs without a voluntary effort, as in the maintenance of body postures or changes in facial expression. In either case, reflex arcs still play an important role. Suppose one touches a hot surface. Immediately, a reflex arc occurs and the hand is moved away. A sensor in the skin (heat or pain receptor) is activated and sends impulses inward along a sensory nerve. The impulses reach a center in the spinal cord where they activate outgoing impulses along nerves to the appropriate muscles. On arrival of the impulses, the muscles are caused to contract. Thus, the same arc of sensor, input path, control center, output path, and effector is operating as in the autonomic response.

As useful as these coordinated reflexes are, they do not encompass all that is included in human behavior. It is the compact but intricately complex brain that makes possible the thoughts and feelings associated with human consciousness. Although scientists are far from fully comprehending the brain, they know that one of its important aspects is that it contains a number of centers linked in incredibly complicated ways and that from these centers come messages that control the most elaborate behaviors. In some fashion also—and this process is not understood at all—there arises in this coordinating machinery of the nervous system the sense of awareness or consciousness that leads to choices

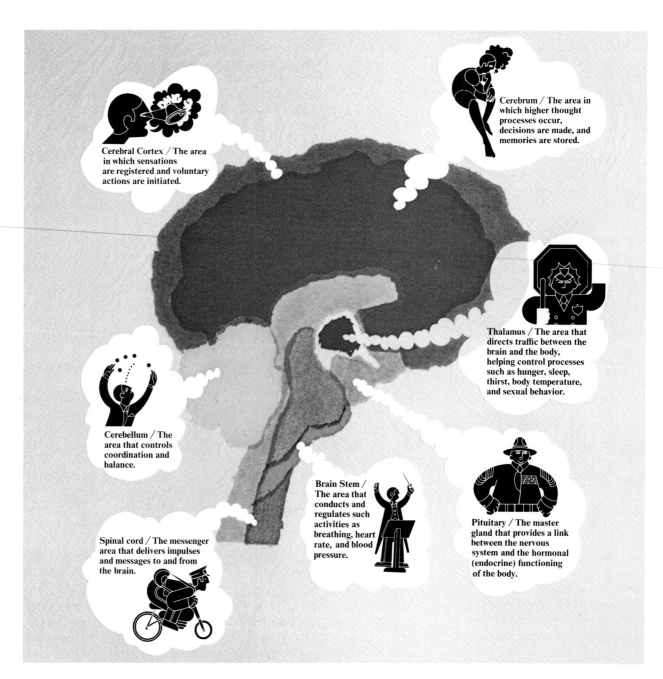

Figure 2.29   The functions of the various parts of the brain are shown here schematically.

that transcend simple reflex patterns. Here in his own brain is the most profound challenge to man's capacity to understand both a complex natural phenomenon and himself.

THE REPRODUCTIVE SYSTEM

One of the most remarkable properties of the human body is its capacity to reproduce itself. Though each human body is mortal and finite in life span, it is part of a lineage that extends back to the beginning of life on earth. The preservation of this lineage is the function of the *reproductive system*. Given so fundamental a role, it is no surprise that this system interacts with everything else that goes on in the body.

In man, as in many other living organisms, generation of a new individual occurs by *sexual reproduction*; that is, it requires the interaction of two separate individuals of opposite sex. Central to the reproductive system are the *gonads*—the *testes* (testicles) of the male and the *ovaries* of the female. The gonads are central because they are the source of the male sperm and the female egg and because they produce hormones that affect the sexual characteristics of the rest of the body. The gonads, however, are not independent—they function under the regulatory control of the pituitary. In fact, the gonads can be thought of as part of the endocrine system. Just as the thyroid gland cannot function without TSH from the pituitary, the gonads require the pituitary because it produces *gonadotropins*—hormones that stimulate gonadal function. Like thyroxin, the gonadal hormones act back on the pituitary to inhibit its output of gonadotropins. This reciprocal interaction between gonads and pituitary is an important part of the regulation of the reproductive cycle, particularly in the female. Moreover, the pituitary is attached to the base of the brain and is partly a neural structure; thus the nervous system also affects the reproductive cycle.

The biological purpose of all sexual reproductive activity is the union of the sperm and the egg under conditions that maximize the chances of successful development of the egg. The male reproductive system provides a large number of sperm and regulates the mechanisms for delivery of these sperm into the immediate vicinity of the egg. The female system provides a limited number of eggs, usually one per month, and a mechanism to receive the sperm and to nurture the egg once fertilized.

The male testes are suspended externally in a sac, the *scrotum*. The testes consist of a large number of winding *tubules* packed together with looser tissue between (see Figure 2.30). Male sex hormone is produced by the tissue between the tubules and is discharged directly into the abundant capillary network. Sperm are produced in the walls of the tubules and collect in their central cavities. The mature sperm move along the tubules of the testes into those of the *epididymis* and hence into the *vas deferens* of either side. These collecting ducts join the urethra just below its emergence from the bladder. At various points of the sperm's road, accessory glands (seminal vesicles, prostate, bulbourethral glands) contribute their secretion to form the *semen*, the fluid that ultimately will be discharged.

The distal portion of the urethra running through the penis can convey either urine or semen. Urine flows through the flaccid penis when the sphincter muscle at the base of the bladder relaxes. Semen is discharged through the erect penis by muscular contraction during orgasm. *Erection* occurs when the male becomes sexually aroused and extra blood is forced into the blood vessels and spongy tissue along the shaft of the penis.

The testes and the accessory glands and ducts make up the male reproductive system proper. Beyond the gonads, however, maleness is conferred on many other parts of the body by the circulating male sex hormone. Hair distribution, depth of voice, muscular development, fat distribution, and behavioral characteristics are not always easily or unequivocally related to reproduction but they clearly are part of human sexuality.

The female ovaries lie in the abdominal cavity on either side of the backbone. Each is partly surrounded by the funnel-shaped opening of its *Fallopian tube*, or *oviduct* (see Figure 2.31). Eggs are produced in follicles that progressively mature during each ovarian cycle of about twenty-eight days. At the time of full maturation the follicle is close to the surface of the ovary, through which it ruptures—discharging the egg or ovum into the Fallopian tube. Like the testis, the ovary produces hormones that move directly into the circulation. These female sex hormones are important in controlling the activities of the accessory sex structures and are produced in different quantities and kinds during the sexual cycle.

The egg normally is deposited in the upper end of the oviduct. Currents convey the egg along its length to the uterus, the site of development of the egg in the event of pregnancy. More will be said of this remarkable organ later (Chapter 13). The uter-

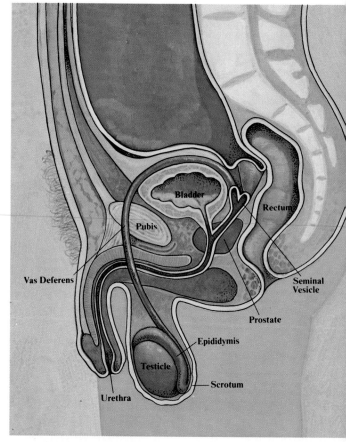

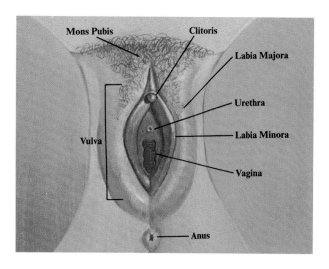

Figure 2.30   (*top right*) An internal view of the male reproductive system.

Figure 2.31   (*above*) The female external genitalia. (*bottom right*) An internal view of the female reproductive system.

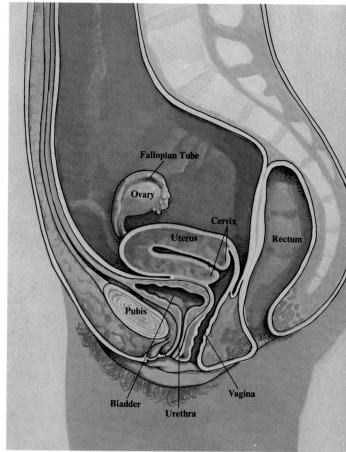

us leads into the vagina, the glandular passageway into which the penis is inserted in intercourse and through which the infant is delivered at birth. Glandular secretions from the uterus, the vagina, and the glands of Bartholin contained in the fleshy folds known as the labia, as well as the products of monthly uterine bleeding, are discharged through the vulva, the external opening of the vagina.

As in the male, the female reproductive system involves more than the gonads and accessory structures. Femaleness is reflected also in development of the breasts, hair distribution, muscular development, and other secondary sex characteristics resulting from the absence of male sex hormone and the presence of female sex hormones.

Thus, reproduction, so essential to the preservation of the human species, is a function of a specific set of organs and activities closely coordinated by endocrine and nervous influences. Knowledge of the nature of these systems is essential to understanding the many subtle and yet profound ways in which sexuality interacts with other bodily functions and influences personalities and society.

A SYSTEM OF CELLS

It is apparent from the many different functions the body performs that there are many different, specialized tissues. The blood vessels and tubules of the kidney must be arranged differently than the blood vessels and nerve cells of the brain or the blood vessels and muscles of the heart. These structural differences are visible not only at the tissue level but at the cellular level as well.

Every organ or tissue of the body is composed of *cells*. Cells are, in fact, the basic unit of all living things. A disease-causing bacterium is a single cell. The human body, on the other hand, has perhaps 100 million million cells. In order to function, each living cell requires nutrients and oxygen and must have its wastes disposed of before they become so plentiful they poison the cell. It is really to serve the body's cells that the respiratory, digestive, circulatory, and excretory systems exist. By means of respiration and digestion, oxygen and nutrients for the cells are acquired. The circulation delivers the oxygen and nutrients to the capillaries, where they can pass through the thin walls of the blood vessels and reach the cells. The circulatory system also collects the waste products of cell activity and transports them to the lungs and kidneys, where they are expelled.

With organs fulfilling so many different functions, it is not surprising that the specialized cells of the body are all quite different. The cells of every system discussed in this chapter have their own characteristics: bone cells are specialized to be stiff and strong; muscle cells to contract; blood cells to transport gases and to perform other tasks; endocrine cells to manufacture and discharge specific hormones; nerve cells to transmit messages that report on the environment or control the activity of muscles, glands, and other organs; male and female sex cells to reproduce the species.

Despite this great diversity, every cell also has certain standard features that identify it as a cell. Even though one sort of cell may be round, another rectangular, and a third long and strung out, all have certain common characteristics (see Figure 2.32). The contents of the cell are enclosed by a *membrane*. Although it is the cell's "skin," nutrients, wastes, and gases can pass through it. At or near the center of the cell is the *nucleus*, also surrounded by a membrane. It contains the chromosomes that enable the cell to reproduce itself by containing all its potential properties encoded in the chemical substances known as nucleic acids (see Chapter 14).

The rest of the cell between the nuclear membrane and the outer membrane contains a thick

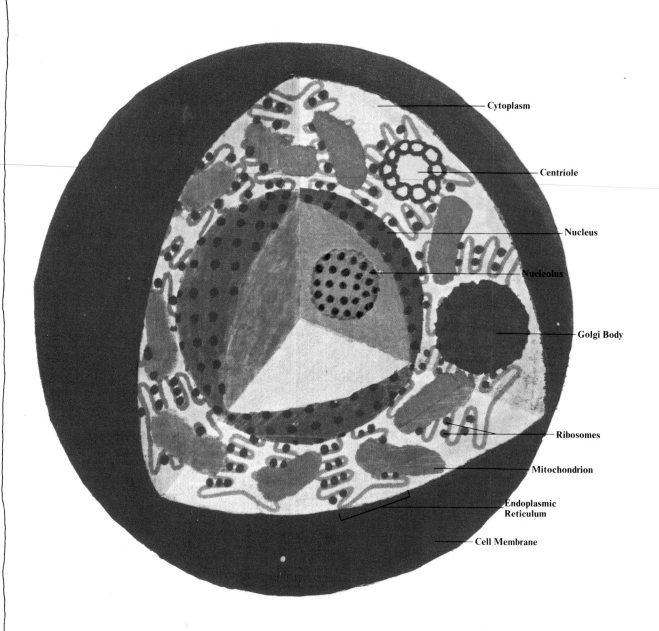

Figure 2.32 The cell. The cell membrane encloses the cell cytoplasm. The cell membrane is semipermeable, which allows certain molecules to pass into and out of the cell. The cytoplasm is a jellylike substance made up of complex membrane systems and intricate proteins. The events that occur in the cytoplasm, such as digestion, respiration, secretion, and excretion, depend on the activity within the nucleus. The nucleus is the governor of cell structure and activity and is the depot of genetic information—the DNA and RNA are contained in the chromatin of the nucleus. The mitochondria serve as the cell's power plants, and the ribosomes, as will be shown in Chapter 14, are the sites of protein synthesis. At the right are examples of various human cells: (*top to bottom*) Normal liver cells, pituitary-gland cells, connective-tissue cells, ciliated cells of the Fallopian tube.

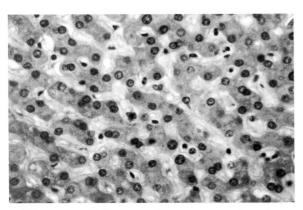

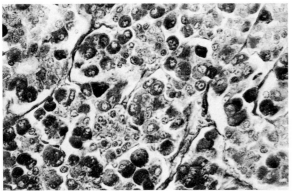

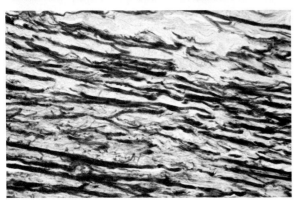

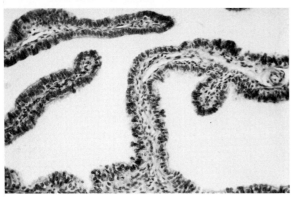

fluid known as the *cytoplasm*. Dissolved in this fluid are many substances—proteins, lipids such as fats, carbohydrates such as sugars, and minerals. The cytoplasm also contains hollow spaces that serve as canals for transporting certain materials, and numerous separate bodies that play essential roles in the life of the cell; all of them are enclosed in membranes. Particularly important are the *mitochondria*, sausage-shaped units that are found in almost all cells. They are often called the power plants of the cell, for they process the nutrients that the cell uses to produce energy with which it can do its work.

At some stage of life every cell is capable of reproducing itself by the simple process of cell division. The cell duplicates its genetic parts, then splits in two. (The process sounds simple when described this way, but it is actually complex and a fascinating subject to be discussed more fully in Chapter 14.) Cell division is responsible for much of what happens when a fertilized human egg cell begins to grow, eventually becoming the fetus in its mother's uterus. Even in an adult human certain cells can still reproduce themselves. Skin cells grow to heal an open wound, leaving a scar. Bone cells heal a fracture. And a partly destroyed human liver can grow back to its full size.

But not all cells can reproduce. Nerve cells, for example those found in the spinal cord or the brain, do not reproduce, which is why certain diseases or injuries of the spine produce permanent paralysis. In the brain, however, certain functions can be taken over by other, undamaged cells, and the victim can relearn them using other brain parts.

MORE THAN THE SUM OF ITS PARTS

It should be apparent by now that in many ways a cell is a miniature version of the body. It requires oxygen and must dispose of carbon dioxide, it consumes nutrients and produces wastes. It repro-

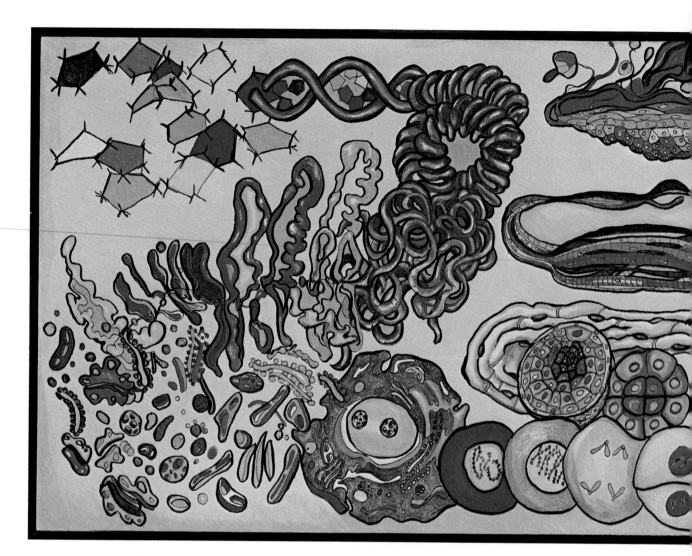

duces itself. And specialized reproductive cells, the male sperm and the female egg, enable the human body to make a replica of itself; therefore, without cellular reproduction, there would be no human reproduction.

At the same time, the human body is a beautifully complex, intricately coordinated system of many highly specialized cells. All the cells of the body depend upon those in the lungs, because all require oxygen. All depend on the red blood cells, which are very efficient carriers of oxygen and carbon dioxide. All cells of the body depend on the muscle cells of the heart, which pumps blood to them. All depend on the cells of the digestive tract

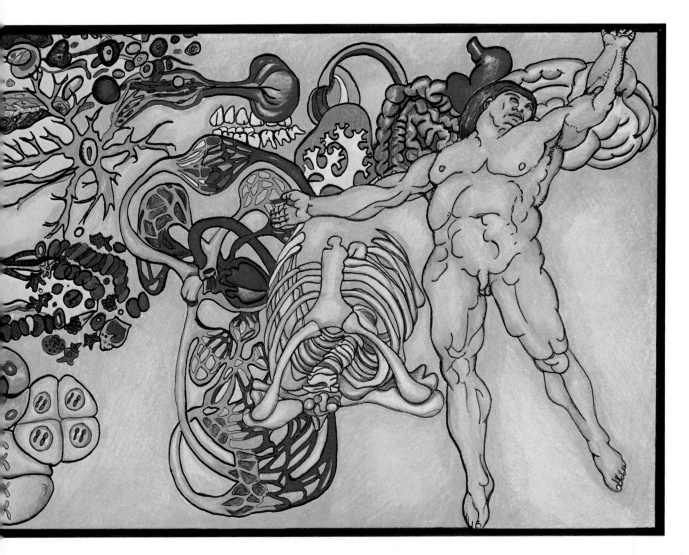

and the kidneys, which collect nutrients and dispose of wastes. All benefit from the controls provided by the endocrine and nervous systems.

Each individual human body is made up of many parts—separate cells, tissues, and organs that could not survive if they were cut off from their very different companions. Put all these parts together, however, and the body becomes a remarkable whole. It is at the same time much greater than the sum of its individual parts, and still completely dependent upon them. Truly, the existence of a person through the medium of his body is an awesome reality deserving, if anything is, of the label "miracle."

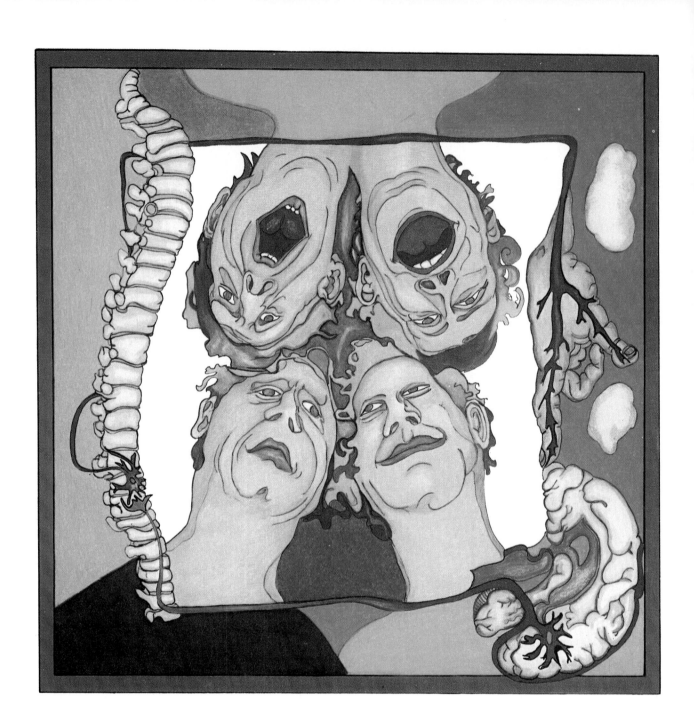

II MENTAL AND EMOTIONAL FUNCTIONING

Computerized robots can be created to duplicate and to exceed human performance — they can even be programmed to laugh and cry. But only humans can actually *feel* and interpret the significance of their feelings. Health is inconceivable apart from the qualities of mind and emotions that enable one to perceive clearly, to feel deeply in congruence with those perceptions, and to grasp the meanings of emotional experiences. ¶ Few health problems are as tragic as the psychoses — they separate the individual, more or less, from the core of his existence and the meaning of his experiences. Conversely, mental health facilitates full, rich perceptions, interpretations, and meanings and thus contributes in the most profound sense to human well-being. Understanding conditions that nurture the development of emotional health are of central importance to all who would seek health. ¶ The study of the human mind, the ways man's thoughts and feelings work, is a new but already complex field. The following three chapters are an attempt to put this entire science into a nutshell — Chapter 3 outlines current studies and knowledge in the physical bases of mental and emotional functioning; Chapter 4 presents the highlights of personality theory and developmental psychology; Chapter 5 condenses the entire fields of abnormal and clinical psychology. By reading these three chapters, one should begin to realize what an awesome possession is the human mind and how very little is actually known about its powers and abilities. Perhaps someday in the not-too-distant future most men will be able to control the workings of their inner organs by will — lowering their blood pressures, slowing their heartbeats, relaxing their muscles with but a thought; psychophysiologists have already found that such control is possible. Neuroscientists believe that the average human being may utilize in his lifetime but a tiny percentage of his nerve cells; perhaps man will learn in the future to make use of greater and greater portions of his brain — and his potential mental power. Although much has been done in the psychological field in the last fifty years, scientists have only begun to explore the outer walls of the palace that is the human mind.

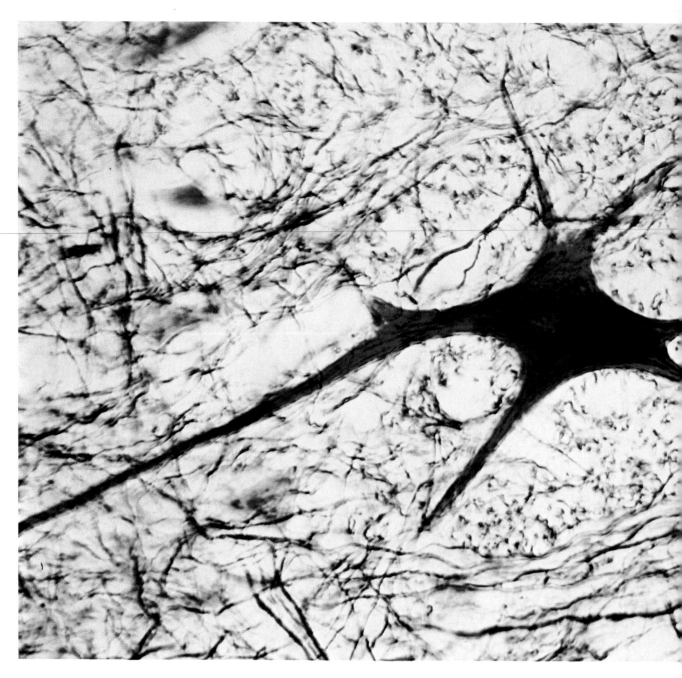

Figure 3.1   A photomicrograph of a nerve cell.

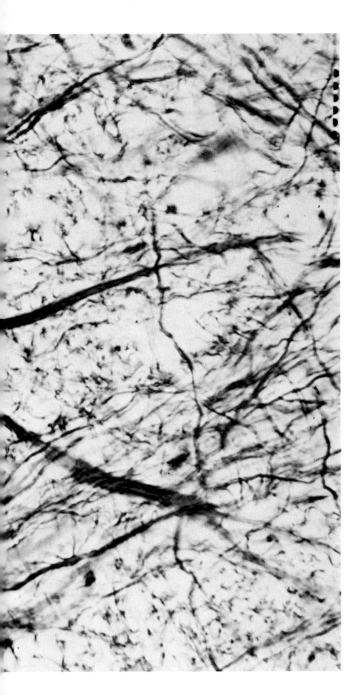

3 Consider the tennis player engaging in a tricky shot or savoring the triumph of a hard-won match; the student absorbed in his homework or worrying about his next test; a businessman reading the morning paper or analyzing the stock market reports; or anyone, whether he walks or daydreams or plays a game of chess, whether he is sick or in health. Whatever one does or does not do involves an incredibly detailed coordination among all the billions and billions of cells that make up the tissues, organs, and systems of his body. This coordination depends on effective, flexible, and yet precise communications.

There are two communication systems on which the body depends. The more primitive one is a *chemical* system: the messages are chemical substances that are distributed by the blood and other body fluids. The chemical substances available in the surroundings of each cell regulate its metabolic activities, and the activity of the cell in turn alters the chemical environment, which then affects other cells, in a sense "informing" them about each other's activities. Besides this general exchange of chemical signals, there also exists a special chemical communication based on hormones—the secretory products of the endocrine system (see Chapter 2)—whose role is to trigger defined activities in specific target areas. This chemical communication system can be seen as similar to the mails; advertising and other general materials are distributed to all kinds

Physiological Basis of Behavior

of addresses—as are the general metabolic messages—while personal letters reach only specified addresses, as do hormones. Note that in this system, as in the mails, the messages are only distributed, never modified.

In contrast, the second communication system on which the body depends is comparable to the telephone system. The messages are basically *electrical*, and the route of distribution is along prelaid cables, linked with one another by relays and switchboards. This second system is the *nervous system*: the cables are the individual nerve fibers, or *axons*; the relays are the *synapses* between neurons; the switchboards are either *interneurons*—nerve cells interposed along a main line of communication—or whole *networks* of neurons. Although it overlaps and sometimes duplicates the chemical system of communication, the nervous system is a more sophisticated arrangement that allows an organism—animal or human—to cope with increasingly fine nuances in its interaction with the environment. It controls all organs and functions of the body and mediates their relationship to both external and internal environments and to one another.

THE PHYSIOLOGY OF THE NERVOUS SYSTEM

The nervous system underlies both *physical* and mental activities of the body. The mental activities include the surge and expression of *emotive* responses as well as the intellectual, or *cognitive*, processes. Many scientists suspect that the emotive and cognitive activities of the nervous system are not basically different from those through which it regulates the body's physical functions, except for the number of nerve cells involved and the intricacy of the nerve-cell networks. Therefore, in order to understand complex functions and malfunctions, such as memory or drug addiction, one must first consider the operation of the smallest units of the nervous system, the neurons, the way they are struc-

tured, and the way they communicate with one another.

The Neuron

The basic unit of the nervous system, as was presented in Chapter 2, is a specialized cell, the *neuron*. The cell membrane of the neuron serves to separate differently charged particles (or ions) from the inside and outside of the cell. When some disturbance occurs at the membrane, it causes the membrane to become leaky, so that the charged particles flow across the membrane, thus cancelling the difference in charge. After the original disturbance is removed, however, the leak in the membrane is soon repaired, and the difference in charge gets reestablished.

The neuronal membrane is shaped essentially like a long, thin sausage skin. A leak occurring in one region of the membrane acts as a disturbance to the neighboring regions, causing them to in turn become leaky, and eventually the leak reaches the end of the sausage skin. As the disturbance spreads away from the point of origin, reduction of charge (actually even a reversal of charge) across each successive point of the membrane is followed by a return of the original charge difference. This sharp sequence of electrical charges is called an *action potential* (see Figure 3.2). Because an action potential reproduces itself as it travels, neural signals can be sent over long distances in the body without getting weaker. Neural signals are thus superior to electrical signals sent over wires, which tend to decrease with distance; the penalty for this advantage is that the signal traveling down a neuron is much slower.

Certain neurons have special molecules, embedded in their membranes, that make them leaky when particular forms of disturbance or energy are applied to them. For instance, there are cells in the eye (photoreceptors), whose membranes contain

Figure 3.2   The action potential. If a neuron is excited with appropriate electrical or chemical stimuli, it causes a change in voltage on the cell membrane. When a critical difference in voltage is reached, an *action potential* is generated. The action potential is a rapid change in voltage that results in a brief reversal of the normal electrical condition (*resting potential*); that is, the interior of the membrane briefly becomes positively charged with respect to the outside of the cell before the resting potential is restored.

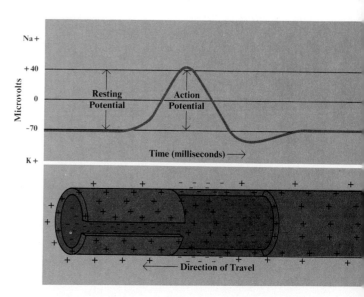

Autonomic Control

by Peter J. Lang

Before Harry Houdini performed one of his famous escapes, a skeptical committee would search his clothes and body. When the members of the committee were satisfied that the Great Houdini was concealing no keys, they would put chains, padlocks and handcuffs on him.

Of course, not even Houdini could open a padlock without a key, and when he was safely behind the curtains he would cough one up. He could hold a key suspended in his throat and regurgitate it when he was unobserved.

The trick behind many of Houdini's escapes was in some ways just as amazing as the escape itself. Ordinarily when an object is stuck in a person's throat he will start to gag. He can't help it—it's an unlearned, automatic reflex. But Houdini had learned to control his gag reflex by practicing for hour after hour with a small piece of potato tied to a string.

In more recent years scientific investigators have studied men with unusual body control. The Russian psychologist A. R. Luria described a mnemonist who in addi-

tion to his remarkable memory could control his skin temperature and heart rate. Merely by visualizing himself as asleep or as vigorously active, he could abruptly alter his heart rate over a range of nearly forty beats per minute. And he could raise the skin temperature of his right hand by imagining it was on a hot stove, while simultaneously lowering the temperature of his left hand by imagining that it was holding an ice cube.

Houdini and the mnemonist run counter to our ordinary conceptions of what the human body can do. Tradition divides human responses into two neat classes—voluntary and involuntary—that correspond to two distinct parts of the nervous system. The fact that we need not control "involuntary" events is a great convenience in day-to-day life. We do not have to take time out from other activities to digest a meal—it happens without our direction. When we wield pen or hammer, our attention is not diverted by the task of moving blood to the relevant muscles. On the other hand, our inability to control these internal events is often discouraging. It would be a blessing if a seasick voyager could calm his stomach at will. And how helpful it would be if a patient with hypertension could lower his own blood pressure.

The first researcher to produce serious evidence that human beings might be able to control their own visceral organs was the

Russian psychologist, M. I. Lisina. In 1958 she reported in this country that she had tried to train her subjects to dilate or constrict the blood vessels in their arms in order to avoid electric shock. At first she was unsuccessful, but when a subject was permitted to watch his own vascular changes displayed on a recording device, he quickly learned how to control them.

A few years later Donald Shearn, working in this country under the direction of the pioneer psychophysiologist R. C. Davis, taught subjects to control their own heart rates. A subject listened to amplified feedback of his heartbeat and learned to avoid a mild electric shock by increasing his heartbeat to a specified rate at scheduled times during the experiment.

In 1962 I started work on the problem of autonomic conditioning in my laboratory at the University of Pittsburgh, and later at the University of Wisconsin in Madison. With Michael Hnatiow, I built an apparatus that permitted a subject to "drive" his own heart. The machine was reminiscent of the driving-skill booths in penny arcades. A subject had to keep the variability of his heartbeat within a specified range. For example, one subject's heart beat about sixty times a minute, with an average of one second between one beat and the next. The subject watched a small spot of light on a screen in front of him. Whenever the interval between two heart-

Adapted from Lang, P. J. "Autonomic Control," *Psychology Today* (October 1970), pp. 37–41, 86.

beats was exactly one second, the light appeared on a vertical line in the center of the screen. When the interval was longer or shorter, the light moved off to the right or left. The subject was told to keep the light within a narrow "road" often less than 90 milliseconds wide—from 955 to 1,045 milliseconds. He soon was quite skilled at keeping the light on the road, and his ability improved with practice.

When we asked the subjects to explain how they had learned, their replies were diverse and inarticulate. This was not unexpected—the English language has almost no words to describe how our bodies feel. I am just as inarticulate in trying to describe the muscles and movements I use in making a forehand shot in tennis as my subjects are in describing how they control their heart rates. In post-experiment interviews our subjects often said that they used idiosyncratic mental routines—counting backward, thinking of emotional events—or small ritualistic movements that they superstitiously believed were causing heart-rate changes.

Other researchers have used operant-feedback methods to demonstrate that a human being can learn to control his own blood pressure, sweat-gland activity, and brain waves. Last year Eberhard Fetz of the University of Washington demonstrated reward learning in a single neuron in a monkey's brain.

Now that we know it is possible to train autonomic functions, we are eager to test the limits of the operant-feedback procedure. We now use a digital computer to process physiological data instantly and display it on a screen for the subject. As soon as a subject's heart beats, he sees moving across the screen from the left a horizontal line that is stopped by his next heartbeat. His job is to make the line stop between two stable, vertical lines positioned by the computer. The computer scores the hits and the misses on a scoreboard. When the subject achieves a certain number of successes the computer compliments him and then automatically readjusts target lines to require more control for success.

The computer is helpful and understanding. A subject who can't succeed at first gets an easier problem to work on until his success rate entitles him to a more difficult game. The machine is programmed to turn off in the event of unusual changes in respiration or muscular activity. Thus, voluntary-muscle "cheating" (such as using chest muscles to control breathing and thus heart rate) is discouraged and only heart-rate changes are reinforced.

Work on voluntary control of the autonomic nervous system has forced psychologists to some profound theoretical considerations. In the first place, the traditional neat di-

chotomy of voluntary and involuntary responses is now out the window. And we must now revise our conceptions of human emotion. For many psychologists the visceral activity of emotion was its primary defining property. In fear, one's mouth goes dry, the pupils dilate, breathing quickens, hands sweat, the heart beats harder and faster. One may deny he is afraid, but supposedly these autonomic signs will give him away. The belief that affect (emotion) is immutably tied to the autonomic nervous system is so well-established that the instrument for detecting autonomic change is called a lie detector. But if visceral responses can be shaped in the same way as any other behavior, the lie detector is no sure route to emotional truth.

This is not to deny that visceral arousal normally accompanies strong emotion. Indeed, the autonomic arousal may itself contribute to the emotions. It is difficult to be calm, even in a safe and comfortable situation, when the heart pounds and the hands sweat. Reducing nervous symptoms directly may help to reduce the anxiety—the function of a tranquilizer. Perhaps one day we can do this voluntarily.

Systematic desensitization, which is one very effective type of therapy for fear, works with analogous principles. A patient is trained to relax muscles all over his body and to remain relaxed while a therapist describes scenes that would ordinarily arouse anxiety in him. Operant-feedback methods may one day permit a patient to calm his own heart rate, blood pressure, and intestinal activities—even his brain waves—while the therapist describes the scary scene.

In our laboratory we are working on an experimental version of systematic-desensitization therapy in which the therapist is actually a digital computer. During treatment the computer analyzes the subject's physiological state continuously and the results may be used to adjust the pattern of his exposure to fear materials. Preliminary work suggests that a machine is in some ways more efficient than a live therapist. We plan to improve the effectiveness of computer therapy by training patients to relax their internal organs as well as their skeletal muscles.

It has been assumed that psychosomatic diseases arise as a result of interpersonal stress, although it is difficult to explain why some individuals who lead relatively placid lives develop disease, while some who lead stressful lives do not. The new visceral-learning data suggest that some body abnormalities may arise through accidental reinforcement learning. A child who is repeatedly allowed to stay home from school when he has an upset stomach may be learning the visceral responses of chronic indigestion. If family arguments always erupt

at the beginning of a meal, the food could reinforce the elevated blood pressure of the antagonists. This process may lay the ground work for many cases of essential hypertension.

A number of investigators are on the autonomic-learning frontiers. They apply research findings to human problems. Bernard Engel of the Baltimore City Hospital uses operant-feedback methods to teach patients to control cardiac arrhythmia. His results are very promising although it is not yet clear that the therapeutic changes he has achieved are due solely to the feedback program. Research groups at Harvard and the University of Tennessee are looking at high blood pressure and disturbances of blood flow to see if they can be brought under voluntary control with operant-feedback therapy.

Francis M. Forster and his associates have reported some success in using analogous methods to treat epileptic patients. One patient who developed seizures when he was exposed to a specific rate of flickering light was treated successfully with a computer-controlled feedback system. In this procedure therapists exposed the subject to flickers at frequencies progressively closer to the critical rate. The computer analyzed changes in the electrical activity of the patient's brain. Whenever his brain waves began to look like those that typically precede a seizure the computer turned off the light and presented auditory clicks to disrupt the seizure pattern. The technique was effective in eliminating the patient's epileptic reactions.

While some researchers have reported dramatic success, it is not yet clear that visceral learning will actually become an important therapeutic method. No one has yet achieved consistent, large changes in cardiovascular or intestinal activity. Most learned changes in human heart rate and blood pressure have been modest—below the level of significant therapeutic effect. And it is doubtful that any learning can overcome autonomic abnormalities that result from physical damage in the organ tissues. Also, it may be that only a few autonomic athletes will be able to achieve important control—early data indicate as much. Work by Jasper Brener and Bob Stern suggests that actors may be able to learn heart-rate and sweat-gland control more readily than ordinary folk. And of course, it is possible that the patients who are unable to control their visceral responses are the ones who develop systemic diseases in the first place.

It is, nevertheless, clear that operant-feedback research has taught us much that we previously did not know about control of the human body. Whether we will be able to use the control to develop practical therapies for emotional disturbance or systemic disease is, I think, one of the most exciting questions in psychology today.

light-absorbing molecules. Light striking such molecules brings about a change in electrical charge across the membrane. On the tongue and in the nose are receptor cells for taste and smell, whose membranes become leaky when molecules of special shapes are fitted into slots on the membrane. Such slots are called *receptor sites*. Furthermore, all neurons have receptor sites for chemicals called *neurotransmitters* that are released by other neurons.

Transmission of Signals Between Neurons

At the end of each neuron are many little bags, called *synaptic vesicles*, that contain the chemical transmitters. When an action potential arrives at the neuron ending, it forces the contents out of some of the vesicles and into the space between two neighboring neurons, called the *synaptic cleft* (see Figure 3.3). The expelled transmitter fits into the corresponding receptor sites in the membrane (called the *postsynaptic membrane*) of the next neuron lying across the cleft and generates a membrane disturbance that will be propagated down its length as another action potential. At the same time, the transmitter that has reacted with the membrane receptor sites is rapidly removed and destroyed, so that the sites are once again available for a new delivery of synaptic transmitter.

The arrangement that allows one neuron to excite another is called an *excitatory synapse.* In other synapses, called *inhibitory synapses*, the expelled transmitter makes it more difficult or even impossible for the postsynaptic neuron to become excited through other (excitatory) synapses. Most neurons have a large number of connections with other neurons, and many have more than 10,000 separate excitatory and inhibitory synapses on their membranes.

Although the properties of the tiny neuron seem far removed from the problems of ordinary life, they do enable one to understand what hap-

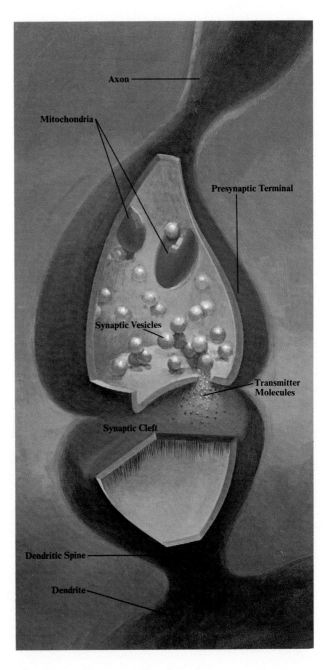

Figure 3.3   The synapse. Note the neurotransmitter being released into the synaptic cleft by the synaptic vesicles.

pens when someone takes drugs. For instance, it takes social and personality theory to explain why a person starts to take a drug, but the main reasons for tolerance and addiction once the drug has been taken are physiological. All the drugs that have an effect on the mind presumably modify transmission across some synapses by interfering with the production, storage, release, or disposal of the transmitter or with the postsynaptic receptor sites on which it was to act.

One transmitter used primarily by certain parts of the nervous system is *noradrenalin* (also called *norepinephrine*). Its involvement in the basis of emotive behavior will be discussed in a later section. An even greater number of neurons in the nervous system utilize another transmitter called *acetylcholine.* This transmitter also is released at the junction between neuron endings and many muscles or glands—the effector organs of the body. Various substances can prevent or reduce the amount of the transmitter acetylcholine released into the synaptic cleft. One example is botulinus toxin, a poison produced by bacteria that grow in improperly sterilized food. When even a small quantity of this toxin is in-

gested, it prevents neurons using acetylcholine as a transmitter from passing signals to other neurons. The results can be fatal.

Interaction Among Neurons

Whatever functions the nervous system is called upon to serve, the basic scheme of neural activity can always be viewed as comprising an *input*, a *central*, and an *output* component (see Figure 3.4).

Primary, or sensory, *inputs* to the nervous system come through the various receptor organs, or sensors, from the outside world as well as from all parts of the body. Thus, one takes in not only sights, sounds, smells, temperature changes, contacts, and so on, but also changes in the temperature and composition of the blood (the chemical communication system), the position or movements of various parts of the body (limbs, head, the visceral organs), and the rhythm of others (heart, lungs). Furthermore, neurons that have received primary inputs from one or another sensor can in turn act as sources of signals to other neurons and thus provide secondary inputs.

Information is sifted and processed in the *central*

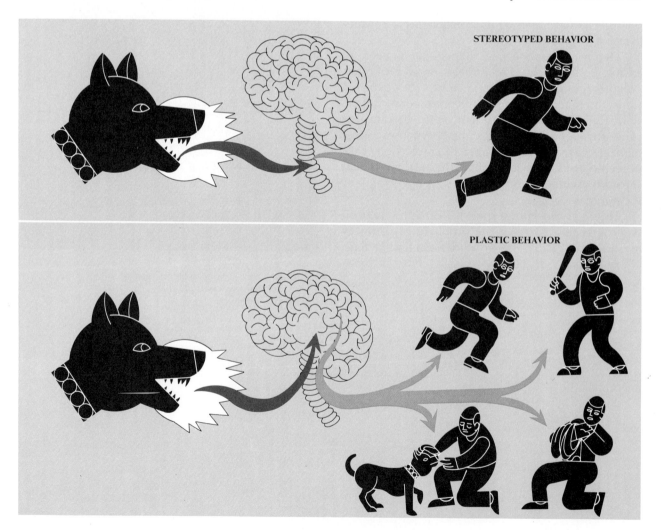

STEREOTYPED BEHAVIOR

PLASTIC BEHAVIOR

component, which corresponds basically to the brain and spinal cord, or central nervous system (CNS). The higher on the animal ladder, the greater the size and complexity of the central nervous system. The number of neuronal links along each chain of communication also increases, as do the number of extensive networks connecting different chains with one another. This increase in nerve-cell numbers and neuronal interconnections is grossly reflected in an increase in the anatomical size and structural complexity of the nervous system. In the human body, it is estimated that the input and output components engage some 3 to 15 million neurons, while the CNS, or central component, comprises 10 billion or more of them. The greater this central build-up, the greater the number of options that the body has available to respond to a given situation. The number of options is actually far, far greater than even the number of CNS neurons because of the possibilities many of these neurons appear to have to branch out and connect with any one or any number of the others.

Once the central nervous system has processed the information it receives from the input system, it sends out directions (the motor *output* component) that will set into motion the body's muscles and glands, that is, its mechanical and chemical *effectors*, whose actions will modify both external and internal environments.

THE NERVOUS SYSTEM AND BEHAVIOR

Interactions among neurons—along the input, central, and output components of the nervous system—are what determine the final response that a person will have to any given internal or external situation. The sum of these responses is called *behavior*. Many of these responses are overt actions involving the relationship of the person to his external environment and can be directly perceived by the person himself and by other people. Other responses, like changes in the composition of the blood or the electrical waves of the brain, might only be detectable with the use of sensitive instruments or may go undetected for lack of sufficient knowledge about their nature.

But behavior also is a form of *communication between individuals*. As such, it uses many different modes: postures and gestures, odors and colors, sounds and, perhaps most obviously, language. As a form of communication, behavior becomes a social as well as an individual phenomenon. Because it starts from inputs deriving from the *outside* as well as the *inside* worlds, an individual's behavior is sensitive to disturbances of *both*. Thus, behavioral inadequacies become social, as well as individual, disorders. The study of behavior helps one to understand what goes on *within the individual*, what kinds of mechanisms operate in the expression of specific behavioral traits, what kinds of stimuli or experiences are responsible for triggering them, and eventually, what physical or mental diseases may cause the behavioral response to be inadequate to the situation that generates it.

Psychologists distinguish different types of behavior, depending on the degree of conscious control involved, and psychophysiologists have attempted to define the physical systems underlying them. In a *stereotyped behavior* (stereo means solid, hence rigid), only one response is possible to a given signal: there are no options. The neuronal chain linking the reception of the stimulus to the output of the corresponding directive is laid out in the body and cannot be modified. Stereotyped behavior is common in the lower animals, but also occurs in man; the simplest example of it is the reflex arc discussed in Chapter 2.

The next higher mode of behavior is *plastic behavior*, in which options are available and the final selection depends not only on the signal (as in stereotyped behavior) but also on the mood and the

Figure 3.4   The difference between stereotyped and plastic behaviors. Both involve input, central, and output components. Where stereotyped behaviors have only one possible output, plastic behaviors may involve a variety of possible outputs.

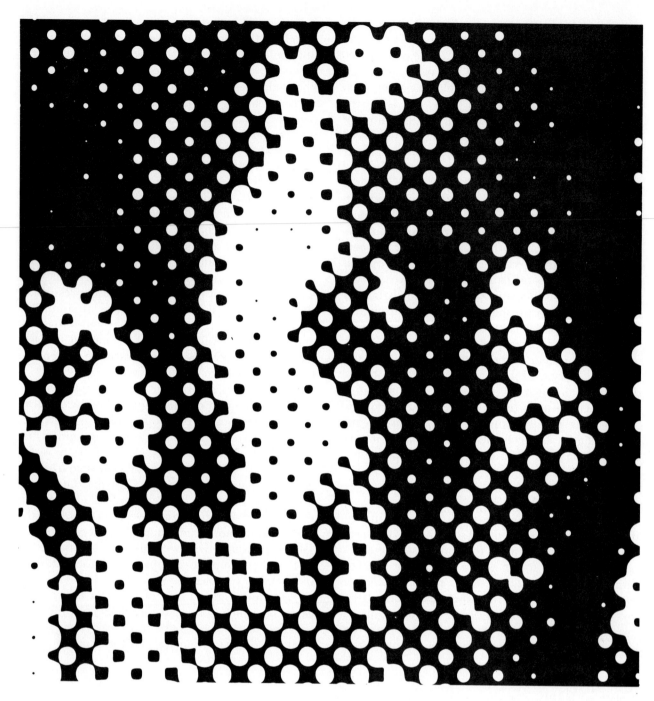

Figure 3.5 (*above*) Look at this picture closely, then look at it from a distance. The eye takes in sensations, which the mind integrates into perceptions. This type of integration can be impeded or altered by fatigue or certain drugs, for instance.

Figure 3.6 (*right*) Visual representation in the brain. (*top right*) An oscilloscope recording shows a "firing" of the neuron when a spot of light strikes the field center; if the spot hits an "off" area, the firing is suppressed. In the second type the cell fires if the light hits outer areas and is suppressed if the light hits the center. (*bottom right*) Simple cortical cells have fields of various types. In all of them the "on" and "off" areas, represented by magenta and orange dots respectively, are separated by straight boundaries. Note that orientations and widths of fields vary. In the cat's visual system such fields generally are one millimeter or less in diameter. (*left*) How the experiment was conducted. One experimenter throws a line of light on a screen in front of the animal's eyes, while another marks the features to which a particular brain cell responds. (Adapted from D. Hubel, "The Visual Cortex of the Brain," *Scientific American* (November 1963), p. 57. Copyright © by Scientific American, Inc. All rights reserved.)

history of the individual. The "mood" can be defined as the individual's *motivational* state at any particular time (see Chapter 4); the nervous system contributes to it through both its emotive and its cognitive activities. The "history" is the sum of all imprints left in the individual by the experiences of the past as the result of memory and learning, two mental processes that involve mainly the cognitive functions of the CNS. The highest form of plastic behavior is that which includes language. Plastic behavior plus language is the privilege of few animal species, and some scientists claim it is exclusive to man. In it, the final activity of the individual is affected by signal, mood, history, *and* the purely cognitive ability to name and relate different entities as abstractions. It is through such abilities, for example, that one can say "lion" without at once jumping up and getting ready to attack or escape.

At the input end, too, one must distinguish between a "passive" reception, or *sensation*, not unlike the stereotype output behavior, and an "active" reception, or *perception*, in which the incoming message is interpreted in terms of the source or the action that produced it and is expanded on the basis of the receiver's expectations. For example, a person receiving certain sensations of roundness, hardness, coolness, and other visual cues will synthesize these cues into the perception of a cup. Or sometimes one hears only half a word or sentence and makes up or presumes the rest. Perception, therefore, involves the signal and its source, the mood (or receptiveness), and the history (or past experiences) of the "receiver," just as plastic output behavior does in the case of the "broadcaster."

BRAIN FUNCTION

It used to be thought that the brain was largely undifferentiated—that no part of the brain was essential for any particular ability and that the parts were interchangeable in their function. Many experiments have confirmed the fact that various functions of the brain—from visual representation to muscular control to highly sophisticated cognitive activities—are localized in specific brain areas.

Visual Abstraction

Scientists are now beginning to understand a little about how man sees shapes and grasps abstract relations. Tiny electrical probes, called *microelectrodes* (tiny needles capable of carrying electrical current), can be placed close to single neurons near the surface of the brain, so that they can register action potentials as the neurons react to incoming signals. When such probes were sunk into the area of cat's and monkey's brains that is linked—through a chain of neurons—to the nerve cells of the eye, it was found that the cells in this brain region produced action potentials only when specific shapes were presented to the eye. For instance, a cell would produce action potentials only when a line was placed in a certain position and would stop producing them if the line was moved or tilted. Another cell would produce action potentials only

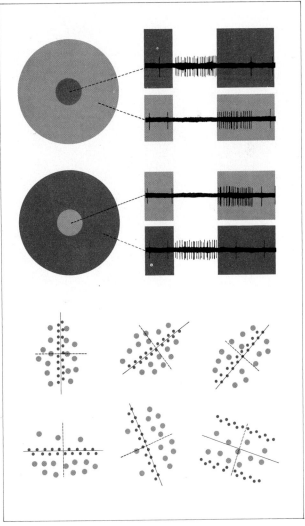

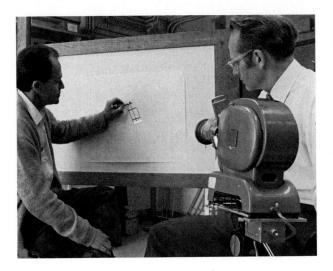

when two lines converging at a certain angle were placed in a specific spot, while yet other cells were triggered only when a line slanted at a specific tilt ended at a certain point.

These microelectrode experiments have brought under observation a part of the process of *abstraction* without which even rudimentary intelligence is impossible. Without being able to tell lines and their tilts and angles, man could not make use of the images formed in his eyes. Cells in other brain areas take the process of abstraction even further. These cells produce action potentials when a certain number of flashes or sounds have impinged on the animal. In other words, these neurons count. One neuron will produce action potentials when four sounds or lights have occurred and stop thereafter; another will produce action potentials after six sounds or lights and then stop.

How do neurons abstract? Taking the visual function as an example, at the back of the eye is a surface (the retina) coated with light-sensitive neurons (see Chapter 19), which are indirectly connect-

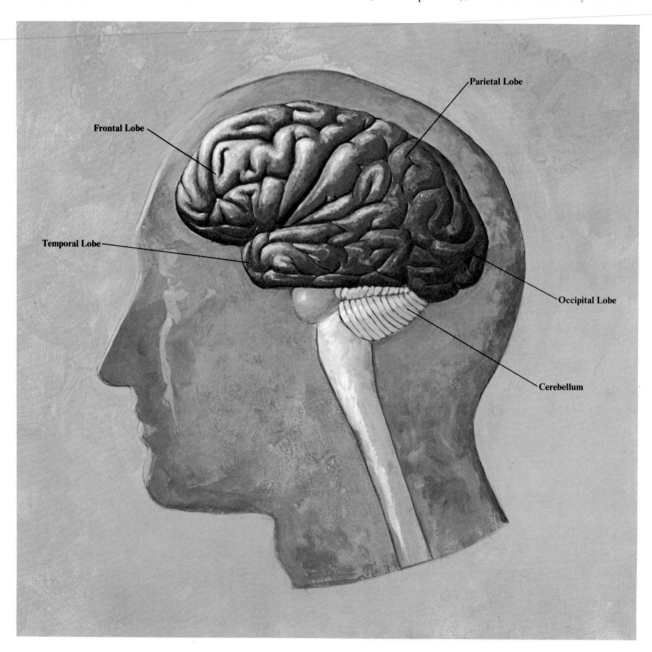

Figure 3.7 The major divisions of the cortex.

ed to neurons in the brain. One cell in the brain may be connected to many neurons in the eye, some excitatory and others inhibitory. A large number of these excitatory cells of the eye, for example, could all be neighbors, lie on a straight line, and be surrounded by inhibitory cells. If a viewed line falls exactly on the line of excitatory light-sensitive neurons, they will *excite* the neuron in the brain. However, if the line falls out of alignment, it will trigger some of the light-sensitive neurons that *inhibit* the brain neuron, and the latter will show no activity even though the line falls on some of the excitatory neurons.

Studies on Epilepsy

Evidence that different parts of the brain perform different tasks also has been confirmed by electrical stimulation of the brain. Stimulation on human patients is most often performed during surgery for epilepsy. Epilepsy is frequently caused by a small piece of brain tissue that begins to produce abnormal electrical activity when stimulated. The abnormal activity then spreads to neighboring pieces of tissue, gradually involving larger areas of the brain, causing loss of consciousness and often uncontrollable body movements.

In one class of epileptics, the seizure always begins with the twitching of some particular body part such as the thumb or foot—the same body part in the case of any one patient. The convulsive movements then always spread in the same order across the rest of the musculature of the body. John Hughlings Jackson, a nineteenth-century English doctor, was able to deduce the way parts of the body were mapped on the surface of the brain by observing such epileptic seizures. As can be seen from a map of the movement areas in the brain (see Figure 3.8), neighboring areas in the representation of the body on the brain surface are not neighbors on the body. For instance, on the surface of the brain, the thumb is a neighbor of the neck. Jackson would then have observed a twitching of the thumb to be followed by contractions in the neck regions. Jackson's deductions have since been confirmed by direct stimulation of the brain.

Because there often seems to be some small

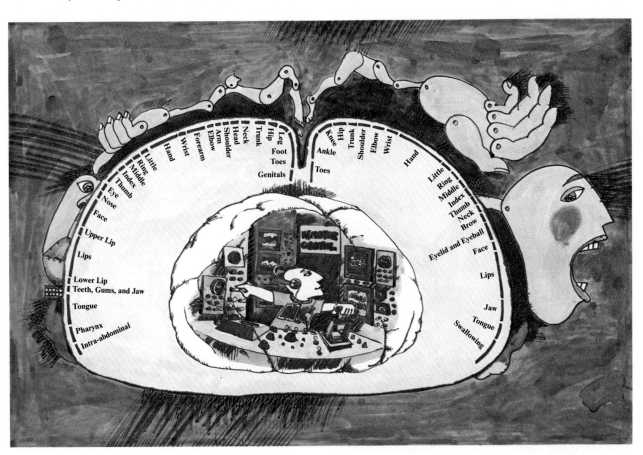

Figure 3.8   Where control of movement in different parts of the body is located in the motor cortex of the brain. (After Penfield and Rasmussen, 1950.)

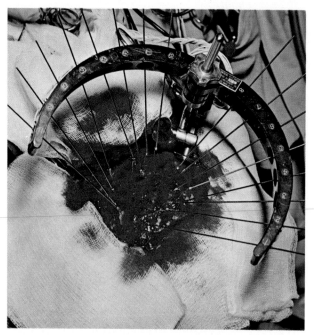

Figure 3.9 Brain operations are performed to determine where abnormalities that cause epilepsy are located and to destroy or remove such areas.

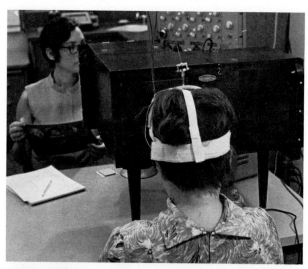

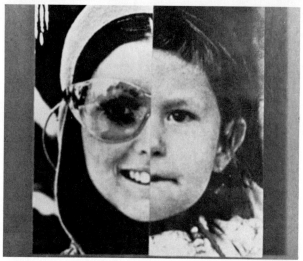

pieces of tissue from which the seizure starts in the epileptic brain, surgeons have attempted to remove these abnormal pieces of brain in order to prevent epileptic seizures from occurring. Such procedures have been quite successful. To know which piece of the brain must be removed, the surgeon opens up the skull under local anesthesia and proceeds to stimulate the brain with small electrodes. When the surgeon's electrode induces the movement with which a seizure always starts, cutting out the small piece under the electrode stops the further occurrence of seizures. The procedure of stimulating the surface of the brain electrically—in fact, the cutting or the burning of brain tissue—is entirely painless because pain (or any other sensation) can be evoked only where there are receptor neurons collecting and conveying messages to specialized parts of the brain. The brain does not have such neurons and therefore is not wired to feel injury to itself.

In some patients the onset of the seizure is represented not by a movement but by a sensation called an *aura*. Some patients have seizures preceded by a specific strong sensation such as that of smell. Others see and hear fairly specific elaborate scenes. Sometimes seizures can be triggered by specific sensations. In one patient, for instance, a seizure could be evoked by scratching the end of one of his fingers. In another case a seizure would occur whenever the patient saw closely spaced horizontal lines; he would thus lose consciousness whenever he came near window screens or certain types of wire fences.

Brain Injury

People involved in an accident may suffer brain damage involving restricted or widespread portions of the central nervous system. Such damage often produces epilepsy, and the damaged area—at times even a whole cerebral hemisphere—may have to be removed by the neurosurgeon before the spread-

Figure 3.10 Severe epilepsy sometimes requires a brain operation in which the two halves of the brain are "disconnected"— the fibers that connect the two halves are severed. Here a housewife who underwent the operation and who is able to function normally in her daily life is given a test. She is shown a face on the screen and then is shown a group of faces and is asked to pick out the one she saw. When she is shown a picture made up of two split faces, a woman's on the left and a child's on the right, the housewife says she has seen only the woman's face. Why? The left side of the brain sees what is in the right visual field and the right side sees what is on the left (see Figure 3.12). Normally this information is then exchanged between the two sides of the brain, but in the housewife's brain the split prevented each side from knowing what the other side was seeing. Because the right side of the brain controls speech, she reported what was in the left visual field.

ing of the epileptic disorder impairs speech or other general intellectual capacities. In other cases, brain damage can be caused by the growth of a malignant tumor, or the occurrence of a cerebral stroke (see Chapter 24). Whatever the cause, destruction of certain parts of the brain can lead to quite specific losses of function.

One example is the destruction of the area of cerebral cortex at the back of the head (occipital cortex) to which the nerve cells of the eye are connected. Such damage causes complete blindness for the side of the visual field opposite to the side of brain injury. This blindness, unlike that caused by eye or optic-nerve injury, can be accompanied by the inability to remember what it was like to see.

There is an area on the surface of the brain underlying the sides of the head (parietal cortex), injury to which can cause various kinds of speech inabilities. Injuries to some parts of this area produce an inability to understand speech; injuries to other parts result in an inability to produce speech. In right-handed people, this area is located in the left hemisphere of the brain; in left-handed people

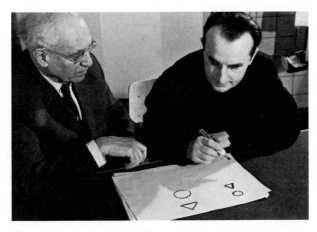

Figure 3.11 Brain injury. The man on the right has received a head wound that affected the area of the brain that helps one to understand spatial relationships; he therefore is confused about such concepts as "above" and "beneath."

Figure 3.12 Visual fields. Normally the right side of the brain perceives the left visual field and the left side perceives the right. If, for example, an injury damages the right side of the brain, the person will see only the right visual field—the left field will be blank.

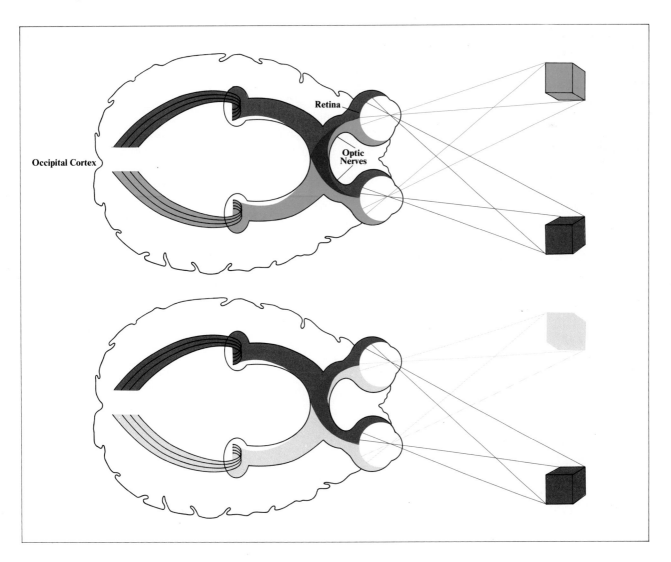

it is on the right. Injury to the corresponding area in the opposite hemisphere leaves speech skill unaffected. Instead, the victim cannot find his way around even in familiar surroundings, cannot draw sensible maps of his environment, and seems to get the spatial positions of parts of common objects mixed up in his drawings. Thus, areas in the two halves of the brain seem to have become specialized. Apparently, this specialization occurs somewhere late in childhood, because before about the age of five either hemisphere can be removed without affecting the ability to speak.

The Neuron and Memory

Whenever a person learns something, there is an alteration somewhere in that vast collection of neurons called the brain. Scientists have shown that whatever it is that changes as a result of learning must change quite slowly for weeks and months after it is learned. For example, people who suffer even slight head injuries often cannot recall anything that occurred just before the injury. If the injury is severe, they cannot recall what happened for many months before it (although some of these memories may return later). They can, however, remember what happened many years before the occurrence. It seems, therefore, that the brain change underlying memory becomes gradually different as it gets older and more resistant to damage.

There is no evidence, at present, that memory processes are clearly localized to specific brain areas. However, the complexity of what psychophysiologists call memory and learning is still so imperfectly understood that certain brain regions may well turn out to play critical roles in some accessory if not central aspects of these functions.

EMOTIVE BEHAVIOR

Emotive activity, such as is commonly encompassed in words like "feelings," "emotions," and "moods," involves interaction between both the neural and the chemical communication systems of the body. As with the other neural activities, three main components are recognizable in emotive activities. The *central* component controlling emotive behavior is thought to be the portion of the brain known as the *limbic system*. Upon this central component impinge *inputs* derived primarily from the other parts of the brain after they have evaluated sensory information from both inside and outside the body. Out of the control centers in the limbic system radiate *outputs*, or directions to the various body organs involved in a specific behavior. In some cases, the directions are relayed, amplified, or further specified by the *endocrine system* as well. The following example will show something about how this system works.

Fight or Flight

If an animal is threatened or if a person becomes angry or scared (feels threatened), a number of processes in the body will prepare the organism for fast action, be it fight or flight. Heart rate and respiration increase to provide more oxygen; blood supply gets reapportioned to service those organs that will be most needed (muscles, heart, brain); fuel such as glucose is mobilized and more rapidly delivered; muscles increase their tone, and senses their alertness. Furthermore, the body assumes postures favorable to action directed to the removal of the threat.

How do these changes come about, and what is the final outcome? The threatening signals, from an external attack or an internal stress situation, are received by a number of different sensors, and the various sensory inputs are integrated in the brain to spell out the message "threat." A special branch of the autonomic motor nervous system, known as the *sympathetic system*, carries the message to various organs, each of which translates the

Figure 3.13 The fight-flight response. What happens in the body when stress is introduced.

neural message into specific instructions appropriate to its own role. In addition, the sympathetic system also brings the "threat" message to the adrenal glands, where it is translated into a new message: "Deliver hormone." The adrenals secrete *adrenalin* into the blood, which conveys it to all parts of the body to further prepare it for action.

But the communication process does not stop there. The activity of the various alerted organs generates in turn new sets of nonspecific chemical messages (metabolic products, glucose and oxygen depletion in the blood, and so on), which the blood again carries around for internal receptor cells to translate into neural messages. These messages, as well as direct neural signals from the organs in action—due, for example, to changes in position—are conveyed back to the brain via the internal sensory neural pathways.

Thus far, the nervous system has performed a "physical" function. If nothing else were involved, the physical portion of the CNS would integrate the "threat" signals from the outside or inside world with the "ready" signals from the alerted organs of the body and coordinate the stereotyped behavior of "rage." The stereotyped behavior of rage constitutes a form of defense response in animals. Postures, facial expressions, smells, growling, and so on, all components of a behavioral communication, may convey a counterthreat to the attacker, trigger in him a similar rage behavior, and either discourage him from attacking or precipitate further aggressive action. Animals usually have only these two options for further defensive responses—attack or escape, fight or flight—and both of them are additional examples of stereotyped behavior.

The choice between the two options is, however, an example of plastic behavior. Furthermore, the threatened animal or person may be involved in some other tasks, and its receptiveness, or alertness, may be decreased. He may have to choose between a "defense" task and the activity in which his current interests are engaged—a matter of "motivation." He may compare the present situation with past experiences—make use of his memory—and decide, for example, that the threat is not serious and should be ignored. In other words, the emotive

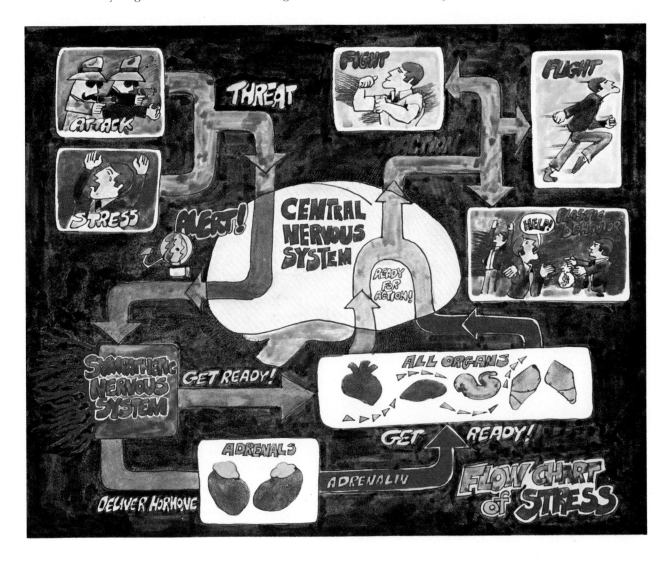

and cognitive portions of the brain get into the act, and the mood and history of the individual will determine whether a new behavior will be evoked and if so, which one.

Switches for Stereotyped Behaviors

As with the fight-or-flight defense behavior, one often makes "instinctive" responses that rely on stereotyped behavior patterns. The *matrix* for each of them—that is, the neural circuitry that underlies it—may have been laid out under genetic instructions during the development of the nervous system or may be acquired later through a series of experiences. These matrices reside in various portions of the nervous system but rarely operate in total isolation from the rest of it. The *switches* that activate them or turn them off may be, and often are, under the control of higher neural centers.

Investigations have been carried out on various types of animals (cats, rats, monkeys) with the ultimate aim of understanding the corresponding mechanisms in man. For example, microelectrodes can be positioned very precisely in a desired brain area and used to stimulate discrete and minute portions of brain tissue or to record their activity. Stimulation and monitoring can even be done by remote control—using radio signals—to avoid the necessity of wires. Microelectrodes, as has already been mentioned, also can be used to destroy selected brain areas by applying greater amounts of electrical current, a highly sophisticated form of microsurgery. Thin, hollow shafts also can be implanted in selected brain areas, through which scientists could inject minute amounts of chemical solutions instead of delivering electrical stimuli.

From these investigations, psychophysiologists have learned of a number of centers that mediate the control of various types of emotive behavior. These centers are located in the limbic system, which is connected with many other brain subsystems—including the cerebral cortex, where many of the cognitive functions reside—as well as with the peripheral sympathetic system that carries the "threat" messages to the various effector organs.

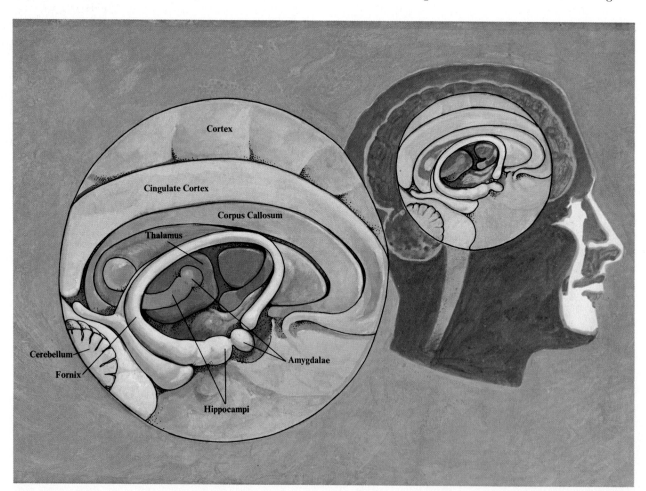

Figure 3.14 The structure of the limbic system. There are varied groups of interconnected structures in the forebrain that have recently received much attention because of their presumed role in regulating the emotional activity of the organism. The structures involved include the amygdalae, cingulate cortex, hippocampus, and septal area. Lesions in those areas have profound effects on emotional reactivity, turning such highly excitable creatures as monkeys and mountain lions into docile pets and converting highly tame laboratory rats into ferocious prone-to-fight subjects (at least for a limited time).

RAGE CENTERS   Within the rear portion of the limbic system are structures known as the *amygdalae*, where the *switch-on* controls for rage behavior are located. Close by the switch-on areas, other tiny areas act as *switch-off* centers through which rage behavior is inhibited. Electrical stimulation of the switch-on centers will induce the typical rage behavior, while destruction of them will prevent such behavior from occurring no matter how threatening a situation is imposed on the subject. The converse is true with respect to the switch-off centers. The existence of these two control centers acting in opposite directions is another example of the antagonistic principle that appears in the operation of so many body systems (see Chapter 2). The *emotive* correlates of rage and related behaviors are anger ("fight") or fear ("flight"), and the balance between these two emotions may well depend on the relative activity of the two antagonistic limbic centers.

These experimental findings already have been applied to man. Both examination and treatment of human patients with unmanageable epilepsy and a past history of uncontrolled assaultive behavior have been carried out by use of electrodes implanted in the limbic centers. A dramatic case is that of a brilliant electrical engineer who suffered from frequent, uncontrollable psychomotor seizures—epileptic attacks affecting both mental and muscular activities—and violent attacks of rage during which he often could not prevent himself from beating and torturing his wife and children. Electrode stimulation of the limbic amygdalae on both sides of the brain evoked pain and the comment, "I am losing control," both characteristic of the spontaneous attacks. In contrast, stimulation of electrode points only one-sixth of an inch away from the previous ones could quickly reverse the patient's emotional state, keeping it changed for several hours. Finally, destruction, through the electrodes, of the first areas caused a transitory depression and, following

that, the elimination of any spontaneous attack since the operation was performed.

PLEASURE CENTERS   Whereas the rear portion of the limbic system controls emergency responses such as rage behavior and emotional responses such as anger or fear, other regions have been found to be involved in different responses. A startling discovery was brought forth by the use of the *Skinner box*, a device with which one could measure the reward value of a signal. An animal placed in a box containing only a lever will press it perhaps ten times an hour. If a food pellet is delivered every time the lever is pressed, a hungry animal learns to perform ten times more frequently. Other "rewards" will induce different increases of the performance rate and thus indicate the relative value to the animal of each type of reward. The lever in the box can be connected to electrodes placed in the brain of the animal in such a way that the depression of the lever delivers a mild electric stimulus through the electrode. In this way, scientists can assess whether or not the stimulation of a particular brain area is "rewarding" or "pleasurable" to the animal.

When scientists explored the midline region of the limbic system by implanting the electrode in one location after another, areas were found that, when stimulated, gave the animal so much pleasure that it would press the lever—and thus bring stimulation—as often as 5,000 times an hour. Thus, direct self-stimulation of these *pleasure centers* was fifty times more rewarding than even the acquisition of food. These centers appear to be located in the same general region that other investigators have found to affect eating, drinking, digestion, excretion, sexual behavior, and other activities with strong "pleasurable" emotive correlates. Placing electrodes in areas nearer the rage centers, on the other hand, appeared to discourage the animal

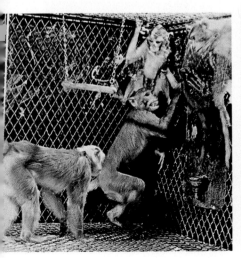
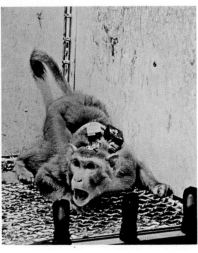

Figure 3.15   Aggression and threat elicited by brain stimulation. The apparatus strapped to the monkey's back receives the signal to deliver current to the brain.

from pressing the lever. These areas, therefore, could be controlling the pleasure centers or even be "punishment" centers antagonistic to them, much as is the case with the rage-control areas.

HUNGER AND THIRST CENTERS   The technique of highly localized, chemical microinjections has been used to show that limbic centers can be activated by a direct application of chemical neurotransmitters, such as acetylcholine and noradrenalin. Experimenters, using the electrical stimulation technique, had uncovered another limbic area acting as a "hunger" center. Upon stimulation of this area a well-fed, sated rat would be made to resume eating at a voracious rate. It has since been shown that the same "hunger" behavior was triggered by the direct delivery of noradrenalin to the center. However, injection of acetylcholine to the same region elicited drinking behavior, with the animal sometimes consuming twice as much in one hour as it usually would in a day.

The simplest interpretation, although by no means the only possible one, is that the same limbic region comprises nerve cells of two types, suscepti-

ble to different neurotransmitters and controlling different drives. Whether that region will perform as a hunger or as a thirst center could then depend on which neurotransmitter is delivered from incoming, and presumably different, networks—a chemical counterpart of the optional concept of plastic behavior.

The Role of Chemical Transmitters in Emotions

Electrical stimulation of the brain (ESB) has been, and still is, a valuable tool for research scientists to probe and affect brain areas involved in behavior control and thus define an electrical basis of behavior. But neurons are normally triggered not by electric shocks but by the delivery, from other neurons synapsing with them, of one or another chemical transmitter. Thus, as confirmed by the experiments on the hunger and thirst centers, one can more appropriately think in terms of a *chemical basis of behavior*. It appears that noradrenalin and other related chemicals are the primary transmitters involved in the emotive functions of the nervous system.

As its name suggests, noradrenalin is closely related to the hormone adrenalin, which, too, is a neurotransmitter in certain animal species. Adrenalin and noradrenalin have been reported to play specific roles outside the brain with respect to stress or threat situations inducing the fight-or-flight behaviors and their correlates, anger and fear.

One series of studies that gave evidence of this role involved the examination of students' behavior in selectively contrived or naturally occurring situations. It has been known for some time that injection into the blood of either adrenalin or noradrenalin provokes a pattern of physiological reactions characteristic of the chemical injected. College students, made deliberately angry, displayed the physiological reaction pattern characteristic of noradrenalin effects. The same subjects, deliberately made

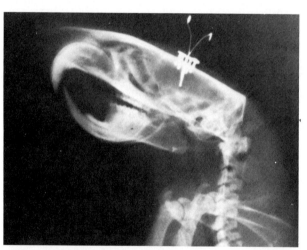

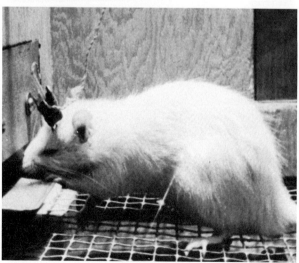

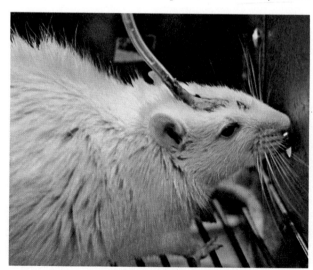

afraid, exhibited the pattern typical of the effects of adrenalin injections.

Similarly, medical students were examined under a stress situation (certification of their hospital internship), where some persons reacted by getting angry and aggressive, others by becoming afraid or depressed. Those who got angry showed noradrenalinlike patterns, while those who got depressed showed adrenalinlike ones. The adrenals secrete predominantly noradrenalin in highly aggressive animals like the lion and predominantly adrenalin in animals who depend primarily on flight for survival (like the rabbit) or who lead highly socialized or domestic lives (such as the baboon or the cat).

Thus it appears that anger or aggressive behavior involves primarily a surge in the blood of noradrenalin, while fear or escape behavior involves a surge of adrenalin—or at least of chemicals mimicking these two substances. The decision as to which chemical is to be released does not lie with the adrenals but with the limbic system.

DRUGS AND NEUROTRANSMITTERS *Pharmacology* is the science that studies the effects and mechanisms of action of drugs on living systems. *Psychopharmacology* is concerned with certain categories of drugs that are "psychoactive," that is, that primarily affect mental functions. That such a specific category of drugs exists is understandable when mental processes are viewed as having a chemical as well as an electrophysiological basis. The effects and social implications of use, misuse, and abuse of psychoactive drugs are discussed at great length in Unit III. What is of particular interest here is the examination of the possible relationship of some of these drugs to neurotransmitters and neurotransmitter action in mental processes.

Years ago, doctors started treating tuberculosis with a drug called Iproniazid. This drug, like many others, was synthetic—manufactured in a chemical laboratory and then tested for pharmacological activities. Some doctors noticed that many of the treated patients exhibited a markedly uplifted, euphoric behavior. This chance observation led to the discovery that Iproniazid and other drugs act as potent antidepressants. It was subsequently found that these drugs inhibit an enzyme whose normal function in the nervous system is to destroy noradrenalin and other similar neurotransmitters. Thus, presumably, the drug might alter the levels of the neurotransmitter and influence networks and centers susceptible to its action.

Similarly, the treatment of patients with high blood pressure by use of the drug reserpine led to the observation that this drug acts as a "tranquilizer," that is, it reduces the anxiety level of the patient. Reserpine is a natural substance, one that is extracted and purified from a plant rather than synthesized in the laboratory. The snakeroot plant rauwolfia, which contains reserpine, had in fact been used in India for centuries as a sedative and a treatment for epilepsy long before its effects were discovered by Western medicine. Yet, the mode of action of reserpine is still only partially understood. It does release adrenalin and noradrenalin from their storage sites in the adrenals or in nerve cells, and presumably this depletion results in a less active performance by neural systems or centers depending on these two neurotransmitters. Reserpine and a number of synthetic drugs that also act as tranquilizers are extensively used in psychiatry to counteract hyperactive states (such as epilepsy, manic phases of the manic-depressive syndrome, and certain forms of schizophrenia).

Drugs exerting an effect grossly opposite to that of the tranquilizers are the so-called *psychoenergizers*, or stimulants; one foremost example is amphetamine. Amphetamine and many other such drugs have chemical structures closely resembling that of noradrenalin. It is probable, therefore, that they

Figure 3.16 (*top left*) Electrodes implanted in the brain of a rat. The electrodes can be used to give an electrical stimulus to the brain or to record brain impulses. (*bottom left*) Rat in Skinner box. When the rat presses the lever it triggers a brief electrical impulse to the brain. When the stimulation is pleasurable, rats have been known to press the lever as often as 5,000 times an hour. (*right*) Neurotransmitters can be delivered directly to a rat's brain through an implanted cannula.

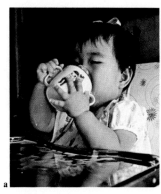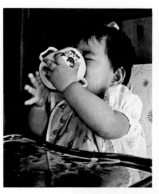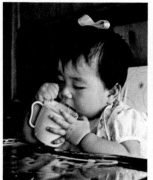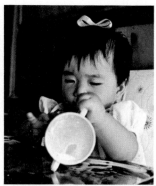

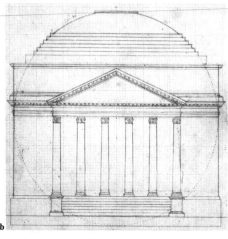

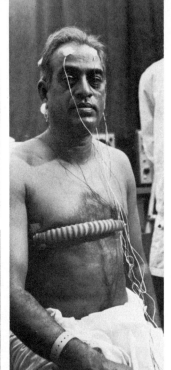

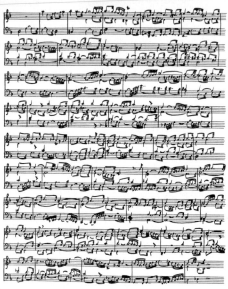

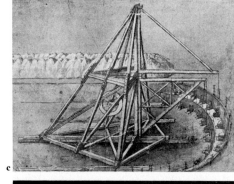

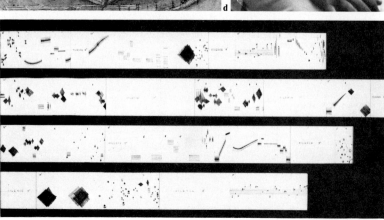

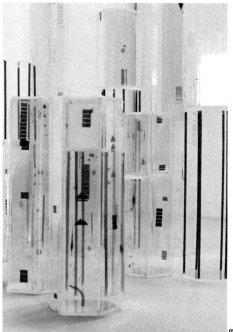

act as analogues to the neurotransmitter either by performing the same tasks, namely "energizing" the same neural centers or networks, or by keeping the transmitter-destroying enzymes so busy that the natural transmitter is protected and thus made more effective. These drugs also are extensively used to combat various forms of depression.

Another group of drugs is called *hallucinogens* because they generate hallucinations (sensory delusions), or *psychedelic* (because they generate mental images), or *psychotomimetic* (because they mimic psychotic states). The group comprises LSD (from a fungus called ergot), mescaline (from the peyote cactus), and psilocybin (from the Mexican mushroom), among others. It is remarkable that, once again, the chemical structures of many of these drugs are analogous to noradrenalin, while others resemble another brain neurotransmitter, *serotonin.*

Why among all these chemical analogues of neurotransmitters do some act as hallucinogens, others as stimulants, and yet others as tranquilizers? This question is not fully understood. It is reasonable to conceive that it may, at least in part, depend on the specific brain structures to which each drug has readier access or a greater affinity.

THE DYNAMICS OF INVESTIGATION

Cognitive or emotive changes and disorders may originate from an alteration of any one of the three major segments of neural activity. New signals from the external world, changes in the body or some of its parts, or products of the integrative processes can equally modify the *inputs* to the emotive centers of the brain. The *centers* themselves may be directly affected by a lesion, by chemical agents that have gained access to them from the blood, or by the cumulative experiences of the organism. The *output* segment, while carrying perfectly "sound" directions, may yet find the executive apparatus of the body defective in some way. Whether the outgoing directives are based on unusual background information, are incorrectly elaborated, or are incompetently carried out, the emotive response will be altered.

Although present knowledge of how the brain works is incomplete, what is known has convinced scientists that the physical state of the brain is of the greatest importance in producing behavior. Many behavior disorders that were once considered to be mental problems are increasingly seen as disorders of physical systems in the brain. For instance, a general paralysis found in some insane persons was once thought to be due to behavioral and character causes but is now known to be due to the invasion of the brain by the organism responsible for syphilis. Further, many patients were confined to mental hospitals in the South because they showed the symptoms of schizophrenic madness; later it was found that their so-called madness was actually a symptom of a form of pellagra—vitamin B deficiency.

The investigation of the physiological basis of behavior is a popular and dynamic area of psychology. The studies currently in progress are far too numerous to be discussed here. However, the importance of this area can in part be evaluated by the public recognition given to new advances in understanding behavior. Hardly a month passes without some report of an important advance in this research area appearing in some newspaper or magazine. As the pressure grows for people to live in proximity to one another, the need to understand behavior and the actions that result from particular stimuli also increases. Man needs help in learning to live in harmony with his fellow man and the environment; an understanding of the physiological basis of behavior is one promising means of providing such help.

Figure 3.17 The wonders of the human mind. (a) The small child must learn even the simplest of behaviors, such as how to drink from a cup. Yet the adult can master a number of such behaviors routinely and can use his mind to create fantastic buildings, musical compositions, and works of art; to invent philosophies, scientific theories, and machines; to save human lives and to enrich them; and even to control his body's internal functioning. (b) This library rotunda at the University of Virginia was designed by the great statesman Thomas Jefferson. (c) One of the many products of the mind of Leonardo da Vinci was this canal-digging machine. (d) India's Yogi Ramamand is wired for monitoring his physiological responses. The yogi is able to slow down his respiration and heart rate. (e) Manuscript page from "The Art of Fugue," Bach's last major work. (f. g) A new method of musical annotation, developed by Lawrence Parque to present his work, "Synapse," which combines music, space, and film in order to present a feeling of what a neuronal synapse is like.

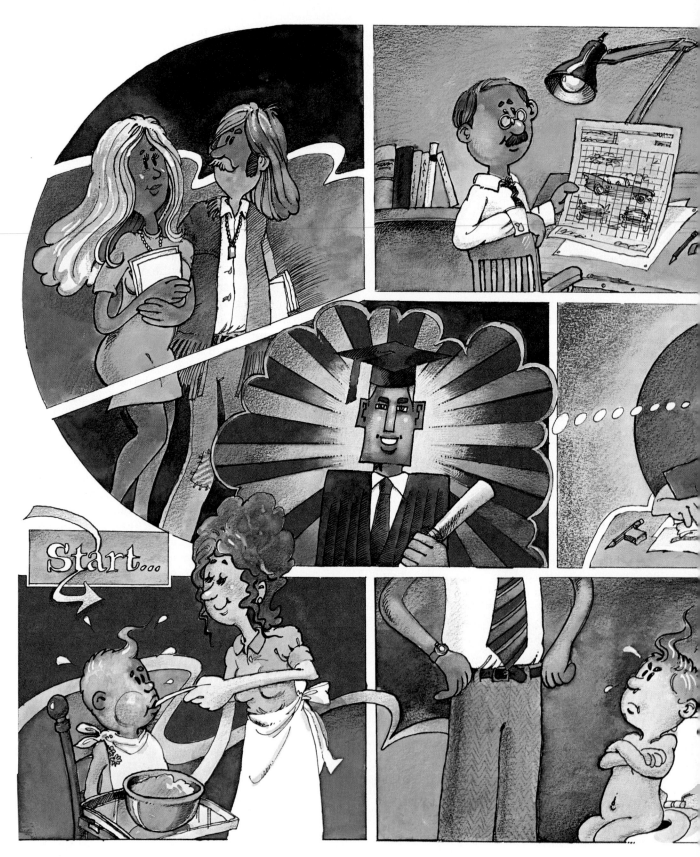

Figure 4.1 Psychological development is thought to occur in a series of orderly stages. What occurs at each stage, differentiating it from other stages, has been the focus of a number of psychological theories. Freud, for instance, saw the individual as passing through periods focusing, in turn, on oral activities, anal activities, love for the opposite parent, sublimation of sexuality, heterosexual love, and adult work.

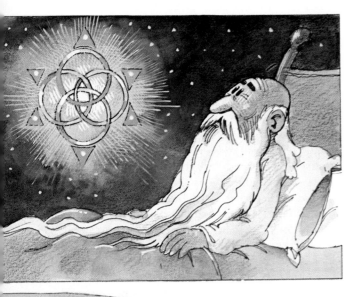

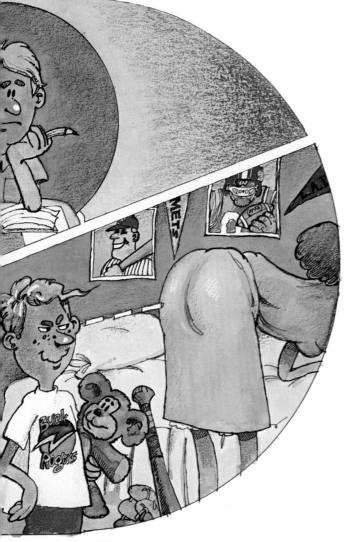

4 Several people can experience the same event and have totally different emotional reponses to it. Each person's response depends on a number of conscious and subconscious variables related to his own past history. The response also depends to a large degree upon his emotional make-up. Emotions can work for a person, as is the case when people perform feats of physical strength and endurance that defy belief. Yet, emotions also can work against man and tamper with his functioning, both physical and mental—as is implied in such common expressions as "he was so angry he couldn't see straight," "paralyzed with fear," "a fit of jealous rage," or "overcome with grief."

Emotional health is as important as physical health for the life of a human being. Chapter 3 presented what is known about the physiological mechanisms involved in emotional health; this chapter will discuss some of the forces that shape healthy emotional development; Chapter 5 will discuss how normal development may go awry.

EMOTIONS

Emotions have both mental (psychological) and bodily (physiological) components. Everyone has experienced bodily sensations that can accompany an emotion—a racing heart, cold or clammy hands, profuse sweating, blushing, tensed muscles, and so on. Such reactions can be observed directly and also can be measured with scientific instruments. The psychological aspect of emotions, on the other

Psychological Development

hand, is not so easy to observe or measure as the physiological one. It can be studied only through reports of the subjective emotional experiences of specific individuals and through observation of subtle behavioral indications. Furthermore, emotions cannot be studied in isolation from other mental components. The term *psyche* (and the adjective psychological) represents the sum of all the *cognitive* and *emotive* events that take place in the nervous system, and each of them is continuously interacting with the others. The development of the human psyche is an extremely complex process that is barely beginning to be understood by psychologists.

The Nature of Emotion

Like all neural events, emotional events have three parts: the stimulus, the evaluation, and the response—or, to use the physiological concepts of Chapter 3, the input, central processing, and output. To understand emotion, one must focus on the central process of *evaluation*.

Psychologist Magda Arnold has defined emotion as "a felt tendency toward something intuitively assessed as good, favorable, beneficial, or away from something assessed as unfavorable, harmful, bad." Thus, the first basis for evaluation is the pleasantness or unpleasantness of the stimulus. If the stimulus is found pleasurable, the person will act to achieve or maintain contact with it; if it is found painful, he will act to avoid it. If the stimulus yields neither pleasure nor pain, the person will be indifferent to it and will take no action. The pressure to take action, whether positive (seeking the stimulus) or negative (avoiding it) is called *motivation*. A person may experience an emotion without being sufficiently motivated to take some action, but the converse is not true—motivation never occurs without an emotional reaction preceding it.

As the psyche develops, evaluation of a stimulus becomes more and more complex. Rather than just two *feelings* (pleasant/unpleasant), many others come into play (good/bad, useful/damaging, urgent/nonurgent, important/trivial, for example). Needs or drives begin to sort themselves out from one another and become individual *motives*, such as the seeking of food, shelter, mates, education, wealth, prestige, acceptance, or the avoidance of disease, physical danger, pressures, censure, responsibility, immediate action. Past experience and cognitive activities begin to set conscious *values*, positive or negative, to such actions as working, eating, playing, taking drugs, seeking or avoiding a policeman, and so on. A person's values are what he assesses as being good or bad in the world. If he does not have what has positive value to him, he may seek to attain it—he has a *goal*. The *emotions* that an individual experiences, then, come to reflect his underlying attitudes—values, motivational strength—and what he succeeds in doing about them. If he likes something he does not have, he feels desire; if he attains it, he feels joy; if something happens that he dislikes, he feels sorrow or unhappiness; if he succeeds in disposing of it, he feels relief; if he sets a goal and fails to reach it, he feels frustration, and so on.

Unconscious Behavior

Most human feelings by which actions are prompted never reach consciousness and are not thought about. If every single act had to be consciously considered and reasoned about, one would be paralyzed. On the other hand, the hazard of acting on a preponderance of unconscious motivation is that it is difficult to alter certain actions even though they are harmful or out of tune with conscious values.

The more values a person develops, the more emotionally differentiated he becomes and the more often he will meet with situations that he will assess as positive by some of his values and as nega-

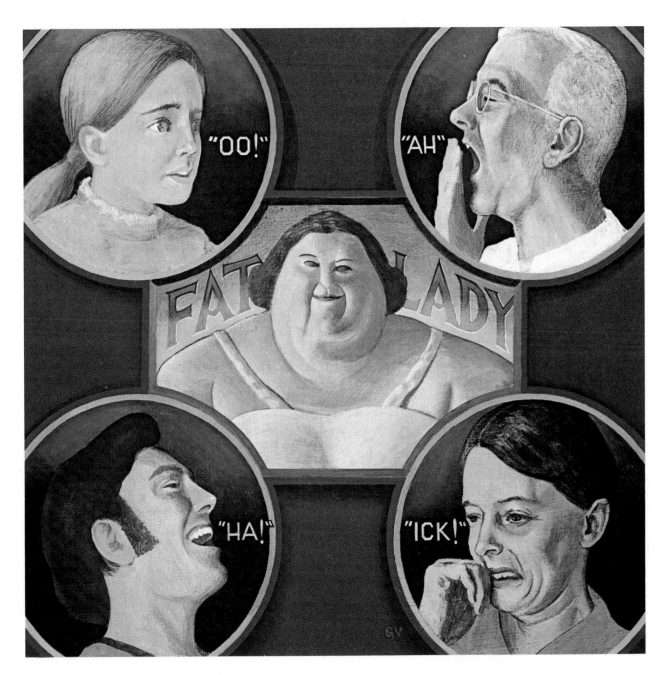

Figure 4.2 Different people respond differently to the same stimulus because of their unique emotional make-ups and their varying values.

tive by others. The psyche runs into trouble when it encounters conflicting motives or sets conflicting goals. No man and no environment are perfect, and so every psyche must encounter such *conflicts*. How often conflicts occur depends on how consistently an individual's emotional development has proceeded and how firmly some motives and values have established their predominance over others. Furthermore, the environment—physical and social—is a constant source of external limitations to any goal-directed action, which assures perpetuation of conflict within, as well as among, individuals.

A conflict often arises between one's conscious values and unconscious motives. Such conflict often remains unconscious even though the person becomes more and more aware of guilt, hostility, or anxiety feelings. This mechanism of *repression* with which the psyche reacts to conflict may extend progressively to any thought or memory that threatens to bring out the repressed feelings again. Instead of eliminating the original conflict, repression creates new unconscious motives that will cause additional conflicts to arise. Many conflicts, however, are susceptible to *conscious resolution*, and most personality theories today offer suggestions on how to seek such resolution, as will be described later.

Emotional Development

The diversification of values that takes place during the development of the psyche involves the acquisition of information. A child, for example, develops his abilities for *symbolic representation*, first as feelings, then as images, later with language; for *discrimination*, telling things apart from one another; for *generalization*, the discovery of things that go together or have a relationship; and for *organization* of the acquired experience. Through these growing abilities, the child forms a more and more explicit model of the world surrounding him, creates a model of his own self in his environment, and becomes increasingly able to anticipate events and take appropriate actions.

Symbolic representation, discrimination, generalization, and organization are but aspects of *cognitive learning*, that is, the perceptual manipulation of information. But cognitive learning cannot be dissociated from *emotional learning*, which guides one to acquiring the information in the first place, and both take place in the psyche together all the time. Emotional learning sets the priorities for what will be learned cognitively. The emotion that accompanies a cognitive process and gives it motivational significance can itself be thought about—a process known as *affective appraisal*. Through this process one can talk about his emotions, speculate as to their meaning, and predict how he might react in a future situation.

Although emotions are importantly involved in the process of learning and can be appraised cognitively, how much are they themselves *a product of learning*? Every human being is a product of two main forces. These two forces have been called by several names: heredity and environment, nature and nurture, instinct and learning, aptitude and training, and so on. Emotional development, like physical or intellectual development, must reflect the interaction of both such forces. The question that generates debate—and an ongoing, at times heated one, at that—is not *whether* but *how much* each force contributes to human development. The following sections will present some of the arguments and theories of current interest.

THE ROLE OF HEREDITY

Victor Hugo once said, "If you would civilize a man, begin with his grandmother." This whimsical and, unfortunately, impractical bit of advice reflects the importance of genetic factors in determining emotional health. Psychological research on newborn infants has shown that babies differ greatly from one another at birth in terms of, for example, motor activity, responsiveness to stimuli, cardiovascular functioning, and ability to be soothed when in a state of distress. Some babies rarely cry, others are demanding and fretful. These and many other innate differences are not necessarily inherited; they could be caused by aspects of the fetal environment or events during birth, but they do appear far too early in life to be attributed to differences in parental care.

Firmer evidence of hereditary differences comes from comparisons of *identical* twins, who have the same genetic make-up, with *fraternal* twins, who are no more similar genetically than any other siblings. On an amazing variety of characteristics—response to music and color, self-confidence, stubbornness, food preferences, brain-wave patterns, smoking habits, susceptibility to physical and emotional diseases—the identical twins are much more similar to each other than are fraternal twins. (Twin studies in relation to the heredity-versus-environment question are further discussed in Chapter 14.)

These observations deal with individual heredity and most commonly relate to genetic characteristics of the physiological aspects of behavior. But psychologists also have examined the relative effects of heredity and environment in terms of the developmental processes that are characteristic of the human species—in other words, as *theories of human development*. American psychology traditionally has minimized the role of heredity in development—to believe that people are genetically tucked into a particular fate runs counter to the American tradition. In fact, the strongest arguments for a genetic mechanism in emotional development have been presented by a group of European scientists who developed, in the Darwinian biological tradition, the science of *ethology*—the study of animals in their natural habitat.

Ethological Theory

Ethologists such as Konrad Lorenz and Niko Tinbergen and writers such as Robert Ardrey argue that much of man's behavior is *instinctive* rather than learned. Most of the ethologists' concepts, however, were formed by studying nonhuman species, so it cannot be certain that they apply equally well to man. It is quite clear that as one climbs the phylogenetic ladder, instinct becomes less and less important. Ethologists recognize this fact but insist that instinct is much more important in man than is commonly thought.

What are some of the ethological findings and their possible implications for man? The German scientist Konrad Lorenz noticed in 1937 that newly hatched geese, if separated from their mothers, would follow any available moving object, including Lorenz himself. Throughout the rest of their lives, they then reacted to Lorenz as they ordinarily would have to a member of their own species. They even made sexual displays to him. This phenomenon, termed *imprinting*, has been studied primarily in birds but also has been observed in dogs, sheep, and guinea pigs. Lorenz also found that there was a *critical period* for imprinting. Animals only attach themselves to an object at one time in their early lives. For ducks it is between thirteen and sixteen hours after birth, for monkeys it is probably sometime before one year of age.

Imprinting is an interesting phenomenon, but does it have any relevance to human behavior? Do human infants go through critical periods? No psychologist would intentionally isolate a human infant—as scientists usually do with animals under study—but some unfortunate infants have been isolated in other circumstances, and psychologists

Figure 4.3 Identical and fraternal twins. Identical twins develop from the splitting of a single zygote; they share the same chorion and placenta. Fraternal twins develop when two egg cells are released from the ovaries at the same time and are fertilized by different sperm; they have separate chorions and placentas.

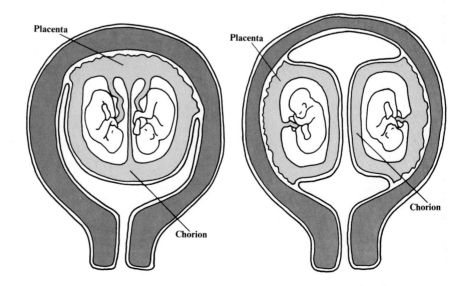

have studied them. Children who had been kept locked in attics or cellars for most of their lives showed clear effects of the isolation they had suffered: their behavior was essentially nonhuman—they could not control their emotional reactions, speak, or even relate to people. Another group of children that have been studied are those who have been confined in institutions, where they usually receive minimal care. Psychologists found that institutionalized children who did not receive proper affection and stimulation manifested unusual symptoms: they were either overly active or severely depressed, they had no appetites, they withdrew from and rejected adults, and they were more likely to die than other children. It is possible that

these children never had the opportunity to "imprint" on a human figure. Other research has shown that infants who are separated from adults at particular ages react most strongly: ages six months to two years, for example, appear to be a critical period for attachment in human infants.

Psychologist Harry Harlow has advanced understanding of attachment and love through his experiments with rhesus monkeys, a species with which humans share several important similarities in early development. Harlow reared his subject monkeys in complete isolation from their true mothers. The infant monkeys obtained milk by sucking from nipples attached to either of two "mother surrogates," one constructed of wire and

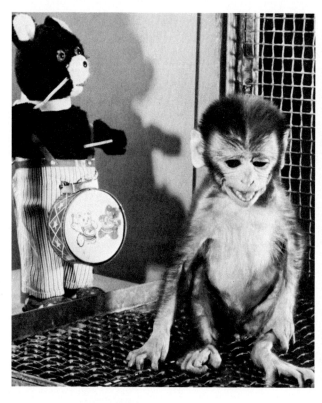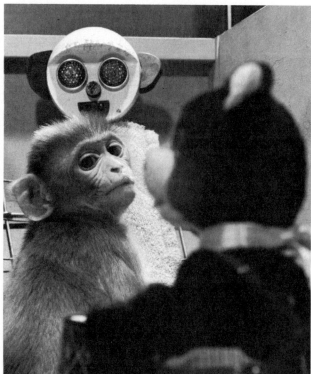

Figure 4.4 Monkeys raised apart from their mothers become frightened when a strange object is placed in their cage. If, however, a cloth mother with whom the monkey was raised is present, the monkey is curious rather than afraid.

the other of soft, cuddly terrycloth. The monkeys were then tested to determine their preferences for the two surrogates and the effects of isolation from the true mother. Results were dramatic. The infants strongly preferred the cloth mother, even when they had been fed exclusively with the wire one. For example, when frightening objects were placed in their cages, their fear was reduced by the presence of their cloth mother but not by the wire one. The monkeys probably preferred the cloth mother because it was more similar to their real mother and, as Harlow suggested, because it supplied "contact comfort."

The monkeys' strong attachment to the cloth mother, an attachment that endured up to two years of separation, sounds very much like imprinting, and it is reminiscent of the attachment of human infants to blankets and teddy bears. But the terrycloth mother did not satisfy all the monkeys' needs. Although they responded affectionately to the mother surrogate, they never developed into normal adult monkeys—by age three they were all socially and sexually abnormal.

Ethological theory contends that there are critical periods for particular responses. Humans are much more complex than other animals, and they may go through a number of "critical" periods in their development. Several personality theories, for example, can be interpreted as suggesting a series of critical periods, or *critical stages*, of development. The most appropriate example is the psychoanalytic theory of Sigmund Freud.

Freud's Psychoanalytic Theory

Psychoanalytic theory is similar to ethological theory in many ways, in particular the acceptance of instinct as the basis of development and the importance of critical periods. Sigmund Freud hypothesized two basic instincts, the *life instinct*, manifested mainly through sexual desire, and the *death instinct*, manifested mainly through aggression. Freud thought that children pass through five qualitatively distinct stages of development in which sexual tension is relieved by stimulation at successive *erogenous* zones such as the mouth, anus, or genitals. Freud's stages are outlined in Figure 4.5.

Freud felt that gratification at each successive stage, but especially through the first five years, is essential for healthy development and that the personalities or characters of people are the result of fixations at early developmental stages. For example, failure to achieve oral gratification gives rise in the adult to an emphasis on oral activities such as chewing, smoking, and talking. Stinginess and stubbornness characterize the anal personality. Failure to resolve the Oedipal conflict, which arises during the phallic stage, results in inability to achieve normal heterosexual relationships.

Erikson's Psychosocial Theory

Freud's theory is based on the idea that man's instincts are in constant conflict with his social environment. Man desires pleasure but society must prevent him from unrestrained hedonism. A later psychologist, Erik Erikson, who was trained by Freud's daughter, Anna, accepts this central tenet of psychoanalytic theory, including the idea that the sexual or life instincts supply the energy for emotive development, but he differs from Freud in two important respects: (1) he finds Freud's conception of the events at the five stages of development too narrow, and (2) he points out that there are other stages later in life that also are important. Erikson's theory is called *psychosocial* rather than psychoanalytic to emphasize his concern with interpersonal (versus intrapsychic) events in human development.

Erikson believes that man progresses through

eight different stages and that the outcome at each stage contributes to the ultimate adequacy of the adult. His first stages strongly resemble Freud's stages and, like them, are each characterized by a potential crisis or conflict of critical importance for the future adult. These conflicts are summarized in the names that Erikson has assigned to each stage. One need not adhere to the basic tenets of Erik-son's theory to grasp the importance of the crises of development he describes. Erickson's stages of development are summarized in Figure 4.6.

The Competence Theory of Robert White

Robert White, a psychologist from Harvard University, has supplied another perspective on Freud's stages of development and Erikson's re-

Age	Stage	Aspects of Development
Birth to about one year	Oral stage	Pleasure centers around the mouth—eating, sucking, spitting, biting, chewing. Adults who fixate at this level may displace their oral impulses by being gullible, possessive, sarcastic, or argumentative, for example.
One year to three years	Anal stage	Pleasure centers around the retention and expulsion of feces; type of toilet training can affect the child's personality—depending on whether the training is too strict or too permissive, the child may become (as an adult) obstinate and stingy, or destructive and messy, or creative and productive, for example.
Three years to six years	Phallic stage	The child discovers and derives pleasure from his genitals; the Oedipal conflict and castration anxiety occur.
Six years to about eleven years	Latency period	To relieve the anxiety stemming from the Oedipal conflict, the child represses his desire for his opposite-sexed parent and identifies with his like-sexed parent, repressing all erotic impulses toward the opposite sex.
Adolescence	Genital stage	Egocentric and incestuous love is replaced by hetero-sexual love and sexuality; the adolescent prepares for adulthood by channeling his drives into group activities and preparation for work and marriage.

Figure 4.5   Freud's psychosexual stages. Freud did not assume that there were any sharp breaks or abrupt transitions between the stages. The adult personality is the result of contributions from all four stages. Freud's stages are descriptive primarily of the male; he was less clear about female stages.

Age	Stage	Result of Success	Result of Failure
Early Infancy (birth to about one year) (corollary to Freudian oral stage)	Basic Trust vs. Mistrust	Trust results from affection and gratification of needs, mutual recognition.	Mistrust results from consistent abuse, neglect, deprivation of love, too early or harsh weaning, autistic isolation.
Later Infancy (one to three years) (corollary to Freudian muscular anal stage)	Autonomy vs. Shame and Doubt	Child views self as person in his own right apart from parents but still dependent.	Child feels inadequate, doubts self, curtails learning basic skills like walking, talking, wants to "hide" inadequacies.
Early Childhood (about ages four to five years) (corollary to Freudian phallic locomotor stage)	Initiative vs. Guilt	Child has lively imagination, vigorously tests reality, imitates adults, anticipates roles.	Child lacks spontaneity, has infantile jealousy "castration complex," is suspicious, evasive, suffers from role inhibition.
Middle Childhood (about ages six to eleven years) (corollary to Freudian latency stage)	Industry vs. Inferiority	Child has sense of duty and accomplishment, develops scholastic and social competencies, undertakes real tasks, puts fantasy and play in better perspective, learns world of tools, task identification.	Child has poor work habits, avoids strong competition, feels doomed to mediocrity; is in lull before the storms of puberty, may conform as slavish behavior, has sense of futility.
Puberty and Adolescence (about ages twelve to twenty years)	Ego Identity vs. Role Confusion	Adolescent has temporal perspective, is self-certain, is a role experimenter, goes through apprenticeship, experiences sexual polarization and leader-followership, develops an ideological commitment.	Adolescent experiences time confusion, is self-conscious, has a role fixation, and experiences work paralysis, bisexual confusion, authority confusion, and value confusion.
Early Adulthood	Intimacy vs. Isolation	Person has capacity to commit self to others, "true genitability" is now possible, *Lieben und Arbeiten* — "to love and to work"; "mutuality of genital orgasm."	Person avoids intimacy, has "character problems," behaves promiscuously, and repudiates, isolates, destroys seemingly dangerous forces.
Middle Adulthood	Generativity vs. Stagnation	Person is productive and creative for self and others, has parental pride and pleasure, is mature, enriches his life, establishes and guides next generation.	Person is egocentric, nonproductive, experiences early invalidism, excessive self-love, personal impoverishment, and self-indulgence.
Late Adulthood	Integrity vs. Despair	Person appreciates continuity of past, present, and future, accepts life cycle and life style, has learned to cooperate with inevitabilities of life, "death loses its sting."	Person feels time is too short; finds no meaning in human existence, has lost faith in self and others, wants second chance at life cycle with more advantages, has no feeling of world order or spiritual sense, fears death.

Figure 4.6 Erikson's eight stages of human development.

finements of them. White suggests that a great deal of an infant's behavior is oriented to nonsexual goals, particularly the pursuit of *competence*. Consider Freud's oral stage, for example. White points out that although the most important event of the period for the child is probably to obtain nourishment through sucking, he engages in many other activities, such as playing and trying to feed himself, that are not strictly "incorporative." White suggests that although early motivation is instinctive and some of it is sexual, much of it is aimed at gaining competence. He points out, for example, that weaning could be a major tragedy in the life of all infants but in many cases is not because of the sense of competence young children gain from drinking from a cup.

White also takes exception to the importance attached by psychoanalysts to toilet training. He contends that the most important events for two-year-olds are learning to walk, learning to talk, getting into things, and learning to play with toys—gaining competence over their world and gaining self-esteem. The negativism of the two-year-old is more a message that says "I want to learn to do it myself" than it is a displacement of bowel training.

Similarly, the phallic stage and especially the latency stage, which Freud's emphasis on sexual energy led him to neglect, contain challenges to competence. White points out that in Erikson's fourth stage, a sense of industry is based mainly on a sense of competence.

Competence is a concept used by White to include the vast range of activities children engage in to master their world—locomotion, language, and the manipulation of objects and people. He believes that research has documented needs for curiosity and exploration and warrants the conclusion that not all motivation is based on tension reduction, as Freud contended. Rather, White believes that people are motivated to make an impact on themselves and the world, even when it means *increasing* tension in their lives.

THE ROLE OF ENVIRONMENT

The allegiance to heredity of the various theories reviewed thus far lies not so much in a definition of what specific psychological traits are inherited but in the belief that there are basic motivational drives—or instincts—that are not to be denied for a healthy emotional development and that there are specific times during development when such fulfillments must occur. They recognize the importance of environmental influences—for instance, the effect of parents—in the shaping of an individual, but only to the extent that they permit or hinder the fulfillment of the instinctual goals.

In contrast, *learning theories* focus on the *ways* in which behavior is learned. They pay little attention to heredity—although they do not deny the potential importance of individual, inherited differences—and no attention at all to any rigid characterization of in-built, instinctual drives. They do, however, share with other theories an appreciation

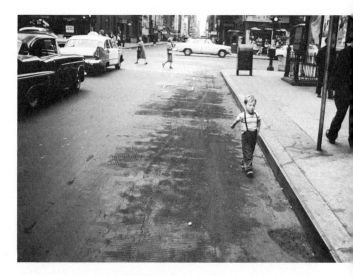

Figure 4.7 The child's need for competence—mastery over himself and over his environment—is the motivating force of his development, according to Robert White.

that the potential of a growing individual for a healthy emotional development may well vary qualitatively or quantitatively over his lifetime and that the early years are of special importance.

Learning Theory

Learning theory contains two main principles: that people associate pleasant or painful experiences with whatever happens at the same time (the *classical conditioning* mechanism) and that behavior that brings reward is increased but behavior that brings punishment is decreased (the *operant conditioning* mechanism). All learning theorists share one common assumption: people are what they are largely as a result of their past history of rewards and punishments, stimuli and responses.

The ways in which conditioning shapes people's lives are many and varied and their effects cannot be underestimated. For example, consider a classic experiment by John B. Watson and R. Rayner. The experiment involved a young boy named Albert. Albert liked white rats and often played with them. In the experiment, every time Albert reached for a white rat, the experimenters made a loud sound that frightened him. Thereafter, Albert was afraid of white rats. He had been conditioned to fear them. Perhaps more significantly, he also feared many things similar to the white rats, including his mother's fur neckpiece. This experiment demonstrates the basic principle of classical conditioning—the idea that when a stimulus that always causes a specific response (conditioned stimulus) is paired with an unconditioned stimulus, the latter will come to elicit the same response. It shows that people can be conditioned to fear things and people irrationally, simply because they have been associated with painful reactions (see Figure 4.8).

The same principle, of course, applies to positive behaviors and pleasurable events. In normal development most children become "conditioned" to love their mothers, because their mothers are almost always there to bring them pleasure and relieve pain or frustration.

In *operant* conditioning, the response depends more on values, because this type of learning is based on the idea that rewarding a response will in-

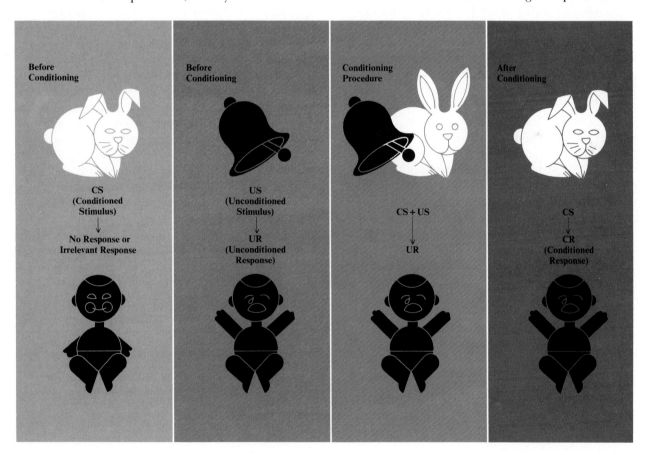

Figure 4.8 Diagrammatic outline of the classical conditioning procedure. Here a child learns to fear a stuffed animal. In order for conditioning to take place the conditioned stimulus must either be presented simultaneously with the unconditioned stimulus or must immediately precede it. Presenting the conditioned stimulus after the unconditioned will not produce conditioning.

crease its occurrence and punishing or ignoring a response will tend to decrease its occurrence. Thus, different events may be reinforcing to different people. For example, some children pulled a lever on a pinball machine when they were reinforced by candies, but other children ate candies in order to play the pinball machine: candy eating reinforced pinball playing and pinball playing reinforced candy eating. As another example, most experiments on negative reinforcement use pain as a punishment, but a masochist might find pain pleasureful. What all this seems to indicate is that the principle of reinforcement does *account* for a large proportion of human behavior but does not really *explain* it — or, more specifically, it does not explain what makes a particular reinforcement effective for a particular individual.

Social Learning Theory

Social learning theory goes farther to explain human behavior than basic learning theory. Research by Albert Bandura and Richard Walters, for example, has shown that much of what constitutes human behavior is the result of imitation, or *modeling*. People tend to do what they see other people do. Children who watch an adult punch and kick a large plastic doll do the same thing when given a chance, especially if the adult is rewarded for his behavior, is nurturant, or is of high power status. Social learning theory agrees with psychoanalytic theory on the importance of parents, but views parents as important because they are convenient models.

Recent experiments have shown that people are influenced by models more than they commonly realize. In one experiment drivers were found to be much more likely to stop and help someone fix a flat tire if they had just observed another driver helping another motorist fix a flat.

Another experiment found that Christmas shoppers were more likely to contribute to the Salvation Army after they had seen another person give than if they watched and no one contributed. Yet other experiments have shown that modeling also can work negatively — when people watch other people refusing to help, even in emergencies, they are less likely themselves to intervene.

Cognitive-Developmental Theory

Learning theory, or *behaviorism*, as it is often called, has had a great impact on American psychology. While American psychologists were testing learning theories, a Swiss psychologist, Jean Piaget, was talking with and studying children. From his observations he constructed a theory of development that stressed what the behaviorists had omitted — namely, the mind, or cognition. Piaget and other cognitive-developmental theorists did not deny that people learn from modeling and from reward and punishment, but they pointed out another fact — that people also learn by thinking. When someone solves a math problem or interprets the behavior of a friend, he learns without reinforcement.

Cognitive-development theory suggests that human development is the result of thinking. It suggests that the main motivating force in life is the need to know. Robert White's ideas about competence come close to capturing the core of motivation proposed in cognitive-developmental theory. People all strive to increase their understanding of, and control over, the world. Competence is a way of being in control. Development is a process of constructing cognitive structures that give men maximum comprehension of their world and allow new information to be fitted into the structures.

In emphasizing the importance of thinking, cognitive-developmental theorists do not neglect the role of emotion in human development. They argue, however, that the most important part of emotion is the way it is interpreted — the cognitive

Figure 4.9 Cognitive theorists base many of their ideas on experiments like this. A four-month-old infant is shown a pattern on a screen. He can keep it in focus by sucking on a pacifier hooked up to the screen. The infant will work (suck) with great energy and interest for a while to obtain the reward of the picture. However, he eventually gets somewhat bored, does not suck as hard, and the picture fades. When a different picture is made available, the energy put into sucking once again increases.

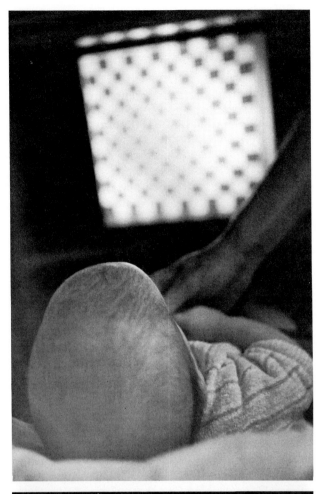

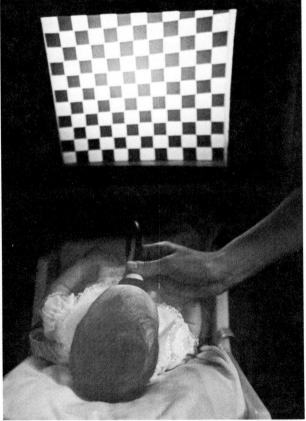

process of affective appraisal. The same bodily sensation or feeling can become any number of "emotions," depending on the circumstances that have created it and how it is labeled. Although this idea may seem a little unusual, several experiments have supported it.

The most famous experiment was by Stanley Schachter and Jerome Singer in 1962. Subjects were injected with adrenalin—the emotion-arousing hormone—were given correct, wrong, or no information about the expected effects of the drug, and were individually exposed to a "stooge" (a confederate of the experimenters) who deliberately behaved angrily with some of them and euphorically with others. The behavior of subjects who had the correct information was independent of the stooge's behavior. In contrast, the misinformed and the uninformed ones mimicked (actually, overmimicked) the particular behavior the stooge had exhibited. Schachter and Singer concluded that the subjects were labeling their emotional arousal in terms of their environmental situation, rather than in terms of the effects of the drug.

Later researchers have replicated Schachter and Singer's original experiment, and other investigators have found independent support for the basic idea. Stuart Valins, for example, found that if he played back a falsely increased heart rate to subjects while they were judging pictures, the subjects rated the pictures as more emotionally arousing than when supplied with true heart rates. Michael Storms and Richard Nisbett found that insomniacs would fall asleep earlier than they used to if told that they had been given drugs that would keep them awake: thinking that their sleeplessness was due to the drugs and not to personal problems helped them to relax and go to sleep.

These and other findings encourage the view held by cognitive-developmental theorists that what one thinks about the way he feels helps him to

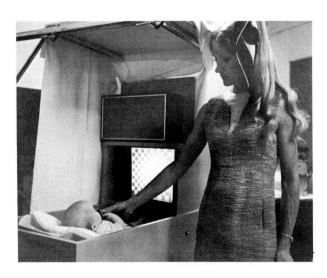

define it as an emotion and that this evaluation can have a great effect on the way he will react. This, of course, fits well with the psychophysiologists' view that the control centers of emotions receive inputs from the cognitive parts of the brain (see Chapter 3).

Enriched Environments

Cognitive-developmental theory holds that environmental enrichment stimulates development. It, of course, is not the only theory that adopts this view. Experiments on enrichment are easier to do than experiments on deprivation, and most of those that have been done show that enrichment — at least within limits — has beneficial effects.

In experiments on the effects of enriched as opposed to deprived environments, laboratory animals, usually rats, are exposed to environments that are stimulating — bright lights, interesting sounds, other animals, various kinds of toys, mazes to solve, and new areas to explore. In experiment after experiment involving various learning tasks, these animals outperform ones that have experienced normal environments. In one experiment, Seymour Levine found that added stimulation, even of a stressful nature, accelerates development. Levine stressed infant rats for three minutes per day by shocking, cooling, mechanically shaking, or just handling them. Using an extensive battery of tests, the experimenter compared these animals with others that had been left undisturbed. Advantages were all on the side of the stressed rats. They grew longer and heavier, opened their eyes sooner, were more resistant to disease, and were less fearful in novel situations. Thus, *mild* stress in infancy appears to be valuable in preparing organisms to cope with future stress.

Experiments on humans also have shown that enriched environments produce profound effects. Bertram White worked with month-old infants in a state hospital. He enriched the environments of some of them by handling them with greater than normal frequency, removing their crib liners for several periods each day, replacing the white crib liners and sheets with patterned ones, and hanging colorful objects over their cribs. These infants were capable of grasping objects held above them at an average age of three and one-half months; infants restricted to normal hospital routine were unable to reach successfully until five months. In a later study, White found that a single colorful object mounted on the crib rails for the first two months of life, followed by the introduction of more elaborate ornaments, produced even more favorable results. Objects were grasped at less than three months.

THE MATURE PERSONALITY

One of the characteristics commonly found in emotionally disturbed people is a faulty self-concept. Conceptions of self are undoubtedly the individual's most important cognitions, and the desire to develop and maintain self-esteem is a powerful motive. The development of self-concepts plays a central role in the theories of Carl Rogers and Abraham Maslow.

Rogerian Theory

Carl Rogers feels that the distinguishing characteristic of the psychologically mature person is that he has a value system derived honestly from his own experiences rather than from the opinions of others. Rogers points out that infants do not have fixed value systems; they clamor for food when they are hungry but reject it when they are not. The infant knows what he likes because his choices are directed by the needs of his body, which are not influenced by parents, church, or Madison Avenue. But the infant also needs love, and he is sometimes threatened by its loss when he behaves in particular ways. For example, he may be severely reprimanded by his mother for playing with his feces. Then,

Figure 4.10 Bertram White studied the effects of stimulation on the development of reaching behavior in infants. He compared institutionalized children (*left*) with no visual enrichment to those with massive visual enrichment (*center*) and found that the massively enriched infants developed reaching behavior earlier. However, infants who had only a few objects mounted on the sides of their cribs (*right*) developed reaching and grasping behavior even earlier than the massively enriched group.

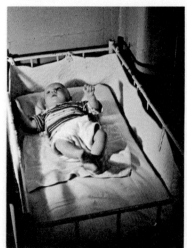
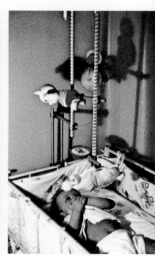

even though the act affords him pleasure, he develops negative attitudes toward it and its originator, himself. As a result, the source of his values is changed from himself to his mother.

The consequence of this developmental process is that most adults have value systems that conflict with their own experiences and their self-concepts. Two separate values may even be contradictory to each other. According to Rogers, it is not surprising that most people are insecure, and it is only when one changes his valuing process that he can hope to change. The individual must develop a self-concept that he values, in Rogerian theory.

The Rogerian therapist tries to treat patients respectfully, so that they can come to the realization that they have worth as individuals. In Rogers' terms, the therapist must give his client "unconditional positive regard" and must have an emphatic understanding of the client's frame of reference. The ultimate goal of such therapy is to make the person's self-concept more congruent with his experiences and values and to teach him to evaluate experiences in terms of the extent to which they are self-enriching and self-fulfilling. This type of valuing process is similar to that of infants in that it is flexible and based on the moment. According to Rogerian theory, the psychologically mature person, like the infant, trusts the wisdom of his body.

Maslow's Humanistic Theory

Because of his emphasis on the positive aspects of development, Carl Rogers has often been called a humanistic psychologist. The contributions of humanistic psychology to the understanding of motivation and emotional development have been most elaborately presented by Abraham Maslow. Maslow placed humanism next to behaviorism and psychoanalysis as a "third force" in American psychology.

Maslow argued that attempts made to derive universal laws about man from laboratory procedures are doomed to failure. Men are unique, he said, and they must be studied individually. His primary concern was to characterize the man who is functioning to the peak of his capacities. Such a man is said to be *self-actualized*.

Maslow's theory is essentially a theory of motivation. He differed from most traditional motivational theorists, who concern themselves with deficits such as hunger and thirst and their satisfaction; he believed that too much emphasis was placed on *deficit needs* and not enough on *growth* needs. Maslow concerned himself with motivation to grow, with gratification rather than deprivation. Unlike Freud, Maslow believed that man is essentially good but that his essential goodness can be spoiled by a bad environment.

Maslow outlined a hierarchy of motives. At the bottom of the hierarchy are "deficit" needs such as the needs for food and safety. Once met, these needs become relatively unimportant for human functioning and the person is free to satisfy higher types of needs. The first "growth" need is "belongingness." Then come the needs for love and self-esteem, in that order. Finally, at the top of the hierarchy, is the need for self-actualization. Maslow believed that the result of failure to fulfill any of the five classes of needs is similar in many respects to the result of an inadequate diet. A person who is not self-actualized is no less sick than a person who is suffering from a vitamin deficiency.

Maslow studied forty-nine "successful" people — people such as Lincoln, Thoreau, Einstein, and Schweitzer — in order to obtain some idea of the characteristics of self-actualized people. From this study, he found fifteen outstanding characteristics; they are listed in Figure 4.11.

Reading through the characteristics of self-actualizers, one will undoubtedly compare himself to the ideal. One might also assume that if he behaves

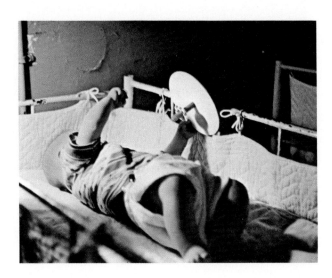

Characteristic	Explanation
1. More efficient perception of reality and more comfortable relations with it	The self-actualized person judges others accurately, detects falseness in others, and is capable of tolerating uncertainty and ambiguity.
2. Acceptance of self and others	He accepts himself as he is and is not defensive. He has little guilt, shame, or anxiety.
3. Spontaneity	Self-actualizers are spontaneous in both thoughts and behavior.
4. Problem centering	The problems with which the self-actualized person concerns himself are not of a personal nature, but instead are outside of himself.
5. Detachment; the need for privacy	Although he enjoys others, he does not mind solitude and sometimes seeks it.
6. Autonomy: independence of culture and environment	He is relatively uninfluenced by local customs.
7. Continued freshness of appreciation	He derives ecstasy, inspiration, and strength from the basic experiences of life. Acts that serve biological functions, such as eating and sexual behavior, are relatively unimportant in the total scheme of things but when enjoyed are done so wholeheartedly. There is no accompanying anxiety to detract from the intense pleasure.
8. Mystic experience	The self-actualizer, much more commonly than others, has experiences during which he feels simultaneously more powerful and more helpless than ever before.
9. Social interest	There is a feeling of identification, sympathy, and affection for others.
10. Interpersonal relations	Relationships with others are few, but they are deep and meaningful. The self-actualizer does on occasion get angry, but he does not bear long-lasting grudges.
11. Democratic character structure	He respects people irrespective of birth, race, blood, and family.
12. Discrimination between means and ends	Most people work only in order to receive the paycheck at the end of the week. The self-actualizer enjoys his work.
13. Sense of humor	He has a sense of humor that is both philosophical and nonhostile.
14. Creativeness	Maslow felt that everybody is potentially creative. He was not referring to great works of art or science, but rather to expressiveness, spontaneity, and perceptiveness in everyday life.
15. Nonconformity	Self-actualized people swim against the mainstream. They are open to new experiences.

Figure 4.11 Maslow's fifteen characteristics of the self-actualized person.

in a manner similar to the description of self-actualizers, he will come closer to attaining the goal of self-actualization. But one should not forget that self-actualization is an ongoing process—it is not a state of being that one can instantly attain.

CRITERIA FOR EMOTIONAL HEALTH

Many psychologists besides Maslow, Rogers, Erikson, and Freud have formulated theories of what constitutes the emotionally mature, mentally healthy person, and although these theories differ in many ways, there are a few qualities that all of them would consider to be characteristics of the mature personality. One such attribute would be the ability to be intimate—to give and accept love and affection. Also considered important is the ability to be sociable—to have friends, to be devoted to and nurturant of those close to one—as long as there is no implication of conformity in the sociability. It also is agreed that some clear, vivid sense of who one is, what one's goals, values, and abilities are, is characteristic of emotional health. Another attribute of the mature person is an interest in and ability to do productive work.

But although psychologists are in general agreement as to such characteristics, they tend to disagree as to how one goes about *becoming* a mentally healthy person. Some, like the behaviorists, say it is wholly a matter of being conditioned to act "correctly." Others, like Rogers, say self-actualization must follow from trusting one's inner impulses and desires as opposed to the impositions of others, coupled with having been given "unconditional positive regard" by the important people in one's life. Still others, like Erikson, say one becomes mature if he successfully works through the crises of each of the eight stages of development outlined in his theory. The cognitive-developmental theorists, on the other hand, place the burden of emotional health on the individual's ability to use his mind to understand the world, himself, and his ability to fit in with or change his environment.

In many respects, each individual must decide for himself what *he* considers to be optimal emotional health and what *he* thinks is necessary to achieve it, based on whatever information he can gather about how human beings can best develop and function. Perhaps he will agree with an existing psychological theory and be guided by it. Perhaps he will formulate his own. Perhaps he will do what most people do, and that is to follow a set of standards given to him by his culture as to what is a "good" or "bad" person.

Whatever the choice, it will be a difficult one to carry out. Emotional health is a continuous process—one that is constantly subjected to stress from the environment, from other people, from oneself. In real life, emotional conflicts are practically unavoidable, but not necessarily unresolvable. The more one evades and represses conflict, instead of identifying and resolving it, the more severe psychological problems he will suffer.

For the adult, the nearest key to maximizing emotional health appears to be in the second component of the emotional event, the *evaluation*. To understand his emotions one must know his evaluations. Uncovering one's true evaluation is often the goal of psychotherapy, because once one realizes the way he really views things, he can go about resolving some of the conflicts arising in his life. One may well want to ponder the advice of psychologist Nathaniel Branden: "If his emotions are to be a source of pleasure to man, not a source of pain, he must learn to *think* about them. Rational awareness is not the 'cold hand' that kills; it is the power that liberates."

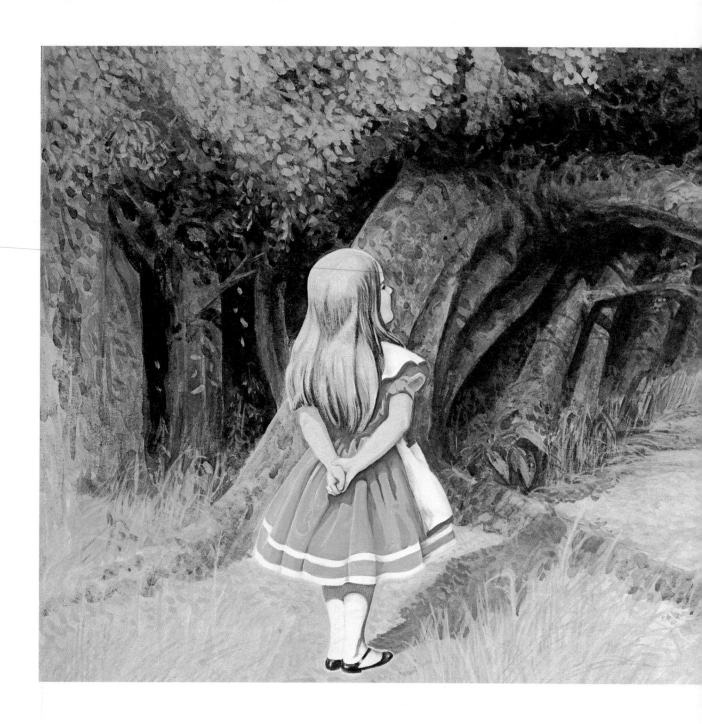

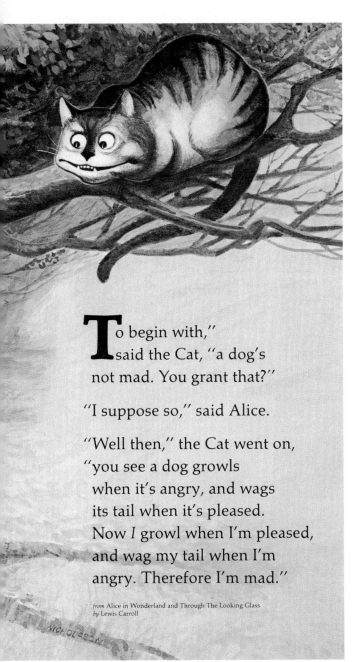

"To begin with," said the Cat, "a dog's not mad. You grant that?"

"I suppose so," said Alice.

"Well then," the Cat went on, "you see a dog growls when it's angry, and wags its tail when it's pleased. Now *I* growl when I'm pleased, and wag my tail when I'm angry. Therefore I'm mad."

from Alice in Wonderland and Through The Looking Glass
by Lewis Carroll

5 A young woman attempts suicide when she learns that her fiancé has been killed while fighting overseas. A forty-year-old man is arrested for exposing himself to a woman at a bus stop. An elderly woman gives away large sums of money to people she has never met but will not give her children a cent; a teen-age boy runs away from home after threatening to kill his father. Are these people mentally ill?

Obviously, it is impossible to pass judgment on these people without extensive knowledge of the circumstances leading to their actions. But even with a thorough knowledge of an individual's life story, one would still be making a *value judgment* as to the state of his mental health.

Mental illness, at least as the phrase presently is used, is a relative term. It refers to the actions or words of those who deviate from what is normally expected from them—socially, psychologically, ethically, or politically. Depending on who is doing the defining, atheists could be considered mentally ill, and so could homosexuals, communists, hermits, vegetarians, or comic-book collectors. Because of this ambiguity, even the professional must examine his own value system when he decides who should be considered ill.

THE PROBLEM OF DEFINITION

Psychiatrist Thomas Szasz has suggested that the term "mental illness" be discarded in favor of more

Mental Health and Mental Illness

accurate, less stigmatizing descriptions of an individual's behavior. Those disorders of thinking and behavior that have known physiological causes—brain injuries, brain diseases, chemical defects, or intoxication—should be regarded as disorders of the brain. Other problems in psychological functioning that have no physiological basis should be totally removed from the idea of illness, according to Dr. Szasz. These other problems result from conflicting personal needs, aspirations, values, and so on, so they should be considered psychosocial or ethical problems rather than physical ones.

Dr. Szasz suggests that the phenomenon now called mental illness be "removed from the category of illnesses and be regarded as the expression of man's struggle with *the problem of how he should live*." Dr. Szasz also points out that the concept of mental illness as it now stands allows people to avoid facing their problems; they assume that because mental illness is considered a disease, it is something over which they have no control—it just happens to them. Under this assumption there are no specific actions that the individual can take to rid himself of the "illness"—it either will go away naturally or will require professional medical treatment. The concept of mental illness does not allow for the fact that an individual may be the source of his own troubles through wrong or conflicting choices or values. It suggests only that human behavior is determined by antecedent injuries to the body, largely outside the control of the individual.

Although the individual may be the source of his own trouble, mental disturbance involves a conflict between the individual and the environment in which he attempts to "live" his choices or values. The suffering of an anxious or depressed individual can sometimes be radically modified just by correcting his external social environment. A child who is sulky and destructive because he is overtly rejected by his parents might seem a changed per-

sonality with the affection and understanding newly given to him in a foster home. It is unfortunate that arthritis or cancer cannot be cured in the same manner.

Indeed, the techniques used today for treating mental illness have little in common with those that doctors use for treating physical illness. In studying and treating people who often have no detectable physical defects, psychiatrists deal with character traits, with interpersonal communications, with the

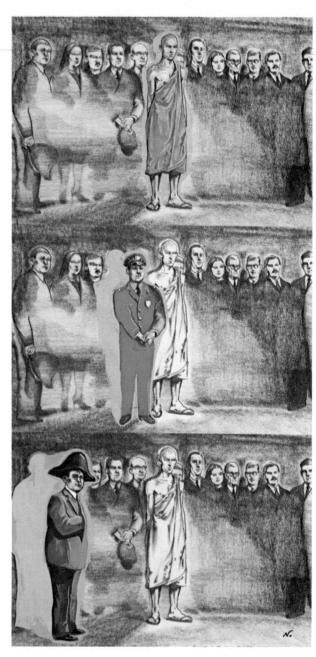

Figure 5.1 Who is deviant? Some would say that anyone who would give up the comforts of middle-class American life to join a strict religious cult is "psychotic." Others might say that anyone who becomes a police officer and thus an agent of the "Establishment" is crazy. Most people would say that any person who thinks he is Napoleon, Jesus, or some other famous figure is mentally ill.

"games people play," with the patient's view of his own existence. And because mental disturbance is really a variety of unhappiness, ultimately the attempt is to help the patient to find some semblance of "the good life."

Unlike bodily changes related to physical illness, the disturbances of personality traits can rarely be measured with precision. Thus, the point at which mental difficulties are to be considered serious enough to be termed "illness" usually is decided arbitrarily. Sometimes an individual decides that his own behavior is unreasonable. He has painful emotions, or he behaves so irrationally that he troubles society, and the threat of community reprisal brings about further personal suffering for him. Such a person may voluntarily seek help and define himself as a sick person.

Another person may not communicate his personal suffering, or in fact, he may not be suffering at all. He might still be considered disturbed or "mentally ill," primarily when those around him believe his unhappiness to be unreasonable or judge his behavior to be irrational and therefore assume he must be troubled or unhappy.

Any behavior, in fact, that one's peers view as strange, peculiar, or interfering with the individual's capacity to adjust in his community may be labeled by them as "sick" behavior. Even an untroubled individual may be labeled ill, though he is not, simply because those around him are suspicious or hostile toward an individual who does not conform to accepted social patterns. Such a situation once happened in the case of a government scientist. Walking to work he stumbled and hurt his ankle. A police officer saw him limping along the highway and also observed that he was sloppily dressed. The scientist was arrested as drunk. When he objected, a doctor was called who proceeded to determine that the scientist was mentally ill. The next day a judge ordered him to a mental hospital. It was two months before the hospital officials decided the scientist was really sane and released him.

It is important to understand that a judgment of unreasonable suffering or behavior is a value judgment frequently based on arbitrary or shifting criteria. What is considered unreasonable in one society may be considered reasonable in another. A dedicated Buddhist in Asia may douse himself with gasoline, strike a match, and burn to death as a means of communicating a deeply felt concern. In his culture he is not considered mentally ill and may, in fact, be admired for this ultimate use of himself to express his behavioral congruence with what he believes and feels is right. In American society, however, a person behaving in such a manner would be viewed as mentally ill, and such labels as "suicidal," "masochistic," and "psychotic" would be applied.

The label of mental illness can be used to humiliate people, reduce their social status, negate their dissent, or deprive them of their freedom. It is therefore important to consider the motives of those who make or influence such labels and to determine whether they represent the power structure of the community, have their own interests at stake, or in fact attempt to reflect the objective interests of the accused individual.

PROBLEMS IN EVERYDAY LIVING

Individuals vary in their ability to cope with the stresses and conflicts in their lives. To the extent that one can handle these problems, he can be considered mentally "healthy"; to the extent that such problems interfere with the individual's personality and his striving to achieve his goals, he may be considered mentally "ill."

To gain a better understanding of the task man sets for himself in working to maintain mental health, one must examine the kinds of problems, stresses, and conflicts that man encounters and the

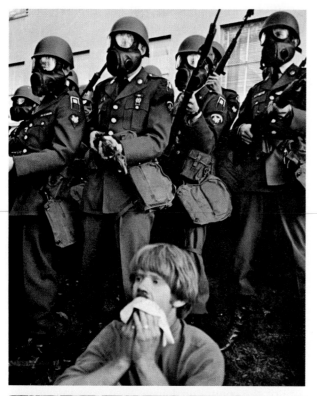

ways in which he can either avoid or resolve his psychological troubles.

Stress

Stress is any stimulus that interferes with the biological or psychological equilibrium of an organism. Behavior depends on how individuals respond to both environmental and internal stress. Most people encounter a considerable amount of stress in their daily lives and learn to reduce it either by changing something about their environment or changing something about themselves. Every person's capacity to "adjust," therefore, is limited by the opportunities he has to change the environment and by his physical and emotional make-up. A given individual can tolerate only so much stress, however. If he is exposed to more than he can withstand, he will experience physical and emotional distress and will be unhappy. Either his feelings of unhappiness or his efforts to alleviate his unhappiness can, under some circumstances, be considered unreasonable by himself or by others.

ENVIRONMENTAL STRESS   A great deal of stress comes from one's environment. The most important environmental stresses are imposed upon individuals directly by other individuals or indirectly by social institutions created by man.

Considerable environmental stress is generated by society's interference with the individual's opportunity to satisfy what he considers to be his basic psychological needs. Everyone needs self-respect, for instance. But black people living in the urban ghetto may feel that the police who summarily halt them on the street and treat them harshly are demolishing their self-respect. Policemen, on the other hand, sometimes find their desires for respect and fair treatment undermined by being called "pigs" and other derogatory names when they view themselves as valued servants of society.

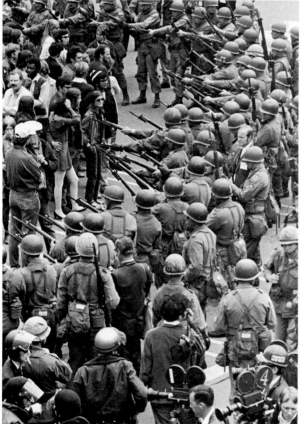

Figure 5.2   Very direct stress can be felt by individuals on both sides during social conflicts.

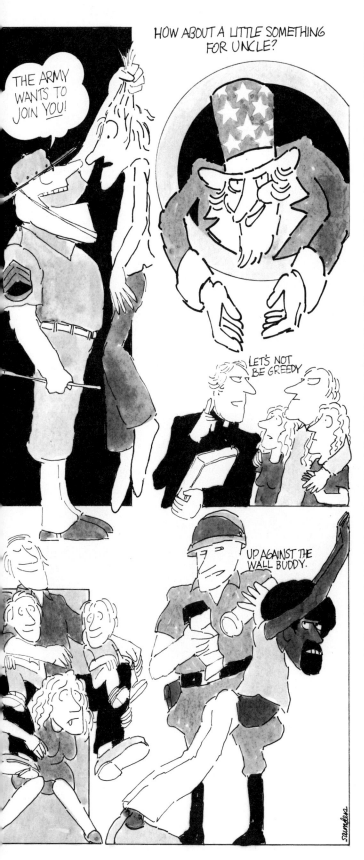

Figure 5.3 There are a number of ways in which society can interfere with the needs and desires of the individual, providing him with another source of psychological stress.

The hardest stress usually falls on minority groups, who are viewed as inferior by virtue of being poor or racially or ethnically different. In such instances the source of stress, while at times a misconception on the part of the minority, usually can be traced directly to the ignorance, apathy, selfishness, or malevolence of those in power. The social system may then take on an oppressiveness of its own, irrespective of the intentions of its creators or even of its present members taken individually. Modern American society is viewed by many as one that is too impersonal and too complex to provide all citizens with the opportunity to achieve sufficient independence, dignity, responsibility, or meaningful work. Such a society can impose *indirect*, but nevertheless powerful, stress upon all of its citizens.

When an individual feels stress from the social system, he is likely to experience considerable psychological discomfort. Sometimes he can detect the source of that discomfort; sometimes he cannot. A young man who is beaten up or humiliated by a street gang has a clear idea who his oppressors are. He may not be able to express directly the aggression he feels, but at least he knows he is angry and knows the source of his anger. On the other hand, if he is eligible for the military draft but has no desire to enter the service, he may be just as angry. But now he finds it difficult to identify a source toward which he can direct his emotions, particularly if he is basically patriotic. His frustrations will engender feelings of aggression that are likely to be directed toward his friends or relatives, or even toward himself. Because he cannot deal with impersonal government bureaucracy, he may have furious arguments with his parents, take up alcohol or drugs, or suddenly drop out of school. Any citizen who believes his society is basically benevolent but who also feels he is being persecuted by that society will have similar reactions. The person who is oppressed but who cannot identify the source of

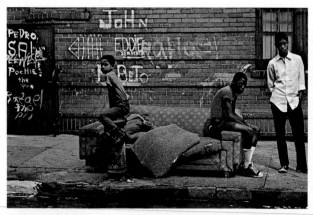

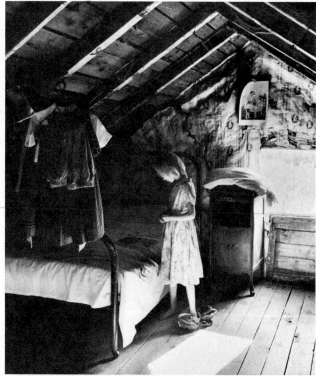

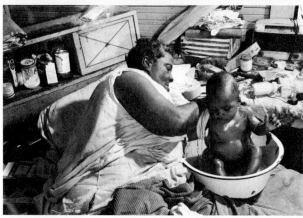

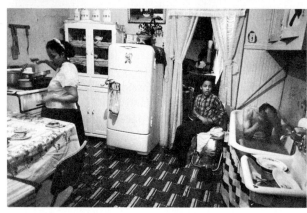

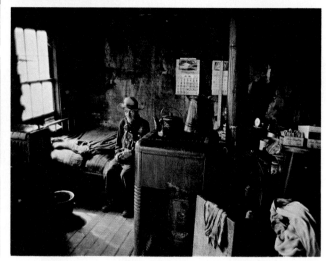

Figure 5.4   Indirect social stress puts a particular
psychological burden on the shoulders of the poor, the old,
and racial minorities.

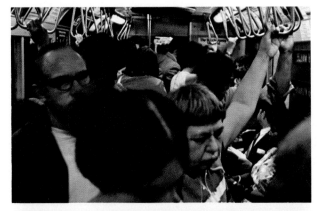

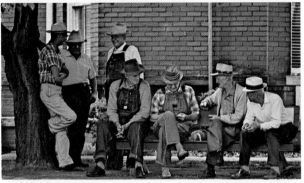

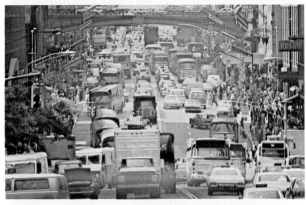

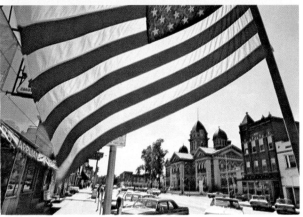

Figure 5.5 Different kinds of stress are felt by persons in different kinds of environments, as in urban versus rural living.

his oppression is likely to react strongly and often in misdirected ways.

People also feel stress from smaller social systems, such as the family, neighborhood, or social clique. As in the larger social system represented by society, stress generated by smaller social systems may be a *direct* one. A parent, for example, may openly abuse or reject his child. An employer may harass or persecute a given employee or discriminate against him. Stress generated in this way may influence an individual even if he is totally or partially unaware of the source of that stress.

Indirect stress also can be generated by a smaller social system. A younger member in a family of outstanding people may worry about his not achieving a comparable stature. A person owning a house in a "plush" residential area may feel pressured to live beyond his means in other respects so that he may be "in" with his neighbors.

INDIVIDUAL STRESS No two individuals experience or react to the same stress in the same way. One person will shrug off an insult; another will be troubled by it and become depressed; a third will find it psychologically devastating and will react violently. There are actually no objective means of measuring the "absolute" severity of a stress. The best one can do is try to obtain some consensus as to how most people, particularly one's peers, would view a given stress and to understand the manner in which the individual exposed to the stress actually perceives or reacts to it. For example, most people would consider the death of a loved one a severe stress; they would consider being spoken to rudely by a stranger a minor stress. Emotional disturbances seem to generally involve sensing of excessive oppression from the outside world.

Very real stress can be imposed upon a person without his being aware of it. But it is not only the person who is stressed who has difficulty in perceiving the source of indirect stress—often those around him cannot see it either. Not infrequently, some people are labeled mentally ill because the community and professionals who apply the label are unaware of the extent of stress that person experiences. In such instances, the person's apparent unreasonableness proves to be much more reasonable once his situation is understood. An elderly man, for example, grew very argumentative when he was told by the manager of the hotel where he lived that his room was being changed. The argument grew so heated that police were called and the man was taken to a hospital for observation, then admitted to a mental institution. Eventually a legal aid organization was able to get him released.

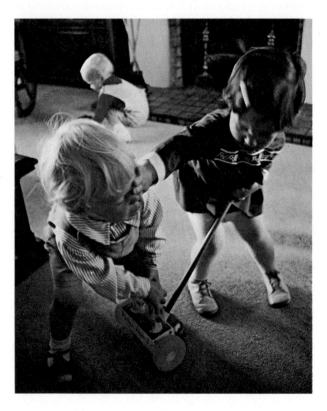

Figure 5.6   Direct stress occurs in the family when family members experience interpersonal conflict, such as that which occurs in sibling rivalry.

The man had a valid reason for protesting his room change—he had a stomach ailment and required his own bathroom, but the manager insisted upon moving him to a room with no bathroom.

A person may, however, perceive his environment as excessively oppressive even when the total stress in his life would not be judged as excessive by those who knew all the indirect and direct stress being imposed on him. An individual who sees more oppression than actually exists may be viewed as having a defect in his perceptual processes, that is, in his ability to integrate external stimuli and internal "standards" in order to correctly interpret the overall message. Every person is constantly receiving messages from his environment, some of which he perceives as friendly, others as unfriendly. A person who is not equipped to interpret environmental messages correctly is quite likely to interpret friendly messages as unfriendly. If a child's parents prevent him from playing with matches, the child may perceive his parents' intentions as malevolent even though his parents mean to be benevolent. A child may not have the *intellectual* or the *experiential* equipment to decipher his parents' communication correctly.

Adults who have limited intelligence or who have obvious defects in their capacity to perceive things (such as deafness) also may interpret their environment as excessively unfriendly. Many psychiatrists believe that those who become emotionally disturbed with no obvious defects have more subtle physiological deficiencies that prevent them from correctly interpreting the messages of their environment. There is, however, no conclusive evidence as yet to support this belief.

Experience also can lead one to sense excessive oppression. If one is deprived of love or is treated cruelly during his early years, he learns to anticipate stress even in a relatively stress-free environment. If an individual is raised in an overly strict home and develops a powerful conscience, he will be plagued by feelings of oppression, even in the most liberated environment. The person who experiences deprivation, rejection, or guilt is likely to project inadequacies and fears onto the external world and will constantly anticipate the possibility of attacks from others. If one subconsciously holds goals or values that conflict, he may experience stress if the conflict is not brought into consciousness and resolved. Whatever the experiential background that may cause it, if a person miscalculates the intentions of those around him, he will react in a way that will appear unreasonable to others. Eventually he will offend his neighbors. They in turn will respond aggressively, and he will have to deal with new, and this time real, oppressive responses from others.

All individuals are inevitably exposed to sufficient internal and environmental stress in their early life so that when they reach adulthood they are at least partly inclined to feel more oppression than actually exists. But people have different kinds of childhood experiences. A person is more likely to distort his perception of the environment in adult life if he has been exposed to a great deal of oppressive stress earlier in life.

At any given moment, then, every individual must deal with stresses that can deprive him of gratification and happiness. Society as a whole can exert either direct or indirect oppressive stress upon any of its individual members. Small social systems, such as family or friends, also can impose stress directly or indirectly. In addition, there is an entire set of stresses that man, in a sense, imposes upon himself by misperceiving his environment or by holding unresolved or unidentified conflicting values. In this set, stress is generated by man's failure to interpret correctly the nature of his position in relation to the social system as a whole, or to the smaller social systems of his family and friends, or

to himself. It is obvious that all these major sources of stress are closely interrelated. Stress from any single source is likely to elicit behavior that will increase stress from the others.

Dealing with Stress

Many psychological theories attempt to describe what constitute appropriate and inappropriate ways of dealing with stress. Psychoanalytic theorists primarily are concerned with the manner in which stressful experiences in early life generate conflict and anxiety from which the individual seeks protection. The person in conflict develops psychological defense mechanisms that help to repress some of his more painful feelings—to keep them out of his consciousness.

Defense mechanisms are automatic responses that help one to alleviate or avoid stress rather than solve the problem causing it. Some of the most common defense mechanisms are *rationalization* (convincing oneself that one's reasons for doing something are different than they really are); *projection* (attributing one's own motives to others or blaming someone else for one's own problems); *denial, withdrawal,* and *avoidance* (refusing to notice or identify stressful situations); *compensation* (making up for a feeling of inadequacy in one area by excelling or overindulging in another); *reaction formation* (attempting to remove something that one is attracted to but that causes one anxiety); and *displacement* (transference of an emotion from the situation that caused it to a less stressful situation).

Although these mechanisms may carry a person through some stages of life in a relatively trouble-free manner, psychoanalysts believe that overdependence on some of these mechanisms makes the individual highly susceptible to maladaptive behavior even when exposed to comparatively minor stress. For example, a man who has rationalized being fired as being the result of poor health may feel extreme anxiety at the thought of a simple visit to the doctor, and he may do everything in his power to avoid his appointment for fear that the doctor will find nothing wrong with him. The fear of being forced to face up to his past rationalization creates a stress where none would normally have occurred.

Psychoanalysts also believe that psychological defense mechanisms induce the individual to repress important feelings or eliminate them from his consciousness. According to this theory, sex and anger are the two critical feelings that must be dealt with if the individual is to achieve mental health. If an individual's defenses do not allow him to be aware of and to deal with these feelings, he will experience conflict and anxiety in his efforts to relate to people in his immediate environment.

Although psychoanalytic theory remains the predominant approach in understanding and treating maladaption to stress, there are several other important approaches. Behavior therapists, for instance, attribute all maladaptive behavior to re-

sponses that have been learned through reinforcement. Those psychologists who are primarily biologically oriented tend to search for physiological or biochemical defects in the patient that cause him to interpret his environment incorrectly and therefore leave him susceptible to even minor stress. Existential schools hold that emotional disorder is based on an individual's failure to acknowledge and act upon his authentic feelings. Another view is that inappropriate handling of conflicts results from irrational values and irrational thinking on the part of the individual.

Most psychologists would say that it is healthy to tackle conflicts and problems directly and to think them out without resorting to defense mechanisms, habit (learned responses), the opinions of others, or irrational thinking. Each new problem must be considered in its particular context and within the framework of one's own particular goals and values. Whenever one holds conflicting goals and values, or he continually avoids his problems or deals with them inappropriately so that they begin to

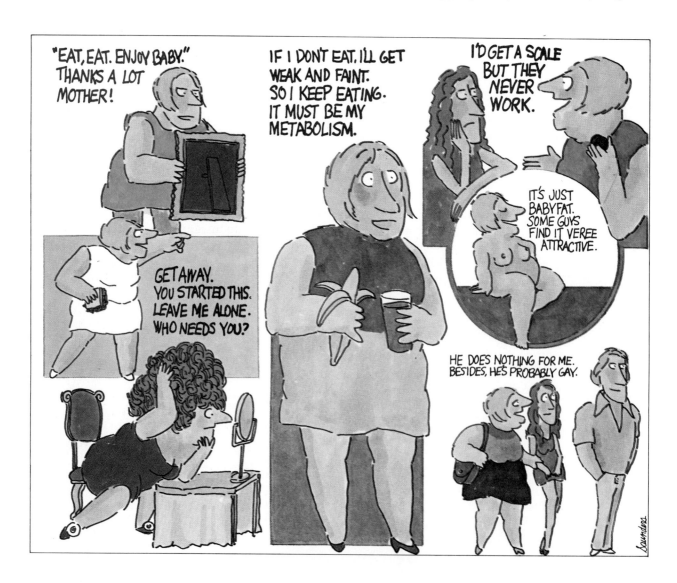

overwhelm him, or his brain suffers physical damage, part or all of his adaptive functioning may break down.

WHEN PROBLEMS GET OUT OF HAND

For centuries physicians and other scientists have been seeking a logical and useful classification of behavior disorders. Yet, human behavior has proven thus far to be too complex to be adequately categorized. No classification of behavior disorders has the same precision or usefulness as related categories or diagnoses in general medicine. Two doctors working in the same hospital may regularly use different criteria for diagnosing schizophrenia. Nor does making a diagnosis dictate any specific treatment. A person labeled schizophrenic may be treated with the same techniques applied to a person labeled neurotic.

The standard practice in psychiatry has been to differentiate between disorders known as *psychoses*, which are characterized by behavior that is so unreasonable as to impair the individual's capacity to meet the ordinary demands of life, and disorders called *neuroses*, which may be characterized by great suffering but still do not impair the individual's ability to retain sufficient contact with reality to function in most areas of his life. In each instance the diagnosis requires knowledge of the patient's environment and a judgment as to whether he is able to cope with this environment.

There are two other somewhat less significant categories of behavior disorders. *Personality disorders* are diagnosed in people who have deeply ingrained maladaptive patterns of behavior that can be thought of as being fixed aspects of their personality. *Psychophysiological*, or *psychosomatic*, *disorders* are diagnosed in persons who develop physical symptoms, frequently involving a single organ system, that are caused by emotional factors. The official diagnostic and statistical manual of the American Psychiatric Association lists hundreds of categories and subcategories of emotional disorders. Rather than attempting to list all of them here, a brief description of only the major disorders will be given.

Neuroses

The neuroses are best understood as manifestations of, or efforts to deal with, anxiety. *Anxiety* is a distinctively unpleasant emotion. It can affect one physiologically with disturbed breathing, increased heart activity and other circulatory changes, muscular disturbances, and increased sweating. Psychologically it may produce a sense of powerlessness, a presentiment of impending and almost inevitable danger, a tense and physically exhausting alertness as if facing an emergency, an all-absorbing apprehension that interferes with solving practical problems, and an irresolvable uncertainty concerning the nature of the threatening evil. Anxiety is to be distinguished from fear in that *fear* is a frank reaction to a real or threatened danger while *anxiety* usually occurs as a reaction to vague, diffuse, or imagined dangers.

Neurotic anxiety is generally manifested either in physical symptoms or in peculiar behavior. Some people chronically feel weak, tire easily, or become exhausted even though they are in excellent physical health. Other anxious individuals may develop nervous-system disorders. Such symptoms as blindness, deafness, loss of the touch sensation, or paralysis can develop even when there is no organic basis for them. When such symptoms are present, the individual is generally considered to have a form of neurosis called *hysterical neurosis, conversion type*. Neurotic behaviors associated with anxiety include *phobias* (intense fear of an object or situation that the patient consciously recognizes as no real danger to him), *obsessive-compulsive behavior* (the persistent intrusion of unwanted thoughts, urges, or actions that the individual is unable to stop even though he

Figure 5.7 People may employ a number of defense mechanisms to keep from facing the truth about themselves.

may perceive them as absurd), and *hypochondriasis* (a preoccupation with the body and with fear of presumed diseases even though the individual is in good health).

Depression

There is one form of behavior usually classified under the neuroses that is so important in the study of general medicine, psychiatry, or human behavior in general that it deserves special consideration: *depression*. Depression is a disorder characterized by sadness, anxiety, insomnia, withdrawal from others, agitated behavior, and a reduced ability to function and work with others. Depression ranges in intensity from a mild feeling of unease and sadness to intense suicidal despair. It may be so severe that it is accompanied by distortions of reality, in which case the depressed individual is labeled psychotic.

Depression is of special interest to general physicians because many patients who go to a doctor do not have a real physical illness but are depressed and are looking for help by complaining about physical problems. The depressed patient may

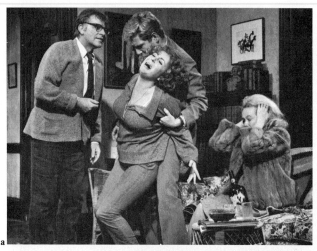

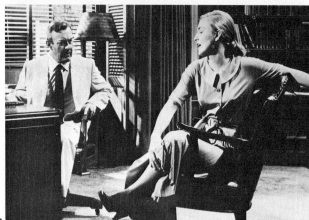

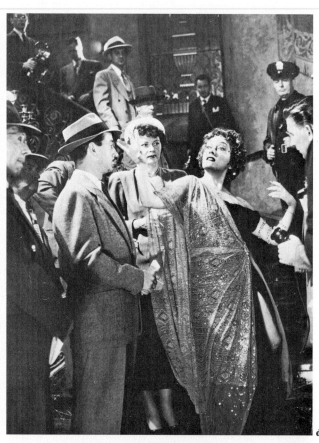

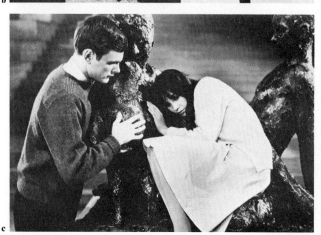

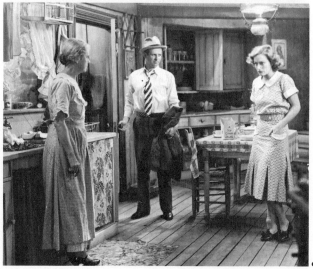

complain about almost any disorder, and it often takes considerable skill on the doctor's part to determine that the patient actually needs help with his psychological problems. Any kind of emotional loss—a loss of a loved one, a loss of one's sense of physical well-being, or a loss of one's status and importance in his community—can be a major factor in precipitating depression. Depression among older people, for example, always seems to be greater in those societies where the aged are not revered and are denied the status and affirmation that they previously enjoyed.

A person who is severely depressed must be considered a suicide risk. Suicide is more common in males, in the fourth, fifth, and sixth decades of life, among individuals of non-Catholic religious faith, and in urban rather than rural areas. Suicide is more likely if the patient states his intentions, if he has made previous suicide attempts, if his insomnia is severe, and when he has experienced rapid weight loss. Suicide also is more likely either when the patient is first becoming depressed or when he seems to be getting better. Physicians have learned that it is therefore important to continue to observe and treat patients who have been severely depressed even when the patient seems to be moving rapidly toward recovery.

Psychoses

Individuals whose perceptions of reality are so grossly impaired that they cannot function properly under normal circumstances are labeled psychotic. Sometimes their behavior seems clearly related to a physical defect, but sometimes it does not.

An anatomical lesion or physiological disorder that interferes with the brain can impair the individual's ability to function effectively in the interpersonal sphere. Such organic disorders can result from circulatory disease, drug intoxication, infection, senility, epilepsy, tumors, mechanical injury, and a wide variety of metabolic disorders, all of which can produce either mild or severe psychological malfunctioning. Organic brain disorders are characterized by five categories of symptoms: (1) impairment of orientation (knowledge of time, place, and person); (2) impairment of memory; (3) impairment of all intellectual functions such as comprehension; (4) impairment of judgment; (5) instability and shallowness of feeling.

There are other psychoses not known to be associated with neurological impairment, the most common of which is called *schizophrenia*. Although no clearly defined brain dysfunction can be ascertained in those labeled schizophrenic, there is some evidence that genetic factors contribute to the disorder (see Chapter 14).

The schizophrenia label is usually applied to individuals who have severely disturbed thinking, moods, and behavior. These disturbances are marked by misinterpretations of reality. Often the person who is called schizophrenic has *delusions*; that is, he holds false beliefs that cannot be corrected by logical argument. Sometimes he *hallucinates*—he perceives external objects when no such objects are present (perhaps he "hears" a long-dead relative or friend). Generally, delusions and hallucinations offer the individual some form of psychological protection; that is, they help him retain his sense of integrity and self-esteem. Most commonly, they involve projections of the individual's unacceptable thoughts and feelings onto others. Mood changes also are characteristic of schizophrenia. The person may respond to an emotional situation inappropriately, like laughing at the news of someone's death. He may withdraw from others, become excessively active, or adopt bizarre gestures or postures. Some element of paranoia—extreme delusions of persecution or grandeur—also is generally present.

Although schizophrenia usually seems to be

Figure 5.8 Neurosis and psychosis have been popular themes in films and literature: (a) "Who's Afraid of Virginia Woolf" provided a glimpse of four neurotic individuals; (b) Joanne Woodward played a schizophrenic with three distinct personalities in "Three Faces of Eve"; (c) the psychoses of two teen-agers, one with a great fear of being touched and the other able to talk only in rhymes, are explored in "David and Lisa"; (d) Gloria Swanson plays the neurotically driven faded star trying to make a Hollywood comeback in "Sunset Boulevard"; (e) in "Possessed" Joan Crawford plays a schizophrenic murderess.

precipitated by some interpersonal or social stress, behavioral scientists have no precise idea what type of stress will initiate a psychotic reaction and what type will initiate a neurotic reaction. Much research has been done in trying to determine just what types of early-childhood and life-situation experiences seem to elicit schizophrenic behavior and what type of person seems to be most susceptible. These efforts have not been notably successful. There has been some suggestion that those who experience symptoms of schizophrenia may have been exposed to more severe stress than those who become neurotic, but actual cases do not always bear this theory out. In general, behavioral scientists do not know a great deal about why individuals who are exposed to what seem to be quite similar stresses react differently.

Another major group of psychoses characterized by a disorder in mood is known as the *affective psychoses*. The mental life of a patient with such a condition is dominated by excessive and inappropriate elation or severe and unreasonable depression. Sometimes, as in the so-called *manic-depressive psychosis*, the patient alternates between these two extreme moods.

Personality Disorders

Because of social and interpersonal stress beginning early in life, some individuals develop characteristic maladaptive reactions to social situations. Sometimes the responses are so consistent that the individual can be classified as having a distinct personality disorder. *Personality disorders* are diagnosed on the basis of persistent behavior patterns such as paranoia, variation in mood, withdrawal, impulsiveness, obsessiveness, drug addiction, or effort to find sexual gratification through activities that are considered abnormal by the community. Diagnosing an individual as having a personality disorder is in large part based on social and ethical criteria. The diagnostic categories are certainly arbitrary and the behavior that society finds sick or deviant can generally be related to social or interpersonal stress. The importance of social and ethical factors is most apparent in two of the commonest personality disorders—hysterical personality and sociopathic personality.

Some individuals, particularly women, characteristically react to minor stress by becoming excited and acting in an emotionally unstable manner. They complain excessively about minor bodily discomforts. They exaggerate their own characteristics to gain attention, frequently in a seductive manner. These individuals are sometimes labeled *hysterical* personalities. What they are doing is trying to control their relations with other people by appearing to be sick. Generally, the hysterical person denies responsibility for his manipulative behavior and behaves as if he cannot help himself.

Hysterical behavior patterns are most common among those who are somewhat oppressed by society and who are denied access to more direct and aggressive means of obtaining gratification; this situation applies most often to women. The woman who is considered hysterical probably learned in early childhood to translate her feelings of helplessness into signs of physical and mental illness in order to gain attention and control others. Such a woman might be the mother who has "spells" whenever her thirty-year-old son who supports her mentions getting married. If she can learn to communicate her needs more directly and if she is permitted to live in an environment that affirms her status as a first-class citizen, her hysterical behavior may diminish markedly.

Individuals having *sociopathic* personalities find themselves in repeated conflict with society. They seem, at least superficially, to be incapable of significant loyalty to individuals, groups, or social values. Their frustration tolerance is low. They often are

by Julian Silverman

There are forms of schizophrenic experience that can be positively and creatively constructive. Karl Menninger, in 1959, put it this way: "Some patients have a mental illness and then get well and then they get weller! I mean they get better than they ever were. . . . This is an extraordinary and little-realized truth."

A handful of psychiatrists have recognized the validity of this observation—Harry Stack Sullivan, John Perry, R. D. Laing, and others. But most psychiatrists find it hard to regard the bizarre disorganization of schizophrenia as anything but ominous, and they see the crazy disturbances as behaviors to be done away with as quickly as possible. When this cannot be done, they prescribe huge doses of antipsychotic drugs.

But there is mounting evidence that some of the most profound schizophrenic disorganizations are preludes to impressive reorganization and personality growth—not so much breakdown as breakthrough. Kazimierz Dabrowski has called it "positive disintegration." It appears to be a natural reaction to severe stress, a spontaneous process into which persons may enter when their usual problem-solving techniques fail to solve such basic life crises as occupational or sexual inadequacy. If this natural process is interrupted by well-intended psychotherapy or by antipsychotic medication, the effect may be to detour the patient away from the acute schizophrenic episode, away from a process as natural and benign as fever. The effect can be disastrous—it can rob him of his natural problem-solving potential.

Anton Boisen was one of the first to recognize the potentially beneficial aspects of psychosis. Boisen was a psychologist and chaplain who went through several brief schizophrenic periods himself. Acute schizophrenic reactions, he wrote, are "not in themselves evils but problem-solving experiences. They are attempts at reorganization in which the entire personality, to its bottom-most depths, is aroused and its forces marshaled to meet the danger of personal failure and isolation. . . . The acute disturbances tend either to make or break. They may send the patient to the back wards, there to remain as a hopeless wreck, or they may send him back to the community in better shape than he had been for years."

As Boisen indicates, while some patients are likely to recover—even benefit—from their psychotic experiences, others may be severely disturbed for the rest of their lives. There has been extensive research in recent years concerning which patients are which; usually this has involved collecting a quantity of data about many schizophrenic patients, waiting to see which ones get better, then rechecking the data to see if the improved patients were in any way systematically different from the unimproved patients.

One of the most common findings is that the patient who improved had a sudden onset of symptoms; he typically went from a moderately effective life style to severe psychosis in a period of perhaps a few days or weeks. Further, there was typically a precipitating event, some life-crisis that immediately preceded the break. On the other hand, the schizophrenic who has been developing his symptoms over a period of years, gradually becoming more withdrawn and out of touch with reality, is more likely to remain in a disturbed condition for many years.

There are other typical characteristics of the "problem-solving schizophrenic." A reaction to personal failure or guilt often starts with high anxiety as the patient searches for any possible way to repair his self-esteem. With increasing emotional turmoil, he takes a highly subjective orientation to the problem and becomes preoccupied, socially isolated, and withdrawn. He feels despair and hopelessness. As Sullivan has noted, he may finally think "that he is dead, that this is the state after death; that he awaits resurrection or the salvation of his soul. Ancient myths of redemption and rebirth seem to appear." Ideas of death-rebirth, world catastrophe, and cosmic importance are common.

The patient may regress to childish behavior. He may go so far as to simulate the womb by wrapping himself in wet sheets. He may become extremely withdrawn—not eating or drinking, not talking, not blowing his nose, staying in bed all day, perhaps with eyes and mouth tightly closed. He might rock back and forth with strange, rhythmic movements. Occasionally he may pass from his catatonic stupor into violent, random excitement. In this state he may hurt himself or others, but only by accident. He is not mad at anyone else. In fact, persistent outright aggression toward others is a bad sign. It is as if such a patient has aborted his schizophrenic trip, has taken the easy way out by blaming his troubles on someone else. Harry Stack Sullivan has vividly described the implications:

"This is an ominous development in that the schizophrenic state is taking on a paranoid coloring. If the suffering of the patient is markedly diminished thereby, we shall observe the evolution of a paranoid schizophrenic state. These conditions are of relatively much less favorable outcome. They tend to permanent distortions of the interpersonal relations. . . .

"A paranoid systematization is, therefore, markedly beneficial to the peace of mind of the person chiefly concerned, and its achievement in the course of a schizophrenic disorder is so great an improvement in security that it is seldom relinquished. . . .

Adapted from Silverman, J. "When Schizophrenia Helps," *Psychology Today* (September 1970), pp. 63-65.

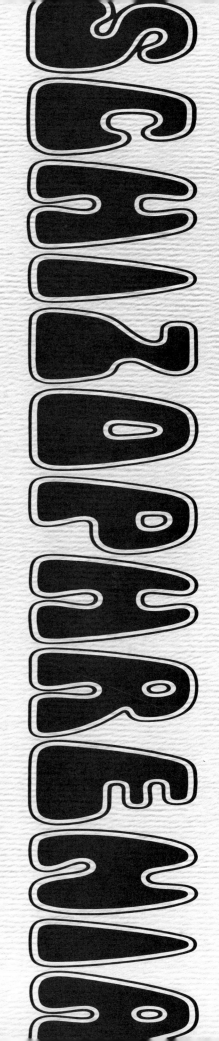

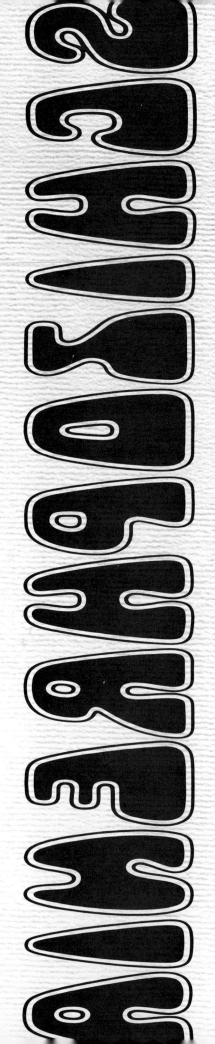

It is for this reason that the paranoid development in a schizophrenic state has to be regarded as of bad omen.''

Phenothiazine drugs—especially chlorpromazine—have made it possible to control the most difficult, craziest patients. But in certain individuals these drugs may interfere with recovery. In a recent study, Drs. Michael Goldstein, Lewis Judd, and their colleagues at UCLA tested schizophrenic patients who had shown reasonably good psychological adjustments before they were hospitalized. The acute nonparanoid schizophrenic patients treated with chlorpromazine actually showed increases in thought disorder over a three-week period, while a similar group of patients, on placebos, showed decreases in thought disorder during the same period. This relationship did not hold in patients with the paranoid type of schizophrenic reaction.

Tranquilizers seem to reduce regressed and agitated schizophrenic behavior, and most psychiatrists take this as evidence of improvement. Unfortunately, regressed and disorganized behavior may be essential parts of schizophrenia's problem-solving process.

Several research studies have shown that chlorpromazine reduces the clarity of ordinary experience, and it disrupts a person's abilities to see alternatives and solve problems. It is no wonder that in schizophrenic reactions that are essentially problem-solving processes, the use of chlorpromazine can make the psychosis worse.

Research has indicated several similarities between the schizophrenia trip and the psychedelic-drug trip, with LSD for example. First of all such tranquilizers as chlorpromazine can make a bad trip worse, possibly in the same way that they interrupt the schizophrenic process. The development of paranoid ideas in a person under LSD is also ominous; they take him away from the ideal subjective orientation to the drug experience. We have also found that persons on either kind of journey have a more undifferentiated perceptual orientation than normal persons. For example, they respond to distracting stimuli, which causes them to perform poorly on reaction-time tasks and on complex perceptual tasks.

Further, acute schizophrenics and persons under the influence of psychedelic drugs are highly sensitive to stimuli. Sights and sounds are experienced as brilliant, intense, alive, rich, compelling. This acute sensitivity of schizophrenia has gone unnoticed until recently because it is very hard to test. Schizophrenics do not respond well to complex directions; they are flooded by so many stimuli, and so easily distracted by minor sights and noises, that on many sensitivity tests (''press this button when you see the light'') they appear unable to perceive stimuli as well as normal persons can.

Only in recent studies have we learned

that certain schizophrenics can detect lights and sounds that are too weak for normal persons to sense. We are beginning to accumulate evidence that supports the acute schizophrenic's description of his over-aroused world. He is overwhelmed by stimulation. He has difficulty in focusing attention for very long. While he is expressing an idea, a whole series of complicating ideas may come to his mind. He may be blocked in the act of speaking or may give up the struggle and go mute.

Apparently the mechanism that filters out nonessential stimuli for the rest of us—the humming of the refrigerator, the rustling of the leaves—has ceased to function in the acute schizophrenic. In this distressed individual, who is groping for any possible answer to a life-crisis dilemma, heightened awareness may allow him to see alternative perspectives for making sense out of the life-crisis situation.

In the highly aroused state the schizophrenic may become aware of thoughts, images, and feelings that would ordinarily be beyond the scope of consciousness. Internal events and ideas may be experienced as vividly as if they were real.

With continued overstimulation, inhibition is built up against very strong stimuli. The individual may now be able to tolerate intense pain; he may not show a startle response to very loud sounds. This paradoxical situation of sharpened sensitivity to weak stimuli and reduced responsiveness to strong stimuli has also been reported in subjects on LSD.

Looked at in this perspective, the familiar symptoms of early schizophrenia—distractability, thought-blocking, withdrawal, loss of spontaneity in movement and speech—all may be understood as defensive reactions to overstimulation.

Some studies show that an acute schizophrenic may improve temporarily after being placed in a dark, sound-proofed room. Apparently the brief interlude of semirelief from overstimulation allows him to drop some of his automatically defensive reactions to overstimulation, at least for a while.

At Agnews State Hospital in San Jose, California, I am working with other mental-health professionals who agree that this type of schizophrenic reaction should be encouraged and supported. With systematic clinical tests, electrophysiological measures, and computer techniques we are attempting to identify those individuals who are on the schizophrenic trip. We are withholding antipsychotic medication from patients who ordinarily would be heavily drugged.

It may be that one day acute schizophrenics of certain types will not go to hospitals but will go instead to asylums or sanctuaries to grapple with their otherwise unsolvable life-crisis problems. One hopes that in this kind of environment the schizophrenic patient who emerges ''weller than before'' will be more the rule than the exception.

described as grossly selfish, callous, irresponsible, impulsive, and unable to feel guilt or learn from experience. These individuals are frequently labeled antisocial personalities. In the extreme, they may be totally without conscience. The psychopathic individual is one who, although he knows the difference between right and wrong, is unable to care. His desire for self-gratification takes precedence over all other values.

The majority of sociopathic individuals come from lower socioeconomic or other oppressed groups. Sometimes it is unclear whether their behavior should be considered an understandable reaction to massive social oppression or a psychological disorder. In general, it is useful to consider the antisocial personality as someone who has more or less abandoned hope that his basic needs will be gratified by the community or those who are close to him. He behaves as if he does not care whether others love him or not. His efforts to free himself from the need for others often lead to behavior that the community condemns as antisocial. Many criminals, particularly murderers, have been diagnosed as sociopaths.

Psychophysiological Reactions

Excessive psychological stress often produces physical symptoms that involve a single organ system. Normal physiological changes that accompany certain emotional states may become so intense and long lasting that an individual develops a physical disorder, largely because of his inability to cope with stress and anxiety. He may not be consciously aware of the emotional state that is contributing to his disorder. These disorders are referred to as *psychophysiological* or *psychosomatic* reactions. Such reactions can disturb almost every bodily system. Behavioral scientists have little idea as to what specific types of stresses may be related to specific physiological dysfunctions. They do know, however, that those who are likely to have backaches, tension headaches, asthma, hypertension, migraine, colitis, or peptic ulcer, or be frigid or impotent are often unable to deal with psychological stress.

HELP FOR PROBLEMS

Because behavior disorders are generated in large part by interactions between the disturbed individual and his environment, the disorder can often be altered either by changing the environment or by changing the disturbed individual himself. Sometimes this process is a reciprocal one in which changes in the environment will make the person feel differently or in which changes in the person will make him more capable of modifying his environment. For the most part, treatment in the mental-health professions focuses upon the disturbed individual. Obviously, though, reducing real oppression originating in the disturbed individual's community or in his interactions with friends and family will improve his plight. Viewed in this light, the field of mental health encompasses almost every aspect of community and family organization. It is possible to speculate about the kinds of social structures and family or peer-group structures that are most conducive to mental health, and efforts to create such structures can in a sense be viewed as treatments of mental illness. Thus, efforts to end racism, poverty, or war can legitimately be considered broad, albeit ill-defined, treatments of mental disorders.

Community Psychiatry

In the last decade, a new movement called *community psychiatry* has directed the attention of behavioral scientists to the problem of preventing emotional disorders. Community psychiatry is concerned with three types of prevention: *primary prevention* consists of measures to reduce the incidence of mental disorder in a community by eliminating its causes and stopping its spread; it involves working with community agencies and other social organizations in an effort to reduce oppressive stress in the social environment. *Secondary prevention* involves reducing the prevalence and severity of mental disorder in a community through early diagnosis and therapy. *Tertiary prevention* consists of measures to reduce residual defects consequent to mental disorder—measures that limit the disability and that are designed to initiate rehabilitation.

The community psychiatrist is concerned with efficient delivery of health services. He is concerned that services are available to those who need them at times of crisis or at critical stress periods in their lives, such as marriage, childbirth, or divorce.

Community psychiatry, because it is provided through public funds, has been criticized by some as a means of converting social misfits into socially useful citizens with no attention to the person's own psychological needs. It is seen as an agent of socialization with the aims of the community, not of the individual, as its goals. Defenders of community psychiatry point out that it attempts to make available for all what private psychiatry delivers to only a few.

Symptomatic Treatment

Much of the therapy provided by mental-health professionals is *symptomatic*: that is, it is designed to alleviate the overt manifestations of the patient's suffering or unreasonable behavior without recognizing or dealing with the stresses that led to the disturbance.

Treatments that influence the physiological and biochemical state of the disturbed individual are among the most effective symptomatic treatments. (Some of the reasons for the effectiveness of drug treatments were given in Chapter 3.) The medical profession has long used such drugs as barbiturates and bromides to help alleviate severe anxiety. Unfortunately, these drugs also cause drowsiness,

which patients find undesirable. In recent years tranquilizers have proven to be effective agents for alleviating anxiety without causing undue sleepiness. It is now possible to give highly disturbed people medication that enables them to function more or less normally in their work and personal relations. Since the advent of the tranquilizing and antidepressant drugs, mental-hospital populations have consistently gone down even though the number of admissions has increased, which means that more patients are coming into the hospital but more are leaving and they are leaving much more quickly.

Although neither tranquilizers nor antidepressants *cure* mental illness, they do seem to have powerful effects upon *relieving* the most painful aspects of anxiety and depression. They are not perfect solutions to these problems, however. Both classes of drugs may have undesirable physical and psychological side effects. They are not always effective and they make a few patients worse. It is quite likely, however, that in the near future these drugs will be improved and other new drugs will make it possible to provide quick symptomatic relief for the most painful and debilitating emotional disorders. (Tranquilizers and antidepressants are further discussed in Chapter 7.)

Other treatments, such as electroshock therapy, insulin-shock therapy, and lobotomy, are now used less frequently. *Electroshock therapy* is the application of a sufficient electrical current to the brain to produce a convulsion; it is still used occasionally for severe depression and certain excited states. *Insulin-shock therapy*, which is the inducement of a coma through large doses of insulin, and *lobotomy*, the cutting of various nerve tracts in the prefrontal area of the brain, are rarely used in the United States any more.

Another group of treatments that primarily are designed to alleviate symptoms can be referred to

Figure 5.9   The situation in American mental hospitals in the past was not always conducive to the patient's recovery. Patients were often treated as animals.

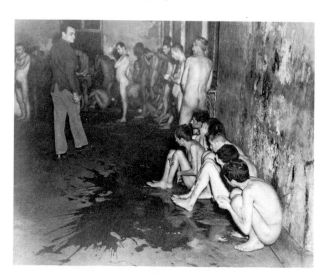

collectively as *behavior therapies*. Behavior therapy is based upon classical models of learning and conditioning. The behavior therapist views all behavior as a response to a stimulus, and he believes that most behavior is learned through the process of conditioning, by which links are established between certain stimuli and certain responses (see Chapter 4).

The behavior therapist tries to help his patient rid himself of troubling behavior by putting the person into learning situations where he can, in a sense, unlearn or get rid of an unwanted response. The therapist also may try to teach the person new and more adaptive behavior by changing the environment so that he is rewarded or receives reinforcement for developing more desirable responses. Sometimes the person is relieved of a troubling fear by being exposed to fear-provoking stimuli under conditions that are incompatible with fear. The person is taught how to relax while being systematically exposed to progressively more frightening imaginary or symbolic representations of the feared stimulus. Eventually he is able to face the actual feared stimulus with little anxiety. An individual who fears snakes may begin treatment by looking at pictures of snakes while in a relaxed condition. He will be exposed to stimuli (always while he is relaxed) that more closely represent the actual snakes until he reaches a point when he can touch and handle snakes.

In other forms of behavior therapy, undesirable behavior can be extinguished by systematically "punishing" the patient during situations when the unwanted behavior might ordinarily be elicited. This method is called *aversive conditioning*. A cigarette smoker who wants desperately to stop smoking and who has tried several times without success may submit to a training program during which stale tobacco smoke is blown into his face each time he takes a puff of a cigarette. Quickly he learns to associate the unpleasant experience with smoking and is thereby reinforced in his efforts to live without cigarettes.

Another form of behavior therapy, based on the operant-conditioning model of B. F. Skinner, attempts to shape behavior by systematically rewarding desired responses. Some psychotics and many neurotics have been changed considerably by being systematically rewarded when they behave in a desirable manner and ignored when they do not.

Psychotherapy

Individual psychotherapy is the major treatment used in American psychiatry and psychology today that aims at more than alleviating the patient's symptoms. The psychotherapist sees the patient regularly, listens to him, talks with him, and through reassurance, skillful use of the therapeutic relationship, insight, and education helps the individual to restructure his whole approach toward life and to function more effectively.

There are many schools of psychotherapy. Most of the psychoanalytic therapies place considerable

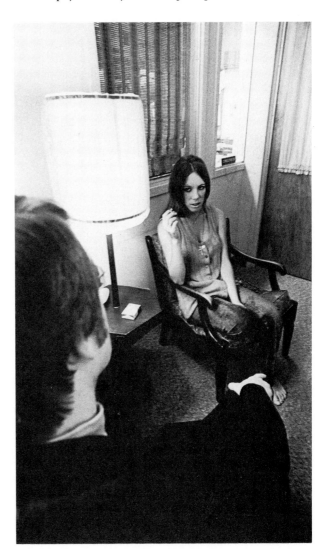

Figure 5.10 Individual psychotherapy is the most widely used treatment for mental illness.

emphasis upon the individual's past life and on stresses in early childhood that may have predisposed him to emotional disturbance. Other therapists, such as those of the Rogerian school, focus heavily upon the client-therapist relationship. Still other therapies, such as existential therapy, reality therapy, or Gestalt therapy, place considerable emphasis upon the patient's life in the present—the means by which he influences and is influenced by his present environment.

Although differing schools of therapy may give greater emphasis to one or another critical factor in the therapeutic approach, all psychotherapies seem to have three common ingredients:

1. *Emphasis on the favorable aspects of the relationship between client and therapist.* All therapists believe that the compassion and honesty that is developed within the therapeutic relationship and the intimacy and models for identification that the therapist provides have favorable effects upon a disturbed individual. All therapies depend upon helping the patient gain a better sense of reality and sometimes helping him find strength through the therapist's concern, wisdom, and even love.

2. *Efforts to help the client understand why he behaves as he does.* All psychotherapies are designed to help the individual learn what factors in his environment and what aspects of his own behavior seem to get him into trouble. The emphasis may be either upon past experiences or current happenings that contribute to emotional disturbance.

3. *Efforts to help the client find alternative modes of behavior.* All psychotherapies involve directly teaching or helping the patient discover for himself that there are alternatives to his current maladaptive patterns of behavior and that these alternatives may allow him to find a more meaningful way of living.

Doubts have been expressed about the effectiveness of individual psychotherapy. Twenty years ago psychologist Hans Eysenck collected evidence on the proportion of patients who in follow-up studies appeared to have been really helped by psychotherapy. On the average, he found that about two-thirds of them could be judged improved, but he also estimated that about two-thirds of similar persons not receiving psychotherapy also improved more or less "spontaneously" through normal interventions from others or the environment. More recent studies have suggested, however, that improvement rates for more carefully specified disorders are higher when the patients receive psychotherapy than when they do not.

FAMILY THERAPY In the past decade, therapists have increasingly moved away from individual psychotherapy and have begun to experiment with treating couples or families as a unit. If one spouse comes to a therapist complaining of anxiety or depression, the other partner soon is invited to join in the therapy so that they can be treated together. If a child is having emotional difficulties, he may be treated together with his parents and perhaps even his siblings.

The family-therapy model adds an exciting and highly practical systems-oriented dimension to psychotherapy. It enables family members to learn how to communicate with one another. It provides each member of the family unit with a clear understanding of the other members' problems. Each person in the family learns something about how others view him, and it is often possible to untangle the twisted web of relationships that have led one or more members in the family to experience emotional suffering. One of the most useful aspects of family therapy is that it quickly exposes the power alignments within the family and allows the therapist to help the family to do something about them.

GROUP TREATMENT There also are a number of techniques that involve treating people with emotional problems in groups rather than individually. So many different varieties of formalized group interaction are popular in American society that it is difficult to decide which should be called group therapy and which should not. Many groups do not claim to have a therapeutic purpose but rather are supposed to provide their members with training in human relations or a better understanding of how to increase one's self-awareness, creativity, and satisfaction in life. These groups include T-groups (for "training"), sensitivity training, encounter groups, and many others. Participants in these groups do not consider themselves patients but are seeking an educational experience that will help them understand their own behavior and the behavior of others. Although there are obvious differences in the goals and methods of training or sensi-tivity groups as opposed to formal therapy groups, both represent techniques that focus upon interpersonal conflicts and that encourage the participant to examine his position within a social system.

Group-treatment techniques, although rarely allowing the patient to experience the deep intimacy of individual therapy, do have certain advantages. The patient learns to see himself as others see him, and the group provides him with a considerable degree of understanding of the motivations and personality styles of others. Each participant has the opportunity to experience and deal with interpersonal stress as it is happening in the moment. Group therapy is most effective if the participants have similar problems and interests.

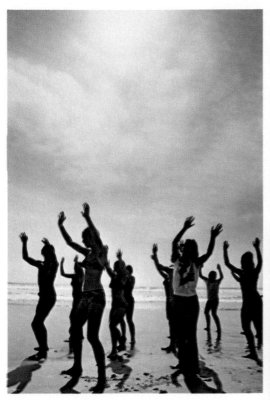

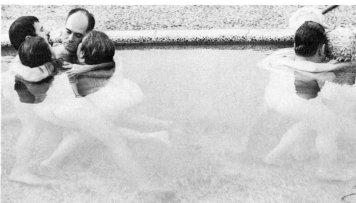

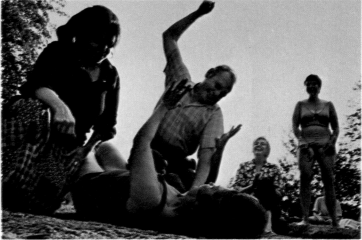

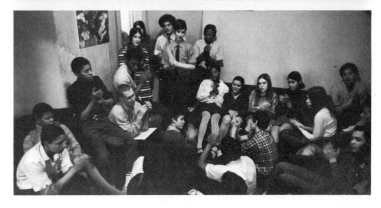

Figure 5.11 Group therapy occurs in a variety of forms designed to help the individual in his interactions with others. It may take the form of sensitivity training sessions, nude marathons, psychodrama, or family therapy, for example.

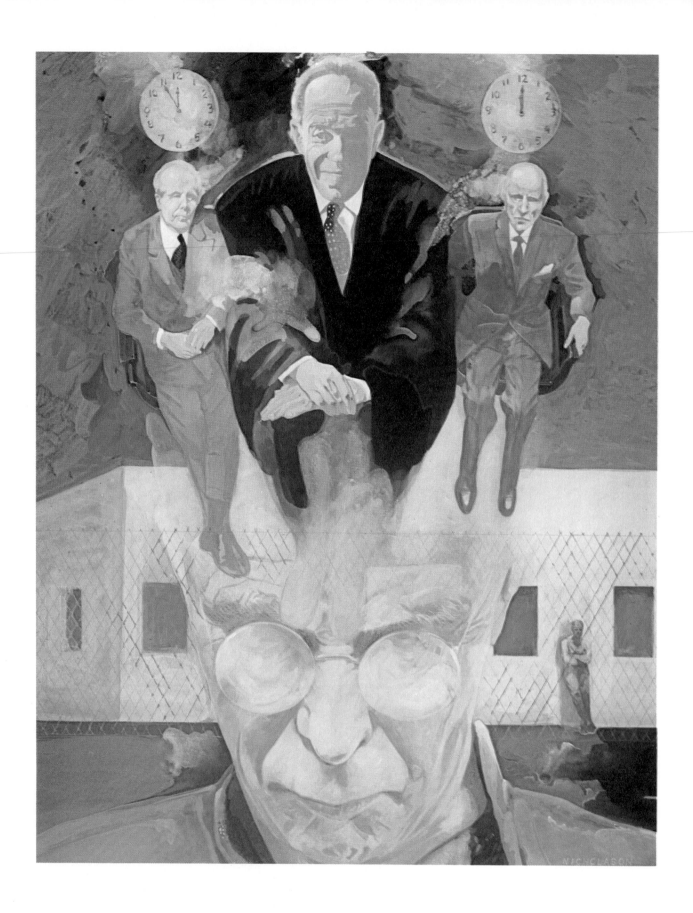

Therapists and Their Training

There are several types of practitioners of psychotherapy, and they are distinguished by the amount and type of training they receive. *Psychiatrists* have a medical degree and generally three years of additional training in the medical specialty of psychiatry; psychologists generally have a Ph.D. in psychology; *social workers* generally have a master's degree in social work. Many other individuals who have training in counseling and guidance serve in therapeutic capacities. Most forms of psychotherapy can be carried out by people who do not have medical training. Professional therapists with warmth, compassion, intelligence, and the ability to understand human behavior can be effective regardless of their training.

Thus the individual beset with personal problems has a choice among sources of help: he may seek it from a general practitioner, a clergyman, a lawyer, a social worker, a neurologist, a psychiatrist, a psychoanalyst, or may even have himself committed to a mental hospital.

Involuntary Commitment

If an individual whom society sees as deviant does not wish to seek professional help or does not consider himself "ill," he may be placed under psychiatric care against his will. The issue of involuntary commitment is a controversial legal and ethical one. It has been argued that the mental patient has fewer rights than a convicted criminal and carries more of a social stigma once he is released. In addition, many persons are placed in mental institutions simply because they are too old or too poor to go anywhere else.

Commitment also has been used as a tool to deprive some people of their freedom and rights for the benefit of other persons. Take, for example, the rich widow who began to give away her fortune to various charities. Worried that she was dissipating funds that they were entitled to, her children succeeded in getting her declared mentally incompetent and in committing her to a mental institution, where she died two years later. Thus although enforced psychotherapy can be extremely helpful to the stressed individual, it also can be fraught with ethical and legal hazards.

It is easy for people who are basically happy, well-adjusted individuals to look down on or even fear those with serious emotional disturbances, which is one reason why mental patients are so often placed in institutions. It is often easier for relatives, friends, associates, or society at large to put the patient out of sight than to face the personal or social injustices that have oppressed him. The question of mental illness is thus not just an individual one but a problem with many ramifications and complications. There can be no simple answer to the question or solution to the problem. Each case must be judged by itself, in light of the little that is known about mental functioning and about the particular individual.

Figure 5.12   The crime of involuntary commitment. More than half of all Americans who enter mental hospitals each year do so against their will. Commitment proceedings in many states ignore the rights of the accused—they require a statement that the person is mentally ill signed by relative or friend, a confirmation by a physician, and a hearing. The physician often has only a few minutes to examine the person, and the confirmation is usually a routine one done on an assembly-line basis. The hearings take an average of five minutes, during which the accused is usually heavily sedated. Reform of such procedures is underway in many states, but many complex issues are involved.

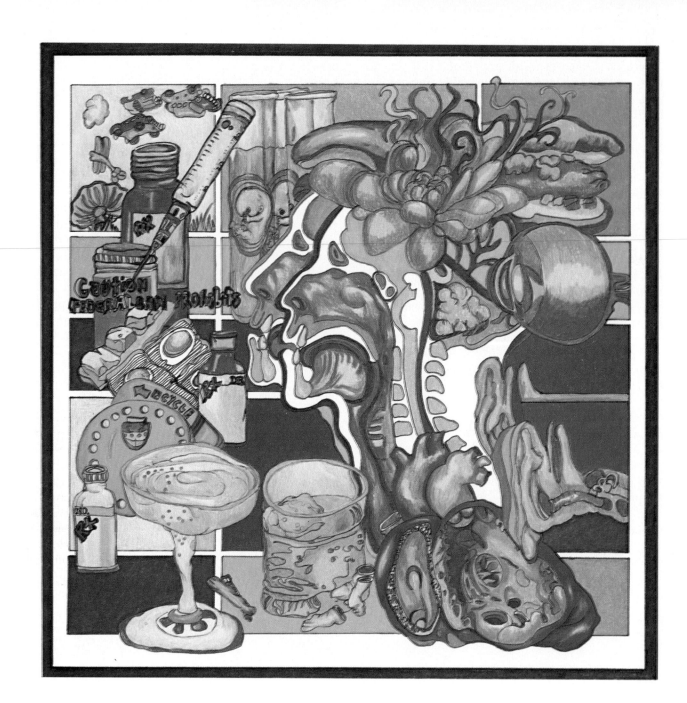

III CHEMICAL ALTERATION OF BEHAVIOR

Mind-altering drugs are deeply rooted aspects of human experience. The question, "Should people use drugs?" seems absurd in light of the fact that virtually all human beings have been, are, and will continue to be users of chemical modifiers of physiological functioning and behavior. The more relevant question is: Who should use what chemicals for what reasons, under what circumstances, and with what results in order to maximize the positive values and minimize the risks? ¶ Such a question cannot be answered without a thorough understanding of what drugs are, how they affect human functioning, and the present role of society in their availability and control. In the space of one unit in a health text book it is impossible to present every aspect of drug use and abuse—in fact, not every aspect is known. What *can* be done is to present a picture of the role drugs play in the American society of today; a compilation of the major psychoactive drugs, their effects and abuses, focusing further on the two mostly widely abused drugs, alcohol and nicotine; and a view of the current situation in respect to drugs and the law. ¶ The final chapter in this unit, "Drugs in Perspective," was contributed by one of the foremost experts on drugs in America today, Dr. Joel Fort. Dr. Fort encourages people to actualize their potentials, to go beyond drugs in their search for meaning in life. But he also condemns those who would punish those who do use drugs; he feels that it is not a crime against the state to do what one wishes to do with one's body. Government now punishes people who sell and use drugs; is it possible that at some time in the future government will be a *source* of drugs and will punish those who do not ingest the substances that will keep them submissive for yet another day? Aldous Huxley predicted such a situation in *Brave New World;* other novelists have used similar themes. ¶ The drug controversy is not something that will be a problem solved in this decade, or even this century. There have always been and will always be individuals who use chemical substances to alter their consciousness. What may change, however, are the attitudes people have about their own drug usage and the approach society as a whole will take toward drugs and those who use them.

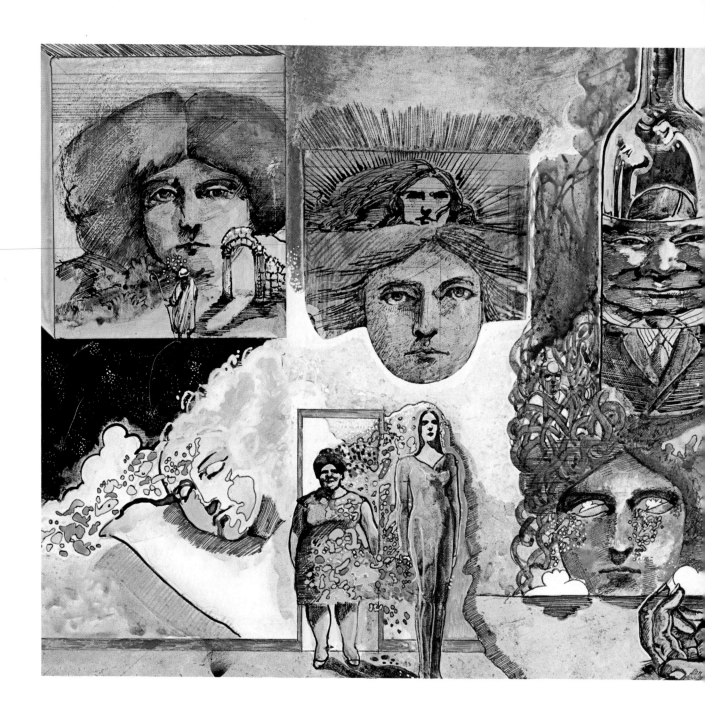

118

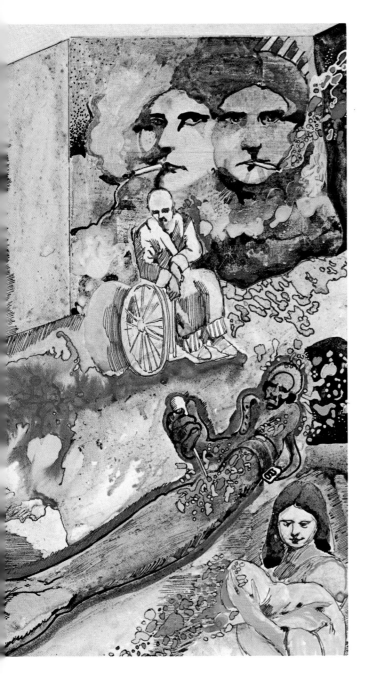

6 Throughout history, man has not been satisfied with himself or with the world as he has found it. He has tried to improve or embellish things, to dress them up, or to build his own images of the world through work, figurative arts, music, architecture, literature—and chemicals that can alter his perceptions, moods, and actions. For many centuries drugs, some of them used to treat disease and alleviate suffering, also have served for pleasure, escape, relaxation, and to add experience and meaning to man's life. As with their other endeavors, in the area of drug use people often make mistakes and carry a good thing too far, failing to control the destructive components. Drugs and those who abuse them are part of man's continuing reality. The challenge, then, is to develop those understandings and circumstances that will result in more and more constructive uses of these substances while, at the same time, discouraging the destructive uses. Judiciously used, drugs can bring better health by fighting disease, relieving symptoms of mental problems, reducing infant mortality, and increasing life expectancy. Nevertheless, as many drug users have discovered, overreliance on such drugs as alcohol, nicotine, or other mind-altering substances is dangerous, for it can cause, obscure, or complicate real problems.

Many people seek drug cures for problems in all areas of their lives, not just the physiological.

The Role of Drugs in the Good Life

They look to drugs for meaning and escape—"Relief is just a swallow away." But the problem itself will remain, even though the person can now ignore or forget it. People may look to drugs for meaning, emotional or intellectual; but the enhanced appreciation or crystalline understanding of a problem fades away with the effects of the drug and often is replaced by an opposite reaction.

What exactly are these substances that can raise one to the heights of joy or lower one to the depths of despair? How have people used and abused drugs throughout history, in all cultures, in all walks of life? What constitutes drug abuse? Why do some people become abusers of drugs when others do not? These are some of the questions to be discussed in this chapter.

PSYCHOACTIVE DRUGS

The word "drug" refers to any biologically active substance that is foreign to the body and is deliberately introduced to affect its functioning. Thus aspirin, penicillin and other antibiotics, antihistamines, and antacids, as well as the mind-altering or psychoactive drugs, are included in this definition.

Any drug can be harmful to the human body if taken in large enough doses, too often, or in an impure form. Any drug, therefore, by harming the body may eventually affect the mind in some manner or degree. There are drugs, however, whose major effects appear to be *primarily* directed to the mind; on being taken into the body, they can temporarily change a person's perceptions, mood, or behavior. They are the so-called *psychoactive* drugs.

Psychoactive drugs will be the focus of discussion here because they are widely used and abused, most often being consumed for relief from psychological or social problems or for recreation. The psychoactive drugs have been highly publicized, often with widely conflicting reports as to their possible benefits and harmfulness. The more facts one

knows about these substances, the better able he will be to decide what role such drugs should or should not play in his life.

The major drugs in the psychoactive category are alcohol, nicotine, caffeine, barbiturates, tranquilizers, amphetamines, cocaine, marijuana, narcotics (opium, morphine, heroin), LSD and other psychedelics, and antidepressants. Such miscellaneous substances as glue, gasoline, antihistamines, morning glory seeds, nutmeg, and others also have exhibited psychoactive properties. Specific information about the effects and abuses of individual drugs will be provided in Chapter 7. This chapter is devoted to overall observations and commentary about these substances and their usage.

THE HISTORICAL PERSPECTIVE

Psychoactive drugs have played some role in every human culture. *Alcohol* is the oldest known mind-altering substance. Archeological evidence indicates that beer was used as long ago as the Stone Age. By about 2000 B.C. beer was a staple in many cultures. It was used to alter mood and presumably as a source of energy.

Another drug that has enjoyed world-wide popularity is *cannabis*, known to various cultures as marijuana, kif, ganja, maconha, dagga, bhang, charas, or hashish. The Chinese Emperor Shen Nung, who lived about 2700 B.C., described his experiences with cannabis and could have been describing the sensations of many today. He entered a dreamy state of altered consciousness and noticed he had disconnected ideas, vivid hallucinations, reverie, and depression. Cannabis also has been used for religious and medicinal purposes for thousands of years and still is in India, Pakistan, and other countries. As late as 1937 the U.S. Pharmacopoeia still listed it for relief of pain or discomfort in various ailments. The drug did not become popular in the West as a mind-altering agent until

Figure 6.1 Many different psychoactive drugs are part of the daily routine of most Americans.

about the middle of the nineteenth century, when some French and American writers and artists began using it.

Opium was used by the ancient Greeks and Romans. Traders probably introduced the opium poppy to China and Persia about A.D. 900 and to India in the early 1500s. It became an important crop in India, and a great deal of it was exported to China. In fact, the opium trade caused two wars in the nineteenth century between China, who wanted to stop it, and Great Britain (at that time the colonial power ruling India), who wanted continued profits from it. For a long time the use of opium continued to be legal and acceptable in China. In the 1920s it is estimated that 25 percent of the adult population of China and Hong Kong were using it, mainly in moderation for social reasons. Under the present Communist government of mainland China, however, the use of opium has declined dramatically, although in Hong Kong, Thailand, South Vietnam, and Iran both opium and heroin are being heavily used and abused.

Opium began to be used in Western nations during the eighteenth century and was an important staple in the East Indies trade. It was mixed with alcohol and sold as *laudanum*, a popular household remedy. Subsequently the active ingredient, *morphine*, was refined from opium. Morphine, used in caring for the injured in the Civil War, and opium in patent medicines, as well as opium brought into the United States by Chinese immigrants, all contributed to the growth of narcotics addiction in this country. Today a chemical derivative of morphine, *heroin*, is the principal narcotic used for nonmedical purposes, while morphine and Demerol are the most popular in medical practice.

Nicotine, in the form of tobacco, was introduced into Europe by Columbus, Raleigh, and other explorers who witnessed the practice of smoking among various tribes of Indians in the New World. Since then tobacco has become one of the most widely used mind-altering drugs throughout the world.

Caffeine in coffee, tea, chocolate, and cola drinks first became popular in about the fourth century, when Asians adopted tea as a drink. Tea and coffee

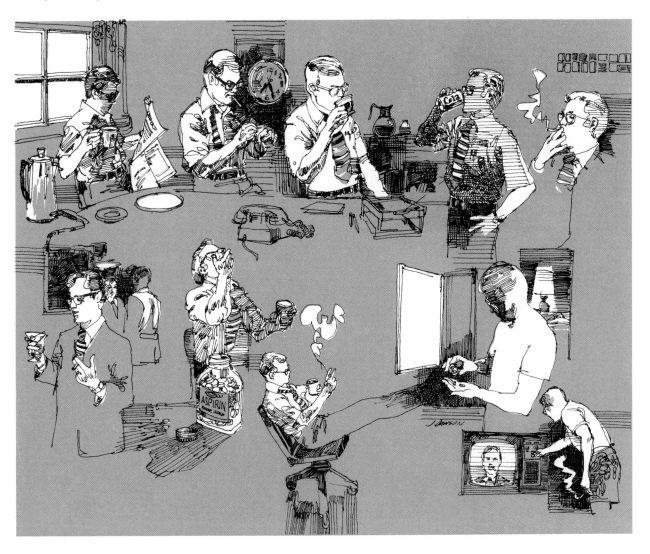

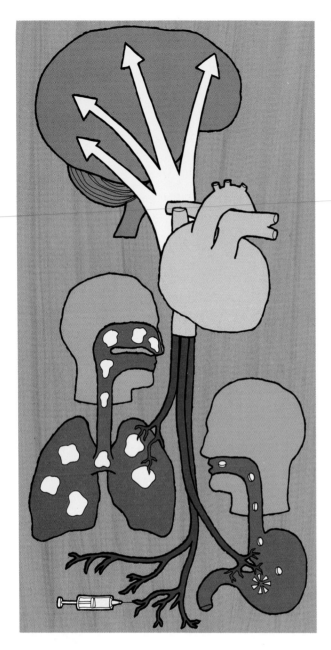

Figure 6.2   Drugs reach the brain by several routes — via the digestive tract if ingested, the respiratory system if inhaled, or the bloodstream directly if injected.

reached Europe in the sixteenth century and were introduced to America shortly thereafter. Coffee is generally acknowledged as the national drink of America, and caffeine is the most extensively used of all mind-altering drugs.

Some other widely used psychoactive substances have had long histories. Cocaine, for example, dates back to the Incas, who used it in religious ceremonies. Other drugs, such as the amphetamines, barbiturates, tranquilizers, and so on, have been chemically synthesized only in the last century, originally for medical purposes.

DRUG ABUSE

Any drug can be used occasionally, and only some use involves regularity, let alone abuse. Some drug experts make a distinction between misuse and abuse. To *misuse* a drug is to use it in amounts or ways that are not medicinally valid. Drug misuse can therefore apply to a wide spectrum of substances, ranging from agents with profound effects on the brain to caffeine, laxatives, headache remedies, antibiotics, and vitamins. A common cause of drug misuse in the United States is the consumption of overadvertised drugs. However, the concept of misuse would include all use of alcohol and nicotine — in fact all nonmedical use of drugs — so it is a vague and far less helpful term than abuse.

Drug *abuse* can be a confusing term because two distinct concepts enter into its definition. From a *medical* standpoint, to abuse a drug is to use it to an extent that produces definite impairment of social, psychological, or physiological functioning of the taker. There are a variety of drugs that can be thus abused, including tobacco, barbiturates, amphetamines, and narcotics (opium and its derivatives or synthetic equivalents). From a *social* standpoint, drug abuse involves a strong cultural and subjective bias, dependent on whether a society at a particular

Figure 6.3   Drugs and the law. Some drugs, such as marijuana, are illegal even to possess. Others, such as barbiturates or amphetamines, do not incur penalties for possession, but sale of them without a prescription is illegal. Other drugs, such as alcohol, do not cause problems with the law unless the user commits a crime under their influence. Penalties for drug-related "crimes" vary markedly from state to state, as is shown in Appendix B.

point in time or space views the use of a particular drug as acceptable or not. Therefore, what is considered normal use versus pathological abuse by this standpoint varies greatly from drug to drug, from quantity to quantity, from situation to situation, and from culture to culture or even among subcultures of the same society.

Under this social definition, in Western society a chronic alcoholic is regarded as a drug abuser, but it is acceptable for someone to occasionally become drunk—an equally clear-cut case of medically defined drug abuse. The use of barbiturates as medically prescribed sleeping pills is socially sanctioned, but taking the same amount of the same drug to induce euphoria in a social situation is considered abuse. Similarly, using a medically prescribed opiate (such as morphine) to relieve depression or tension rather than for alleviating physical pain is classified as flagrant drug abuse. Most narcotic addiction in America actually is legal medical addiction of persons with terminal cancer or other chronic, severe pain. Few would consider this an abuse.

The period in time or the number of users also may determine what a society would choose to qualify as drug abuse. In the early 1960s the use of LSD was limited to small numbers of intellectuals and research workers in the United States. Perhaps because they heard little about it, the members of American society accepted the use of LSD as a research tool for revealing certain aspects of mental processes. When use of the drug spread from experimentation in the laboratories to widespread underground use among college and high-school students in the mid-1960s, however, use became equated with abuse. Within a short time the manufacture or sale of LSD was not only condemned but became a federal crime and sale or possession a crime in most states.

Another common definition of drug abuse is any *illegal* drug use, which would have to include the most extensively used illegal drugs, alcohol and nicotine, by those under twenty-one or eighteen. To avoid the problems inherent in the social and legal approaches to drug abuse, this book will uti-

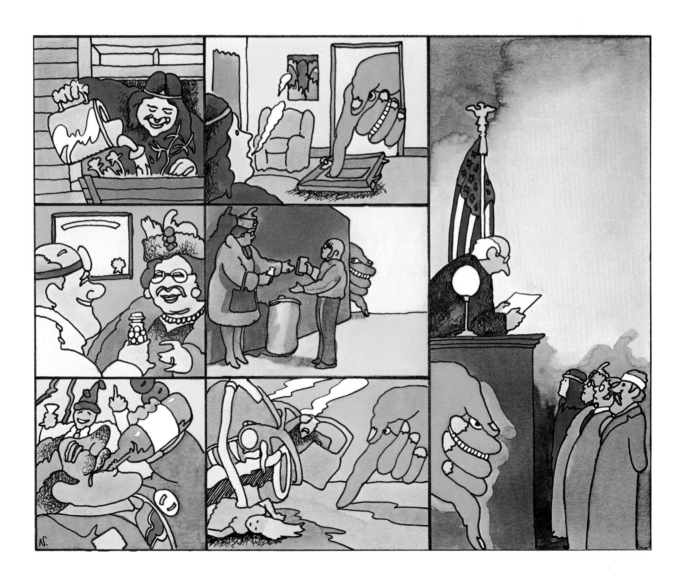

lize an objective definition: *drug abuse is excessive use of any drug that measurably damages health or impairs social or vocational adjustment.*

HAZARDS AND COSTS OF DRUG USE

The risks of drug taking are hard to measure objectively or to balance against potential benefits. Nevertheless, the risks do lend themselves to measurement in a number of ways. Economically, for instance, one can calculate not only the dollar cost of the drugs themselves but that of the legal penalties involved in their use. Likewise, the cost of drug taking can be measured in terms of time—the time lost from school or work while in the drugged state or recovery from it, or the time spent in hospitals, clinics, or jails as the result, for example, of alcohol intoxication or of being apprehended for possession of illegal substances. More basically, the hazards of drugs can be measured in terms of addiction, mental disorder, disability, death, crime, impaired functioning, and so on.

The psychological risks of drug use also can be evaluated subjectively in terms of decreased freedom and autonomy, decreased alertness and self-control, and loss of goals. Death and serious illness also may result from overdosage or individual idiosyncratic reactions to drugs.

Habituation

According to committees of the World Health Organization and the American Medical Association, one of the major hazards in the use of drugs to alter perception, mood, and behavior is that one may reach a state in which he becomes compelled to continue the use of the drug in order to maintain the state of well-being produced by it. At this point the user is said to be *psychologically dependent* on the drug—he is *habituated* to it. When deprived of his drug, the habituated person becomes restless, irritable, uneasy, or anxious. Unlike the physically de-

pendent drug user (who will be discussed later), however, the person whose dependence is only psychological does not suffer a withdrawal illness.

It has been pointed out that under this definition millions of Americans are habituated to their spouses, to television, and to hobbies as well as to a wide variety of drugs, including caffeine, tobacco, alcohol, marijuana, barbiturates, amphetamines, and so on. Whether such psychological dependence is a problem can only be determined on an individual basis.

Tolerance

One characteristic of persistent drug use is that the taker often develops *tolerance* to the drug, which means that the body becomes adapted to it from daily use of large and increasing amounts and requires ever-increasing doses to exhibit the same responses that a smaller dose used to elicit. It is a frequent experience, for example, that half a glass of wine or liquor can make a person drunk the first time he drinks it, whereas he will gracefully guzzle down half a bottle at a later stage of his social-drinking career.

Tolerance also means that one can withstand larger and larger doses without the acutely damaging effects. For example, the long-term heroin or alcohol addict can tolerate dosages that would be fatal to the new or a moderate user. In addition, tolerance imposes a heavy financial and social burden on the user of an expensive drug.

Addiction

The term "addiction" has been used in so many ways that the World Health Organization has recommended that it be discarded and the term "drug dependence" used in its place. The latter term is meant in the sense of *physical dependence*, to be distinguished from the psychological dependence involved in habituation. Physical dependence takes roughly six or more weeks and results from an alteration in the physiological state of the user. Besides developing tolerance, the body now requires continual administration of the drug in order to avoid an extremely painful syndrome known as the withdrawal illness or abstinence syndrome. Tolerance and withdrawal syndrome always accompany physical dependence.

Withdrawal is a temporary physical illness that occurs when someone who is physically dependent on a drug no longer receives it or has a sharp reduction in the amount the body has chosen to toler-

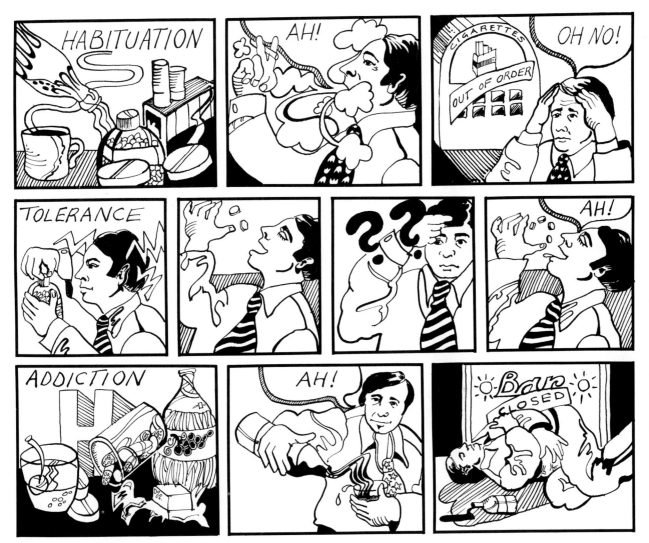

Figure 6.4 With habituation, denial of the drug causes the person to be irritable and nervous. As one develops tolerance to a drug, he finds that he must take larger and larger doses to achieve the desired effect. Tolerance can occur with either habituation or addiction. With addiction, denial of the drug results in a withdrawal illness.

ate. The delirium tremens attacks (DTs) of the alcoholic represent his withdrawal syndrome: Convulsions, hallucination, nausea, vomiting, and tremors (shakes) are some of the principal symptoms. In some cases, death can result.

Addiction is a measure of the degree to which the use of the drug pervades the total life and activity of the user. Fortunately, although almost anything can produce psychological dependence, physical dependence can occur only with depressants: alcohol, opium and related narcotics, and sedatives such as barbiturates. The narcotics carry with them the greatest risk of addiction, followed by alcohol and barbiturates. Thus only some use of drugs involves abuse, and only a segment of abuse involves addiction.

CAUSES OF DRUG USE AND ABUSE

Although the accessibility of a drug, individual curiosity, and even chance all play a role in determining who will and who will not use drugs, other factors, social and psychological, are the most important. Different people will respond differently to their first exposure to the same amount of the same drug, and they also will take different lines of action with respect to their subsequent use of that or other drugs. To account for these individual differences, experts have explored three main areas that might influence use and abuse of various drugs: *psychological* factors, *social* factors, and *pharmacological* factors (the effect of the chemistry of the drug on the physiology of the individual).

There is no agreement among psychiatrists, pharmacologists, and sociologists as to which of these factors is most important in causing drug use. Most drug specialists, for example, believe that social factors are of the greatest significance in producing drug *use* while psychological factors are the major forces causing drug *abuse*.

Psychological Factors

According to drug authority Joel Fort, "The most important determinant of the drug effect is the personality and character structure of the person consuming the drug, including mood, attitude, and expectations. . . . what comes out of the mind-altering drug experience primarily depends upon what you are as a person." The *effect* experienced in taking a drug is in turn one of the many determinants involved in the *motivation* toward continuing to use it.

Motivation in taking drugs can vary from a simple desire for pleasure or euphoria, relaxation, or socialization to a need for escape from reality, boredom, or pain. Some persons, especially with LSD-type drugs, say they take drugs to find meaning or identity, increase their creativity, expand consciousness, or discover new ideas and perceptions under their influence. In one recent survey of ninety-one American and European artists known to have used psychedelic drugs, sixty-four said that the drugs had influenced their art in content, technique, and approach, and only a few said that drugs had not influenced them at all. Some musicians also claim to be more creative or at least more able to perform under the influence of certain mind-altering drugs. Controlled investigations of creativity in individuals under the influence of drugs, however, have failed to substantiate the belief that psychoactive drugs stimulate creative performance. In these studies the subjects frequently reported their own perception of an enhanced performance even after the drug had worn off, but objective examination of their products and performances found no basis for these subjective feelings of improvement. There is little doubt, however, that many drugs are quite effective in producing all sorts of vivid perceptions, and some produce a rush of thoughts, occasionally with new insights.

In trying to determine the more complex, underlying motivational factors that influence a particular individual user to become an abuser, behavioral scientists have come up with a number of theories, none of which is completely satisfactory.

Some researchers feel that people who abuse drugs have an underlying emotional immaturity or inadequacy that seems to be relieved by taking drugs. These investigators contend that the emotional disorder ultimately would become apparent to some degree, whether or not drugs were used. This theory has largely replaced an older school of thought, which held that all abusers (compulsive users of drugs) are morally weak or sinful people who simply overindulge themselves. It does not follow, however, that all people who have emotional disorders would become drug abusers. The general social and psychological factors previously discussed all play a role, as does the availability of alternatives to light or heavy use of drugs. If the individual is so psychologically constituted that he can cope with the stresses and strains, frustrations, and disappointments of living, it is less likely that he will come to depend on drugs in an effort at self-treatment.

It may be that specific types of emotional disturbance determine, at least in part, what drugs will be used. One may conceive that persons suffering from anxiety, depression, or delusions would seek drugs that would most effectively relieve anxiety, or alleviate depression, or suppress delusions. In fact, efforts have been made toward classifying opiate, alcohol, and amphetamine abusers into seemingly distinct psychological categories, or to build psychological "profiles" of an alcoholic or a narcotics addict. If successful, such efforts could at least establish a correlation between certain drugs and the type of emotional disorder of their abusers, irrespective of whether one is responsible for the other or vice versa.

Anxiety, for example, can be viewed as the expression of an unresolved conflict between drives and inhibitions. Alcoholics are said to relieve their conflicts by acting out their drives, such as aggression, dependency, and sexuality. Alcohol, as well as barbiturates, is thought to reduce anxiety by reducing the inhibitions of such drives. Narcotics addicts, on the other hand, may achieve a similar relief from anxiety by reducing the drives instead of the inhibitions. Narcotics addicts are viewed as more passive, avoiding rather than seeking aggressive acts. Interestingly enough, many people who abuse narcotics are often reluctant to turn to alcohol as a tension reliever, even though it is far more socially acceptable.

In summary, the most popular theory today about the psychological causes of drug abuse is that most abusers have psychological disturbances that are both profound and extensive. This theory holds true whether the drug is a narcotic, a barbiturate, alcohol, or amphetamine. Whether these same profound and extensive psychological disturbances existed before the drug abuse and, in fact led directly to it is not yet an established notion. It also is conceivable that compulsive use of drugs exaggerates preexisting emotional disorders so much that an undetectable or clinically insignificant emotional disorder can become pronounced and severe after repeated exposure to a drug. Finally, a possible role of the drug itself in producing rather than merely enhancing emotional disorders is still not being ruled out.

Sociological Factors

Social and cultural factors are obviously significant in promoting drug use and abuse. A growing school of thought contends that one's life style contributes even more extensively than his psychological make-up in determining who will and who will

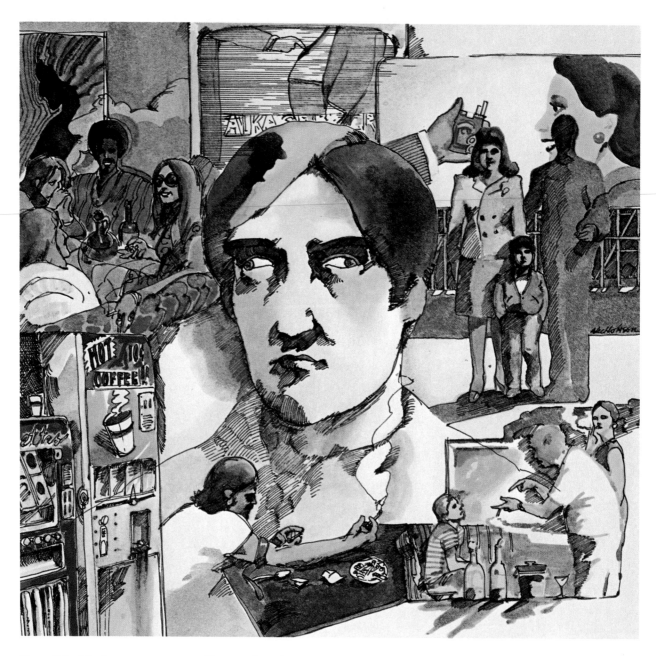

Figure 6.5   Whether or not a person will use or abuse drugs is determined by a combination of psychological, sociological, and pharmacological (physiological) factors that vary from individual to individual.

not take and abuse specific drugs and that life style is by and large the product of cultural environment. More specifically, what has been called the most drug-ridden society in history enters the process of determination in many ways: by providing the exposure to drugs (through advertising and the example of others), by selecting the socio-economic or subcultural group one will tend — or be restricted — to associate with, and by establishing what kind of pressures it exerts on its members.

The fact that people use any drugs at all is culturally determined. Direct observation of other persons and exposure to advertising subtly condition the individual to seek and accept drugs as ways to solve a variety of problems. "Tired? Take ———." "Trouble sleeping? Take ———." "Tense and nervous? Take ———." "Got a cold? Take ———." It really is no surprise, then, that millions of Americans feel that there is a pill, drink, or cigarette for every problem.

In American society, as in others, children get their cues to appropriate behavior by observing, emulating, and modeling themselves after the adults in their world. To a large extent, then, young people who use or abuse drugs are merely doing in their own way what they see the important adults do in their lives at home, in schools, or in films or TV.

Physicians and the *pharmaceutical industry* also must assume a share of the responsibility for drug abuse. Physicians are carefully trained in the tradition of "pharmacological magic." Some of them will tend to prescribe drugs even when they are not required, simply because many patients expect medicine and will feel cheated without it.

Subcultural groups, whatever the parameters by which they are characterized, have often exhibited their own patterns of drug use and abuse. The invasion of drug abuse into new subcultural groups is

another aspect of society's role in promoting drug use and its conversion to abuse — the kind of psychological pressures that a society applies to some, or all, of its members. Many young people today seem to turn to drugs as a means of coping with a world that seems to thwart all their efforts to satisfy their basic needs, from the right to equal opportunities to the development of a sense of self-esteem and identity.

Drugs can be used as a *way to rebel* against what are perceived as the forces of oppression. Those who, at least initially, use drugs as a form of rebellion necessarily choose from among those substances that society has condemned by making them illegal, in the past alcohol and tobacco and more often now, marijuana.

Other persons may use drugs as *a way out* of the "system." In looking for a way out, they sometimes choose drugs that will take them further away from reality and ostensibly closer to their "inner selves." LSD and similar psychedelic drugs have had some popularity in this respect because they induce states of altered perception, thought, or feeling that convey to the individual a sense of "meaningfulness" and "truth."

For many, however, the frustrations from attempting to cope with social pressures are accompanied by attempts at solving one's own problem of personal identity, and drugs can be used as *a way into* specific experiential or social groups. As one drug user said, "Until a couple of months ago I really felt alone, like on the outside of the world looking in. Now baby, I'm in. It's a real groove to be in a gang. Sure we use drugs. It's like glue, beautiful glue to hold us together."

In their desire to belong, many people succumb to *peer-group pressure* — the need to do whatever "everyone else" is doing. In order to be accepted into the group, the individual often is drawn to experimenting with the group-sanctioned drug, whether it be alcohol, tobacco, barbiturates, amphetamines, narcotics, marijuana, diet pills, or glue, even when that substance might ordinarily hold no particular interest to him. Peer-group pressure alone may account for most of the drug experimentation among the young. One of the tragic problems of experimentation is that toxic or even lethal overdoses can result from ignorance, impurities, or careless use of drugs. Furthermore, experimentation with drugs can always lead to abuse. And for those who have not yet learned who or what they are, the need to use the drug over and over again in order to maintain their identity through the group may become even more important than the particular effects of the drug itself.

Many drug authorities believe that these social factors play the major role in drug abuse, blending with emotional problems. Thus, depending on the drug, anyone can get "hooked." Many addicts and other drug abusers are being treated today without psychiatry on the basis of this approach.

Pharmacological Factors

To what extent does the drug itself play a role in the possibility of its misuse or abuse? It is obvious that some substances are more likely to be abused than others. One possible factor is the drug's capacity to produce tolerance and physical dependence. Some of the possible physiological relationships involved were discussed in Chapter 3. It is known, however, that one reason many people continue on a particular drug is simply fear of the withdrawal symptoms they will experience if they quit. One researcher has advanced the theory that the addict's craving for his drug can be traced to the relief it gives from withdrawal distress, not to psychological or sociological factors. Another researcher has postulated that physical dependency becomes a basic biological drive, replacing sexual or aggressive impulses with which the individual may have been unable to cope.

But the pharmacological properties must be seen as only secondary in mind-altering drug responses. Although no specific genetic or constitutional basis has been found to distinguish the potential drug abuser from the nonabuser, many people would eagerly seize upon a physical explanation in order to avoid looking within themselves or their society for an answer.

Interaction of Factors

There is agreement among drug experts that there is no single reason for a person to begin using drugs, no single pattern of abuse, and no single inevitable outcome. In short, drug abusers are a heterogeneous group, all susceptible to many factors that are responsible not only for sustained drug use but also for relapses. A variety of psychological and social factors may interact—in certain circumstances one set of factors may predominate, in other circumstances an alternate set of factors may be the main one. These factors may be important not only in initiating the drug abuse but also in preventing continuing abstinence from the drug. A person desperately trying to stop using drugs may induce tensions in other family members as a result of changes in his behavior and may eventually revert to drug use again just to restore the "family balance" developed during the previous drug use.

Cultural attitudes about narcotics addicts, alcoholics, and drug abuse in general further increase the difficulties. General rejection as a "freak," "junkie," "fiend," or "head"; recrimination; and the absence of alternatives may create pressures so great that the drug abuser may find it easier to return to his old bar or his drug-taking friends where he is accepted, the use of the drug is accepted, and the drug is available. His "cure" would then be over, at least for the moment.

BEYOND DRUGS

Those who are concerned about the use or abuse of psychoactive drugs may, by education, by personal example, and by providing alternatives, be able more and more successfully to move individuals beyond drugs. But, most important of all, they should direct their efforts to eliminate in rational and human ways the psychological and social pressures that are at the base of drug use and abuse.

Certainly racial discrimination, poverty, and social injustices create an atmosphere conducive to drug use as a method of escape. Among middle-class youth, boredom and alienation may lead one to find drugs attractive in a society that has institutionalized their uses. But as anyone who has ever gotten bored with drugs or "outgrown" them

knows, there are many other pleasures that can equal or surpass the satisfactions that drugs may give: self-actualization and personal accomplishment, giving and receiving affection, the arts in their many forms, learning, nature, or contributing to constructive social change, for instance. Dependence on drugs draws individuals into themselves and limits their participation in society, thereby reducing their opportunity to bring about changes that are necessary to progress.

Until a society is prepared to provide all its citizens with the opportunity to satisfy the important human needs without having to resort to social, recreational, or escapist drug use, it must be ready to accept widespread drug use and expect destructive drug abuse. American society has not yet matured to the point of understanding the real drug problems, the human problems that underlie them, or the complex solutions that would have to be applied to move beyond drugs.

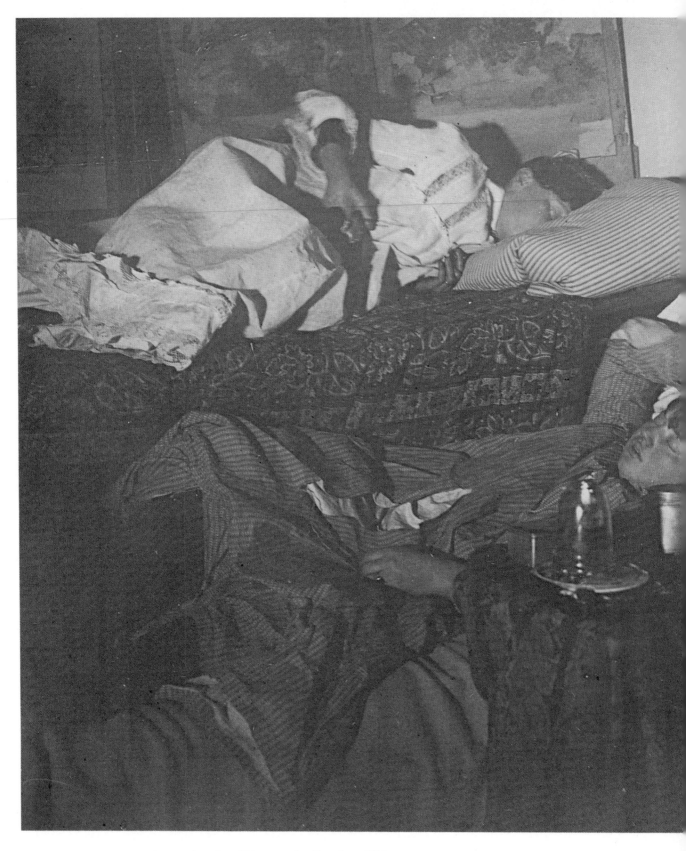

Figure 7.1   A white woman in an opium den, Chinatown, San Francisco, 1892.

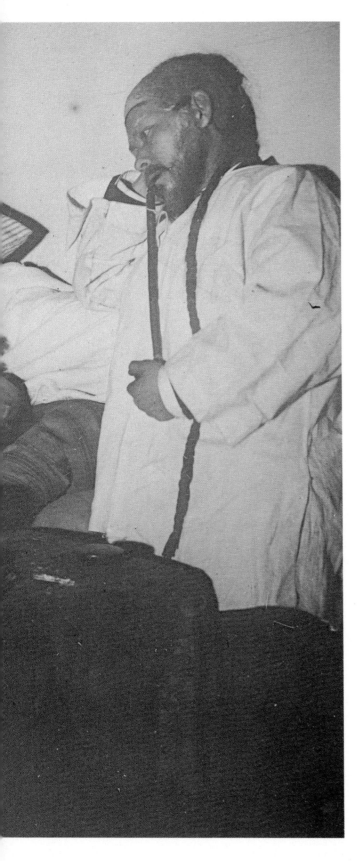

7 Psychoactive substances generate a number of opinions; there are those people who praise them to the skies, and others who condemn them completely. A coed from a major Midwestern university said she took heroin because "it's the greatest high ever." But an underground newspaper in California reported what heroin addicts look like: "You see the faces. Strung out people. People wasting away, dying before your eyes." The ancient Chinese debated as to whether cannabis (marijuana) was a "giver of delight" or "liberator of sin."

People do not usually heed other people's recommendations and opinions, however, and they probably do not pay enough attention to out-of-context or moralistic warnings. What they need are facts about the nature and effects of the most commonly used psychoactive drugs.

The majority of the commonly used psychoactive drugs can be divided into six major categories: (1) depressants (sedative-hypnotics and opiates), (2) stimulants, (3) psychedelic-hallucinogens, (4) cannabis (marijuana), (5) tranquilizers, and (6) antidepressants. Figure 7.2 contains comparative information on the effects, dosage, use, abuse, and other aspects of these major substances used for mind and mood alteration.

Common Drugs of Misuse and Abuse

Name of Drug or Chemical	Slang Names	Usual Single Adult Dose	Duration of Action (hours)	Method of Taking	Legitimate Medical Uses (present and projected)
Sedatives	Downers		4	Swallowing pills or capsules	Treatment of insomnia and tension; induction of anesthesia
Barbiturates	Barbs	50–100 mg.			
Amytal	Blue devils				
Nembutal	Yellow jackets, dolls				
Seconal	Red devils				
Phenobarbital	Phennies				
Doriden (glutethimide)	Goofers	500 mg.			
Chloral hydrate		500 mg.			
Miltown, Equanil (meprobamate)		400 mg.			
Alcohol	Booze, hooch, juice	1½ oz. gin or whiskey, 12 oz. beer	2–4	Swallowing liquid	Rare; sometimes used as a sedative (for tension)
Whiskey, gin, beer, wine					
Narcotics (opiates, analgesics)					Treatment of severe pain, diarrhea, and cough
Opium	Op	10–12 "pipes" (Asia)	4	Smoking (inhalation)	
Heroin	Horse, H, smack, junk	Variable—bag or paper with 5–10% heroin		Injecting in muscle or vein	
Morphine		15 mg.			
Codeine		30 mg.			
Percodan		1 tablet			
Demerol		50–100 mg.			
Methadone	Dolly				
Cough syrup (Cheracol, Hycodan, etc.)		2–4 oz. (for euphoria)		Swallowing	
Stimulants	Uppers				Treatment of obesity, narcolepsy, fatigue, depression
Amphetamines	Pep pills	2.5–5.0 mg.	4	Swallowing pills or capsules or injecting in veins	
Benzedrine	Bennies, cartwheels				
Methedrine	Crystal, speed, meth				
Dexedrine	Dexies				
Cocaine	Coke, snow	Variable		Sniffing or injecting	Anesthesia of the eye and throat
Preludin					
Caffeine	Java		2–4		Mild stimulant; treatment of some forms of coma
Coffee, tea, Coca-Cola		1–2 cups or 1 bottle		Swallowing liquid	
No-Doz, APC		5 mg.		Swallowing pills	

Source: Adapted from Joel Fort. *The Pleasure Seekers: The Drug Crisis, Youth and Society.* Indianapolis: Bobbs-Merrill, 1969.

Figure 7.2 Comparison chart of major substances used for mind alteration.

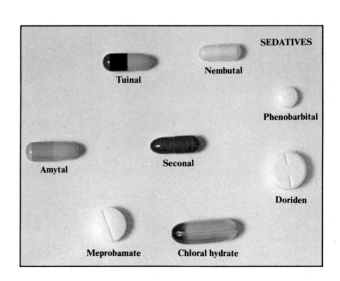

Potential for Psychological Dependence (habituation)	Tolerance Potential	Potential for Physical Dependence (addiction)	Overall Abuse and Toxicity Potential*	Usual Short-Term Effects (psychological, pharmacological, social)**	Usual Long-Term Effects (psychological, pharmacological, social)
High	Yes	Yes	High	CNS depressants; sleep induction; relaxation (sedation); sometimes euphoria; drowsiness; impaired judgment, reaction time, coordination, and emotional control; relief of anxiety-tension; muscle relaxation	Irritability, weight loss, addiction with severe withdrawal illness (like DTs); habituation, addiction
High	Yes	Yes	High	CNS depressant; relaxation (sedation); sometimes euphoria; drowsiness; impaired judgment, reaction time, coordination, and emotional control; frequent aggressive behavior	Diversion of energy and money from more creative and productive pursuits; habituation; possible obesity with chronic excessive use; irreversible damage to brain and liver, addiction with severe withdrawal illness (DTs), possible death
High	Yes	Yes	High	CNS depressants; sedation, euphoria, relief of pain, impaired intellectual functioning and coordination	Constipation, loss of appetite and weight, temporary impotency or sterility; habituation, addiction with unpleasant and painful withdrawal illness
High	Yes	No	High	CNS stimulants; increased alertness, reduction of fatigue, loss of appetite, insomnia, often euphoria	Restlessness, irritability, weight loss, toxic psychosis (mainly paranoid); habituation
Moderate	Yes	No	Minimal	CNS stimulant; increased alertness; reduction of fatigue	Sometimes insomnia, restlessness, or gastric irritation; habituation

*Excessive, often compulsive use of a drug to an extent that it damages an individual's health or social or vocational adjustment, or is otherwise specifically harmful to society.

**Always to be considered in evaluating the effects of these drugs is the amount consumed, purity, frequency, time interval since ingestion, food in the stomach, combinations with other drugs, and, most importantly, the personality or character of the individual taking it and the setting or context in which it is taken. The determinations made in this chart are based upon evidence with human use of these drugs rather than upon isolated, artificial-experimental situations or animal research.

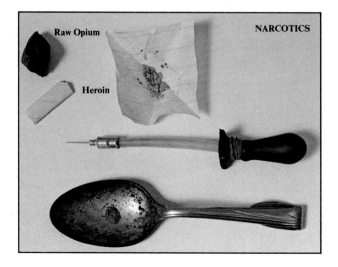

Raw Opium Heroin NARCOTICS

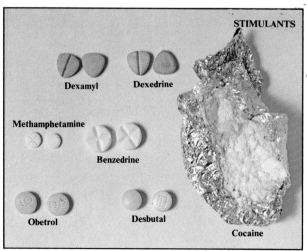

STIMULANTS

Dexamyl Dexedrine Methamphetamine Benzedrine Obetrol Desbutal Cocaine

Name of Drug or Chemical	Slang Names	Usual Single Adult Dose	Duration of Action (hours)	Method of Taking	Legitimate Medical Uses (present and projected)
Nicotine (and coal tar) Cigarettes, cigars	Fag	1 cigarette	1 – 2	Smoking (inhalation)	None (used as an insecticide)
Hallucinogens LSD Psilocybin STP DMT Mescaline (peyote)	Acid, sugar Mushrooms Cactus	150 micrograms 25 mg. 5 mg. 5 mg. 350 mg.	10 – 12 6 – 8 12 – 14	Swallowing liquid, capsule, pill (or sugar cube) Smoking Chewing plant	Experimental study of mind and brain function; enhancement of creativity and problem solving; treatment of alcoholism, mental illness, and the dying person
Cannabis (marijuana) Hashish	Pot, grass, tea, weed, stuff, hash, joint, reefer	Variable – 1 cigarette or pipe or 1 drink or cake (India)	1	Smoking (inhalation) Swallowing	Treatment of depression, tension, loss of appetite, and high blood pressure
Tranquilizers Librium (chlordiazepoxide) Phenothiazines Thorazine Compazine Stelazine Reserpine (rauwolfia)		5 – 10 mg. 10 – 25 mg. 10 mg. 2 mg. 1 mg.	4 – 6	Swallowing pills or capsules	Treatment of anxiety, tension, alcoholism, neurosis, psychosis, psychosomatic disorders, and vomiting
Antidepressants Ritalin Dibenzapines (Tofranil, Elavil) MAO inhibitors (Nardil, Parnate)		10 mg. 25 mg., 10 mg. 15 mg., 10 mg.	4 – 6	Swallowing pills or capsules	Treatment of moderate to severe depression
Miscellaneous Glue, gasoline, and solvents Amyl nitrite Antihistamines Nutmeg Nonprescription "sedatives" (Compoz) Nitrous oxide		Variable 1 – 2 ampules 25 – 50 mg. Variable	2	Inhalation Swallowing	None except for antihistamines used for allergy, amyl nitrite for some episodes of fainting, and nitrous oxide for anesthesia

Source: Adapted from Joel Fort, *The Pleasure Seekers: The Drug Crisis, Youth and Society*. Indianapolis: Bobbs-Merrill, 1969.

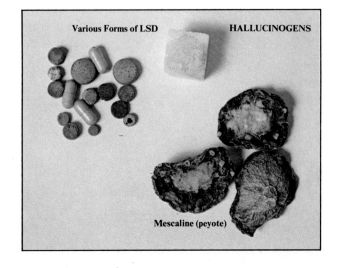

Various Forms of LSD   HALLUCINOGENS

Mescaline (peyote)

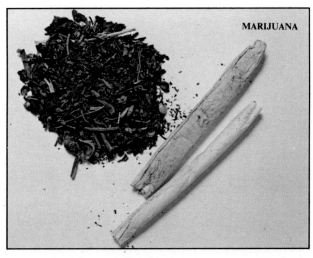

MARIJUANA

Potential for Psychological Dependence (habituation)	Tolerance Potential	Potential for Physical Dependence (addiction)	Overall Abuse and Toxicity Potential*	Usual Short-Term Effects (psychological, pharmacological, social)**	Usual Long-Term Effects (psychological, pharmacological, social)
High	Yes	No	High	CNS stimulant; relaxation (or distraction)	Lung (and other) cancer, heart and blood-vessel disease, cough, etc.; habituation; diversion of energy and money; air pollution; fire
Minimal	Yes (rare)	No	Moderate	Production of visual imagery, increased sensory awareness, anxiety, nausea, impaired coordination; sometimes consciousness-expansion	Usually none; sometimes precipitates or intensifies an already existing psychosis; more commonly can produce a panic reaction
Moderate	No	No	Minimal to Moderate	Relaxation, euphoria, increased appetite, some alteration of time perception, possible impairment of judgment and coordination	Usually none; habituation; occasional acute panic reactions
Minimal	No	No	Minimal	Selective CNS depressants; relaxation, relief of anxiety-tension; suppression of hallucinations or delusions; improved functioning	Sometimes drowsiness, dryness of mouth, blurring of vision, skin rash, tremor; occasionally jaundice, agranulocytosis, or death
Minimal	No	No	Minimal	Relief of depression (elevation of mood), stimulation	Basically the same as Tranquilizers, above
Minimal to Moderate	Not known	No	Moderate to High	When used for mind alteration, generally produces a "high" (euphoria) with impaired coordination and judgment	Variable—some of the substances can seriously damage the liver or kidney and some produce hallucinations

*Excessive, often compulsive use of a drug to an extent that it damages an individual's health or social or vocational adjustment, or is otherwise specifically harmful to society.

**Always to be considered in evaluating the effects of these drugs is the amount consumed, purity, frequency, time interval since ingestion, food in the stomach, combinations with other drugs, and, most importantly, the personality or character of the individual taking it and the setting or context in which it is taken. The determinations made in this chart are based upon evidence with human use of these drugs rather than upon isolated, artificial-experimental situations or animal research.

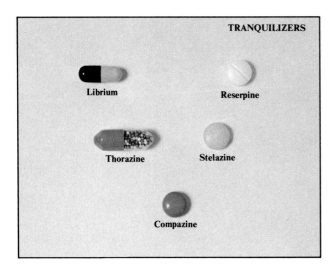

TRANQUILIZERS

Librium

Reserpine

Thorazine

Stelazine

Compazine

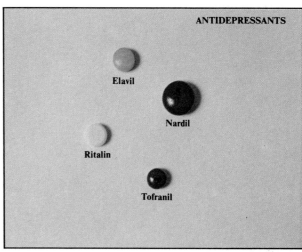

ANTIDEPRESSANTS

Elavil

Nardil

Ritalin

Tofranil

DEPRESSANTS

Depressants slow down or reduce the activity of the central nervous system, particularly the brain. Among the most common central-nervous-system depressants are alcohol; sedative-hypnotics such as barbiturates, chloral hydrate, paraldehyde, Doriden, and meprobamate; the opiates, including heroin, morphine, codeine, Demerol (meperidine), methadone, and opium; volatile chemicals like gasoline or toluene (glue); and general anesthetic agents such as ether or nitrous oxide (laughing gas). In small doses they produce sedation or sleep, in larger doses they can produce coma and death.

Alcohol, the most widely used of all central-nervous-system depressants, will be discussed separately in Chapter 8, but throughout this chapter the reader should be fully aware that alcohol, too, is a drug and is one of the most widely used and abused mind-altering substances.

Sedative-Hypnotics

Next to alcohol, the most widely used group of depressants are the *barbiturates*, which are synthetic drugs in the sedative-hypnotic class. In the United States pentobarbital (Nembutal), secobarbital (seconal), phenobarbital, and amobarbital (Amytal) are the most commonly used and abused barbiturates. These drugs are similar chemically and pharmacologically but differ in speed of onset and duration of action.

A number of nonbarbiturate sedative-hypnotics affect the central nervous system in much the same way as barbiturates or alcohol, even though they have different chemical structures. Chloral hydrate, paraldehyde, thalidomide, Doriden, and meprobamate (popularly known as Equanil or Miltown) are the best-known drugs in this group. Most have come into widespread use only in the last decade. In general these other sedative-hypnotics have much the same side effects, disadvantages, and dangers as the barbiturates but have fewer advantages to offset their greater expense.

EFFECTS The behavioral effects of sedative-hypnotics are quite similar to those of alcohol and include variable amounts of anxiety reduction, changes in mood, slurring of speech, muscular uncoordination, and eventual drowsiness or sleep. As with alcohol, there is great variation in the amount of impairment of cognitive and motor functioning, depending on the task and the individual. Low doses rapidly produce drowsiness in most people. When these drugs are deliberately taken for altering awareness or for social reasons, the individual can avoid some of the sedation and keep awake despite heavy doses, particularly as tolerance develops.

The barbiturates and other sedative-hypnotics are widely used for such medical purposes as the treatment of insomnia, control of epileptic seizures, and daytime sedation. They also are used in combination with such other drugs as stimulants and analgesics (pain killers) to balance or potentiate their physical effects.

Sedative-hypnotics are usually swallowed but may be injected (using injections prepared pharmaceutically). Most barbiturates have a sedative (relaxing) effect when taken in doses of about 50 milligrams several times a day, and they have a hypnotic (sleep-inducing) effect at doses of 100 milligrams or more. Most nonbarbiturate sedative-hypnotics require comparable dosages to achieve the same effects.

ABUSE Although accurate figures are hard to come by, it is estimated that abuse of sedative-hypnotics exceeds that of opiates. Common aspects of such abuse are habituation, tolerance, and addiction, leading to impaired health and social maladjustment.

The patterns of sedative-hypnotics abuse range from infrequent sprees aimed at gross intoxication to prolonged, compulsive daily use of large quantities accompanied by a preoccupation with securing and maintaining adequate supplies. The original contact with the drug is usually either through prescription or through an illicit drug subculture. In the medical patient, abuse may develop gradually, beginning with prolonged use for insomnia and progressing through increased nightly doses topped with a few capsules at stressful times during the day. Eventually the drug may become a major focus of the user's life.

If the user keeps his daily barbiturate consumption at or below 400 milligrams, he probably will not become physically addicted but may suffer from a variety of side effects including drowsiness, hangovers, nausea, dizziness, and headaches.

All sedative-hypnotics, including alcohol, can lead to the classical physical addictive syndrome that includes tolerance and the suffering of withdrawal symptoms if the drug is removed. Daily heavy use of sedative-hypnotics amounting to 500 milligrams or more of barbiturates or equivalent doses of the others usually produces addiction. Tolerance of up to fifteen times the usual sedative dose can rapidly develop.

Barbiturate or alcohol addicts who are deprived of their drug undergo acute withdrawal symptoms, more severe than those associated with opiates. The symptoms begin with nervousness, trembling, and weakness and if untreated develop into generalized epileptic-type seizures with loss of consciousness and a toxic psychosis with delusions and hallucinations. The most severe symptoms of untreated withdrawal last about four days and can be fatal.

Like the severe alcoholic, the barbiturate abuser usually cannot function adequately in his daily activities, often becomes mentally confused, and frequently is obstinate, irritable, and abusive. This behavior is in marked contrast to that of the opiate addict, who usually remains passive and able to function moderately well.

As a means for self-destructive behavior, barbiturates and such other sedatives as meprobamate, chloral hydrate, and Doriden clearly pose a major health problem. The high incidence of addiction, suicides, and accidental deaths attributable to the improper use of barbiturates is a matter that should be of great concern to the medical profession and the public. It is estimated that barbiturates account for 20 percent of acute poisoning cases admitted to general hospitals and for 6 percent of suicides and 18 percent of accidental deaths – figures exceeded by no other poison.

Barbiturate overdose currently is the most frequent method of suicide among American women and accounts for more than 3,000 known deaths a year. In addition, many temporarily disabling illnesses are due to ingestion of less than lethal doses. Moreover, many accidental deaths result from the combined use of barbiturates and alcohol, neither of which would have proved fatal by itself. Both drugs have depressant effects on the brain; they have an additive effect and halt breathing as they progressively depress CNS functioning.

Opiates (Narcotics)

Heroin, morphine, codeine, and opium are all known as the opiate alkaloids. These drugs and Demerol, methadone, and others are usually classified under the term *narcotics* and are widely used both medically and illicitly. Most of the opiates can be administered in a variety of ways: heroin is commonly injected or sniffed, morphine is taken intravenously, and opium is smoked or swallowed.

Opium is a juice derived from the opium poppy. Its active ingredients are *morphine* and *codeine*. Other narcotics are derivatives of these ingredients or are artificially synthesized drugs. Morphine is the primary ingredient of opium and is most widely used for medical purposes. Although *heroin* ("horse," "H") is derived from morphine, it is barred from medical use in the United States and is the most popular of illicitly used opiates. On a weight basis, pure heroin is about two and one-half times more potent than morphine, although street heroin averages only 3 to 5 percent pure.

The opiates are primarily central-nervous-system depressants and have a high potential for habituation, tolerance, and addiction. The usual starting dose of heroin is 3 milligrams, but tolerance can increase the user's needs within several months to doses of 1,000 milligrams. Thus heroin addiction can become a very expensive habit, costing the user 50 to 100 dollars or more a day.

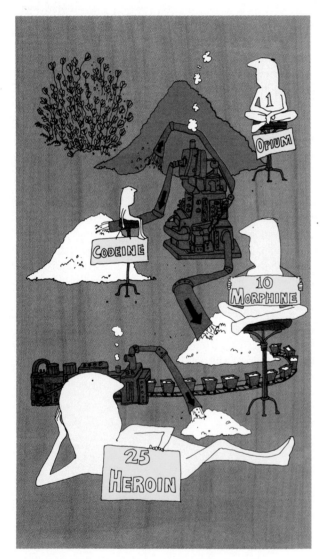

Figure 7.3 The opium poppy and its derivatives. Codeine and opium are refined from the poppy. Codeine is a very mild narcotic. Morphine is refined from opium and is about ten times more potent. Heroin is refined from morphine and is about two and one-half times as potent as morphine. The quality of the narcotics purchased from pushers in the United States is about 10 percent pure.

EFFECTS The initial effects of the opiates are relief of tension and anxiety, decrease in physical drive, drowsiness, and analgesia. Some users experience a sense of well-being and euphoria, but others, particularly if they are not anxious or in pain, experience distinct unpleasantness. Therapeutically, the opiates are effective in reducing pain, depressing respiration, sedating, controlling diarrhea, and suppressing coughs. The exact biochemical mechanisms by which the opiates produce these effects are not known.

ABUSE The history of opiates illustrates some of the the complexities of drug abuse. Opiate ingestion for medical and social purposes was prevalent in China for centuries with no discernible addiction problems. After the Portuguese introduced tobacco smoking into China, however, a variety of psychoactive substances, including opiates, were experimented with utilizing this more efficient mode of administration. The more potent effects of smoking opium became apparent, and subsequently it appears that opium use and addiction became more widespread in eighteenth-century China.

When morphine and the hypodermic needle were introduced in the 1850s, this more potent opiate and still more efficient method of administration were heralded as an effective treatment regimen for opium addiction. Only with time was the even greater addiction liability of morphine recognized. Similarly, at the turn of the century heroin was expected to be the "heroic" cure for morphine addiction and, so named, was introduced. Again, there was a lag before heroin's extreme addictive potential was acknowledged.

The chronic use of opiates often leads to the classical addiction syndrome. The typical abuser is characterized by constricted pupils, skin rashes, nausea, vomiting, dizziness, and constipation. With larger single doses, depressed respiration is pro-

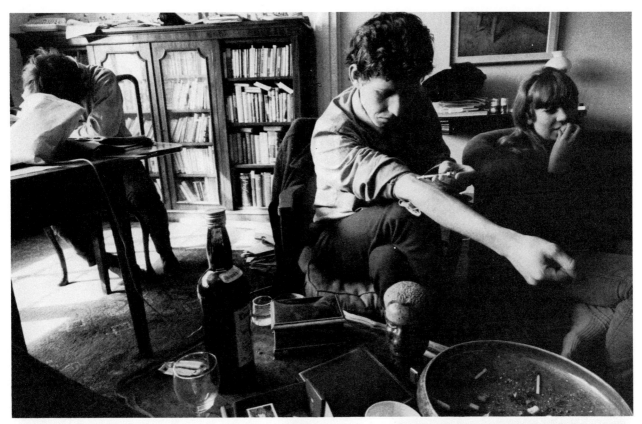

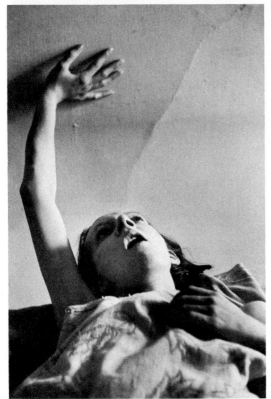

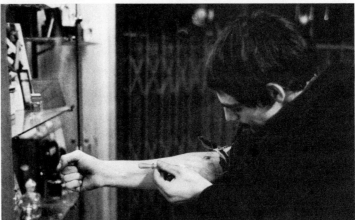

Figure 7.4   Heroin use. (*top*) In a drug treatment center in London, one young addict undergoing gradual withdrawal of the drug concentrates on mainlining his allotted dose. (*left*) A young woman undergoing withdrawal illness. (*above*) A man shooting-up outside a London drugstore where he gets heroin legally with a prescription.

nounced and sleep ensues. Opiates can thus aggravate respiratory ailments such as asthma, sometimes resulting in death.

The opiates have more potential for addiction than alcohol or the sedative-hypnotics; nevertheless, only a minority of those Americans who are exposed to opiates either medically or on the black market continue to use them to the point that they become addicted.

It has been estimated that about 1,000 persons die a year in New York City as the result of accidental overdoses of heroin (and about 1,000 from alcohol overdose). Those that are accidents occur primarily because of variations in strength of black-market drugs and because of fluctuations in the individual's tolerance level. Other deaths linked to opiate addiction involve suicidal or murderous overdose or related problems such as serum hepatitis or bacterial endocarditis.

Short of overdose, there are no known permanent effects on the body's organs that result from opiate abuse. The user can, however, develop serum hepatitis, heart disease, skin abscesses, and other medical disorders from using unsterilized needles, and the addict suffers from constipation, loss of appetite, weight loss, impotence, and sterility, all reversible.

The symptoms accompanying withdrawal from morphine or heroin can be excruciating to the addict, although they are less severe than with alcohol or the barbiturates. Such symptoms as running eyes and nose, yawning, and perspiring appear about four to six hours after the last dose. As these symptoms increase in intensity, weakness, depression, nausea, and vomiting also occur. Heart rate and blood pressure increase. The addict suffers from intestinal pains and diarrhea. His skin breaks into goose pimples, a condition users describe as "cold turkey." His back muscles, bones, and extremities all ache severely. These symptoms reach their peak within twenty-four hours and are mostly over by forty-eight hours. With the extremely diluted heroin that is usually available in the United States, this abstinence syndrome is not nearly as bad as with 50 to 75 percent pure heroin.

STIMULANTS

The most commonly used CNS stimulants are caffeine, nicotine, amphetamines, phenmetrazine (Preludin), and cocaine. Nicotine will be covered primarily in Chapter 9; the discussion here will focus on caffeine, amphetamines, and cocaine as representative of the stimulant group of drugs.

Caffeine

Caffeine is the main active ingredient in coffee, tea, cocoa, cola drinks, and over-the-counter preparations for overcoming fatigue, such as No-Doz. Although caffeine is a potent CNS stimulant, the low doses normally consumed produce only mild side effects. Because the forms in which the drug is marketed are readily available and relatively inexpensive, and because of its relative harmlessness and the strong social support for its use, caffeine is the most widely used of all the psychoactive drugs by Americans of all age groups.

The nicotine in a cigarette is roughly comparable to the amount or effect of caffeine in a cup of coffee. Thus the amount of nicotine normally consumed acts as a mild stimulant. Both caffeine and nicotine rapidly produce tolerance and habituation, but not physical addiction.

A normal dose of caffeine from a single cup of coffee or tea relieves drowsiness and muscle fatigue, stimulates thinking, and promotes more sustained physical and intellectual activity.

Caffeine abuse occurs with overconsumption of the common caffeine-containing beverages (such as six or more cups of coffee daily). Physical effects of excessive caffeine include insomnia, restlessness, irritability, and aggravation of both peptic ulcers and high blood pressure. One can develop both tolerance and habituation to caffeine, although daily moderate use of the drug does not seem to impair functioning in any way.

Amphetamines

The amphetamines are synthetic drugs, chemically resembling the neurotransmitter noradrenalin (see Chapter 3). They include Benzedrine ("bennies"), Methedrine (methamphetamine, "speed"), and Dexedrine ("dexies"). Users call them "uppers." A moderate dose of an amphetamine given to one person is likely to produce some combination of an elevation of mood, a sense of increased energy, decreased appetite (phenmetrazine, or Preludin, has been marketed as a diet pill), irritability, and anxiety. Amphetamines are not physically addicting but they can produce tolerance and habituation.

In low doses amphetamines increase alertness, well-being, and wakefulness and decrease fatigue and appetite. They can also sometimes improve performance in activities requiring extreme physical effort and endurance, such as athletics or military combat, but because they speed heart rate and raise blood pressure, they are dangerous when used for this purpose. Although physical reaction time is shortened and motor coordination is improved, there is no improvement in intellectual function as far as comprehension, problem solving, and judgment are concerned. Nevertheless, if one's intellectual performance is diminished because of fatigue, amphetamines can have a positive effect.

Those who use amphetamines to stay awake while driving are taking a great risk because the drug's effects often wear off abruptly. The user may quickly become drowsy and may even fall asleep. Prolonged use or large doses of amphetamines is nearly always followed by mental depression and fatigue. Side effects can include headaches, dizziness, agitation, confusion, and delirium.

Amphetamines are used much less often than caffeine but are more abused. One nonmedical pattern of use involves ingestion of low oral doses for limited periods of time by students cramming for exams, fatigued executives, military personnel, and truck drivers.

Another type of use involves oral ingestion of average (5 to 10 milligrams daily) doses of amphetamines over long periods of time. This pattern generally is followed by people who are trying to control their weight or who are chronically fatigued and enjoy the wide-awake, alert feeling they get from amphetamines. In a relatively short time, tolerance develops and the dosage must gradually be increased. For some individuals this pattern of use may ultimately lead to paranoid psychosis, manifested by unfounded suspicions, hostility, hallucinations, and delusions.

Intravenous injection of large doses rapidly leads to abuse. An individual may have an injection occasionally, or he may have a *run*. During a run the user injects the drug every few hours for a period of several days, during which he may eat little and remains awake continuously. Immediately after each injection the user experiences a generalized pleasurable feeling, termed a *flash*, or *rush*. He feels invigorated and perhaps euphoric for several hours. When he begins to feel irritable and uneasy he is compelled to take another injection in order to avoid discomfort and to recapture the pleasure of the initial rush. A run ends when the user either runs out of the drug or becomes too disorganized or paranoid to continue. He then sleeps for twelve to eighteen hours or even longer if the run has been unusually long. Upon awakening, most users are lethargic and some are depressed. Taking the drug again relieves the lethargy and depression, and the cycle begins anew.

Although no withdrawal symptoms per se follow amphetamine abuse, there usually is some physical discomfort associated with the abrupt cessation of high-dose amphetamine use, the prolonged sleeplessness, and the irregular eating. Intravenous use

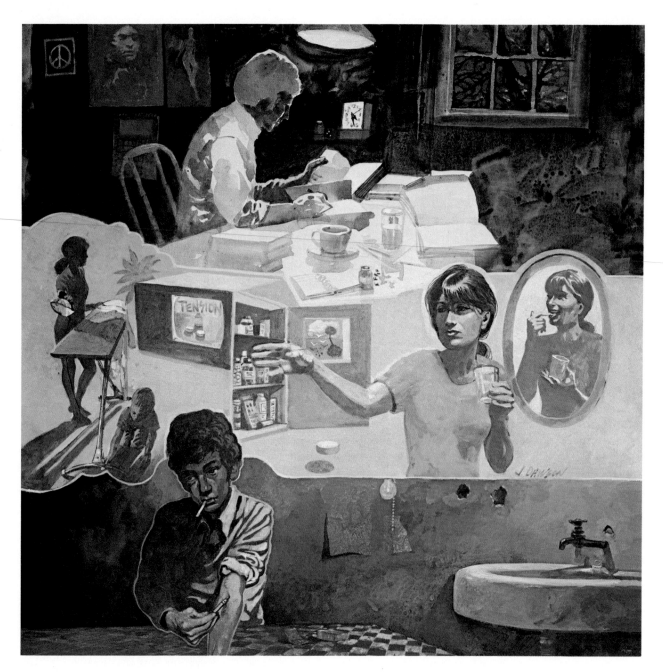

Figure 7.5 Patterns of amphetamine abuse. Three distinct
patterns emerge in comparison of types of abuse, varying
according to the frequency and amounts of drug taken.
Infrequent use of small amounts characterizes the first type.
Daily use of small to medium amounts can be seen in the
second type. Long periods of intravenous use of large
amounts characterize the third type.

may cause fatalities through burst blood vessels, stroke, and so on in addition to the general dangers of needles, such as serum hepatitis, bacterial endocarditis, and most recently, malaria (due to sharing needles with infected Vietnam veterans).

Chronic amphetamine use, though it does not produce physical dependence, does produce other harmful effects in the individual and to others in his life. It can gradually erode personal, social, and work relationships until the user can focus on nothing but procuring and using the drug. This progressive exclusion of formerly meaningful activities closely resembles the classical addiction syndrome of the opiates.

In one respect intravenous amphetamine use can be a stepping stone to other drugs. People who go on a run frequently try a variety of depressants to counteract the discomfort they feel when the run is over. They often find that barbiturates or heroin not only help them come down, but also produce pleasurable effects of their own. With time, heroin use can become more frequent.

Cocaine

Cocaine ("coke") is a drug extracted from the leaves of certain plants, but it also is synthesized in the laboratory, as are all amphetamines. Cocaine has never been extensively used in the United States, primarily because it costs so much, is not readily available, and has strong side effects. The drug has some popularity among street users and middle-class professionals. Cocaine is the most potent of the stimulant drugs, but its effects, uses, and abuses are similar to those of the amphetamines.

The effects of cocaine are much stronger, although shorter in duration, than those of amphetamines. Cocaine is extremely potent in altering mood and is probably the strongest antifatigue agent. Medically it is sometimes used as a local anesthetic because it can block nerve conduction. In order to be effective, cocaine, unlike amphetamines, must be sniffed or injected — oral ingestion is ineffective because the drug is poorly absorbed from the gastrointestinal tract. Prolonged use can perforate the wall between the nostrils, producing a constant nasal congestion in the user that nasal sprays cannot alleviate.

Abuse of cocaine follows a pattern similar to that for amphetamines. Use usually does not begin for medical purposes but specifically for the purpose of getting high. The drug is initially introduced through sniffing it in a powdery form known as "snow," but the habitual user, upon developing tolerance, often switches to intravenous injections, sometimes combined with heroin to produce a "speedball."

Psychological dependence, which can occur with any drug, is more marked with cocaine. Chronic use can result in a general systemic poisoning, characterized by mental deterioration, weight loss, agitation, and paranoia. The most serious cases of cocaine poisoning from excessive doses involve headaches, nausea, vomiting, hallucinations, rapid heartbeat, dilated pupils, chills or fever, irregular respiration, convulsions, coma, and sometimes death (the same results can be produced by large doses of amphetamines taken at one time).

PSYCHEDELIC-HALLUCINOGENS

This category is actually a wastebasket one that contains a variety of drugs also referred to as psychotomimetics, or psychotogenics. Included in this group are lysergic acid diethylamide (LSD-25 or LSD for short), phenylethylamine derivatives (peyote or mescaline), the indole derivatives (psilocybin, DMT), the piperidine drugs (Ditran), phenylcyclidine (Sernyl), and others.

There is no sharp line that separates these drugs from other classes of psychoactive drugs. Under certain conditions or at certain high dosages a variety of other drugs, including alcohol, can induce illusions, hallucinations, delusions, paranoia, and similar alterations of mood and behavior. The feature usually used to distinguish the LSD-type drugs from other classes is their great likelihood of inducing these effects, the intensity of the effects, and the duration of the experience.

Although marked tolerance can develop with frequent use, these drugs cause little compulsive drug-seeking behavior and no physical dependence. Mescaline, LSD, and psilocybin have a cross-tolerance to each other and are generally similar in their effects; therefore, they may exert their effects through a common, yet unknown, mechanism (see Chapter 3). Because LSD is the most well known of the drugs in this category, it will be discussed as a representative example.

LSD Effects

The ingestion of even one-millionth of an ounce of LSD, or "acid," which is odorless, colorless, and tasteless, will produce noticeable effects in most people. An average dose of 150 to 250 micrograms produces slight dizziness, weakness, nausea, dilation of the pupils, and particularly such perceptual alterations as distorted time sense, intense visual experiences, heightened auditory acuity, and *synesthesia*—the blending of two senses so that the person "hears" colors or "sees" sounds. Psychological symptoms include the flooding of consciousness with numerous thoughts in new combinations, rapid changes in mood, a feeling that one's body is distorted, and dissociation of oneself from external reality. These effects usually occur in sequence. Physical changes come first, then the perceptual alterations, and finally the psychic changes, although there is considerable overlap among these three phases.

The sort of experience one will have with LSD, particularly in lower doses, as with other drugs, is determined in large part by the user's own personality, what he expects of the drug, recent events in his life, the setting, and other psychosocial factors. Because many of the effects are so different from one's usual sensations and perceptions, users often find it difficult to describe their experiences in words.

Severe panic reactions ("bummers" or "bad trips") and other untoward effects sometimes occur with this class of drugs. Although the probability of a bad trip is reduced by emotional stability, relaxing surroundings, proper dosage, screening, and a trusted guide, a tranquil trip cannot be guaranteed. LSD users report having hundreds of good trips with pleasurable and ecstatic experiences before inexplicably having a bummer replete with monstrous perceptions and delusions of being trapped forever in the drugged state. These unexplained bummers are more common with high doses and impure drugs. Accidental overdoses occur because the purity of black-market LSD varies widely and the extremely small amounts in each dose require skillful measurement. A person experiencing a bad trip can be treated by placing him in a serene, nonhospital and nonjail setting, providing psychological support, and "talking him down." Thorazine also may be helpful. Treating bummers with drugs, however, must be done with great caution because the person may have thought he was using LSD when in fact an entirely different drug was used.

There is a disturbing incidence of abuses resulting from use of LSD. Acute (short-term) and sometimes prolonged psychotic reactions and "flashback" phenomena occur in both occasional and chronic users. *Flashbacks* are the brief, sudden, unexpected perceptual distortions and bizarre thoughts of an LSD trip that occur after the pharmacological effects of the drug have worn off (perhaps months or years after the last ingestion). In some individuals LSD can precipitate serious

Figure 7.6 Drawings done by a man under the influence of LSD. (a) 20 minutes after first dose: Drug has not taken effect. (b) 85 minutes after first dose, 20 minutes after second dose: The subject sees the model correctly but has difficulty in controlling the wide sweeping movements of his hand. (c) Two and one-half hours after the first dose: Outlines of the model seen normally, but very vividly and in changed colors. The subject states: "I feel as if my consciousness is situated in the part of my body that is now active. (d) Shortly after third drawing: "The outlines of the model are normal but those of my drawing are not. I pull myself together and try again: it's no good. I give up trying and let myself go at the third attempt." (e) Shortly after third and fourth drawings: "I try again and produce this drawing with one flourish." (f) Two and three-fourths hours after first dose: "The perspective of the room has changed, everything is moving . . . everything is interwoven in a network of color . . . The model's face is distorted to a diabolic mask." (g) Four and one-quarter hours: He is in a euphoric mood; intoxication is less marked. The subject attempts to draw a portrait similar to his first one. "If I am not careful, I lose control of my movements." (h) Five and three-quarter hours: "It is probably because my movements are still too unsteady that I am unable to draw as I normally do . . . The intoxication is wearing off, but I can both feel and see it ebbing and flowing about me (now it only reaches to my knees); finally, only an eddying motion remains." (i) Eight hours: The intoxication has now worn off, apart from a few small waves (for example, sudden distortions of faces from time to time). The subject feels bewildered and tired. "I have nothing to say about the last drawing, it is bad and uninteresting."

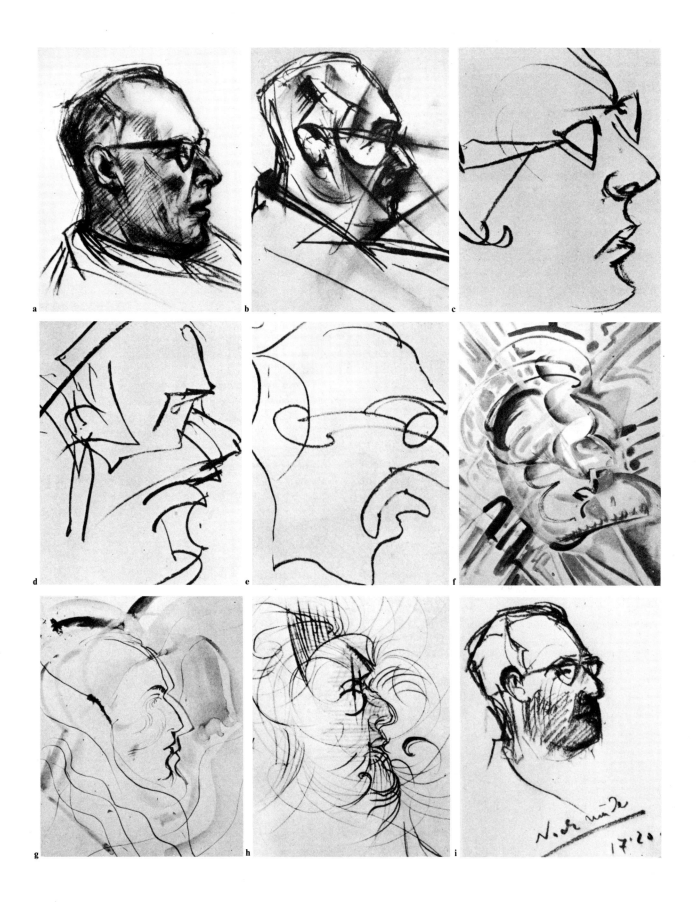

depressions, paranoid behavior, or chronic psychoses. Fatal accidents and suicides have occasionally occurred with the use of LSD. Some studies have implicated LSD as an agent causing chromosomal breakage, an idea discussed in Chapter 11.

Other Hallucinogen-Psychedelics

Although LSD is representative of the effects of the psychotomimetics, the use and effects of similar drugs vary in many ways. Again, it must be emphasized that the effects, especially with low doses, depend to a large extent on nondrug factors such as the expectations, mood, attitudes, and personality of the individual, the setting, and so on.

Mescaline, in the form of peyote buttons from the Mexican cactus, is the ceremonial drug of the (Indian) Native American Church. It also is in vogue with drug users who value "natural" drugs and who shun the synthetic drugs such as LSD and amphetamines as products of technology and hence too much a part of the establishment. Synthetic mescaline has somewhat different effects than the natural type.

Ditran and related drugs have a profound effect on the transmission of impulses within the central nervous system. Accordingly, they produce considerable confusion and disorientation and greater intellectual impairment than most other LSD-type drugs. *Sernyl* differs from the other psychotomimetics by markedly reducing sensory input, thus creating various degrees of sensory deprivation. *Dimethyltryptamine* (DMT) and *diethyltryptamine* (DET) have many characteristics similar to LSD but differ in that their onset is more rapid and their duration of effects is one to four hours. Because of their intense but brief effects, these drugs often go by the name of "the businessman's trip." In contrast, *dimethoxy-methylamphetamine* (DOM or STP) can induce a longer trip than LSD. Similar effects also can be obtained from morning glory seeds, nutmeg, datura plant (jimson weed), and many other botanical products. Most users find these sources unsatisfactory because of such side effects as nausea, vomiting, and diarrhea.

CANNABIS (MARIJUANA)

Marijuana and hashish are the main active drug preparations derived from the hemp plant *Cannabis sativa*. Cannabis is grown around the world, and its components or derivatives are known by various names. *Hashish* is the concentrated resin of the leaves of the cultivated female plants. It is thus more potent than crude marijuana although using smaller amounts of it will produce the same result as larger quantities of less pure forms of cannabis.

The active ingredient in hashish and marijuana belongs to a class of chemicals called the tetrahydrocannabinols (THC). The amount of THC in a given preparation determines the potency of that preparation. THC has recently been produced synthetically, but it is difficult to prepare and is therefore too expensive to be widely available either legally for research or illegally on the black market.

Marijuana does not fit neatly into any of the established drug categories. In average doses (such as the amount inhaled from smoking one or two "joints"), it acts partially as a sedative-hypnotic, somewhat like alcohol, and partially like a stimulant, as well as having some unique properties of its own.

Short-Term Effects

A common effect of moderate doses of marijuana is to alter one's perception of sounds, colors, spatial configurations, and other sensory phenomena. As with most mind-altering drugs, there is wide variability in these perceptual changes, and there are marked differences among individuals in their awareness and interpretation of them. These differences are significantly influenced by the user's expectations of how marijuana will affect him and

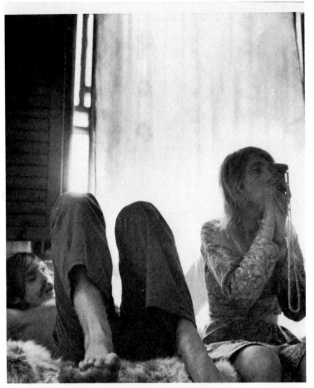

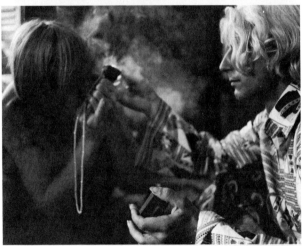

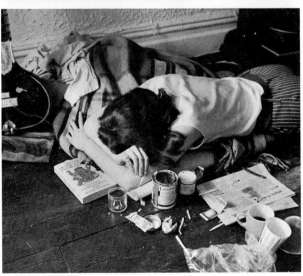

by his previous experience with the drug. The chronic user may get a "high" from low-potency marijuana, whereas the neophyte may feel nothing with the same dosage.

The effects of cannabis preparations on mood and personality are variable, as with other drugs. There may be an initial slight apprehension, then pleasant lassitude interspersed with euphoria. Later, sedative effects take over, and sleep is common. The changes in behavior induced by marijuana may follow a cyclic pattern of waxing and waning rather than a smooth "dose-effect" curve.

The acute physical effects of marijuana are minimal, but include slight increases in heart rate and dilation of blood vessels in the conjunctiva of the eye (creating characteristic reddened eyes). The exact sites and mechanisms of action in the brain are unknown.

With higher doses of THC, as with most psychoactive drugs, the behavioral effects are determined more by the drug properties per se and less by such psychosocial factors as the individual's personality and circumstances. With these higher doses, and occasionally with low doses in particularly susceptible individuals, the changes just described may be markedly exaggerated. Subtle alterations of sensory input become gross distortions, and the user may feel inundated by a myriad of sensory cues from his environment. Extensive disintegration of the thought process may prohibit the individual from thinking clearly. In contrast to LSD-induced bad trips, in which perceptual disorders often predominate, thought disorders, particularly of a paranoid nature, seem to be more frequent with marijuana overdoses.

Such effects lead some users, especially neophytes, to think they are losing control over their minds and becoming "crazy." The user's mood changes from the usual relaxation and tranquility to a state of anxiety and panic.

Figure 7.7 The smoking of pot to many young people has become an enjoyable social activity; for others it is a means of relaxation or escape. There are perhaps as many reasons for using marijuana as there are users.

Long-Term Effects

The long-term effects of cannabis consumption are inadequately understood, but seem to be minimal. This ignorance is partially due to the lack of systematic studies. In addition, as with other drug abuses, it is difficult to devise ways of evaluating other factors that might produce related changes in chronic cannabis users, factors such as poor nutrition and deprived socioeconomic conditions.

Nevertheless, scientists can reasonably predict on the basis of experience with other drugs that long-term heavy use of marijuana will lead some susceptible individuals to a persistent impairment of certain cognitive functions, such as immediate memory, the temporal integration of past and present events with future goals, and sustained attention. Similarly, a few vulnerable long-term excessive users of marijuana are likely to show persistent changes in mood and in their usual sensory abilities, especially regarding time perception. Bronchitis may occur from the smoking process. Only a minority of chronic users will have these mental and physical disorders, none of which has been proved to actually occur in conjunction with marijuana abuse.

Although cannabis is nonaddictive, probably a small percentage of chronic marijuana users will increasingly center their lives around the drug, gradually excluding other activities that were once meaningful and satisfying to them.

TRANQUILIZERS

Like barbiturates, *tranquilizers* reduce excessive excitability in the nervous system and are useful in medical treatment of a variety of symptoms. In addition, however, they suppress anxiety and irritability without making the patient sleepy, thus leaving him alert enough to work and function almost normally. Tranquilizers have specific value in treating psychoses, a property the sedative-hypnotics lack. Furthermore, tranquilizers have minimal potential for habituation, and they are nonaddicting.

Tranquilizers are used in severe emotional illnesses to reduce or eliminate hallucinations and delusions, calm the emotions, and slow motor activity. When given simultaneously with narcotic or hypnotic drugs, they intensify the effects of those compounds. Although tranquilizers do cause the user to feel better and calmer, he does not experience the euphoria associated with many of the other depressant drugs. Tranquilizer users may occasionally suffer side effects ranging from faintness, dermatitis, and discoloration of the skin to hypotension (low blood pressure), allergic jaundice, and epileptic-like seizures.

Although tranquilizers do not cause physical de-

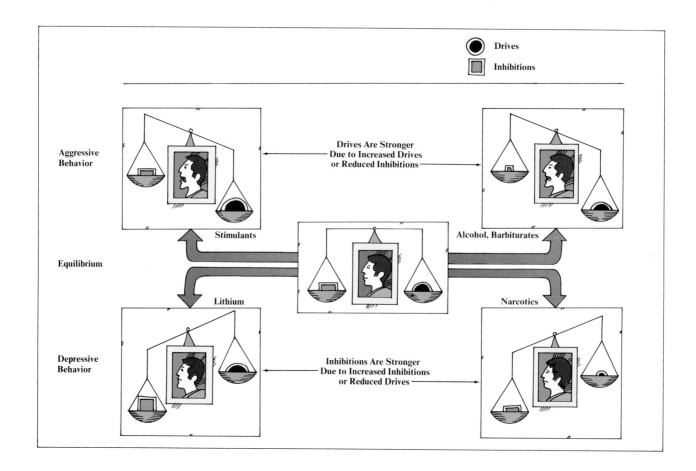

pendence or tolerance, some individuals who use phenothiazine tranquilizers such as Thorazine experience toxic side effects, including skin rash, light sensitivity, muscle rigidity, hepatitis, and general blunting of their emotions. Other harmful side effects can result from use of the tranquilizer *reserpine*, which can cause drowsiness, nausea, diarrhea, depression of fertility and potency, and suicidal depression.

OTHER PSYCHOACTIVE AGENTS

A number of important medical advances recently have been made in developing drugs that directly act on psychological depression. The *antidepressants*, or mood elevators, include the monoamineoxidase (MAO) inhibitors and the tricyclics (imipramine). The MAO inhibitors have a number of dangerous side effects and have been largely replaced by the less toxic tricyclics. In certain individuals, these drugs elevate mood and increase activity and drive when taken for days or weeks (rather than an immediate effect). Although their exact mechanism of action is unknown, they seem to be more effective in treating individuals who demonstrate severe depression unmixed with such other components as anxiety, hostility, and hyperactivity. The more these components are involved, the less effective antidepressants seem to be.

A speculative, and certainly oversimplified, way to attempt interpreting these effects could be to consider the anxiety-generating conflicts between drives and inhibitions, already discussed (in Chapter 6) with respect to alcohol and narcotics. Severe depression, such as is observed in the depressive psychosis, may be conceived as related to abnormally low drives, which could be strengthened by the antidepressant drugs with an overall beneficial ef-

fect (see Figure 7.8). Where abnormally low drives are accompanied by strong inhibitions, raising the drive level could increase their conflict with the existing inhibitions and therefore generate even more anxiety; in these cases, antidepressants would prove to be an ineffective, or even adverse, treatment.

The *lithium salts* are among the newest drugs for the treatment of disorders in mood. Unlike the antidepressants, they are clearly effective in improving the patient with mania who has exaggerated euphoria and excessive self-confidence and tends to be hyperactive. In addition, lithium can be useful in treating manic-depressive disorders in which the individual oscillates between extremes of mania and severe depression.

AN ENDLESS LIST

Within a few years it will probably be necessary to revise this summary of misused and abused psychoactive compounds because many new drugs will have become available. The pharmaceutical industry and the medical profession are attempting to find substances that will do a better job of treating behavior disorders than those on hand today. Perhaps some of the undesirable side effects of the current drugs will be circumvented. Some new substances or new derivatives of older ones may open further areas for therapy.

Almost inevitably, though, some individuals or groups will utilize these drugs for other than medical purposes, so that the wrong use and the overuse of medically active drugs, as well as those not used medically, will still remain a problem. The solution of this problem, like many others fostered by technological advances, lies not in the elimination of the technological advances but in improving the wisdom of both the individual and the society.

Figure 7.8 The mood balance. One theory of how drugs have their effect and of why different people choose different drugs lies in the balance between a person's drives and his inhibitions. Following this theory, those who wish to increase their drives take stimulants while those who wish to release their inhibitions imbibe alcohol, both providing aggressive behavior. Passive or depressive behavior is brought about by increasing inhibitions (lithium) or decreasing drives (narcotics).

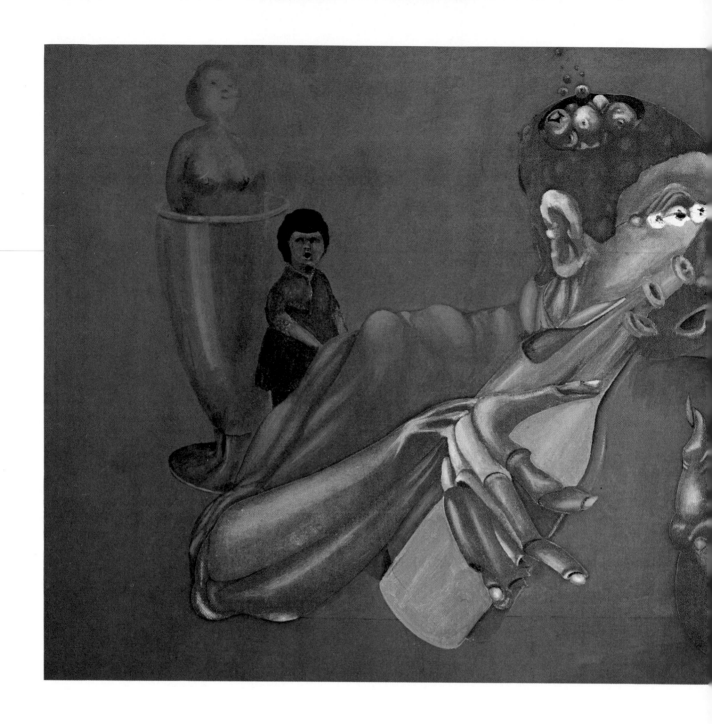

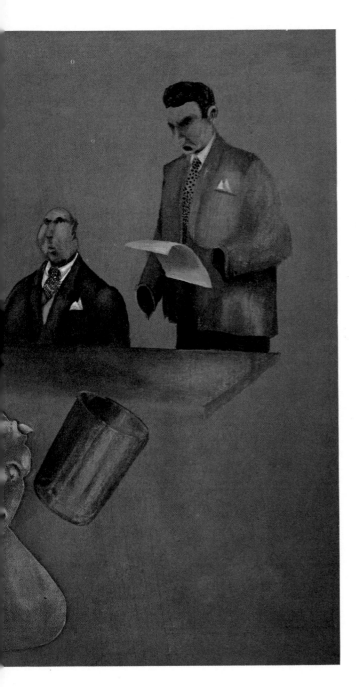

8 Abuse of alcohol is one of the biggest health and social problems in the United States today. It is estimated that there are 9 or 10 million persons whose drinking is associated with serious problems, including about 7 million who are alcoholics. More than 50 percent of the fatal accidents and a high proportion of the injuries occurring on the nation's highways involve drivers or pedestrians who have had too much to drink. Alcohol use often is associated with crime, poverty, and other social problems. Alcohol also contributes to physical illness, mental illness, and family conflicts. Why, under these circumstances, do people drink?

When used in moderation, alcohol can reduce anxiety and tension and bring on a feeling of relaxation and well-being. These effects help explain why alcohol has had an accepted place in so many human societies. Nevertheless, few societies have been able to enjoy the benefits of alcohol without complications that are inherent in the intoxicating properties of alcohol, a drug that can adversely affect any user temporarily and upon which many drinkers become dependent.

What does alcohol do to the human body? What factors influence the variations in human response to the effects of alcohol? How does society affect alcohol consumption, and what consequences does it suffer from alcoholism? Can people be helped to recover from problem drinking or alcoholism? These are a few of the questions that will be examined in this chapter.

SOURCES AND TYPES OF ALCOHOL

Alcohol is the common active ingredient in such varied beverages as wine, beer, hard liquors (gin,

Alcohol Abuse

whiskey, brandy, rum), and cordials. It is prepared from a number of natural products, including fruits, cereals, and grains. Some methods for making it have been known since before the beginnings of recorded history.

The different forms of alcoholic beverage vary greatly in strength as measured by the concentration of alcohol they contain. The most common alcoholic beverages—beers, wines, and distilled spirits—are made by different processes. Beer and ale are derived from various cereals by a brewing process and generally contain from 3 to 6 percent alcohol. Wines are made by fermenting the juice of grapes or other fruits. Table wines that are often served with meals have a natural alcohol content of from 9 to 12 percent. Other varieties, such as sherry, port, and muscatel, are reinforced by the addition of distilled alcohol to bring their alcohol content up to as much as 18 to 22 percent. The strongest alcoholic beverages, such as gin, whiskey, brandy, or rum, are manufactured by distilling brewed or fermented products so that liquids containing from 35 to 50 percent alcohol are recovered. Ounce for ounce, the amount of pure alcohol in most distilled liquors is ten to twelve times greater than that in beer.

The term "proof" indicates the concentration of alcohol in a beverage. Proof can be converted to percent by dividing the proof number in half. Thus, 80-proof whiskey is 40 percent alcohol, and 100-proof whiskey is 50 percent alcohol. Every ounce of 100-proof whiskey, then, contains one-half ounce of pure alcohol.

In order to relate what is known about alcohol's effect on man to the everyday experiences of drinking and to determine what effect a particular drinking episode will have on the behavior of a particular person, several factors must be considered. These factors include the pharmacological properties of alcohol, an individual's physiological reactions to alcohol, his absorption rate of the alcohol, his rate of consumption, the alcoholic strength of the beverage, his body weight, his motivation for drinking, his prior experience with alcohol, and the impact of the family and society's drinking customs and beliefs on his orientation to alcohol.

THE PHYSIOLOGICAL EFFECTS OF ALCOHOL

Alcohol is a systemic drug, carried by the bloodstream to act on the central nervous system with both psychological and physiological consequences. Pharmacologically alcohol is an anesthetic, a tranquilizer, and a depressant. It may seem at times that the drug is a stimulant because it can spark conversation and activity in a social setting. But in fact, such mood changes are induced because alcohol depresses the part of the brain that controls impulsive behavior, judgment, and memory. It also depresses other parts of the brain involved in sending out instructions to the body, which results in the most measurable of alcohol's effects, impairment of motor coordination. It is not yet known precisely how alcohol acts on the brain cells. Recent studies, however, tend to link alcohol intoxication to alcohol's effects on the chemical transmitter acetylcholine, while others suggest an interference with the transmitters noradrenalin and serotonin.

Alcohol can produce confusion and hallucinations under certain circumstances, even in moderate doses. Prolonged heavy use may bring on temporary or permanent psychotic conditions. Furthermore, as with other depressant drugs, daily alcohol intoxication along with tolerance produces a state of physical dependence. The intensity of the withdrawal symptoms when alcohol is stopped reflects the degree to which the individual is dependent. A "hangover" following a few hours' intoxication is regarded by some as a state of mild withdrawal. There is nothing mild, however, to the seizures and hallucinations or delirium tremens

(DTS) that can accompany the abstinence syndrome or withdrawal illness in alcohol addicts.

Besides its effects on the nervous system, even in moderate doses alcohol can affect the cardiovascular system by increasing the heart rate and dilating blood vessels near the skin. This vasodilation gives the drinker an illusion of feeling warmer although he is actually losing heat more rapidly from his body. There is some evidence that alcohol may contribute to the constriction of the coronary arteries, especially in chronic heavy drinkers; it may therefore be dangerous to someone with heart disease. Alcohol also increases secretion of the saliva and stomach acid and is a mild diuretic. Alcohol in distilled liquor can irritate the stomach and contribute to digestive disorders, such as gastritis.

Prolonged heavy use of alcohol often brings a high rate of serious illness. Large quantities of alcohol increase fat deposits in the body, particularly in the liver. Because alcohol supplies calories it is often used in place of food, but it does not supply essential vitamins and amino acids. Furthermore, because it supplies a significant amount of calories, it has a tendency to depress the appetite. As a result, a variety of disorders and illnesses are frequently associated with chronic drinking, including vitamin deficiency and cirrhosis of the liver.

Alcohol Absorption and Blood Alcohol Level

As a psychoactive drug, alcohol is unique in that its effective dose is much greater than with other intoxicants. For example, full effects of LSD are observed upon ingestion of ten-millionths of an ounce, or about three-tenths of a milligram. Mescaline

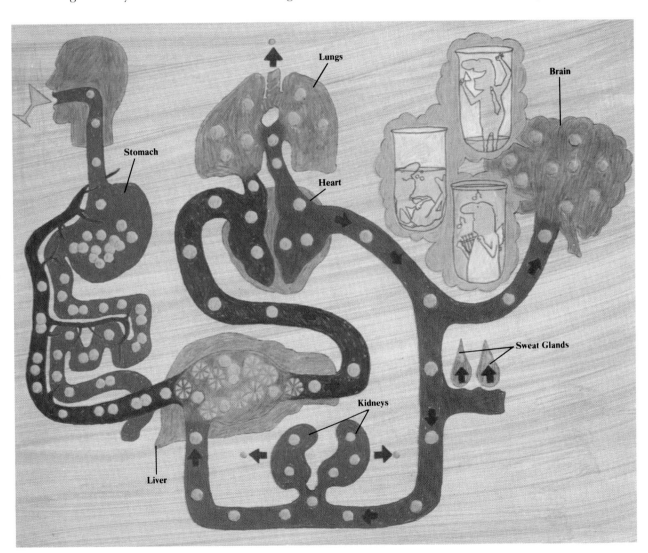

Figure 8.1 Alcohol flow chart. Once the alcohol gets into the bloodstream it is carried to all parts of the body. Some of the alcohol is lost through expiration, sweat, and excretion. The amount that finds its way to the brain depends on a number of factors, but if the level gets too high it can cause unconsciousness or even death.

and barbiturates need roughly 1,000 times larger amounts (about 300 milligrams) than LSD. With alcohol, intoxication follows an ingestion of about 50 to 100 grams (two to four ounces), that is, 200 to 300 times more than with mescaline and almost a million times more than with LSD. This difference is primarily because most of the alcohol ingested does not reach the brain. The body absorbs alcohol into the bloodstream partly through the lining of the stomach and partly through the small intestine. Once in the blood, between 80 and 90 percent of the alcohol is broken down in the liver and other tissues, eventually to carbon dioxide and water; the rest may circulate through the brain before being eliminated through the kidneys or sweat glands.

The *blood alcohol level*—the concentration of alcohol carried by the blood to the brain—determines how much effect the drug will have on a person's behavior. Whenever the rate at which alcohol is absorbed into the blood is greater than the rate of breakdown and elimination, the excess of unaltered, nonoxidized alcohol is able to reach the brain, where it produces its intoxicating effect.

The body oxidizes alcohol at a fairly constant rate, with variations depending largely on the size of the liver, which in turn is somewhat dependent on body weight. For example, the liver of a man weighing 150 pounds would oxidize about .3 ounce of pure alcohol an hour—roughly the alcohol to be found in .6 ounce of 50 percent whiskey or seven ounces of 4 percent beer. A smaller, lighter person, with a correspondingly smaller liver, would have a

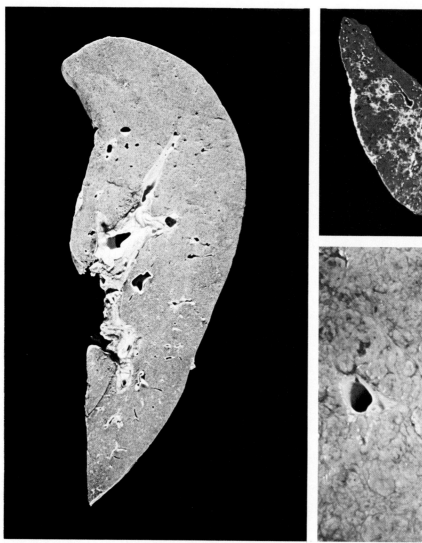
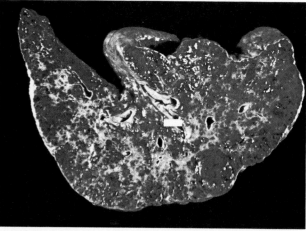
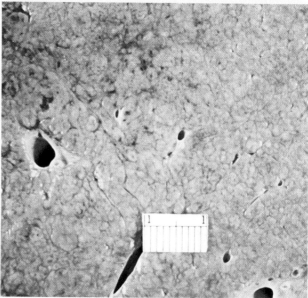

Figure 8.2   (*above*) Normal human liver. (*top right*) Cirrhotic liver. Cirrhosis of the liver, which is usually caused by heavy, prolonged consumption of alcohol, can also result from a substandard diet. The condition is characterized by hardening of the liver due to the formation of scar tissue. (*bottom right*) Close-up of a cirrhotic liver. The scar-tissue cells interfere with the functioning capacity of the liver. The condition is nonreversible, but its progress can be slowed by discontinuing the consumption of alcohol and correcting the dietary inadequacies.

higher alcohol level in the blood reaching his liver and possibly an even higher level in the blood leaving the liver.

Although there are individual variations, most people will experience little noticeable effect at a concentration of up to .02 percent (two parts per 1,000) of alcohol in the blood. Some recognizable sensations will generally occur between the levels of .03 and .05 percent. These sensations may include lightheadedness, a sense of relaxation and well-being, and release of some personal inhibitions, often leading the drinker to say a few things he might not ordinarily say or do a few things he might not ordinarily do. By the time the blood concentration reaches .1 percent there is major depression of sensory and motor functions. The drinker may stagger slightly, fumble objects, and have some trouble saying even familiar words.

If his alcohol concentration reaches .2 percent, the drinker will usually be both physically and psychologically incapacitated; at .3 percent the drinker is in a stupor, and concentrations above .4 percent lead to coma. A concentration of .6 or .7 percent would cause suffocation and death. Fortunately, such a high concentration rarely occurs because most drinkers lose consciousness before they consume that much alcohol or because the alcohol irritates the stomach and the drinker vomits before absorption of a fatal dose occurs.

Blood alcohol level depends on the amounts and modalities in which alcohol is *consumed*, the rapidity with which it is introduced, or *absorbed*, into the bloodstream, the volume of blood into which it is *diluted*, and the rate at which it gets *removed* from the bloodstream. Many factors influence each of those four aspects.

TYPE OF BEVERAGE It has already been noted that distilled liquor contains a greater percentage of alcohol than beer or wine. One ounce of pure alco-

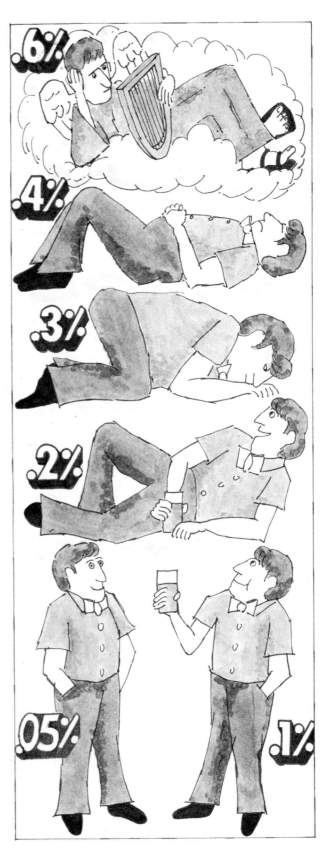

Figure 8.3 Blood alcohol levels and their effect on the drinker's behavioral state.

hol could be ingested from a two-ounce shot of 50 percent (100-proof) whiskey, from five ounces of reinforced wine, from ten ounces of natural wine, or from two twelve-ounce bottles or cans of beer. The alcohol content of each beverage, then, is very important in determining what effect a certain drink will have.

BODY WEIGHT   The concentration of alcohol in the blood obviously depends on both the amount of alcohol absorbed and the volume of blood into which it is absorbed. Blood volume is related to body weight. If it is assumed that a 200-pound person has roughly twice as much blood as a 100-pound person, all other factors being equal, the heavier man can consume twice as much alcohol for the same final concentration of alcohol in the blood and hence the same effect.

This factor is critical in determining the intoxicating properties of given amounts of alcohol, yet it is one that is seldom taken into account when a group of people are drinking. Quite apart from sentiments about the equality of the sexes, because women generally do not weigh nearly as much as men, most women cannot safely drink as much as most men. Again, all other factors being equal, body weight—not sex—is the primary determinant of one's being able to "drink like a man."

RATE OF CONSUMPTION   In order for alcohol to reach the brain and have an effect on behavior, it must be consumed and absorbed more rapidly than it is oxidized. Absorption rates depend partly on rates of consumption. An ounce of alcohol in whiskey (two ounces of liquid) can be downed in an instant, but even the veteran drinker will take at least a few minutes to get down the equivalent amount of alcohol in two bottles of beer. Differences in consumption time become more significant when larger amounts of alcohol (and liquid) are involved. The rate of consumption (but not absorption time) is influenced by custom and by the setting where drinking takes place. For example, on some occasions one sips a drink slowly but on others one may be urged to chug-a-lug.

RATE OF ABSORPTION   The rate of absorption is significantly affected by what is in the stomach when one is drinking. When people drink on an empty stomach, such as at late-afternoon cocktail parties, there is usually nothing present in the stomach to slow down the absorption process. Therefore, absorption takes place rapidly enough to produce a noticeable effect even from relatively small amounts of alcohol. On the other hand, alcohol that is consumed with food, especially after a large meal, will be absorbed much more slowly. In fact, the half-ounce of alcohol sipped from an after-dinner cordial may well be broken down almost as rapidly as it is absorbed. The same would be true of an after-dinner beer because people tend to drink almost any liquid more slowly after a meal than before. There is some evidence that beer contains substances that may slow absorption time slightly and that the common carbonated sodas with which whiskey is often mixed may slightly accelerate the absorption process.

Other Biochemical Factors

There are additional factors affecting the individual's response to alcohol that should be mentioned, although they are perhaps the least understood. In some cases at least, they may involve permanent or temporary differences in the efficiency of the absorption and/or the breakdown processes. Some people are particularly sensitive to alcohol, and for them even small amounts produce unpleasant reactions. Such people, and in fact no one, should be encouraged or pressured to drink merely for the sake of conformity. Many people seem more susceptible to alcohol's effects when they are extremely fatigued or have been recently ill. Such people find they simply cannot drink the way they usually do without experiencing uncomfortable effects.

A serious complication of alcohol use occurs when people drink at the same time that they are taking other kinds of drugs. Alcohol itself is a powerful drug. When two drugs are taken at the same time they often produce an effect that is different from that which either of them produces alone; in fact, if their actions are directed to the same body systems their combined effect is often more powerful than might be expected from adding the independent effects. For example, both alcohol and phenobarbital (a barbiturate) are depressants. The combination of the two depressants, each in doses well below the lethal level, can kill a person. Occasionally there is a lot of publicity about the death of a prominent person who took what ordinarily would be a nonlethal dose of a barbiturate while under the influence of alcohol. Nevertheless, and in spite of the sometimes unpredictable consequences of mixing various drugs, far too little attention is given to the potentially serious outcome of drinking while a person is taking almost any form of medication, including numerous over-the-counter remedies that contain drugs with sedative or depressive properties.

A factor currently under study that may alter some notions about the intoxicating properties of alcoholic beverages is the presence of generally minute amounts of substances other than alcohol that can have toxic effects on the drinker. These substances are called *congeners*. Congeners exist in many varieties of alcoholic drinks and appear to be by-products of fermentation or of the processes by which liquors are aged to achieve taste, color, and bouquet. Beverages vary widely in their congener content; vodka and gin have the least, while bourbon and brandy tend to have the most. Congeners do not contribute to the specific drug effects of alcohol, but they themselves may cause their own set of toxic symptoms, including hangovers. Congeners may help explain certain individual variations in sensitivity to different alcoholic beverages.

PSYCHOLOGICAL EFFECTS OF ALCOHOL

As with the other mind-altering drugs, the effect on the mind of average doses of alcohol depends mainly on the underlying personality and character of the user interacting with the setting and the drug. The psychological effects of alcohol include two distinct but related categories. First, there are effects on overt behavior, including perception, reaction time, the performance of motor tasks and skills, and processes of learning, remembering, thinking, reasoning, and solving problems. Second, there are the effects on emotional behavior, such as fear, anxiety, tension, hostility, or the feeling of euphoria.

Numerous studies have demonstrated that alcohol, even in small amounts, has a deleterious influence on task performance. The effect of given amounts of alcohol on skilled performance increases with the complexity of the task, the unfamiliarity of the task to the performer, and the inexperience of the performer with drinking. Even small amounts of alcohol may affect simple tasks if the performer is inexperienced both in drinking and in carrying out the task at hand.

There is an insidious paradox in alcohol's effect on man because this effect can be beneficial and harmful at the same time. Even at a concentration of about .1 percent, while the drinker feels more relaxed and has become less tense, he loses some of his dexterity, speed of motor responses, tactile perception, and auditory and visual discrimination. At the same time, however, he has the illusion that his reactions, perceptions, and discriminatory powers are better than normal. This false sense of well-being compounds the effect of alcohol by misleading the drinker into believing that he can safely undertake dangerous tasks (such as driving) or that he can make decisions demanding discriminatory judgment.

There are many psychological and cultural factors that may affect the degree of influence alcohol may have on any one individual. These factors include the individual's personal motives for drinking, his family's orientation and use of alcohol, his own previous experiences with it, and the customs and beliefs of his culture about alcohol.

As is the case with all aspects of human behavior, there is, of course, a fundamental relationship between man's physiological and psychological responses to alcohol. For example, the intensity with which a drinker may experience his physiological reactions to alcohol can be partly influenced by such psychological factors as experience with drinking and expectations. Conversely, a physiological factor such as fatigue can affect psychological responses to drinking.

Motivation

Social groups or individuals who are seeking to maximize the psychopharmacological effects of alcohol—that is, people who drink for the effects that alcohol produces—have learned to adjust their choice of beverage and their speed and time of consumption to produce the desired effects. On the other hand, those whose drinking is more related to the symbolic meaning of alcohol usually select beverages and circumstances that minimize the intoxicating effects of alcohol. For example, a man who really wants to get drunk, whether it is to forget things that are bothering him or to celebrate something, will often choose distilled whiskey and will drink it rather rapidly. Someone else who just wants to be polite at a party may drink wine or beer, or a mixed drink with low alcohol content, or a strong drink but nurse it along slowly.

Role of Experience

Another factor that appears to influence the effect of alcohol on the individual is the amount of prior

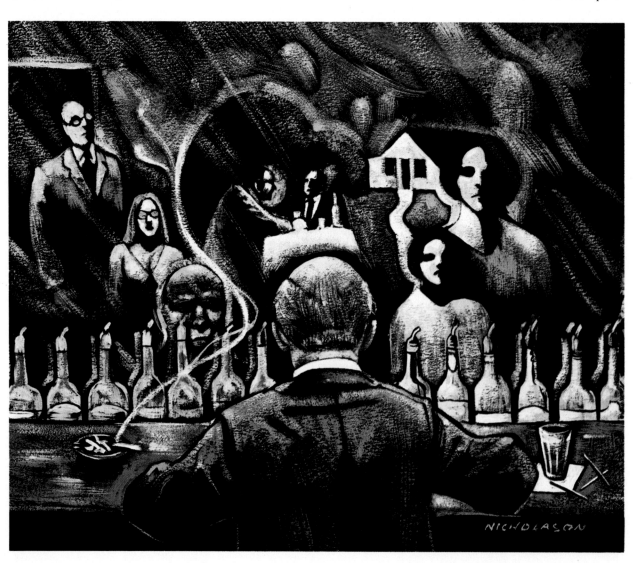

experience the drinker has had—his previous exposure to the sensations produced by alcohol and his interpretation of them. When all other factors are kept constant, the individual who is experimenting with alcohol for the first time or who has had little prior experience is apt to display more variable and less pleasant responses than the experienced drinker. This difference may be explained partially by the strangeness of the sensations and a tendency for some people to hyperreact to various kinds of new experiences. It also may reflect an attempt on the part of the drinker to conform to what he assumes his reactions should be.

Some people appear to be more intoxicated when drinking than might be warranted by the amount of alcohol they have consumed. Conversely, as people become experienced drinkers they often learn to compensate for some of the alcohol-induced behavioral responses. They can appear to be more sober than might be expected from their alcohol consumption. These differences are essentially psychological adaptations to the experience of drinking. At the physiological level, people appear to have some capacity for adapting to the irritating properties of alcohol. A novice taking a strong drink for the first time may throw it up—a reaction not too different from that of children who experiment with tobacco. All these differences should not, however, be confused with the phenomenon of alcohol-induced *tolerance*.

Tolerance to alcohol, like that to other psychoactive drugs, is built over a prolonged period of drug abuse. Progressively higher amounts of alcohol are "tolerated" with no recognizable signs of depressant action. The mechanisms underlying the build-up of alcohol tolerance—or of alcohol addiction—are not known, nor is it established whether they involve a "desensitization" of the target nerve cells or an improved machinery for alcohol breakdown. Some investigators have suggested that the body may learn to meet persistently higher blood alcohol levels with an increase in the enzyme or enzymes necessary to dispose of the excess alcohol. If, then, the abnormal blood levels are abruptly reduced, as would occur upon "going dry," the excess enzymes are no longer kept in check by the products of alcohol breakdown, may turn against physiologically important substances, and thus create the conditions for the withdrawal syndrome.

Drinking and the Family

For most people the question of drinking or abstaining and problems of alcohol are most intimately experienced within the family. Several studies have found that the family is the most frequent setting and family members the most frequent companions at the time of earliest exposure to alcohol and that about half of those who drink report some experiment or taste by the age of ten. There also is a high correlation between young people and their parents in regard to the types of beverages used, frequency of drinking, and amounts consumed. Within the family most individuals also acquire the sense of security or inadequacy that may influence the psychological meaning of alcohol for them and their future motivations for drinking.

Drinking Customs

The prevalence of problem drinking also is related to differences in customary beliefs and patterns of alcohol use. Conditions that favor the rapid absorption of sufficient alcohol to affect behavior are associated with higher rates of intoxication and increased exposure to alcoholism. Such conditions are generally found in societies where most drinking is done on an empty stomach and involves beverages with a high alcohol content in relatively undiluted form. Such conditions tend to prevail at the typical late-afternoon American cocktail party. Not only is the buffering effect of food missing, people

Figure 8.4 The psychological factors involved in the effect, use, and abuse of alcohol may include prior experience, expectation, family background, motivation, and customs and beliefs.

tend to drink more rapidly when they are not eating and when they are standing rather than seated. Lower rates of problem drinking tend to be found where customs favor drinking of beers or low-alcohol wines and where the conditions of drinking impede rapid ingestion or absorption.

DRINKING IN AMERICAN SOCIETY

Within this century, with the exception of the period of national Prohibition, a gradual but steady trend toward the use of alcohol by more and more people has been recorded. In a recent study of American drinking practices it was estimated that 100 million Americans above the age of fifteen, in-

cluding about eight out of ten adult men and six of ten adult women, use alcoholic beverages. Perhaps 90 percent of those who drink appear to use alcohol without noticeable danger or damage to themselves or others except when they drive after drinking, but the drinking habits of at least 10 million people cause distinct problems. This last group includes the estimated 7 million who are alcoholics and others who often are temporarily incapacitated through incidental intoxication from safely or effectively carrying out their various activities.

Drinking Among Youth

Until concern about marijuana, LSD, and campus rebellion stole the limelight, drinking among young people consistently caused friction between the generations. There have been widely prevailing beliefs that drinking is the cause of most difficulties in which youths may find themselves. The mass media have both reflected and contributed to these unfounded assumptions.

In American society drinking has long been permitted only for adults. In most states the sale, purchase, or use of alcoholic beverages to or by persons under the age of twenty-one is illegal. Only three states, New York, Louisiana, and Tennessee, have set the legal age at eighteen, and a few states have set the age at twenty. Some states have made exceptions by permitting those between eighteen and twenty-one to drink beer with only 3.2 percent alcohol or to drink if they are married or in the armed forces. But, by and large, supported by temperance-group political action, prohibition prior to age twenty-one prevails. Kentucky, which many years ago changed the voting age to eighteen and now considers an eighteen-year-old a legal adult, still prohibits drinking until one is twenty-one years old.

Occasional drinkers appear to be as numerous in the age group eighteen to twenty-one as at any

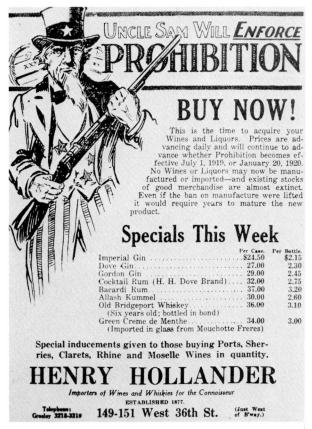

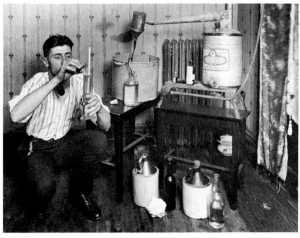

Figure 8.5 During prohibition it was illegal to manufacture or sell alcoholic beverages in the United States, although it was not illegal to possess them.

period of life, despite the legal prohibition proclaimed against them. Available evidence also suggests, however, that the frequency of drinking and the amounts consumed by young people are only exaggerated by the notoriety often given to conspicuous episodes.

Several studies suggest that there is a direct relationship between the force of sanctions against drinking and the occurrence of frequent, heavy, or problem drinking among young people. In colleges where drinking is permitted, it has been found that most students drink but that relatively few get into difficulties because of their drinking. Because they do not have to leave the college in order to drink, fewer students incur the risks of drinking and driving; because they can drink when they please, fewer seem impelled to drink heavily whenever they drink. On the other hand, schools that rigidly enforce rules against drinking, although they may limit somewhat the number of students who will drink, contribute to situations in which those who do drink experience difficulties more frequently. Such students must often drive in order to drink. As one student noted, "When you go to the trouble of driving fifty miles to get a drink, you don't just have two drinks."

Adult example, attitudes, and restrictions have enhanced the attractiveness of alcohol for young people as a symbol of adult status, of rejected authority, or of "forbidden fruit." As a result, these attitudes have probably been more effective in stimulating the kind of drinking that involves risks than they have been in controlling the incidence of drinking. Restrictive regulations also have been consistent with much of the education about alcohol—education required by the laws of every state. Until quite recently such alcohol teaching, like marijuana teaching, so insulted the credulity of students that it appears to have inspired experimentation in the very behavior it was intended to discourage.

During the last few years, concern about alcohol use among youth has been replaced by concern about other drugs. The number of admissions for acute alcohol intoxication at student infirmaries has dropped markedly in the last few years. It is not known to what extent the use of amphetamines, marijuana, and other drugs has affected alcohol use. Serious users of other drugs might have diffi-

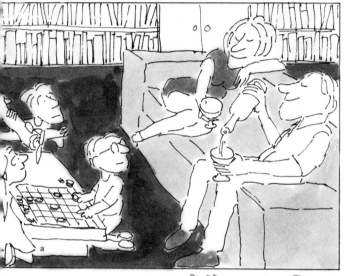

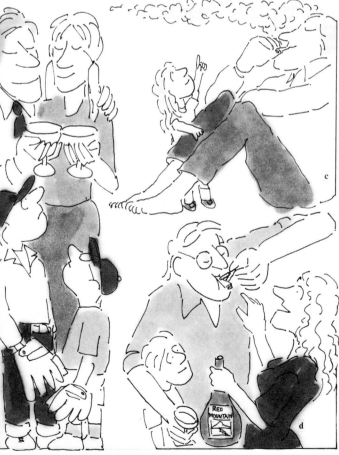

Figure 8.6 Youth and alcohol. (a) Children whose parents drink may (b) follow their parents' pattern and drink; (c) reject their parents and avoid alcohol, even to the extent of choosing a drug representing parental rejection, such as marijuana; or (d) use both alcohol and marijuana, accepting both the parents' life style and that of his own generation.

culty tolerating alcohol at the same time. There is some evidence that alcohol is deliberately mixed with other substances by persons seeking a unique effect. Pot parties seem to have replaced beer parties for some occasions. Yet it does not appear that the use of other drugs has resulted in any marked decrease in alcohol use.

An interesting comparison can be made between the apparent symbolic meanings of alcohol and marijuana. Alcohol has been used as a means of asserting adulthood and being like adults; many young people have patterned their alcohol preferences after those of their parents. Marijuana, on the other hand, seems to appeal to the current generation of youth, principally because it is their "own thing." Compared with alcohol, there is no significant adult pattern of marijuana use. Smoking pot seems for some to be a symbol of emancipation from the customs and values of the adult world. For some young people, however, the use of both drugs involves an element of rebellion.

Intoxication and Society

Whenever a society permits the use of alcohol, some drinking to the point of drunkenness occurs, and, in some drinkers, inhibitions against antisocial behavior are weakened. In some societies intoxication generally occurs only in connection with certain ceremonial events, and provisions are made for protecting the drinker from himself and protecting society from his drunkenness.

Drunkenness is common enough and hardly requires a detailed description. The intoxicated person is euphoric, talkative, lacks inhibitions, and frequently is aggressive. His speech is slurred and his movements are uncoordinated so that he even has difficulty walking. If he becomes very drunk he may go into a stupor and become unconscious. Although rare, it is possible for a severely intoxicated person to die as a result of depression of respiration and heart action.

The severity of the "hangover" one feels after getting drunk is related both to the amount and duration of the drinking and the mental and physical conditions of the individual. One may feel nauseated, vomit, be weak and nervous, and have a headache. His heart may beat quite fast, and he may have difficulty thinking. Fortunately, the hangover usually lasts less than thirty-six hours.

In the United States drunkenness became a cause of public alarm when men with no stable community ties began appearing drunk in public places. Communities justifiably feared the potential violence of these men while under the influence of alcohol. When efforts to control drunkenness by promoting moderation or prohibiting drinking failed, communities turned to jailing those who became drunk in public. Today between one-half and two-thirds of the efforts expended by local police, courts, and jail personnel go into dealing with public intoxication and related offenses. A significant number of those jailed or imprisoned for criminal acts against people or property, crimes such as murder, homicide, theft, burglary, and rape, have been drinking excessively. A large number of accidental deaths and suicides also occur following heavy drinking.

Most of the hundreds of thousands of men who are repeatedly arrested, convicted, and jailed for public intoxication, only to be released and then arrested again in a continuing cycle, are alcoholics. Recently the constitutionality of arresting and jailing an alcoholic for public intoxication has been challenged as "cruel and unusual" punishment. Although the U.S. Supreme Court in 1968 failed to support this contention, the nature of the court's decision suggests that some change is bound to take place soon. In the meantime, efforts are underway in many communities to provide centers for detoxification and treatment in place of jail terms for the chronic public drunkard.

Drunkenness is by no means confined to the

public offender. In fact, most intoxication today occurs in men and women who live with their families, hold jobs, and maintain stable community ties. In the past these persons often were protected when drunk, unless intoxication occurred so frequently or with such dire consequences that the drinker lost his family, his job, or both.

The problems created by people under the influence of alcohol in public or otherwise have been compounded as society has become more technological and as more and more jobs and activities require exacting skill and judgment. The more demanding the job, the less satisfactorily workers may be able to perform while under the influence of alcohol or while suffering the aftereffects of intoxication. In a fast-moving, highly mechanized society it is impossible for most people to escape everyday activities that will not be affected by immoderate alcohol use.

The most vivid example is the case of personal transportation. In the days of the horse-drawn vehicle, the drunken driver was rarely a threat to anyone but himself and his horse. But the automobile and truck are far more dangerous. In 1968, the Secretary of Transportation reported that the use of alcohol by drivers and pedestrians in the United States lead to about 25,000 deaths and at least 800,000 accidents a year. Many innocent victims suffer loss of life, limb, and property. Drinking also leads to a high proportion of accidents in private aircraft, in the home, and in industry. More difficult to estimate but surely a matter of great concern is the role played by alcohol in dulling the judgment of administrators, executives, politicians, and government officials whose daily decisions involve the well-being of countless other individuals.

ALCOHOLISM

Although intoxication in a privately protected environment may occur occasionally without causing undue harm, any intoxication that coincides with the need to drive, work, or make decisions may lead to serious consequences. When intoxication occurs repeatedly, invariably causing problems of personal health or interfering with psychological or social functioning of the individual in his family, job, or community, the drinker can be considered an *alcoholic*.

The definition of an alcoholic includes both social and medical concepts. Repeated use of alcohol can lead to habituation—psychological dependence —and to addiction—physical dependence. Habituation is probably the cause of the greatest number of situations harmful to both self and others. The alcohol addict is usually so impaired in his abilities to function in normal activities that his range of social interactions is considerably more restricted; often, however, the losses to himself, his family, and society are much greater.

The economic loss due to alcoholism, although not really measurable, must include costs related to such diverse factors as crime, accidents, medical and custodial care, absenteeism, and the loss of potential wages. A significant nondollar cost also is involved because of the constant threat to the safety and security of the wives, husbands, children, and fellow employees of alcoholics; the innocent victims of motor-vehicle accidents caused by intoxicated drivers or by vehicles improperly assembled by alcohol-incapacitated workers; and the citizens who bear the cost imposed by alcoholic employees in business, industry, and government and whose taxes support costly but as yet ineffective efforts at the control and prevention of alcohol problems.

What Causes Alcoholism?

There are no completely satisfactory theories about the causes of various types of problem drinking. Researchers have looked into liver metabolism, the function of the central nervous system, hormonal imbalances, vitamin and nutritional deficiencies,

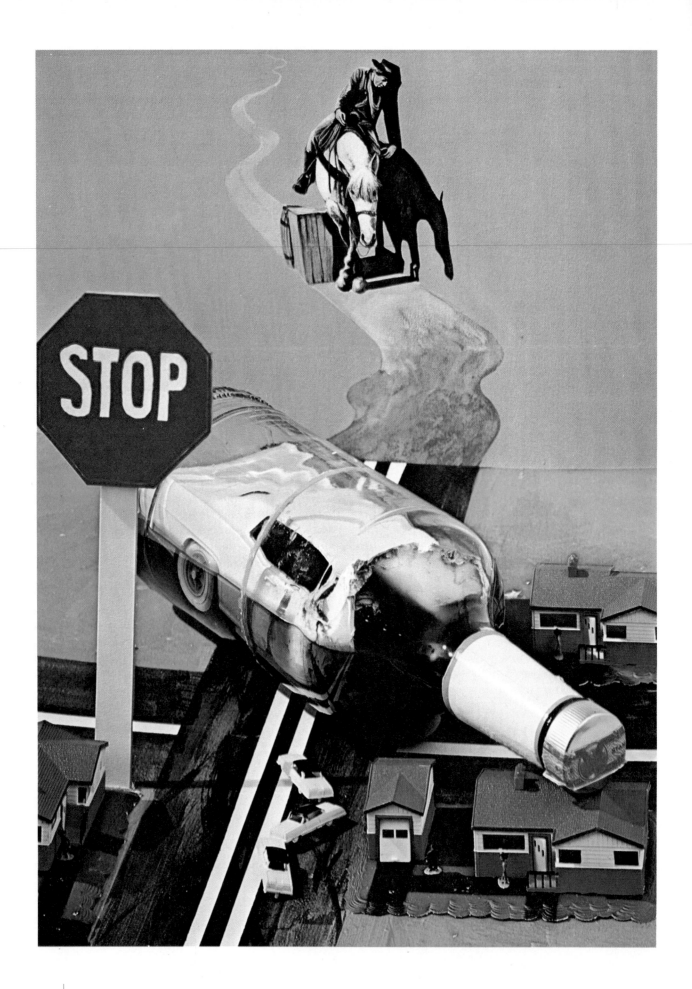

personality disorders, and the role of culture. Most authorities now agree that alcoholism is caused by several interrelated factors that vary from person to person.

Although the existence of specific biological deficiencies or sensitivities has not been identified, the possibility of such factors contributing to alcoholism cannot be ruled out. A number of psychological traits have been identified in individuals who drink excessively, however.

Alcoholics tend to be people who experience greater extremes of psychological discomfort than most other people; they have deep-seated feelings of inadequacy or are frequently anxious and depressed. Alcoholics do seem to have in common the fact that they often experience unbearable psychological or social stress and that drinking provides temporary relief. Yet repeated intoxication invariably causes physical, psychological, or social problems that, in the long run, can only increase the very stress the alcoholic seeks to reduce by drinking and may help to perpetuate his drinking.

It should be stressed that alcoholism is not necessarily determined by the amount or frequency of alcohol consumption. There are people who, by sipping small amounts of alcohol regularly throughout the day, may consume more alcohol over time than the average alcoholic. Yet the pattern of consumption of these drinkers is such that they will rarely, if ever, achieve a high enough concentration of alcohol in their blood to produce noticeable effects on their thinking or behavior. These people drink because of the mild tranquilizing effect of their pattern of consumption, because of social customs, or out of a mistaken belief in alcohol's medicinal value.

Alcoholics, on the other hand, are seeking the intoxicating effect of alcohol, whatever their pattern of alcohol use. Some alcoholics go on binges but are sober most of the time, while others follow regular patterns of drinking, perhaps drinking heavily every night, or only on weekends or holidays. Some, once they start drinking, seem compelled to continue until they reach a peak level of effect; others seek to maintain an alcohol-induced euphoria for as long as possible.

Definitions and diagnoses of alcoholism are not precise. Alcoholism has long been a stigmatized condition. As long as they are able, the alcoholic and often his family and friends may try to deny or hide his condition from others. Denial is a common response of alcoholics who must rationalize their continued drinking. Family and friends may conceal the problem to prevent the alcoholic from losing his job and respectability. It is estimated that in the United States there is one alcoholic for every fifteen to twenty people who use alcohol.

Alcoholics are found in all walks of life, all educational and income levels, occupations, and regions of the country. There are significantly more men than women alcoholics (probably four to one) but the relative rates for women seem to be rising. Because alcoholism for most people becomes visible only after a fairly long period of exposure to high levels of alcohol consumption, there are more alcoholics in their forties and early fifties than in younger age groups. Much problem drinking occurs in men in their twenties and thirties, however, and a trend toward earlier recognition of alcoholism is apparent. Decreasing rates in the age groups past fifty reflect the fact that alcoholics have high mortality rates and that there may be some alcoholics who simply stop drinking.

Dramatic differences in rates of alcoholism are found among certain ethnic groups that have had distinctive cultural patterns of alcohol use, as would be expected from the earlier discussion of the influence of custom and belief on an individual's drinking habits. Americans of Italian, Jewish, and Chinese heritage, whose cultural backgrounds have

Figure 8.7 Technological progress has made intoxication a much more serious problem than it was even sixty years ago because of the possible damage that can be done by an individual working or driving under the effects of alcohol.

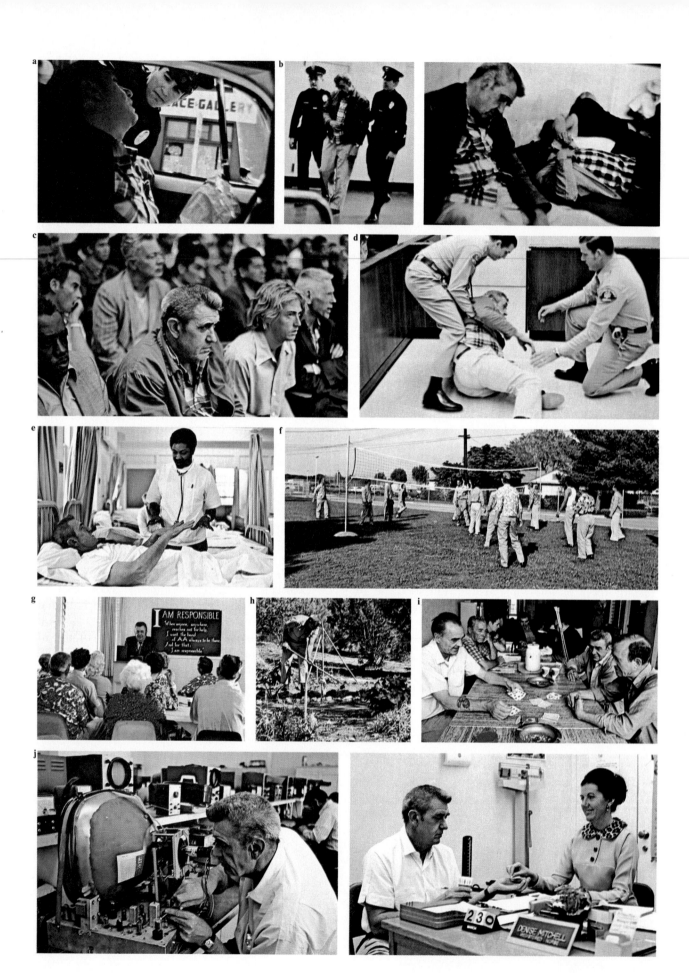

accorded deep-seated nutritional (Italian), religious (Jewish), and cultural (Chinese) meaning to the moderate use of low-alcohol-content wines while imposing strong sanctions against intoxication, have had low rates of alcoholism. In contrast, Irish and Anglo-Saxon Americans, who came from cultures where men were encouraged to use whiskey frequently in order to experience its intoxicating effects, have had unusually high rates of alcoholism. As these groups became assimilated into American culture, however, their rates of alcoholism tend to become more comparable.

These studies suggest that cultural customs and controls and parental practices are significant factors in determining the frequency of alcoholism. Nevertheless, such factors alone cannot explain why, given common drinking practices, some people become alcoholics and others do not.

Treatment

The alcoholic requires support at all levels, ranging from family members to the attending physician. The treatment of alcoholism requires a broad-gauged approach capable of dealing with the physical consequences of prolonged drinking while the alcoholic is helped to understand the social and personality factors that have contributed to his alcoholism problem.

Ideally, treatment programs should provide medical, psychological, and social-work resources and should involve the support and participation of the alcoholic's family, employer, and other significant persons. The organization Alcoholics Anonymous (AA) provides an important resource of therapy for alcoholics. Services of Alcoholics Anonymous are completely free and are based on mutual support and understanding of the problems of alcoholism through personal experience. Contact

with AA can be made anywhere in the United States. There are special meetings for spouses of alcoholics, Al-Anon, and there is also an organization known as Alateens in which teen-age sons and daughters of alcoholics meet to help each other. Many physicians have found that Antabuse (disulfiram), a tablet taken daily that produces a toxic reaction if any alcohol is consumed, can help their alcoholic patients maintain sobriety while receiving other treatment. Group and individual psychotherapy, social-work services, vocational counseling, operant conditioning, and other traditional and innovative approaches should be used in combination with AA and Antabuse. The emphasis should be on full acceptance of the problem drinker as an ill human being who needs long-term specialized outpatient help.

FACING THE PROBLEM

Although intoxication, incidental and chronic, has long presented problems for societies, the consequences of intoxication have increased as the demands of a more and more complex society have created roles requiring physical dexterity, mental alertness, and decisive actions. On the one hand, the more complex the society, the more pressures it places on individuals who use alcohol for temporary (and illusory) relief. On the other hand, the more complex the society and demanding its roles, the less tolerance it affords for individuals whose physical and mental functioning are compromised by alcohol. This dilemma is one that contemporary society faces not only with respect to alcohol but with respect to a wide range of other behavior-altering drugs. It presents a challenge to the coming generations to develop intelligent and effective methods of utilizing the benefits of alcohol and other drugs without incurring their liabilities.

Figure 8.8 Rehabilitating the alcoholic. After being arrested (a) for drunk driving, the alcoholic is escorted to the jail (b) and placed in the drunk tank until he is sober. (c) In the Los Angeles County court (which processes more than 200 drunk driving and other alcohol-related arrests each day) he awaits trial. While standing before the judge (d) he suffers an attack of the DTs. He is taken to the county hospital (e), where he is examined by a staff physician. After his release from the hospital he is sent to the Long Beach (Calif.) Rehabilitation Center for treatment. (f) He participates in recreational therapy. After a period of time the patient is sent to ACTON, another rehabilitation center (g) where he attends an AA meeting. The sign "I Am Responsible" serves as a reminder that the patient *must*

take responsibility for his actions. The patient is encouraged to develop hobbies and interests that will give his life meaning and help him release energy in an acceptable form. (h) Patient caring for his garden at the center. As the patient progresses he is placed in situations that give him more freedom (i) and help him gradually move back into the society, which he previously tried to escape through continuous alcohol-induced oblivion. At a state-supported rehabilitation program (j) the patient studies TV repair—the instability of the alcoholic to cope with societal pressures often is derived from repeated failure as a provider. The patient returns regularly to the center for counseling and Antabuse medication.

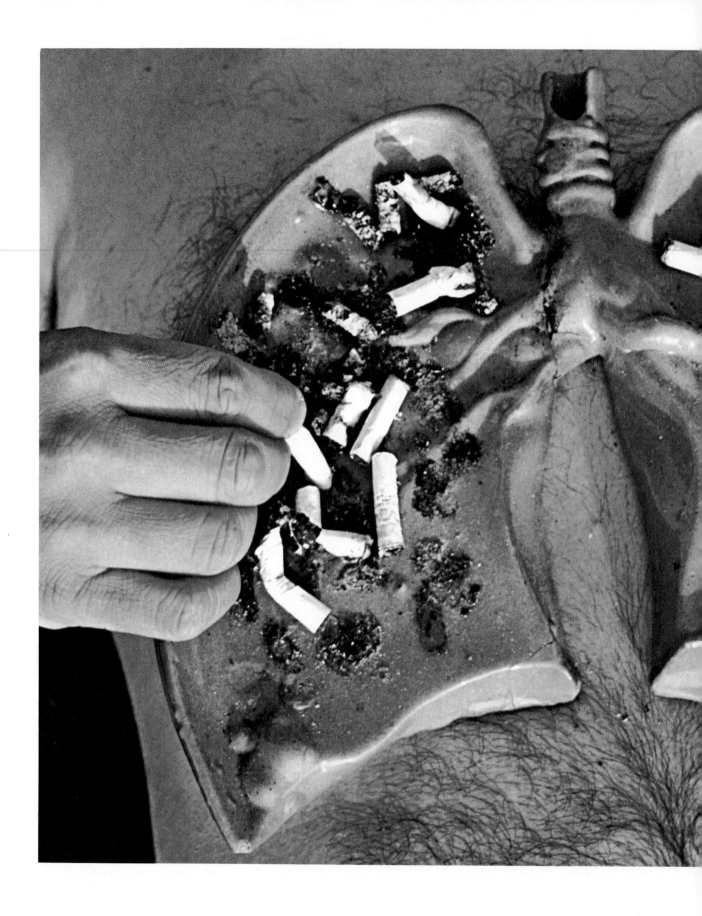

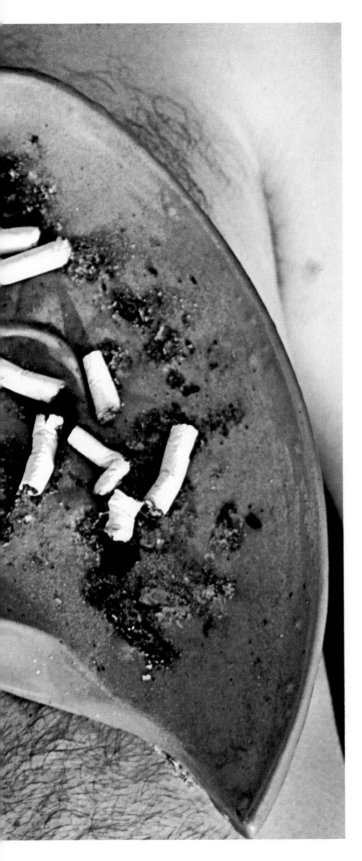

9 On January 11, 1964, the Surgeon General of the United States presented his committee's report on the health hazards of cigarette smoking. And for the first time, Americans began to realize the gravity of the problem. The committee had considered the results of many different investigations, in animals as well as in human beings, and had evaluated a large number of comprehensive epidemiological studies involving millions of people of all backgrounds in the United States, Canada, and Great Britain. Some of the major studies were *retrospective,* comparing the smoking habits of patients suffering from certain diseases with those of healthy "controls" of the same age and sex. Others were *prospective,* following the health histories of many individuals in different population categories until the study was terminated or the subject had died. The conclusion was reported by the Surgeon General in no uncertain terms: "Cigarette smoking is a health hazard of sufficient importance in the United States to warrant appropriate remedial action." Since 1964, hundreds of other similar studies carried out in all parts of the world have removed any lingering doubts on the harmful and at times tragic effects of smoking on the human body.

The most disheartening aspect of this conclusion is that man has brought this misfortune onto himself, and yet, although now aware of it, he still is reluctant—for psychological, social, political, and economic reasons—to turn the tide.

Smoking and Health

THE MAN-MADE EPIDEMIC

Before the invention of the cigarette-making machine, about one hundred years ago, cigarettes were homemade and were smoked by a few rugged individualists. But the machine spawned an industry that was turning out cigarettes at the rate of 4 billion a year at the turn of the century. By the 1920s, yearly cigarette production hit 80 billion. By 1970, smokers were puffing away their lives and polluting the air with the help of some 538 billion cigarettes. In the same seventy years, lung cancer grew from a relatively rare disease to the killer of more than 55,000 Americans in 1969. Bronchitis, emphysema, cancer of the kidney, pancreas, and bladder, and heart disease also have been on the rise, thanks in part to tobacco smoking.

Studies in which selected groups of people (physicians, war veterans, industrial workers, and so on) were studied for as long as ten years dramatically revealed the body-damaging, life-shortening effects of excessive cigarette smoking. Cigarette smokers were found to have a 30 to 80 percent greater overall mortality rate than nonsmokers, all death causes considered, and the rate differences depended on how much or how long the subjects had been smoking. The mortality rate for women, which is generally lower than that for men, also has increased in proportion to the extent to which they have taken up smoking. Mortality rates were almost normal for cigar and pipe smokers, although these smokers were more susceptible than total abstainers to lip and certain other cancers. The studies also showed that chances for a longer life increase if the smoker stops or cuts down his smoking.

The excessive mortality rate observed in cigarette smokers was caused by a variety of diseases, but 80 percent of the increase was tied to lung cancer, bronchitis, emphysema, other respiratory ailments, and heart disease. Lung-cancer incidence was eleven times greater, death from pulmonary diseases six times more frequent, and coronary artery disease almost two times more numerous than for nonsmoking subjects (see Figure 9.1). Non-smoking, lifetime members of the Seventh-Day Adventists experienced almost no lung cancer, even though their jobs and areas of residence exposed them to a wide variety of other environmental pollutants. Conversely, in Iceland, where air pollution is low, a sharp rise in lung cancer followed the large increase in cigarette consumption that took place in the post-World War II years. Thus, the dramatic difference in lung-cancer incidence between smokers and nonsmokers is much more directly related to cigarette smoking than to air pollution. This fact is not surprising, considering the extent of self-contamination to which a smoker deliberately subjects himself. Smoke from a typical nonfilter cigarette contains about 5 billion particles per milliliter, 50,000 times as many as an equal volume of polluted urban atmosphere.

From the increased mortality rate ascribed to

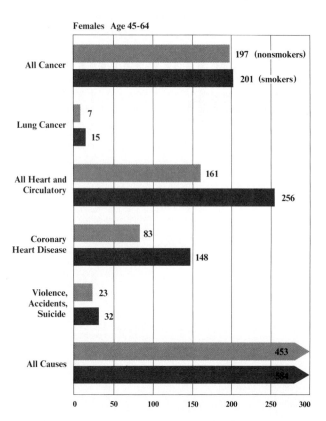

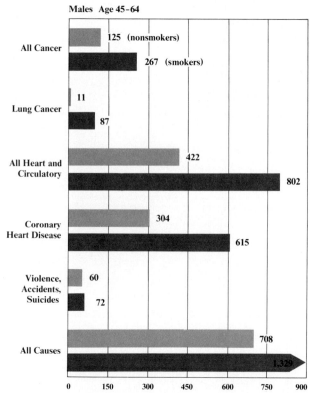

smoking, it is quite obvious that smokers are their own worst enemy. Recent data indicate that these harmful effects also can be passed from a smoking women to her unborn child. Seven large independent surveys involving thousands of pregnancies revealed that smoking mothers have twice as many stillbirths and spontaneous abortions and two to three times as many premature babies as nonsmokers. Furthermore, babies born to women who smoke during pregnancy are one-fourth to one-half pound lighter than babies born to nonsmoking mothers. British physicians calculated in one of these studies that one out of five babies lost would have been saved if their mothers had been nonsmokers. The way by which tobacco smoke affects the fetus is not known; it has been suggested the oxygen supply to the fetus may be reduced by carbon monoxide (one of the gases found in cigarette smoke) poisoning the red blood cells, or by nicotine constricting the arteries and reducing placental blood flow.

Heavy smokers also are much more likely to be ill, miss work more often, and are generally less competent to lead a fully productive life. According to the National Center for Health Statistics, in 1965 two-pack-a-day smokers lost 65 percent more workdays than nonsmokers and showed impaired work performance twice as often. Of the 400 million workdays lost by the nation, whatever the causes, 19 percent would have been avoided if the cigarette smokers were not more prone to illness—or if they had not been smokers. To this loss of work, time, and wages, one must add the cost of increased medical and hospital bills and the major impact on human living for which no financial estimates can be calculated.

COMPONENTS OF CIGARETTE SMOKE

To help determine what portions of tobacco smoke are responsible for the various diseases associated with cigarette smoking, chemists have meticulously broken down the smoke into its components and then tested the various fractions on laboratory animals. Thus far, they have identified more than 1,200 different toxic chemicals, and the number is still growing. When it burns, the average cigarette produces about one-half gram of smoke, 92 percent in the form of gases (a number of them known to be toxic) and 8 percent as ash, nicotine, a tar-rich condensate, and a "wet particulate matter" comprising hundreds of different substances.

The tarry condensate was resolved by the chemists into three fractions, acidic, basic, and neutral. In animal tests, the neutral fraction showed by far the highest carcinogenic, or cancer-causing, activity: upon further fractionation, it was found to contain *benzopyrene*, one of the deadliest carcinogens known, and many other chemicals of the same family. The acidic fraction from the tarry condensate contains phenol and other materials that, it has been suggested by some cancer researchers, could *activate* a "dormant" cancer cell into growing and spreading but are not themselves carcinogens.

Nicotine, the "drug" characteristic of tobacco, was found to occur in the basic fraction of tarry condensate. It is not a carcinogen. Rather, it has been linked circumstantially to some of the other smoke-supported diseases.

Nicotine is an agent affecting primarily the nervous system. Like other drugs of this category, it produces habituation and tolerance but—unlike depressant drugs—no physical addiction. It is known that nicotine mimics some of the effects of the neurotransmitter acetylcholine, enhancing transmission when applied at low doses and blocking it at the higher dose range. A number of the body's responses to inhalation of nicotine are viewed as consequences of the synaptic effects of the drug. For example, nicotine is known to increase the heartbeat fifteen to twenty-five beats per minute while constricting blood vessels in the extremities. Thermographs taken of smoker's hands and feet

Figure 9.1 Death rates of cigarette smokers versus nonsmokers by selected diseases related to smoking (rates per 100,000 person-years).

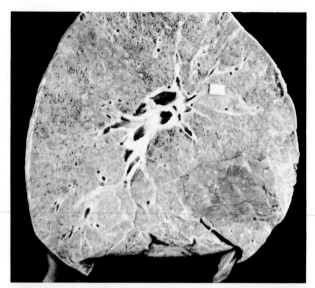

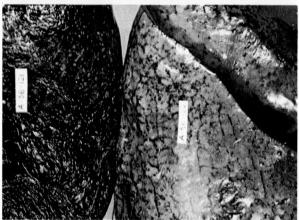

dramatically show the decline in temperature in fingers and toes after a cigarette is smoked. Other effects of the synaptic action of nicotine are suspected to take place at the level of the smooth muscles regulating the constriction of the bronchioles—an important component of respiratory disorders.

SMOKE AS A DISEASE AGENT
Lung Cancer

When the tar-rich condensate from cigarette smoke, or its fractions and subfractions, is applied to the skin, lungs, and other tissues of mice, rats, or hamsters, the compounds it contains produce cancer in the experimental animals. Recent experiments showed that lung cancer could be produced in dogs made to smoke seven cigarettes a day through incisions in the trachea for a period of more than two years. Among dogs that smoked filter cigarettes or half the number of nonfilter cigarettes, some did develop abnormal cell changes in lung tissues that pathologists suspect would eventually lead to cancer. However, the dogs that smoked more of the nonfilter cigarettes showed more of these changes.

One of the most comprehensive studies of the effects of cigarette smoking on human lung tissue was carried out in 1964 at the Veteran's Administration Hospital in East Orange, New Jersey, where autopsied lung tissue from several thousand individuals was thoroughly examined.

A significant finding was the high incidence of *hyperplasia* among heavy and moderate smokers. In hyperplasia, the *basal cells* that underlie the bronchial lining become irritated and begin to pile up in layers, usually five or more deep. The next most noticeable difference in the respiratory passageways of smokers is the loss of ciliated *columnar cells*. These cells include fine hairlike projectons, or cilia, on their surface. The cilia wave back and forth and usually keep harmful materials out of the lungs. Following the loss of the ciliated cells, the remain-

Figure 9.2 (*top*) Cut surface of a normal human lung. (*center*) Heavily carbon-pigmented lung typical of smoker's or coal miner's lung is compared to a normal lung surface. (*bottom*) This carbon pigmentation occurs more in urban populations and industrialized countries and appears even in the lungs of nonsmokers.

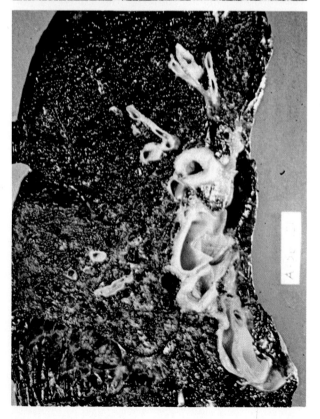

Figure 9.3 The process of hyperplasia.

ing cells flatten out and enlarge to take on the "squamous" structure invariably found in patients with lung cancer.

Most pertinent to lung cancer itself was the appearance of disordered nuclei in the affected lung cells. Cells of this type are seen in *carcinoma in situ*, a localized cancer that may break through to the underlying basal cells, proliferate, and spread throughout the rest of the body. Hyperplasia, the loss of ciliated cells, and the abnormal nuclei were prevalent in patients who died of lung cancer. The researchers also found that among ex-smokers these three conditions had regressed, suggesting that in the premalignant state, at least, the lung cancer process may be reversible. Lung cancer and its incidence are further discussed in Chapter 23.

Coronary Artery Disease

From among the hundreds of different chemical compounds found in cigarette smoke, most pathologists indict nicotine and carbon monoxide as the two major villains in promoting coronary artery disease. Generally, nicotine increases the demand of the heart for oxygen. Furthermore, as lung function is impaired by smoking, the heart must work harder to utilize the remaining air sacs. Its job is further complicated by the constriction of blood vessels in the extremities brought about by nicotine. A normal heart can sometimes stand such

strains, but they can be fatal to an individual who has recently had a heart attack.

Bronchitis and Emphysema

The familiar hacking cough and large amount of mucus coughed up by cigarette smokers are now known to be the early symptoms of two serious diseases—bronchitis and emphysema. These conditions are thought to result when various chemical components of cigarette smoke break down vital tissue in the bronchi or the lungs. In bronchitis, the threadlike cilia that normally flush toxic substances out of the air stream are destroyed or paralyzed, resulting in increasing irritation; the airways of the bronchi are narrowed, breathing becomes difficult, and the affected individual chokes on the excess mucus that is formed. In emphysema, the same conditions occur, with the added disadvantage that the alveoli lose their elasticity or burst. These two chronic disorders are discussed more fully in Chapter 25.

Other Related Problems

The death rates for cancer of the mouth, larynx, and esophagus are significantly higher for smokers than for nonsmokers, and these cancers affect cigar and pipe smokers as well as cigarette smokers, probably because of the heat and chemicals fed directly into the mouth through the pipe stem or

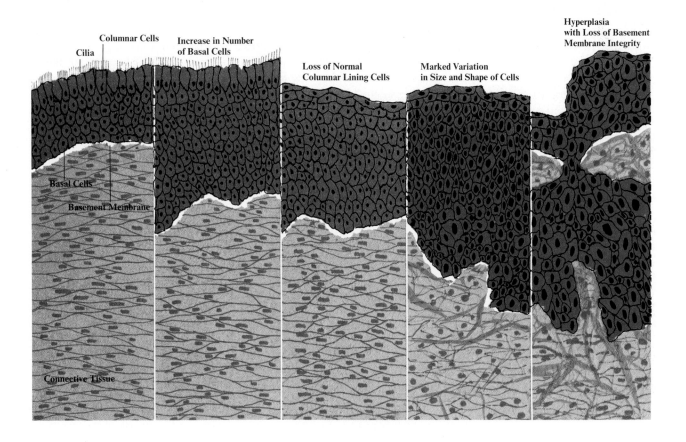

cigar. The lips, tongue, and mucous membranes of cigar and pipe smokers are especially vulnerable to *leukoplakia*, a whitish thickening that is considered to be an early form of cancer.

Together with lung cancer, cancer of the esophagus and trachea has risen sharply since 1935, along with a similar increase in tobacco consumption. Researchers also have linked bladder cancer to cigarette smoking; pack-a-day smokers are twice as likely to die from the condition than are nonsmokers. An increased incidence in cancers of the pancreas and kidney may also be the result of excessive smoking.

Studies conducted in the United States, Great Britain, and Canada show that three to four times as many smokers die from *peptic ulcer* than nonsmokers. Ulcer patients find that smoking increases their pain and that the drugs usually employed to treat the condition lose their effectiveness. It is suspected that smoking does not cause ulcers as such but that it in some way intensifies or perpetuates them.

Sinusitis, an irritation of the sinus cavities (air cavities within certain bones adjacent to the nasal cavity), is not usually considered a serious disease, but it can be distressing and disabling for anyone who has to live with it. Fortunately, the patient can get rapid relief when he quits smoking, because the hot gases and particulate matter of cigarette smoke are known to aggravate the condition.

PROFILE OF THE SMOKER

When cigarette manufacture first became a major industry at the turn of the century, the typical smoker was a middle-class working man who perhaps believed smoking made him seem more manly. For women and children, strictures against smoking were akin to moral law. Women who smoked were considered fast, loose, and capable of almost any depravity. For children, smoking was even more of a stigma: the first step toward a rotting brain and stunted growth. The cigarette was considered a "filthy weed" fraught with undertones of impending disaster for the human race.

During the 1920s, men of all professions and backgrounds turned to the cigarette. The flappers joined them; they considered smoking to be a fashionable mark of sophisticated decadence. It was not until the late 1930s that advertising began to build shining images for cigarettes and the people who smoked them. Smokers were the heroes of the day: fighter pilots, soldiers in the foxhole, tank drivers, doctors, and good-looking nurses.

After that, the word was trumpeted on the radio, in newspapers, and on billboards across the country. With television came visual proof that cigarette smokers were "the good guys." The smoker was a tough-skinned, handsome cowboy driving a herd of cattle across the Western plains. The right cigarette became a sexual lure, attracting bikini-clad beauties off their surfboards into the waiting arms of handsome young men. Another cigarette advertiser conferred a kind of medical certification on smoking, pointing out that more doctors smoked their cigarettes than any other leading brand.

In the 1950s and 1960s advertising campaigns were aimed heavily at the youth market, particularly college students. Sophisticated travelers flying thousands of feet in the sky received complimentary cigarettes with their meal aloft, and children sang songs insisting that bad grammar is less important than the taste of a "good" cigarette.

As a result of this drum-beating, more and more men, women, and children became smokers. By the fall of 1964—right after the Surgeon General's report—one-half of American men and one-third of the women smoked daily, a total of 50 to 60 million smokers. Nearly 49 percent of the young men between seventeen and twenty-four smoked, along with 34 percent of the women in that age group. Between the ages of twenty-five and thirty-four there was a sharp upsurge to 60.7 percent of the men and 43.5 percent of women. From that age upward, considerably less men and women smoked.

The statistics of the mid-1960s also showed that a greater percentage of low-income individuals with poor educational backgrounds smoked than the higher-paid, better-educated segment of the population. Nevertheless, the better-educated, higher-paid men smoked more cigarettes per day than the other group. Men and women who lived on farms smoked consistently less than those who lived in the city.

WHY PEOPLE SMOKE

Generally, adolescents begin smoking and most adults continue smoking in large part because many other people smoke and because the use of nicotine and other drugs is institutionalized in society. More than 50 million Americans smoking an average of twenty cigarettes per day represents a lot of social reinforcement, and 300 million dollars per year in cigarette advertising also "helps." To smokers, smoking is relaxing and pleasurable: something to do with their hands; a means of communication, role playing, and filling time; a brief "lift"; a comfort; a sensory pleasure. This pleasure, coupled with the fact that smokers try to cope with many of their interpersonal relationships

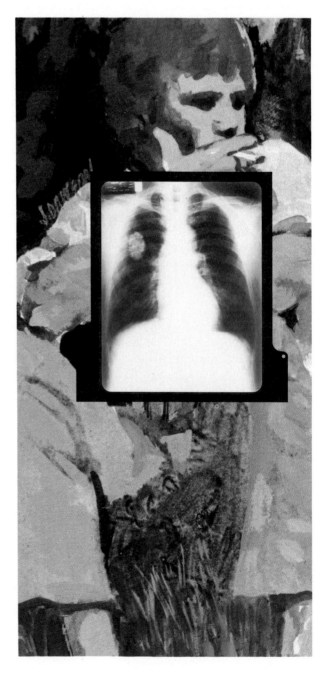

Puff after puff, smoke after smoke you'll live Life.

you'll love Life!

and emotional problems (tension, gratification of needs, and so on) through smoking, produces a profound psychological dependence.

The peculiar effects of nicotine and the convenience of cigarettes together make smoking an "ideal" drug abuse. The initial effect of nicotine is mildly stimulating—a lift—but the lingering effect is felt as mild depression setting up the need for the next cigarette, which can be conveniently carried, lit, and held.

Other important factors related to the taking up of smoking includes parents' smoking, peer smoking, low academic achievement, boredom, lack of alternatives, and adult role playing. To many adolescents, smoking represents a sort of puberty rite and is symbolic of independence from parents and teachers.

SOLUTIONS TO THE SMOKING PROBLEM

Many of the things that can be done to deglamorize smoking, reduce starting, and reinforce quitting have already been initiated, such as the elimination of television and radio advertising of cigarettes and the required label warning, "The Surgeon General has determined that cigarette smoking is dangerous to your health."

In the United States, the trend seems to be taking a turn for the better. Between 1966 and 1970, more than 13 million Americans successfully quit smoking. The dropoff—for whatever the reason—reduced the percentage of male smokers to 42 percent and women smokers to 31 percent in 1970, compared to 52 percent and 34 percent respectively in 1966.

How such a reduction in smoking might improve the national health is suggested by what happened following the decision by thousands of doctors in England and Wales to give up smoking ten years ago. Among the doctors who stopped smoking, the rate of lung cancer dropped 35 per-cent, while the rate remained steady in the rest of the population.

Still, there is much more to be done than telling someone why he should stop smoking, if a national campaign is to be truly successful. The health reasons for not smoking are obvious, but generally they do not discourage the abuse. Young smokers, for example, are not particularly frightened by threats of major illness that may not strike for thirty or forty years. They may be influenced more by findings showing that breathing is harmed no matter what age is involved. Every phase of lung function is impaired when cigarette smokers and non-smokers of the same age are compared. The airways are narrower and gas transfer is reduced, so that less oxygen gets to the blood and body tissues.

There are many economic, social, and political forces that make the quick elimination of cigarette smoking unlikely. The 600,000 farm families who produce the 2 billion pounds of tobacco consumed every year experience lung cancer at the same increasing rate as the rest of the population, but will statistics convince them that they should change their occupation? Will a congressman from a tobacco-producing state agitate for the elimination of cigarettes if it means political suicide?

The federal government finds itself on both sides of the fence. On one side it pays out money to underwrite an aggressive antitobacco crusade, and on the other it props up tobacco manufacture with agricultural subsidies. And, although it is the U.S. Department of Health, Education and Welfare that is designated to attack cigarettes, federal agencies—including HEW—benefit from the more than 2 billion dollars that the government receives every year from tobacco taxes. Similarly, hard-pressed state and local governments collect their own cigarette tax money, amounting to approximately 2 billion dollars a year.

Other major beneficiaries of the tobacco culture

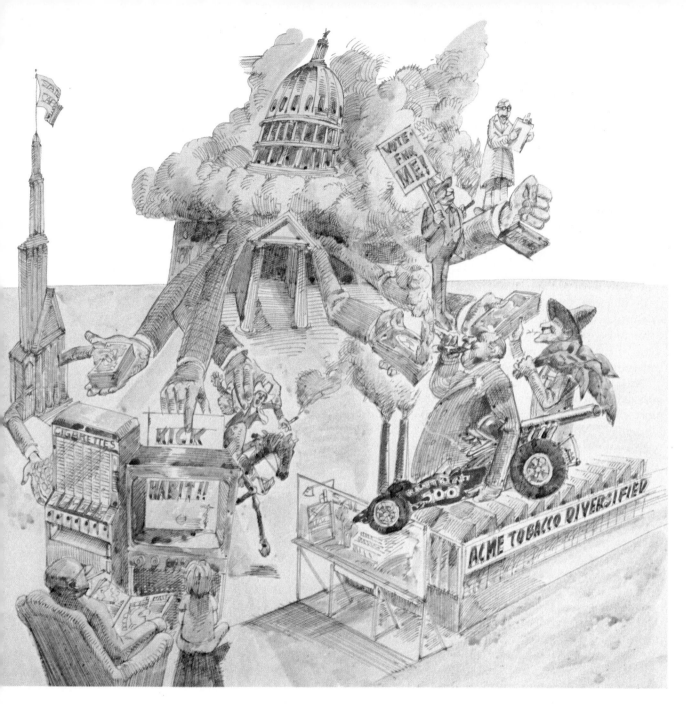

Figure 9.4   Government has an ambiguous role in the perpetuation of cigarette smoking. While financing antismoking campaigns and banning cigarette advertising, it subsidizes the tobacco industry.

are the advertising men who so energetically sell it, the magazines, newspapers, and billboard owners who prosper through cigarette advertising, the thousands of people who manufacture, ship, and sell cigarettes, and the distributors and vending machine operators who together grossed more than 8 billion dollars from cigarettes in 1970 alone.

Pervading this aggregation of pleasure seeking, vested interests, economic pressures, and personal greed is the obstinate insistence of the tobacco industry that there is no link between cigarette smoking and ill health. At the same time, the fact that the industry did invest the time and money to develop a new line of filter cigarettes suggests that they must have put the filters there for some purpose. Whether it was the pressure of public opinion or thirty years of medical findings that prompted them to do so, the approach has at least reduced some of the smoking hazard, according to most of the studies carried out throughout the world.

Any attempt to reverse the course of the self-inflicted epidemic growing out of cigarette smoking must start with the individual. He can stop smoking himself or help other people stop smoking. In the process, the economic and political factors may give way to the more important factor of improved health.

For Those Who Smoke

For those who feel that they cannot bring themselves to give up smoking immediately or completely, HEW has a scheme that has already worked to reduce health problems in numerous cases:

One should choose a cigarette with less tar and nicotine. For many of the reasons discussed in this chapter, cigarettes with reduced tar and nicotine levels might be less harmful. Periodically HEW publishes lists, prepared by the Federal Trade Commission, that detail the tar and nicotine content of leading cigarettes. In addition to improving health, there is some evidence that the low-nicotine brands may help reduce the urge to smoke.

One should not smoke a cigarette past the halfway point. Tar and nicotine accumulate in the butt end of the cigarette as it is smoked. Smoke from the first half of the cigarette contains only 40 percent of the total tar and nicotine, with the remainder concentrating in the other end. If one smokes only half the length of a cigarette before putting it out, he will inhale fewer toxic substances than if he smoked more of it.

One should puff less. By taking fewer puffs on a cigarette, a smoker will draw less harmful material into his respiratory system.

One should try not to inhale. When smoke enters the lungs it does the most damage. Inhaled smoke also promotes the cardiovascular changes that bring on heart attacks and high blood pressure.

One should try to cut down. Smoking fewer cigarettes a day is a nondrastic step in the right direction of giving them up altogether. A smoker should pick a time of day when he promises himself not to smoke. It could be before breakfast or perhaps while driving to work. It also helps to put cigarettes out of easy reach.

The Bigger Picture

In the long run, smoking is more than an individual problem. It affects so many people adversely at such tremendous cost to their health and pocketbook that it has created a nationwide problem.

More and more national governments are confronting the problem, but it is obvious from several studies that people will not stop smoking simply because the government tells them that cigarettes are harmful. Much more effective, if the American experience is any indicator, are private and government-inspired educational programs coupled with controls on advertising, labeling, and distributing. The tobacco industry could conceivably share in the task by developing less hazardous types of cigarettes. Some types of filters do part of the job, but there remains the distant technological possibility that tobacco researchers might be able to process tobacco in such a way that it becomes relatively harmless. It is perhaps futile to suggest that advertisers soften their cigarette sell, but they bear much of the moral responsibility for creating nations of smokers.

A recent report prepared for the World Health Organization by C. M. Fletcher and Daniel Horn stresses that any large-scale approach must focus on educating the young with well-documented evidence illustrating the health hazards connected with smoking. They suggest that it would be relatively easy to build information about smoking hazards into health, science, physical education, or social studies courses at an early age. Parents also must participate in the educational process by heeding the information already available on the hazards of smoking and influencing their children directly by giving up smoking themselves. Physicians can play a major role, say Fletcher and Horn, by checking on the smoking habits of their patients, advising them to cut down or stop whether their health is already impaired or not.

What role can the nonsmoker play? First, he can recognize that the 250,000 to 300,000 excess deaths per year from smoking plus the vastly increased disability and suffering are national social and health problems ultimately affecting the welfare of all. He may then feel more disposed to openly express his antismoking views and thereby contribute to the gradual erosion of the traditional acceptance and reinforcement of smoking. He can campaign for the rights of nonsmokers. For example, increasingly smokers are being asked not to smoke or to put their cigarettes out in closed rooms, airplanes, and other such places.

All of these approaches may help create a new psychosocial environment in which smoking becomes universally acknowledged as the "nation's leading preventable cause of disability and death," as former Surgeon General William H. Stewart described it. The new environment may in turn create an increased public demand for stricter controls on the promotion, manufacture, and sale of cigarettes.

When one bears in mind how many other health hazards exist in the world, it is rather remarkable to learn from the World Health Organization report the real magnitude of the cigarette smoking problem. Fletcher and Horn note that

> smoking-related diseases are such important causes of disability and premature death in developed countries that the control of cigarette smoking could do more to improve health and prolong life in these countries than any other single action in the whole field of preventive medicine.

Conceivably the combination of education and informed legislation will put man in the position where he can begin to curb the epidemic that he himself created.

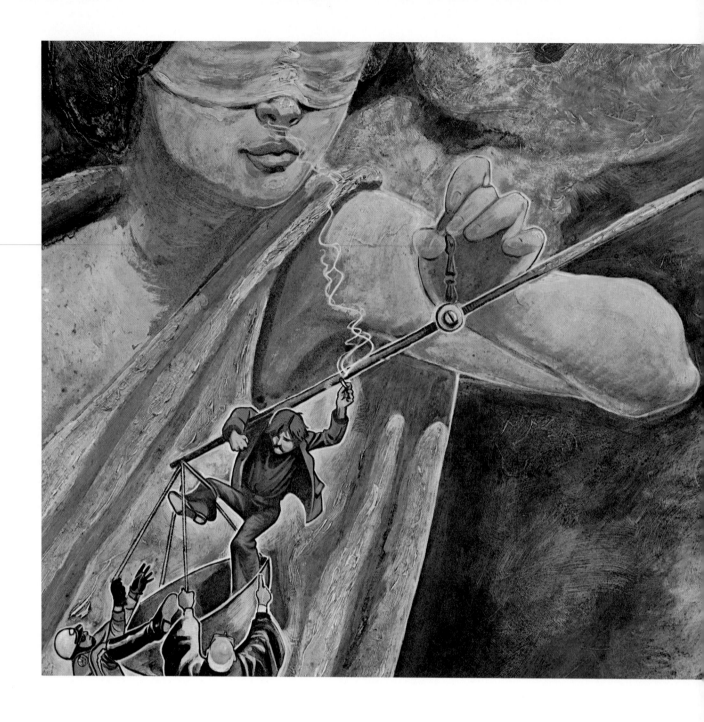

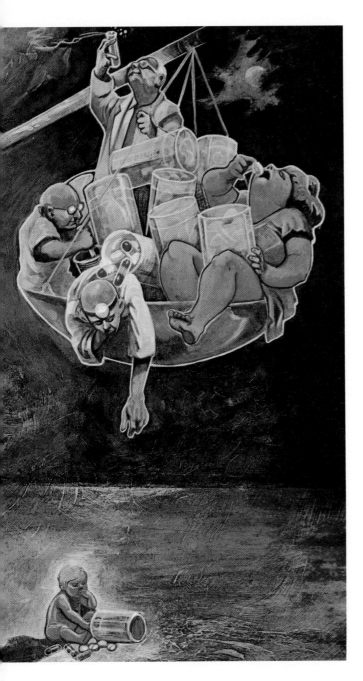

10

There seems to be no single, simple solution to the problem of drug misuse and abuse. Society's attempts at trying to solve drug problems or pretending to solve them are reflected in the laws governing drugs in the United States and elsewhere in the world.

Complete prohibition by law does not halt use. In 1919 the United States outlawed, by constitutional amendment, the manufacture, transportation, and sale (but not possession) of alcoholic beverages. Instead of giving up alcohol entirely, however, most adult Americans got it from bootleggers. Violations of and disrespect for the law were so great, in fact, that in 1933 the amendment was repealed as a bitter failure.

Furthermore, there is almost unbelievable inconsistency, lack of logic, and injustice in drug laws. A man can be sent to prison for life in some states merely for possessing marijuana (on a third offense), although there is ample evidence it is not as harmful to the body as alcohol or the compulsive use of tobacco. One may legally get high on alcohol without risk of arrest, as long as one does not drive recklessly, collapse in public, assault others, and so on. Yet one cannot get high on marijuana without violating the law, even though alcohol is addicting while marijuana is not.

The line between legitimate, socially acceptable medical administration of a drug and its illegal use

Controlling Drug Use and Abuse

may be a fine one. Administration of morphine under physician's prescription to deaden pain after an operation is not a crime. But if a patient becomes addicted to morphine while hospitalized and seeks more of it afterward to keep himself on an even keel, he is immediately considered a criminal.

Barbiturates, tranquilizers, and stimulants also are socially acceptable, but when an individual who has no medical need for them buys them without prescription, he, too, is considered a criminal drug abuser. In contrast, LSD might potentially be useful in treating alcoholism and certain other mental disorders, but even medical use is prohibited by law except in rare instances.

This chapter, then, will look at the broad problem of drug control, concentrating on the psychoactive substances, as do all chapters in this unit. Who abuses these drugs, and how do people get them? What laws aim at controlling them? And finally, how may the most severely addicted, the heroin users, be treated?

PATTERNS OF DRUG USE AND ABUSE

The fact that drug controls are being debated day after day at all levels of government reflects the epidemic status of drug use and abuse in America today. The epidemic persists in the tenements of Harlem, permeates small midwestern towns, and flourishes up and down the long coast of California. Now the junkie is no longer just the underprivileged black or Mexican-American. He, the pill abuser, or the alcoholic may just as easily be a well-to-do young man or woman from the middle or upper class. Marijuana use particularly has spread to hundreds of thousands of professionals and subprofessionals who represent substantial income and "solid" community standing.

School district officials in San Francisco, New York, Chicago, and other large cities are worried over the fact that in 1970, half of all high-school seniors had used illegal drugs other than alcohol and nicotine by the time they graduated, and 95 percent had used illegal alcohol, tobacco, and marijuana. Uppers, downers, pot, smack—high-school students know the vocabulary and think they know what the drugs can do to them.

Although the illegal drug culture originates in the large cities on each coast, it has a way of sending major ripples into the national mainstream. The ripples spread in a number of ways: through personal contacts between drug dealers and users, at rock concerts, glamorization in underground newspapers, and the sensationalism advanced by their overground equivalents. This spread of drug use reflects youth's ability to move quickly to be where the action is, peer-group pressure, and a natural curiosity inspired by continual discussion of drugs in the media and in social groups. Each drug has its own profile of use and abuse, as will now be described.

Heroin

Estimates of the number of heroin addicts range from 250,000 to 400,000, not including the tens of thousands of addicted American soldiers in Vietnam. About half of the American heroin addicts live in New York City, about 25,000 in California, and the rest are scattered throughout the country, mainly in the largest cities. The heroin abusers are mostly men in their twenties and thirties from minorities and the lower socioeconomic level. In American society, where heroin has been driven underground and the price artificially inflated, their addiction means that each of them requires from 350 to 500 dollars a week—a staggering 20,000 dollars a year. Additional hundreds of thousands occasionally use it or other illegal narcotics.

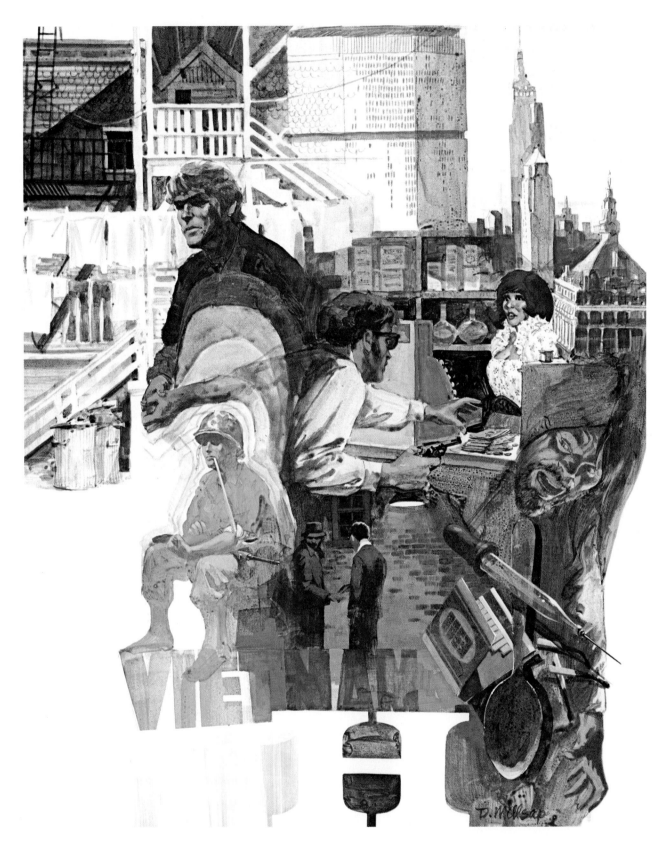

Figure 10.1 Today narcotics abuse is not confined to minority-group members in the ghetto but can be found among GIs in Vietnam and middle-class young people. Heroin addiction does not automatically lead to crime. Nevertheless, drug tolerance requires more and more of the drug, requiring more and more money. It is the need for money that often drives the heroin addict to crime or prostitution.

Heroin has become the "GI's other enemy" in Vietnam, one that according to many American officers is getting to be more threatening than enemy firepower. According to 1970 estimates, 30,000 to 40,000 servicemen who had never used heroin before are heroin abusers, and the numbers have been skyrocketing even higher since the autumn of 1970. The drug is openly available to American troops at less than one-tenth of the price it would cost in the States, as well as in a twenty-fold purer form. Most of these men will return to civilian life as full-fledged heroin addicts, condemned to a life of street addiction and crime that they are totally unprepared for.

Pills

There are somewhere between 5 and 10 million users of amphetamines in America. About 100 billion amphetamine pills are produced each year, and more than half are diverted into the illegal drug scene. Amphetamines are abused by hundreds of thousands of people, including older middle-class men and women getting such pills as Dexedrine or Benzedrine on prescription and young black-market users of methedrine ("speed freaks").

Some 10 million persons take barbiturates and other sedatives as sleeping pills or as tension relaxers, and amphetamine abusers sometimes use them to balance a super-high. The pharmaceutical industry makes enough barbiturates each year to provide forty pills for every man, woman, and child in the United States. Because they are prescribed so widely by physicians, they are exceedingly common in the middle-class drug-taking community, and with their ready availability on the black market they also are quite popular as "downers" in the youth drug culture. It is estimated that there are several hundred thousand barbiturate and other sedative abuser-addicts in the United States. Most are over thirty. Barbiturate overdose is the most common form of adult suicide in America.

Alcohol and Nicotine

Considering the sheer impact of the destroyed health, drunk driving, ruined careers, broken families, and associated misery that it has inflicted on society, alcohol is undoubtedly the most troublesome drug that has ever plagued mankind. In the United States, 90 million people drink regularly, and 7 to 9 million are addicts, or alcoholics. More than half of the 55,000 highway deaths each year are attributed to alcohol. In volume of sales, alcohol exceeds any other drug on the open or underground market. Alcohol users represent all social, economic, and occupational groups and all ages from the low teens (even though illegal) upward.

Nicotine is consumed in tobacco smoked by some 60 million Americans of all levels and ages. Although cigarette smoking is a major contributor to a number of diseases, tobacco is socially acceptable, encouraged, and available to everyone, including those under eighteen for whom it is illegal, with few restrictions.

LSD-type Drugs

In the mid-1960s, LSD was favored by the hippies and by some of the mystically and intellectually inclined. LSD use appears to be declining now, although it may simply have gone underground. Ongoing users of the LSD family of drugs number around 100,000 and are mainly in their twenties. From 5 to 6 percent of college students admit that they have tried LSD or related psychedelic-hallucinogens at least once, and probably as many as 1 million Americans have used such drugs at least once. As with heroin, the degree of experimentation among high-school students is higher than for college students. About 150,000 American-Indian members of the Native American Church use peyote (mescaline) as part of their religious cermonies.

The Marijuana to Heroin Controversy

by Carmen James Pace

Over the years there has been much speculation regarding an association between the use of marijuana and addiction to heroin. While many professionals in the field of drug addiction no longer associate the two drugs causally, some do postulate a cause-effect relationship between the two. The lay public has widely adopted the view that the primary danger of marijuana use is that it almost invariably leads to heroin addiction.

My experience as a psychotherapist and psychiatric social worker suggests that this is not the case at all. Based on clinical work with marijuana users and heroin addicts and discussions with college students who regularly use marijuana, I have found that the two drugs satisfy quite antithetical personal needs. Thus they appeal to individuals who seek completely opposite effects from their drug experience.

I reached this conclusion after counseling hospitalized heroin addicts and spending several years in contact with drug users through various outpatient psychiatric clinics and in my private practice of counseling and psychotherapy. Most of the heroin addicts I worked with were inner-city blacks, while most of the marijuana users—and comparatively few of the heroin addicts—were lower, middle, and upper-middle-class whites.

It is not uncommon to hear critics of marijuana exclaim triumphantly that most heroin addicts used marijuana prior to using heroin. In questioning heroin addicts, however, I found that those who did start on marijuana switched to heroin not because they liked marijuana and wanted something similar and more potent, but precisely because they did not like marijuana. Although most of the several hundred heroin addicts I dealt with had used marijuana prior to using heroin, comparatively few claimed to enjoy the marijuana "high."

Furthermore, the overwhelming majority of heroin addicts explained that they had used marijuana only once or twice and never again. This fact suggests that most of these addicts probably did not even experience the effects of marijuana because they never learned how to smoke it. Marijuana, after all, is not smoked in the same manner as a commercial cigarette or pipe tobacco. One must learn how to smoke it before one can experience the marijuana-induced euphoria. Even those who do learn how to smoke marijuana usually realize no effect until the drug has been used several times. Hence, it would be difficult to maintain that marijuana creates a craving for heroin since most heroin addicts have realized no effects from their use of marijuana.

But what of the heroin addicts who, in their preheroin days, used marijuana enough to learn how to smoke it and to achieve some reaction? I found that these men were able only to muster a half-hearted "It's okay," or "It's all right," in praise of the

Adapted from Pace, C. J. "The Marijuana to Heroin Controversy," *Union College Symposium,* Vol. 4, No. 9. (Winter 1970/71), pp. 32–34.

drug. The majority of heroin addicts on whom marijuana had an effect reported an uneasiness with the drug or a fear of it. The men seemed to fear the loss of control over mental processes that they felt the marijuana brought about. Their most commonly expressed concern was that marijuana "messes with your mind." They also considered it "freaky" and said it gave them "crazy" thoughts.

Why don't heroin addicts like marijuana? To try to answer that question, one must be aware of what both drugs can do to the user. Marijuana is classified as an hallucinogen. Although manifested to a much milder degree, most of the phenomena associated with the LSD "trip" are present in marijuana-induced euphoria. The user senses that consciousness has been heightened and that his perception has been altered. Frequently his perceptions of space and time are distorted. Often there is a feeling of clearer thought and deeper awareness of immediate happenings. Increased sensitivity to sound and a merging of senses (synesthesia) are not uncommon. At times, there is a feeling that the senses are being flooded by stimuli. The overall effect of marijuana—and to an even greater extent, of LSD—is a sense that the doors of perception have opened, revealing new worlds of experience.

The typical heroin addict, however, does not wish to open the doors of perception; he wants to close them. He wants to contract consciousness, not expand it. Heroin is the vehicle for what sometimes amounts to a nearly complete loss of involvement in the external world. Feelings of anxiety ebb, to be replaced by sensations of warmth, calm, and relative inner peace. The external world fades and becomes hazy. Even when he is not high on the drug, the heroin addict's life is such that his perception is so narrowed that what happens around him becomes little more than a blur. When he isn't high, he is trying to score, to obtain more heroin. The activity of trying to score is so intense as to preclude almost all introspection, fantasy, and general awareness that is not directed toward the goal of obtaining more heroin. Consequently, scoring and being high interact to create a narrowing of perception of external as well as internal sensations, since thought and fantasy are minimized.

The need to blur or eradicate thought and fantasy was suggested by a number of my experiences with addicts. While working with a group in an art class, I found that only rarely did one of the members attempt anything creative. Most copied photographs or magazine pictures. Some even traced other pictures. They seemed to avoid all imaginative activity.

This need to keep the mind void was emphasized by several addicts when I questioned them regarding their tolerance for introspection and fantasy. One patient discussed his inability to read a particularly vivid novel about drug use. He explained that at a certain point he was forced to close the book because he was becoming too anxious as he read, that the novel stimulated associations and fantasies too fearful to bear. Another patient who was unable to complete the book offered the same explanation.

One man I counseled talked of his intolerance for fantasies during masturbation. When he masturbated, he used as a stimulus a picture of a woman rather than his imagination. He said that this was common among hospitalized male heroin addicts. He was also adamant in maintaining that it is "bad" to let yourself create "pictures in your mind."

In discussing their reasons for returning to heroin, relapsed addicts emphasized their need to shut out external stimulation. At first, they claimed that boredom was the principal reason. When confronted in group or individual therapy, however, they were willing, if reluctantly, to discuss their true thoughts and feelings. As they talked, the addicts revealed a growing obsession with personal problems, whether financial, marital, or vocational. This concern had generated intolerable tension and anxiety, so it was a need to escape from these thoughts and feelings, rather than boredom, that drew the users to heroin.

Of all the regular marijuana users I have known, comparatively few have even tried heroin. None has become addicted to it. Those I knew who tried heroin did so sporadically over a period of months before abstaining from its use for good (or at least until now, and that covers several years). They refrain from heroin in spite of the fact that they have relatively easy access to it. They do so, it seems, because they have no liking for heroin's effects and because they fear the addict's life, which turns him into a frantically driven outlaw.

Almost all the marijuana smokers, however, have used and enjoyed the effects of LSD. In most instances, marijuana preceded the LSD but all who used LSD continued to use marijuana and to enjoy its effects. Those who are satisfied with the hallucinogens avoid the regular use of heroin because they have no craving to limit their perception. Instead, they seek the increased awareness and giddy euphoria of marijuana as well as the more intense feeling of functioning on new levels of consciousness provided by LSD.

Even as I write this article [October 1970], a vigorous debate is in progress in New York State regarding the question of whether marijuana and heroin are causally linked. According to one news report, a U.S. Attorney has opposed legalization of marijuana on the grounds of a "statistical link" between the two drugs, to the effect that most heroin addicts had first used marijuana. Such an argument is spurious and misleading, to say the least. For example, almost all addicts probably used alcoholic beverages before they took up heroin. Are we to draw from this the conclusion that drinking liquor causes heroin addiction? One could go on. All heroin addicts probably took aspirin, ate ice cream, kissed their mothers, and did any number of things in common earlier in their lives. Did these activities lead to the addiction?

Another problem with the statistics presented is that they usually give only half the story. They tell us that almost all heroin addicts first used marijuana; they rarely tell us how many habitual users of marijuana went on to heroin addiction. My experience leads me to the conclusion that very few marijuana users proceed to heroin. And when they do, the succession has nothing to do with their past marijuana experience.

One argument sometimes used to link marijuana as a dangerous predecessor of heroin is that buying marijuana brings the user into contact with those who sell the harder drugs. This argument is basically weak because, the quality of our times being what it is, anyone attending high school or college or living in the inner city who wants hallucinogenic or opiate drugs will find them readily available.

I am not trying to make a sales pitch for marijuana. As I stated earlier, use and enjoyment of marijuana does seem significantly linked to the subsequent use of the dangerous drug LSD.

Whether or not a person will abuse a drug, and the drug he will choose to abuse, depends on his own personal needs. The universal need of the marijuana smoker, I believe, is for a consciousness-expanding experience. That need is quite the opposite of what the heroin addict seeks, a contraction of consciousness.

Marijuana

On a world-wide basis, marijuana is used by an estimated 250 million people in its various forms. Dr. Stanley Yolles, former director of the National Institute of Mental Health, estimates that 25 million or more Americans have tried the drug once and that a million are probably confirmed "pot heads" who have built marijuana into their way of life. The armed forces estimate that about 30 percent of the troops in Vietnam smoke marijuana regularly, but many returning GIs insist that the actual proportion is at least twice that. Various surveys show that 50 percent of high-school juniors and seniors and college undergraduates admit marijuana use; and some children at the sixth-grade level admit having smoked pot at least once. Although most marijuana users are under thirty, an increasing number of older housewives, lawyers, doctors, businessmen, policemen, and artists are using pot as well as cocktails in their socializing.

Although marijuana cultists talk about pot as a replacement for alcohol, more drinkers use marijuana than nondrinkers. One major study of marijuana use concluded that although many marijuana smokers tended to take an antiestablishment point of view, most users were "reasonably conventional" in their attitudes and behavior.

DRUG TRAFFIC

The term "drug traffic" usually refers to illegal activity, involving either legally permitted drugs that are improperly manufactured or sold or ones that are entirely illegal. However, it also could include all production and distribution of mind-altering drugs, including alcohol and tobacco.

Alcohol and Cigarettes

Alcohol and cigarettes are usually purchased from retail outlets selling the products legally. Although most of the traffic is aboveboard, there is still considerable bootlegging and illegal selling of alcohol, especially in the South and Southwest. It is estimated that the 75 million gallons of illegal spirits produced in the United States every year cost federal and state governments 1.5 billion dollars in lost tax revenue. Criminal aspects of the alcohol traffic involve illicit production and smuggling to avoid taxation, bribery of regulatory agents and police, illegal sales to minors or intoxicated individuals, and drunk driving.

The multimillion-dollar illegal cigarette traffic is mainly limited to smuggling from states where cigarette taxes are low—such as North Carolina—to highly taxed states, such as New York.

The Pill Traffic

According to drug policemen, about half of the more than 20 billion doses of barbiturates, stimulants, and tranquilizers produced in the United States end up in the illegal drug traffic. The leakage can occur anywhere in a chain of distribution that includes the pharmaceutical manufacturers, wholesalers, physicians, dentists, drugstores, veterinarians, researchers, and the individual users. Some drugs are synthesized in illegal laboratories or smuggled in from Mexico and other countries, or they may be sold to illegal distributors by salesmen, pharmacists, or physicians. A particularly profitable and common technique is for a pharmaceutical firm to ship large amounts of pills to a distributor in a foreign country. From there the pills are smuggled back to the United States and sold illegally at a large profit, though a lesser one than occurs with the heroin traffic. Both amateurs and organized crime are involved in this pill-smuggling racket.

LSD-type Drugs

LSD, STP, mescaline, and psilocybin traffic is a much less formal, generally amateur endeavor, but several illegal manufacturers do make large profits on them. The user may resort to natural sources of these drugs, such as the mescaline-containing peyote cactus or the *Psilocybe mexicana* mushroom. People with the right equipment and some competence in chemistry can manufacture LSD from its chemical building blocks, or, more easily, they produce the amphetamine derivative STP. On the illicit market, the psychedelic-hallucinogens cost anywhere from one to five dollars a "trip." Because the dose is so small (the equivalent of 30,000 doses could be put in one aspirin tablet), a little LSD goes a long way. It has been distributed through the underground in hundreds of bizarre ways: on the backs of postage stamps, in sugar cubes, in cookies and crackers, and on the tip of a handkerchief.

Marijuana

Most marijuana is smuggled from Mexico into California; smaller amounts come from Morocco, Ne-

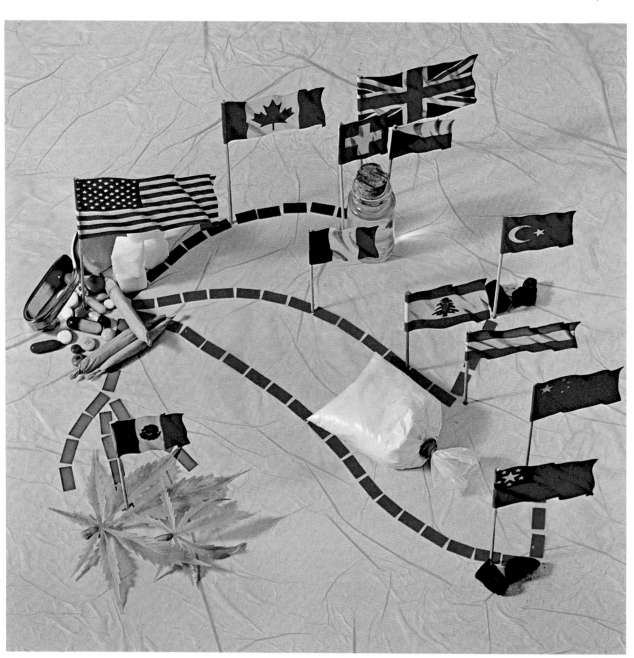

pal, and South Vietnam, and some is cultivated within the United States. When marijuana was primarily used by blacks and Mexican-Americans, organized crime had a stake in this lucrative traffic because it overlapped with the distribution of heroin. In the 1960s and 1970s the Mafia and other groups have been phased out by the amateur and semiprofessional distributors who may even abhor the profit motive. Some believe that their trade is socially useful, that the drug is beneficial, and that attempted controls by the federal government are ridiculous in scope and purpose.

No one knows what the marijuana traffic grosses annually, but crude estimates put it at hundreds of millions of dollars. Marijuana is not nearly as profitable to sell as heroin, from which an investment of a few thousand dollars can escalate to a million dollars in profits after repeated cutting. A full tobacco can or "lid" of marijuana might cost ten dollars to the small-time dealer and can be sold for fifteen to twenty-five dollars. One lid contains about one ounce, enough marijuana to make about thirty marijuana cigarettes, or joints.

Students or "street people" operating as medium-scale distributors may buy a kilo (a kilogram, or 2.2 pounds) of marijuana from a big distributor for anywhere from 160 to 200 dollars; they can then break it up into "dime bags," which sell for about ten dollars apiece. These bags usually contain about three-quarters of an ounce. A total 200-dollar investment could then net about 450 dollars. Often people will sell just enough to pay for their own supply.

Narcotics

Most illegal opium products, including heroin, are produced in Thailand, South Vietnam, Burma, Laos, and the People's Republic of China; Turkey, Lebanon, and Syria; and Mexico. In the United States, the Mafia or Cosa Nostra is alleged to be the chief heroin distributor. Heroin dissemination usu-

ally originates with wholesalers in the big cities and then radiates out through an assortment of middlemen to the neighborhood pusher and his clients. By that time the once-pure drug may have been diluted to about 5 percent of it original strength. The addict can buy enough of the impure product for a fix in a little envelope or "bag" that costs between five and twenty-five dollars, depending on the part of the country in which it is purchased.

Profits are huge in the heroin trade. Twenty pounds of the drug can net a grower about 300 dollars in Turkey, while the retail income produced can be as much as a quarter of a million dollars. Raw opium is converted first into its active ingredient, morphine, then into heroin in chemical plants near the point of origin, then packaged and smuggled into the United States and other countries by many different routes. It is estimated that about 3,300 pounds of heroin enter the United States annually.

DRUGS AND THE LAW

Drug-abuse legislation in the United States has been based on an escalating policy of punishment of the "dope fiend" and, if that does not work, more punishment. The attitude has been reinforced as the number of addicts grows higher and society insists that addiction is a sure sign of criminal behavior—not a potentially solvable medical problem. Until recently, federal, state, and local legislative units attempted to badger the drug-taker by passing ever more repressive laws. They also extended the laws to other drugs that happened to inspire social hysteria. Where narcotics were once the targets of drug-abuse legislation, the dragnet has expanded to pull in users and traffickers in barbiturates, stimulants, and marijuana.

Drug legislation in the United States is a fairly recent development. In the mid-nineteenth century, everybody's favorite aunt might have been an opium taker. The narcotic could be purchased legally in pharmacies and in general stores, and

Figure 10.2 Drug traffic routes. One route for opium and its derivatives begins in Red China (*bottom red line*). From there raw opium travels to Burma, where it is transported to the rest of Asia as either raw opium, morphine, or heroin, and then to the U.S. as morphine and heroin. The second opium route stems from Turkey (*top red line*). After the conversion of raw opium into morphine in Iran, the next stop is Lebanon. The opiates then arrive in France (Paris and Marseilles), where the final processing of pure heroin takes place before transporting it to the U.S. Once in the U.S. various distributors cut the pure heroin

with either milk, sugar, quinine, or less pure ingredients. The legal and illegal traffic of "pills" is basically within the U.S. However, some supplies are shipped legally to other countries such as Mexico and then reenter the U.S. illegally. LSD, originally produced in Switzerland, also now comes from England, Canada, Italy, and Czechoslovakia (*black line*). Usually in a liquid state to start, LSD's most widely used forms of supply are sugar cubes, capsules, crackers, pills, and powders. Marijuana is mostly grown in Mexico and smuggled across the border into the U.S. in the form of bricks and lids (*green line*).

cough medicines and patent preparations of the day were heavily laced with it, often combined with alcohol. Every snake-oil salesman and traveling medicine man peddled opiates to cure an endless variety of human ailments, ranging from arthritis to impotence.

By the turn of the twentieth century the narcotics users (sometimes addicts) became more visible. Many were victims of the opium-base patent medicines. In 1901 a special committee of the American Pharmaceutical Society warned that public consumption of narcotic drugs had become a serious problem. Five years later, the federal government passed the Food and Drug Act of 1906. Its chief effect was to force food and drug manufacturers to list the amount of alcohol and other habit-forming drugs on the labels of their products. But an individual was still free to buy whatever medicine he pleased and to take it for whatever ailed him.

The Harrison Narcotic Act of 1914 made the government and the physician intermediaries between society and dangerous drugs. "Dangerous" according to the definition of the day meant that they were unsafe for self-medication because of their addictive properties or other harmful effects. For the first time the law required a prescription for such drugs—mostly narcotics. Over the years the dangerous list has been extended to include other potentially harmful drugs, such as penicillin, sulfa drugs, stimulants, and barbiturates. Prohibition of alcohol from 1919 to 1933 was in many ways the most far-reaching and unsuccessful drug law. The Marijuana Tax Act and similar state laws intensified the process of criminalization.

In 1951, the Boggs Act shifted the focus entirely away from physicians. Stiff sentences were meted out for the possession or sale of narcotics or marijuana (which was considered a narcotic in all state laws). Under the provisions of the Boggs Act, first-offense convictions for narcotics possession brought a sentence of two to five years with the possibility of probation. Second offenders could expect a sentence of five to ten years without probation or the possibility of a suspended sentence, whereas three-time losers could look forward to ten to twenty years without probation or sentence suspension.

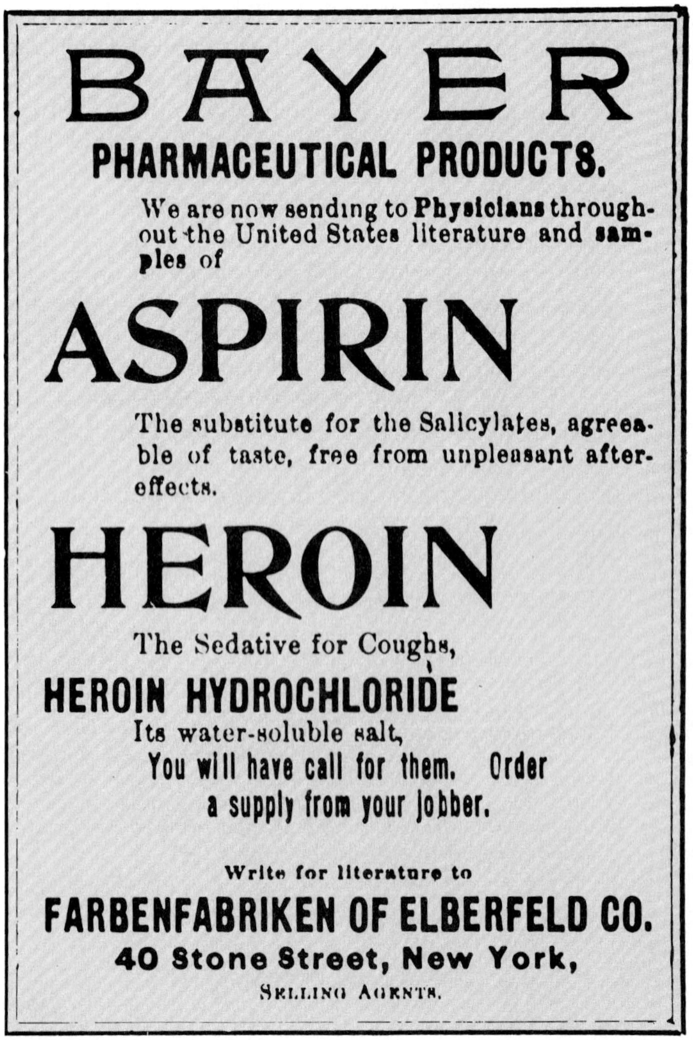

Figure 10.3 Narcotics were active ingredients in many patent medicines sold around the turn of the century.

The laws got still stiffer with the passage of the Narcotic Drug Control Act of 1956. Sentences were increased at all levels on a rising scale leading to a mandatory ten to forty years (with no concessions) for third offenders. If a pusher sold heroin to someone under eighteen, he could get the death penalty. Judges and parole boards no longer had any discretion about the length of imprisonment, and the long sentences left little room for rehabilitation even if it was available. Most states built their own drug-control laws around the federal statutes, in many cases exceeding the original's severity.

In 1965, the government passed the Drug Abuse Control Amendment to strengthen the federal role in controlling the increasing traffic in sedatives and stimulants by imposing stricter regulations on the illegal manufacture and distribution of these drugs. In 1967, LSD and similar drugs fell under the same regulation. Until 1968 this federal law specifically excluded simple possession of these drugs as a crime concentrating, as did Prohibition, on sale.

The Marijuana Act of 1937 had been prodded by several years of national hysteria in which the product of the hemp plant received even wider scare publicity than heroin. Even though marijuana had not been scientifically determined to be addicting or significantly harmful (and still has not been except for individual variation), the law was easily passed by an uninformed Congress preoccupied with other matters. In any case they did not worry about losing any votes, since, at the time, the chief users of marijuana represented relatively impotent segments of society: jazz musicians, a few intellectuals, Negroes, and Mexican-Americans.

The Trend Changes

As the drug culture of the 1960s expanded from alcohol, tobacco, and marijuana to include LSD, mescaline, barbiturates, and stimulants, the long arm of the law also clamped down on them. Although they were undoubtedly health hazards, they were dealt with much less severely than marijuana, a far safer drug. At the same time, minimal restrictions on the new drugs were extended to the drug manufacturer and the pharmacist.

During this time there was a noticeable change in sentiment about the drug problem and what should be done about it. People began to discover that the drug users were not only social undesirables (the junkies, hippie "freaks," felons, and ghetto dwellers), but the apple-cheeked sons and daughters of middle-class America. Governor's sons were picked up for smoking pot, high-school valedictorians primed themselves with stimulants, and bouncy cheerleaders sought the hazy content of the downers. When the legislators saw the extent of drug use in these polite corners of society, they wondered if it was really appropriate to send a handsome young football player to prison for ten years because he smoked a marijuana cigarette or tried LSD. The drug problem became part of the youth problem and made the covers of *Time* and *Newsweek*. It was only then that many of those who had shouted loudest for the blood of the drug user in the past began to suggest that drug-abuse legislation might deserve a second look.

On December 28, 1970, President Nixon signed into law the Comprehensive Drug Abuse Prevention and Control Act, a new schedule of federal drug penalties designed to replace and update the older narcotics laws and to meet the needs of the drug epidemic of the 1970s.

Under the new law, illegal possession of narcotics, such as opium, morphine, and heroin, or of cocaine is punishable by imprisonment of up to one year and/or a maximum 5,000-dollar fine for a first offense. Second and subsequent offenses are punishable by up to three years imprisonment and/or a maximum fine of 10,000 dollars.

Illegal drug distributors or those who have narcotics in their possession for the purpose of sale face up to fifteen years in prison and/or a 25,000-dollar fine for a first offense with a mandatory parole period of three years. For any subsequent offenses the penalties are doubled. The new Act comes down especially hard on adults over eighteen years old who sell or give a narcotic to a person under twenty-one years old. In such cases a first offense can net the pusher up to thirty years imprisonment, and he can be jailed forty-five years or more for subsequent offenses. Individuals who make a continuing business of illegal drug distribution face ten years to life for a first offense along with a 100,000-dollar fine. For a second offense, the fine and ten-year sentence are doubled.

The Drug Abuse Act of 1970 extended the penalties on illegal distribution and possession of barbiturates and stimulants to manufacturers, processors and their suppliers, wholesale druggists, individual pharmacists, hospitals, clinics, public health agencies, and research laboratories. They all must now keep accurate records of all these drugs received and dispensed. The law also imposes stricter controls on the marketing of barbiturates and stimulants and could eventually lead to the imposition of production quotas by the federal government for the more commonly used pills.

For LSD and other hallucinogenic drugs the new drug law is as harsh on the drug pusher as it is for heroin, barbiturates, and sedatives, but it is much less severe on young first offenders. On a first offense for possession, a person under twenty-one years old may be placed on probation and his conviction can be erased from official criminal records if he meets the requirements of a probationary period. Second and subsequent offenses are punishable by three years imprisonment and a 10,000-dollar maximum fine.

Until December 1970, federal law said that possession with intent to sell or sale of marijuana was a felony, punishable by a mandatory two to ten years in jail for a first offense and twenty to forty years for further offenses. A young marijuana offender could thus become ineligible for a driver's license, could not enter a profession such as medicine, law, or teaching, and could not obtain a passport. His record would also make it very difficult for him to find a responsible job in business or industry.

With the new law, the penalties are still severe for traffickers in marijuana, but individual possession for sale or giving away of marijuana is now a misdemeanor, rather than a felony. Minimum mandatory penalties also were eliminated by the new law and reduced significantly to a maximum of one year for a first offense and three years for subsequent offenses. Fines range from 5,000 to 10,000 dollars. Also, for a first offense, a person under twenty-one years of age may be placed on probation in lieu of sentencing, after which the official record of arrest, trial, and conviction can be erased. Although most states continue to treat marijuana as a felony and as if it were a narcotic, they are now being forced to lessen the severity of sentences in line with federal statutes. A listing of state drug laws and penalties is provided in the Appendix.

Local judges now have considerably more leeway in determining how seriously a marijuana offender should be punished for his crime. Drug policemen are increasingly disregarding marijuana use, much as they ignore the illegal alcohol and tobacco use by those under twenty-one or eighteen.

One controversial aspect of the new federal bill is the "no-knock" provision, which, with a few restrictions, allows police to search premises for illegal drugs without the ordinary warrant and without knocking (wiretapping homes suspected of involvement with illegal drugs had previously been authorized). The main provisions of the federal law specify five classes of drugs whose use, possession for sale, and sale are illegal. Class I drugs carry the

Figure 10.4 Help for addicts. (*top left and right*) Young addicts take part in a confrontation session at Odyssey House, a privately supported rehabilitation center in New York City. The boy and girl on the right are eleven and fifteen, respectively. (*bottom left*) The addicts are kept busy doing work around Odyssey House. (*bottom right*) An Odyssey House staff meeting at which the problems of one young addict are discussed.

most severe penalties and are regarded as the most dangerous; included in this category are morphine, heroin, marijuana, LSD, mescaline, and other drugs outlawed for medical use. Class II drugs include opium, cocaine, medically used narcotics, and injectable methamphetamine. Class III drugs are the barbiturates, amphetamines, and "mild" narcotics such as codeine. Class IV drugs include chloral hydrate, meprobamate, and the milder barbiturates. Class V drugs include the medically useful psychoactive drugs with the lowest abuse potential, such as tranquilizers, for which the penalties are the mildest.

This new legislation gives unusual powers to the U.S. Attorney General (rather than to the Secretary of Health). He makes the final decision as to which category a new drug belongs in on the basis of its "potential for abuse." Although he is to consult a scientific panel that he designates, he is not required to follow its advice. It is feared by many drug experts that emotional, political, and even economic criteria may now play an important role in classifying drugs.

TREATMENT

When abuse of narcotics occurs, treatment, short-term and long-term (rehabilitation), is necessary to overcome the effects of drugs and to allow addicts to lead normal lives. Some suggestions for the

treatment of alcoholics are given in Chapter 8. This section will be devoted principally to programs used for those who are addicted to narcotics, especially heroin. For all forms of drug abuse a comprehensive, flexible approach is desirable with the stress on long-term outpatient care.

In the United States, treatment for heroin addiction has been almost nonexistent, often involving "cold-turkey" withdrawal in jails or hospitals, incarceration in the U.S. Public Health Service installations at Lexington or Fort Worth or in state and federal prisons, or extended medical and psychiatric care in a hospital or clinic. Various self-help groups, such as Synanon and Daytop, based on Alcoholics Anonymous principles, try to provide a more intensive and supportive environment for rehabilitation.

The Public Health Service Hospitals were originally established to treat merchant seamen addicted to drugs. Since then, most of the hospitals' population has been made up of addicts voluntarily seeking admission but usually leaving within thirty days rather than the recommended five months. Since 1935 more than 80,000 "patients" have been admitted to the USPHS hospitals, with most of them receiving no specific therapy beyond gradual withdrawal of the drug, followed by psychiatric evaluation and often by job training or group therapy.

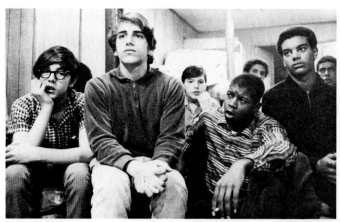
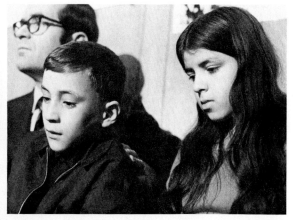
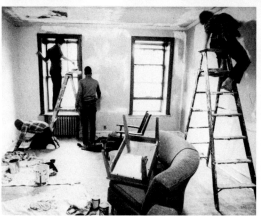
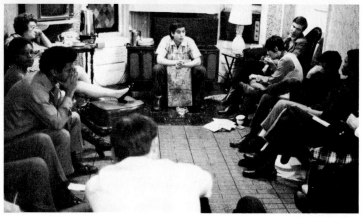

Figure 10.5 Drug treatment at Vista Hill Hospital. This treatment orientation includes extensive evaluation to determine the underlying emotional problems that contribute to the person's need for drugs. Turning to self-destructive drugs often brings these disturbances to the surface and, for some, is an overwhelming cry for help. This clinical approach requires long periods of time to unravel the puzzling problems that lead to drug abuse. The patients admitted to Vista Hill do so voluntarily—however, it is often an alternative to jail or the California Youth Authority. The treatment program includes group therapy, which is led by a psychiatrist. While group therapy can help the patient to express his feelings and thoughts, Dr. Don Schwerdtfeger, a staff psychiatrist, feels its most important functions are to teach the patients constructive social interaction and to allow the psychiatrist and staff to view and evaluate the patients so that accurate diagnoses can be made. A major concern, however, is that because part of the patient's problem is an inability to accept or relate to authority, with a psychiatrist in the room the person's conversation and actions may be so guarded that group therapy is of little diagnostic value to the doctor. He relies more on nonverbal communication (facial expression, gestures, physical confrontation), actions, and conflicts that take place during "nontherapy" hours of the day for indications of the patient's true feelings, fears, etc. Traditional psychodrama, in which defenses are torn down and feelings are forced out, is not the goal of the psychodrama at Vista Hill. "We are dealing with people who have weak defenses—they are fragile, supersensitive kids. They don't need to *express* emotions, they need to learn how to *control* them and channel their tremendous energies in constructive, rather than self-defeating directions. You wouldn't fix a broken vase by smashing it—these kids are in pieces and our goal is to help them glue themselves together." These kids are violently outraged and rebellious—the patient-staff water fights are tremendously helpful in breaking down barriers. The rage that is bursting inside of the kids can come out in a nondestructive, acceptable form. The group sessions with the parents of the Vista Hill patients give the doctors an opportunity to discuss openly and realistically the problems of the patients and the fears and hang-ups of the parents. As the parents learn to confront the entire syndrome of the drug problem through interaction with other parents and the psychiatrist, the psychiatrist has the chance to determine whether the patient, once he leaves Vista Hill, should return home or go to a halfway house, school, or correctional institution that might offer a better chance for growth and acceptance than would the home environment. The parent must be ready to admit and understand that his child's drug problem is a syndrome that he (the parent) is definitely a part of. Therapeutic drug treatment is central to the rehabilitation program. Many of the patients are totally intractable and unable to handle the everyday tasks of living unless the "steam" is taken out of their impulses by large doses of tranquilizing medication. Privileges must be earned; the rules are strict, but from these limitations the patient learns something that he has probably never experienced before—responsibility for his own actions and behavior.

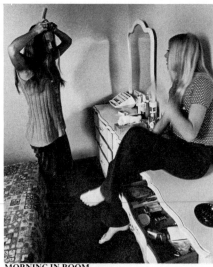

MORNING IN ROOM

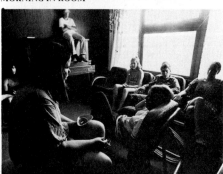

PSYCHODRAMA

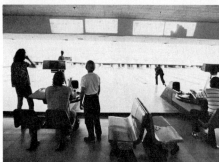

BOWLING

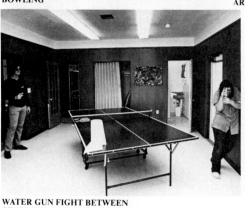

WATER GUN FIGHT BETWEEN STAFF MEMBER AND PATIENT

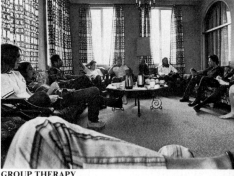

GROUP THERAPY

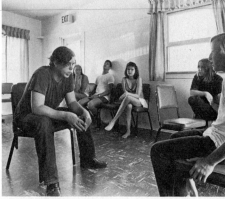

PSYCHODRAMA

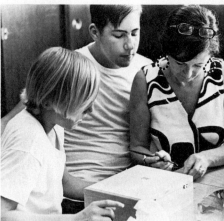

ARTS AND CRAFTS

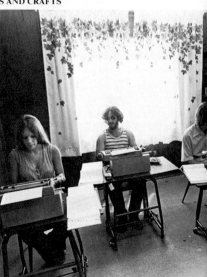

OCCUPATIONAL THERAPY

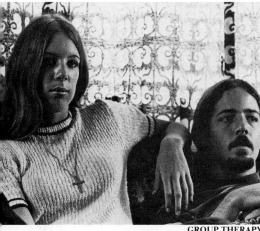

GROUP THERAPY

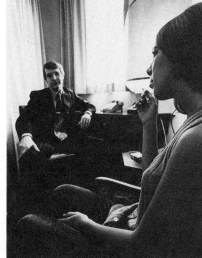

INDIVIDUAL THERAPY

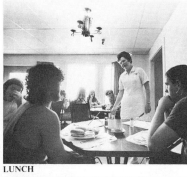

LUNCH

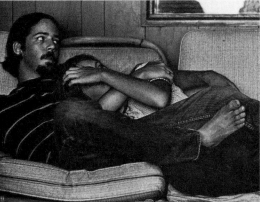

LEISURE TIME

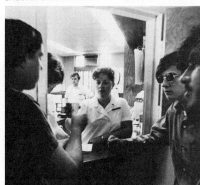

DRUG MEDICATION

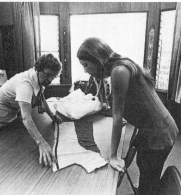

OCCUPATIONAL THERAPY

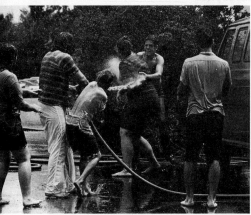

WATER FIGHT BETWEEN STAFF AND PATIENTS

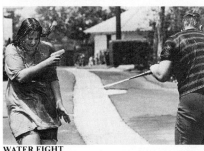

WATER FIGHT

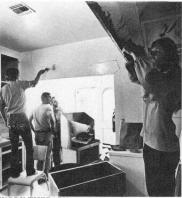

WORK THERAPY

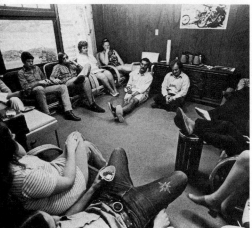

RAP SESSION BETWEEN
STAFF AND PATIENTS

PATIENT WITH PARENTS

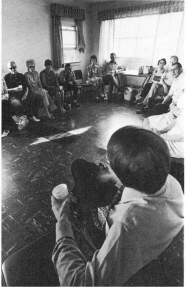

SESSION WITH PARENTS
AND STAFF PSYCHIATRIST

There are few effective after-care or treatment programs in the community and little in the prison-hospital, so the relapse rate is high.

The California Rehabilitation Center (CRC) was established in 1961 within the state prison system to treat addicts found guilty of misdemeanors or felonies under civil-commitment proceedings. The "patients" live at the center for about fifteen months, during which time they work, get vocational training, have group therapy, and if they desire, receive a full academic course through high school. Once the patient is released, he is tested about once a week to see whether he has returned to drugs. If he has, he must go back to CRC. He remains under supervision of parole officers for many years. The relapse rate is more than 50 percent, and in some years about 90 percent.

Since 1966, New York State has been running a similar civil-commitment program for the treatment of addiction. The program is administered by the State Narcotic Control Commission, conducts basic clinical and statistical research on addiction, operates methadone maintenance rehabilitation and after-care centers along with a program of education, care, and community referral. It is still too early to say how this new comprehensive program is faring, but it appears that the methadone maintenance programs are producing the best "heroin-free, crime-free" results. The criterion for cures, used to establish uniform reporting of cure statistics, is the patient's ability to live for at least one year without heroin and without committing any crimes.

Synanon was first established in California in 1958 as a private antiaddiction society. The organization, which has now expanded to other states, is entirely made up of and managed by long-time residents, including addicts, alcoholics, and others, aided by volunteer doctors and other professionals. The addict seeking admission is first screened by a committee, and if he is admitted his character and compulsion to take drugs are broken down by group pressure using an intense "game" and around-the-clock living supervision. If he does not respond, he is expelled; if he does, he can move up into the higher levels of the society. As of January 1971, Synanon listed approximately 1,500 drug-free members in its society, although it does not provide data on its failure or client-rejection rate.

Other antidrug self-help groups such as Addicts or Narcotics Anonymous, Daytop, and the Family provide close interpersonal support, alternatives to drug use, and motivations for abstinence. As with group and individual psychotherapy, it is difficult to evaluate how effective they are in rehabilitating addicts.

Methadone Maintenance Treatment

One of the most active and promising programs now under way to help heroin addicts involves the use of the long-acting narcotic drug called methadone. Methadone itself is addicting but because it is a long-acting orally active narcotic, it produces few of the problems found with heroin, can be taken once a day, and is inexpensive. Methadone has been used as a pain-killer in Europe and the United States since World War II and for the withdrawal treatment of heroin addiction since the 1950s. In 1964 Drs. Vincent Dole and Marie Nyswander of Rockefeller University found that they could keep addicts off heroin by slowly building up a daily maintenance level of methadone that blocked the effects of heroin and had little euphoric effect itself. Since the Dole-Nyswander studies, which still continue, the methadone treatment has been introduced in hospitals and clinics and by private doctors in many cities, with the largest and most ambitious programs currently located in New York City and Washington, D.C. Use of the methadone treatment involves a program of various therapies—vocational, recreational, emotional, and so on—one of which is the administration of the drug.

In the New York program and others like it, the heroin addict comes daily to drink down a dose of methadone in a cup of orange juice. Within weeks he has lost his craving for heroin and is able to stop the criminal activity he was forced into to support the expensive habit. In most maintenance programs he then continues indefinitely to take 60 to 120 milligrams daily. Regular urinalyses are done to detect any use of heroin, other narcotics, amphetamines, or barbiturates.

The cost for each person treated is about 500 to 1,500 dollars a year, compared to yearly prison costs of 5,000 to 10,000 dollars. While on methadone, the ex-heroin addict can live an essentially normal life, working or going to school without the worry of where the next fix is coming from.

Drs. Dole and Nyswander note that about 82 percent of the first 700 patients treated in their clinic are still participating in the program and leading socially acceptable lives. Smaller programs in California and other states report similar results. About 8,000 former heroin addicts are now involved in more than 100 methadone programs in the United States.

To prevent individual physicians from treating heroin addicts in their offices with methadone, the FDA and Federal Bureau of Narcotics and Dangerous Drugs have set up new guidelines for the use of methadone requiring that the drug be given only under conditions of close supervision and scientific evaluation, usually in hospitals and clinics.

Among the potential problems associated with methadone is possible death through overdose, particularly when combined with other depressants such as alcohol, heroin, or barbiturates. Other objections to methadone treatment, however, are philosophical. Many opponents feel that methadone is simply a tool for making ghetto "rebels" into "useful" members of society, thus making the alienated individual conform to the rules of society without solving the underlying causes of his addic-

tion. In addition, any program that requires lifelong addiction is held in suspicion by many.

Methadone maintenance represents only one method for helping heroin addicts; it should be used with discrimination and individualized, with the addict participating in the decision. When used, it should be as one part of long-term, comprehensive services all with the goal of moving the former heroin addict toward freedom and independence from drugs, including methadone (which can and should be gradually decreased as soon as the individual on maintenance has achieved a social reorientation) and independence from government programs or psychiatric help.

Cyclazocine and Naloxone

Cyclazocine and Naloxone are long-acting opiate antagonists that are being used experimentally in the treatment of heroin addiction. If an addict is gradually built up to a daily dose of 4 to 6 milligrams of cyclazocine, the effects of heroin will be completely blocked as long as the drug is used. The results are at present inconclusive.

TOWARD A SOLUTION

In seeking a solution to the drug problem, one must remember that the direct result of antidrug legislation in the United States for the last sixty years has been to turn the drug abuser into a criminal. The pattern has been: make a law against the possession or sale of a harmful or possibly harmful drug, then jail those who run afoul of the law and hope they learn their lesson. This approach does not take into account the degrading atmosphere of prison and the wholesale association with hardened criminals and a large number of other addicts that may push the addict toward real crime. Prison can in no way be considered a solution to whatever problem motivated the person to become a drug abuser. Aside from probation, no real attempt is made to see that the prisoner's drug problem is al-

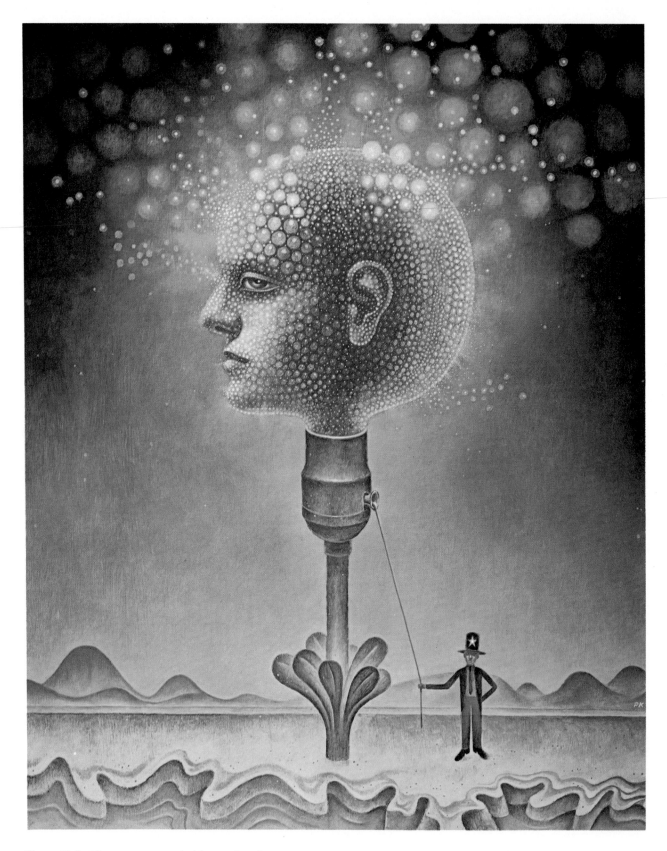

Figure 10.6   If government can legislate against drugs,
may it some day *require* people to take them?

leviated when he returns to the streets, so the record of criminal law and prisons in rehabilitating drug addicts or abusers is extremely poor.

With marijuana, the situation is even more counterproductive. Possession or sale of this drug has been treated with the same vehemence as heroin. Millions of people, most of them young, have been criminalized by laws passed by uninformed and emotional politicians. Whether he is a prisoner or not, a young marijuana smoker is still living outside the law. Because he finds that marijuana is not the horror politicians, police, and the AMA say it is, he loses respect for the marijuana law, for all laws, and for the "establishment."

In his book, *Marijuana—The New Prohibition*, which stresses legalization as the only solution, Stanford law professor John Kaplan contends that if "pot" laws have any benefits, they are far outweighed by the damage they have done to American society and American justice. The current approach, he says, ties up courts and police in a hopelessly enlarging enforcement effort, breeds disrespect for the law, spreads suspicion between children and their elders, and turns a large segment of the younger generation into criminals. He claims that in California alone during 1970 it cost about 72 million dollars to prosecute more than 70,000 marijuana offenders, monopolizing one-fifth of the time of probation officers and judges.

Legalization of marijuana has been endorsed in many quarters as one way to reduce the criminalization of the young associated with the drug. Others object, however, saying that legalization would only confer social acceptance on another health hazard, as it has for alcohol and tobacco.

Others believe that real (honest, comprehensive) education about drugs is the best way to reduce drug use among the young. The goals would include helping them to make more rational and discriminating decisions about drug use, demythicalizing drugs, and providing positive alternatives to drug use. A successful teaching effort would require community support and the backing of health professionals, the educational establishment, prominent citizens, and the youth themselves.

In San Francisco area elementary schools, a program now under way emphasizes a human ecology approach in drug education. This program starts with the concept of what ingestion of a foreign chemical into the body means—what it means when mother takes an aspirin, what it means when daddy smokes a cigarette. This approach moves pill-taking away from the concept of taking something illegal to taking any potentially harmful chemical into the body.

Recently, the federal government focused more strongly on the educational approach to controlling drug abuse by initiating a massive teacher-education program throughout the United States. Its purpose is to give teachers and the schools the primary responsibility for drug education and to separate it from an approach based on law enforcement.

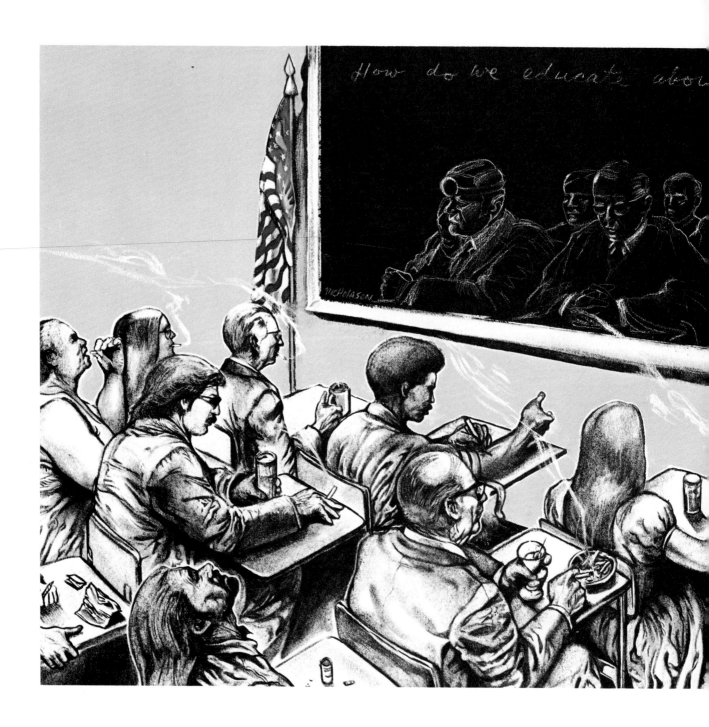

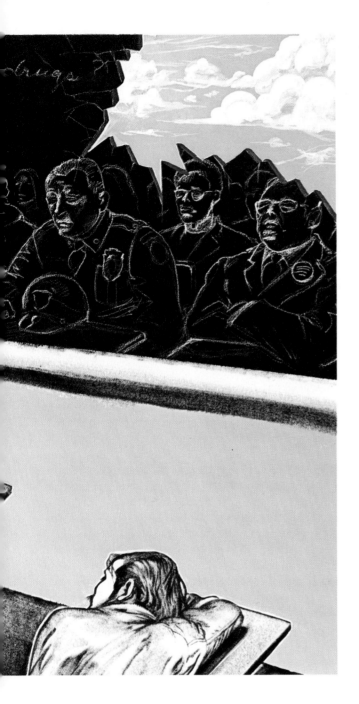

11

As has been shown in the preceding chapters, the use of such mind-altering substances as caffeine, nicotine, alcohol, marijuana, and opium is far from a new phenomenon but rather has a history of many thousands of years during which men and women have sought artificial paradises, escape, relaxation, and pleasure. What *is* new is the tremendous attention drug use and abuse are receiving from society, politicians, and mass media. The increasing pervasiveness of drug use in practically all segments of society and the multiplicity of substances used by the average consumer have alarmed many people.

None of the consciousness-changing substances are totally harmless, inherently beneficial, or necessary for human life. All have some risks and all, including the barbiturates, amphetamines, and tranquilizers, have some benefits under appropriate conditions.

DRUGS AND SOCIETY

There are many reasons why people use drugs, including the fact that the United States has become a society in which the use of mind-altering substances is institutionalized and people are conditioned to relate to other human beings or to deal with all pains, problems, and troubles through the use of drugs. To many, young and old, drugs are "where it's at," the quickest way to alleviate the pain of being unable to cope in a complex or painful environment. This is an age of advanced technology, with the majority of the population fearing

Drugs in Perspective

loss of identity and lacking inner-direction. With so many drugs readily available, it becomes understandable why increasing tens of millions of people are finding life more acceptable by drinking, smoking, dropping pills, injecting, and sniffing.

Drug use and abuse are human problems and are symptomatic of much in the individual's life and of the society in which he operates and with which he seeks to cope. Because there are many kinds of drug problems involving many different drugs, any solution will have to be multifaceted.

Expectations and evaluations of the capacity of drugs to produce both good and evil vary widely. Many people attribute all bizarre, criminal, antisocial, or unacceptable behavior to the effects of certain substances that they define as "the drugs"; conversely, many other people see instant happiness, genius, and solutions to all problems in certain drugs. The manufacturers and the ad agencies guarantee sexual pleasure, eternal youth, and joy from alcohol, tobacco, and pills. In actuality, with average or moderate doses the major factors in a drug response are the personality of the person using the drug and the environment in which the drug is taken.

The most severe problems associated with drug use and abuse come not from the direct effects of the drugs but rather from the effects of the American system that attempts drug "control." Thus the crimes most people attribute to the effects of heroin are not from the heroin, which tends to make people drowsy and passive, but rather from the artificially inflated price and the need to steal or prostitute oneself in order to obtain the large sums of money required to buy a "fix" on the black market. Even long addictive use of heroin, morphine, or other narcotics produces no permanent damage to the body, no mental illness, and no criminal behavior as a *direct* result. The destructive effects of an arrest record, of imprisonment or institutionali-

zation, and stigmatization as a "head," "freak," or "junkie" are fairly obvious but rarely are balanced against the real or imagined destructive effects of the drug that these policies are supposed to eliminate. What is missing almost entirely from the drug scene is context, perspective, logic, rationality, and an ethical framework.

THE DRUG CREDIBILITY GAP

The American system, which holds a laissez-faire attitude toward alcohol and tobacco while applying increasingly severe criminal penalties to both user and trafficker in other drugs such as marijuana and heroin, has been notoriously and obviously unsuccessful and destructive in its antidrug efforts. Responsibility for this approach and its failure lies with those political and administrative leaders of the United States who often prefer to aggrandize their own careers and deal in images, committees, commissions, and press releases rather than with the complex realities of modern life.

Sensationalism

The most common technique of communication used by politicians, journalists, and organized medicine is the one-dimensional, viewing-with-alarm, out-of-context statement. As a striking illustration, suppose that a given drug were described with the following statements, all of them correct. The drug has been used for many decades by hundreds of millions of people, but it is not known how this substance works on the body and brain to produce its effects. Further, several thousand children in the United States die or are disabled each year from accidental overdose of the drug. Finally, this drug has been found to produce birth defects in lower animals. Confronted with such statements, many people would become enraged, ready to demand criminal penalties against anybody involved with distribution and use of such an obviously dangerous substance. If, however, they also were told that the drug is aspirin, they would be much less likely to respond hysterically. Instead, they would realize that a few facts had been carefully and deliberately selected out of context to make it seem that the substance is uniformly harmful and should be carefully restricted.

Similarly, if one were to hear a doctor with lengthy experience in treating skid-row alcoholics talk about all alcohol users as derelicts having severe liver and brain damage, hallucinations, and delusions, one would immediately recognize the distortion, and the doctor's statements would have no further credibility. It is strange, however, that when this technique is used with marijuana, heroin, or LSD, people often uncritically, naïvely, gullibly, and harmfully accept what the communicator says, particularly if he has a prestigious title.

LSD and Chromosomal Breakage

A more complicated example is the alleged damaging effects of LSD on chromosomes. Following an initial "scientific" article by an obscure geneticist in early 1967, the mass media began to focus considerable attention on this question. Evoking memories of the 1963 thalidomide disaster in which a widely used tranquilizer was found to produce malformed babies, these statements caused a strong current of fear, and few people were willing or able to impartially examine the actual evidence. A leading magazine put out a cover story on the evils of LSD, dominated by uncaptioned, unidentified photographs of deformed babies and of people in a state of fear. The article had such statements as: "If you take LSD, your child may be born malformed or retarded"—a meaningless statement because the second half of the statement is invariably true, so that any substance substituted for LSD in the first half, whether it be milk, nicotine, or aspirin, would not change the validity of the statement.

Although many articles appeared subsequently in the scientific literature detailing studies that found no chromosomal, genetic, or birth abnormalities from LSD, these studies usually failed to receive any attention in the popular press. Most people's impressions remained formed by the initial widely publicized study. The first study was based on an examination of only three samples of white blood cells exposed to high concentrations of LSD with no germ (sex) cells or embryos involved, no control group, inadequate methodology, and a strong bias expressed by the author who admitted that he set out to prove the harmfulness of LSD. Studies done with large samples and with high scientific standards have not found that LSD increases chromosomal breakage over the amount of breakage normally observed.

Some of these studies involve examination of white blood cells after their exposure in test tubes to varying concentrations of LSD, while others are concerned with chromosomal changes found in people who have taken street LSD. Complicating such interpretations is the fact that not only do black-market drugs contain a wide range of impurities, but drug identification and dosages are uncertain. Much of what is consumed as LSD is actually amphetamine, mescaline, or something else, so that neither users nor scientists later studying them know exactly what has been ingested. Furthermore, most drug users take a multiplicity of drugs during the same period of their life, sometimes simultaneously, which makes it almost impossible to attribute a given psychological or physical effect to a drug such as LSD rather than to some other drug or their combination.

Several studies with lower animals, including mice, rats, and hamsters, found that certain concentrations of LSD injected into the abdomen early in pregnancy produced a high rate of fetal abnormalities. Thus it seems fair to say that pregnant animals, human or otherwise, should avoid injections of LSD into their abdomen, uterus, or placenta during the first trimester (three months) of pregnancy. The broader picture is that during the gestation period almost all drugs can interfere with normal embryonic development (see Chapter 14). In any case, a direct effect of a drug on the fetus is quite different than an effect on germ cells or their genetic constituents. No studies have shown chromosomal changes in germ plasm from LSD or have elucidated distinctions between LSD use by the father rather than the mother, use five years before, one year before, or during pregnancy, use once versus many times, or use in varying doses.

Furthermore, chemicals closely related to LSD such as morning glory seeds and psilocybin mushrooms have been used for about twenty generations in parts of Mexico, and LSD itself has been used by probably more than a million people since its properties were accidentally discovered in 1943.

Unsubstantiated statements, or outright lies, whether about alcohol, marijuana, heroin, or LSD, are distinctly counterproductive when they are found out. They lead to increased rather than reduced drug use as the listener comes to disbelieve even what a more responsible and knowledgeable source of information would say about certain risks involved with drug use. Disillusionment and alienation, disrespect for law and for authority—all increase in proportion to the big-lie technique.

The honest and responsible preventive-health message that should have been communicated about LSD and birth defects is that if a pregnant woman decides to use potent mind-altering drugs, or other insufficiently known drugs, she should avoid doing so in the first three months of pregnancy, and she also should avoid exposure to any form of radiation, viruses, and other sources of possible injury, simply because the fetus is particularly susceptible to damage during this period.

TOWARD ELIMINATING DRUG HYPOCRISY

Moral or rational persons and societies would not minimize or ignore any aspect of the drug problem but would seek to relate to all of it in a humane and effective way. What use, for example, is it for a man to be saved from heroin only to die from alcohol, or saved from marijuana only to die from nicotine, coal tars, arsenic, cyanide, formaldehyde, and other toxic agents in tobacco?

Current policy is prone to "throw out the baby with the bath water": as part of the hysterical overreaction, marijuana research is stopped, just as private medical treatment of heroin addicts is barred, thus closing off many positive alternatives. Fortunately, such policy has stopped short of excluding narcotics from medicine, where they are one of the most valuable drugs and a boon to anyone in severe pain. Nevertheless, many doctors have been so frightened about the exaggerated dangers of addiction that they avoid giving sufficient doses of narcotics to those in great pain.

Another irrationality among many in the drug world is the extensive overprescribing and undersupervising of sedatives, stimulants, and tranquilizers by physicians. These drugs are a significant component of the drug-ridden society and are among the most prescribed and most refilled prescriptions. Devoting most of its attention to marijuana as it opposes all reforms of the drug laws, the American Medical Association has neglected to condemn the excessive production of these drugs or the prescribing of them, often in large quantities and for vague complaints, without thorough history-taking and physical examination.

Federal and state controls on these drugs are a mockery, with each patient being able to get as many as six prescriptions filled for any amount during any six-month period from any (or more than one) doctor; with drug companies able to manufacture as much as they want to; and with as much as half of the supply being diverted into the black market. The reason people have paid less attention to this aspect of the drug problem is that it is mainly among respectable, white, middle-class adults who are not thought of as deviants, pill heads, or junkies, even when they consume large amounts of codeine, morphine, Demerol, or narcotic cough syrups.

The full context of drugs includes not only the psychoactive ones, from alcohol to heroin, but also aspirin, antibiotics, antihistamines, and many others that when used selectively and appropriately are of great benefit to mankind, even though they always entail certain risks and possible side effects. The patient must therefore bear responsibility for the misuse or abuse of the medicinal kinds of drugs when he demands a pill or injection simply because he has heard or read something about it, or when he threatens to go to another doctor if his request is not granted.

The customs by which alcohol, tobacco, caffeine, and aspirin are accepted as safe recreational or medicinal substances (rarely thought of as drugs) and by which other pleasure-giving or recreational drugs are rejected are hypocritical if not absurd, illogical, arbitrary, and unworkable. Granted, the fact that people use and abuse alcohol and tobacco is not a logical reason to use any other drug. But it *is* logical to demand that abuse of alcohol and tobacco as well as pills be given the highest priority in press releases, public statements, appropriations, and programs related to drugs. Under standards for food and drug safety, and on the basis of present knowledge, neither alcohol nor tobacco could gain cultural or scientific approval if they were newly introduced in America.

Standards of abnormality, deviance, sickness, evil, and criminality are highly subjective and often hypocritical. People train themselves, and are conditioned, to ignore and deny unpleasant realities or inconsistencies and to stampede as a nation of sheep toward criminal law as the "solution" for what others define as "problems." Thus wiretapping and no-knock forcible entry into homes suspected of containing illegal drugs are publicly accepted, and sometimes more attention is given to marijuana than to murder.

Although increasing nonenforcement of marijuana possession laws can be expected—just as the laws prohibiting alcohol or tobacco for those under age twenty-one or eighteen are rarely enforced—what is called for most urgently is decriminalization of the user. Use of mind-altering drugs, understood to occur for a multiplicity of reasons, is best dealt with by education, prevention, and provision of positive alternatives rather than by modern equivalents of burning witches at the stake or throwing the mentally ill into snake pits.

THE FUTURE OF DRUG USE

People use alcohol, heroin, and other such substances because drug use is institutionalized, because they seek pleasure, escape, and individuality, because they lack hope (and imagination), and because the drugs have taken on symbolic significance that goes well beyond their pharmacological capabilities. Drugs also are used and abused to seek meaning, identity, insight; to attempt to relate to and touch others; and to cope with dependency, inadequacy, and anxiety. Rhetoric will not provide solutions, and arrogance of users or of tradition-bound professionals only intensifies the difficulty.

It can be expected that more and more people will use more and more drugs, including more risky ones, rather than face their problems and tackle the sources of their discontent. Increase in drug use will continue as long as society—and the people within it—finds itself incapable of dealing with ambiguity, complexity, and truth. Yet such an

THE PLEASURES AND HAZARDS OF DRUGS

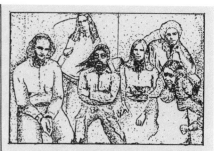

★ ★ ★ ★ ★ ★ ★ ★ ★ ★ ★ ★ ★

I would be far happier if my own teenage children would, without breaking the law, smoke marijuana when they wished, rather than start on the road of so many of their elders, to nicotine and ethyl alcohol addiction. Dr. R. D. Laing, quoted in **Drugs for Young People: Their Use and Misuse** by Kenneth Leech and Brenda Jordan

He really becomes a fiend with savage or "cave man" tendencies. His sex desires are aroused and some of the most horrible crimes result. He hears light and sees sound. To get away from it, he suddenly becomes violent and may kill. **FBI warning against marijuana quoted in Marihuana Reconsidered by Lester Grinspoon**

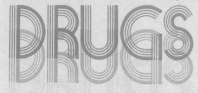

Look, Time, Holiday, Esquire, Saturday Evening Post and *Playboy* have had one or more feature stories [on drugs and the psychedelic movement] each since 1960 . . . These articles not only sell magazines, they also sell LSD. The blackmarket operators in LSD have benefited from millions of dollars' worth of free advertising. I am not implying by this any *intent* on the part of popular magazines or newspapers, of course. Their job is to report the news, even if in reporting it they also help to create it. From an article by Frank Barron in **LSD, Man and Society** by Richard C. DeBold and Russell C. Leaf

At least part of the meaning of LSD today is this: that chemical technology has made available to millions the experience of transcendence of the individual ego, which a century ago was available only to the disciplined mystic. From an article by Frank Barron in **LSD, Man and Society** by Richard C. DeBold and Russell C. Leaf

In a survey of drug use on two eastern campuses . . . administered a self-rating questionnaire in the classroom to 287 students, all but one of whom completed it. The investigators recognized the limitations of this sample, because it did not include absentees and drop-outs. From their data they characterized a typical marihuana user as "a liberal arts student, who reported somewhat looser religious ties than his non-drug using classmates. Many marihuana users classified themselves as agnostics or atheists, or reported preferring an Eastern religion such as Zen to the one their parents professed. Half the marihuana smokers expressed dissatisfaction with their school, in contrast to 20 percent of the nonusers." From **Marihuana Reconsidered** by Lester Grinspoon

The lessening of inhibitions and repression, the euphoric state, the feeling of adequacy, the freer expression of thoughts and ideas, and the increase in appetite for food brought about by marihuana suggest therapeutic possibilities . . . Summary of the 1938 Mayor's Committee on Marihuana Report quoted in The Marihuana Papers edited by David Solomon.

Obviously, the popular discovery of marihuana as a safe euphoric was imminent. Why the public emergence of that fact represented such a problem to authorities is a tantalizing question. It is hard not to speculate (as some prominent sociologists have done privately) that the upsurge of the use of marihuana in the thirties was opposed primarily by pressure groups in both the federal government and the newly revived liquor industry. The suggestion that the ban on marihuana might have been in part a result of a powerful liquor lobby does not seem improbable when one considers that a substantial public shift to marihuana might have created considerable competition to the sale of alcoholic beverages. From **The Marihuana Papers** edited by David Solomon

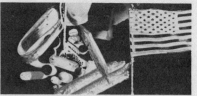

But what about a person who has become addicted, say, to heroin? Is there any hope of cure? Some doctors would say, "No"; and we have to admit that there are many facts to support them. The relapse rate for heroin addicts after going through hospital cures is very high indeed. One doctor who has had three hundred heroin addicts as patients says that in only a few cases can he claim that an addict has kicked the habit. This is a depressing prospect. From **Drugs for Young People: Their Use and Misuse** by Kenneth Leech and Brenda Jordan

increase need not be inevitable. It is perfectly possible to compete in the marketplace with the culture of alcohol, tobacco, and marijuana; to work toward the value of moving beyond drugs; and to make what drug use does occur as selective and discriminating as possible. Even if the broader pattern of increasing dependence on mind-altering substances for pleasure, relief of tension, and socializing does eventuate for the majority, one can still attempt to reach and change a significant minority to make them free, alert, involved, and self- (rather than drug-) confident.

For those who view with alarm the dangers of drugs, it is important to look not only at how drugs really work, but at the broader context of the other risks and dangers of life, including war, hydrogen bombs, cancer, accidents, fire, and so on.

For those who defend alcohol, cigarettes, pot, and the rest, it is important to understand that insofar as a drug brings pleasure, it does so only sometimes and is only one of many potential sources of pleasure, satisfaction, and meaning in life. Such sustaining values as love, interpersonal relationships, sexual pleasure, music, art, nature, sports, knowledge and learning, and continuous development of one's potential are alternatives to drugs. Parents, teachers, politicians, and other role models must make these alternatives increasingly known and available to children and must demonstrate them in their own life styles. Much more than a generation gap, there is today a hypocrisy gap that can only be bridged by living lives of consistency, practicing what is preached, and showing that people can relate to each other, be happy, and become civilized without depending on chemicals, legal or illegal, natural or manufactured, burned or swallowed.

Among the approaches to solving the many drug problems, emphasis should be placed on decriminalizing personal use or possession while concentrating criminal law and enforcement on behavior harmful to others—such as drunk driving—and on major traffickers in *all* unacceptable drugs. Honest educational programs should be instituted, to be presented by specially trained classroom teachers starting in elementary school. Comprehensive out-patient rehabilitation programs for alcoholics, cigarette smokers, heroin addicts, LSD bad trippers, and other drug abusers need to be provided; and more fundamentally, an attack must be made on the roots of alienation, and alternative sources of hope and pleasure must be made available. The more that going to school or work is made a mind-expanding experience, the less likely are people, young and old, to turn to chemicals for real or alleged consciousness-changing effects.

Besides asking "why not?" about use of drugs, simply because they are not as "dangerous" as arsenic or a gun, people need to begin to ask, "why?" Whether or not one chooses to use drugs of any kind should be an independent, inner-directed, free decision in the total context of one's life and the context of choices available, rather than an automatic response or a counter-reaction to someone else's use or views of drugs. Improved family and school communication in an atmosphere of mutual trust and respect, openness, and love will certainly help to bring about this independent choice.

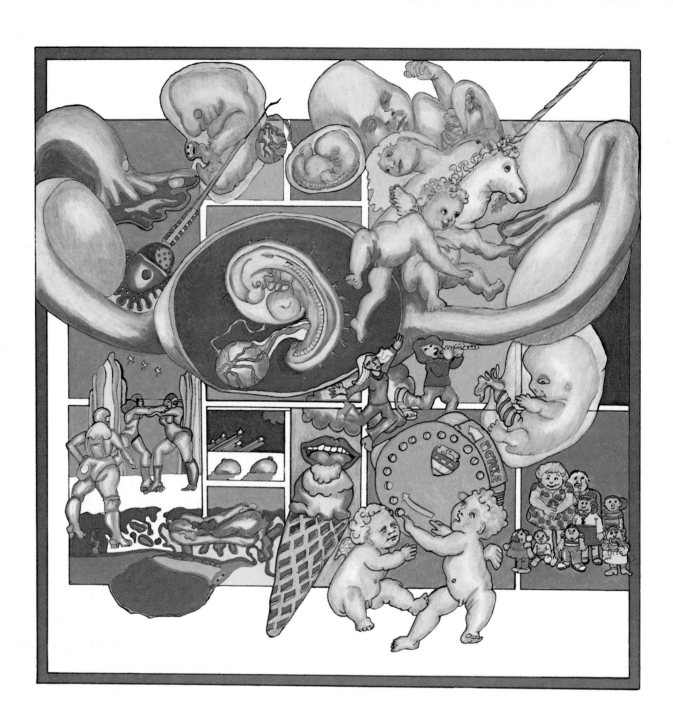

IV FAMILY HEALTH

Man's sexual nature has preoccupied his attentions and dominated his activities to a greater extent than any other aspect of his existence. It has served variously to facilitate individual health and to inhibit it: to some, sexuality has provided deep fulfillment; to others it has brought profound suffering. Patterns of the expression of sexuality vary widely among human cultures, from extreme suppression in some to extreme openness in others. Understanding one's nature as a man or a woman and understanding one's sexual needs are vital to optimum health. ¶ Sexuality brings with it a responsibility—the possibility of producing a new human being through procreation, pregnancy, and birth. The joys of motherhood have been praised throughout history, but today's expectant mother often is fraught with anxiety over the possibilities of having a child with birth defects. Like sexuality, the process of reproduction must be fully understood before superstitions and fears will be allayed, and knowledge of heredity can provide prospective parents with at least some inkling of what their children will and will not be like. ¶ Sexuality also implies marriage in most societies. But is marriage a necessary part of human society, particularly that of modern America? Is the new trend toward group marriages and "living together" without legal sanctions a sign of the future demise of marriage as it is known today? These are a few of the questions discussed in Chapter 15, "Marriage in American Society." ¶ Most people today do get married, and they do have children, with or without full knowledge of the physiology of sex and reproduction and the mechanisms of heredity. Since the advent of "Dr. Spock," child psychology has been a popular and controversial subject among middle-class Americans. Just exactly how much do parents affect their children's psychological development? What makes a good or bad parent? Should everyone be a parent? These topics are the focus of Chapter 16. ¶ Sexuality, marriage, parenthood—these are all aspects of "family" life, the fundamental level at which humans interact with one another. The kind and quality of such interaction can have a profound effect on an individual's well-being, both psychological and physiological.

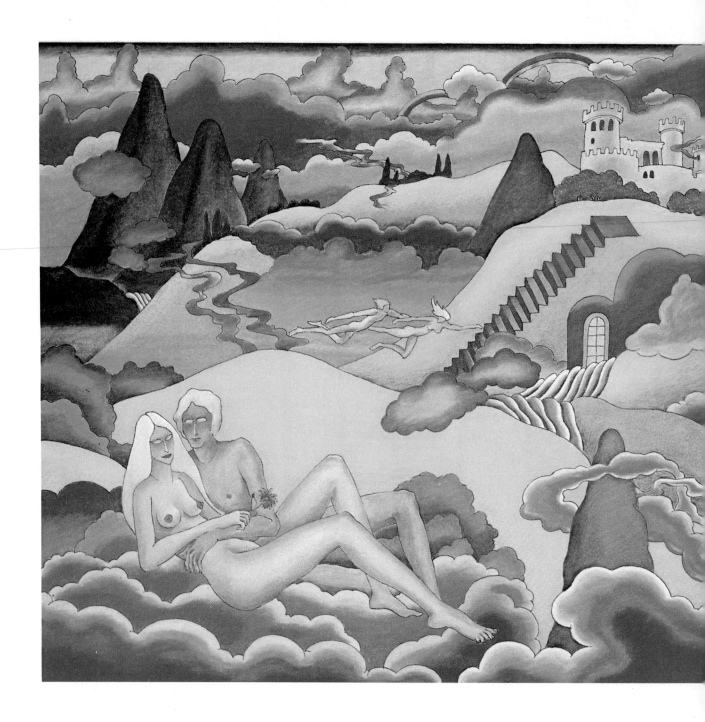

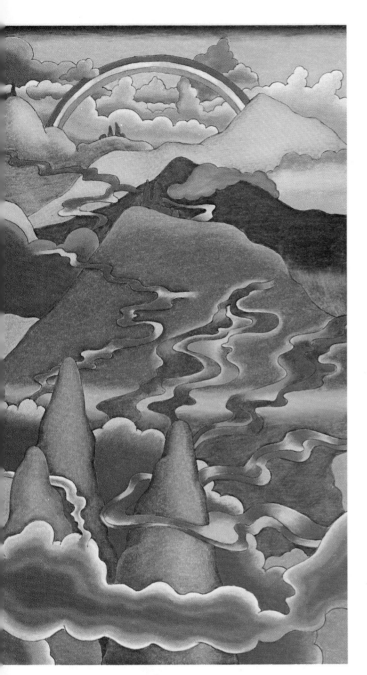

12

Until recently the restrictive sexual mores of American culture inhibited the study and dissemination of information about human sexual functioning. Physiologists and behavioral scientists were encouraged to study such aspects of sex as anatomy, the process of fertilization, courting behavior, and mating patterns, but scientists who chose to investigate coitus were scorned and ridiculed. Fortunately, a few pioneers in the field paved the way, and as a result there is now a more relaxed attitude toward such studies. The information that is slowly being uncovered about the physiology of erotic sensations now provides the basis for a more thorough understanding of human sexual nature. In addition, psychiatry, psychology, and behavioral science have contributed increased knowledge of the psychological aspects of sexual behavior. This chapter will present current views of human sexuality from both the psychological and physiological viewpoints.

PSYCHOSOCIAL ASPECTS OF SEXUAL BEHAVIOR

From the moment the doctor announces the sex of a newborn baby, society begins the long process of teaching that individual "to act like a female" or "to act like a male." The first teachers of these lessons are the parents. Without realizing it or doing it on purpose, they often teach their sons to be independent and their daughters to be submissive. In addition to teaching the child how to act, they will teach it to expect different things from women than from men. This social conditioning, or socializa-

Human Sexuality

tion, continues through childhood and youth. Young adolescents who have never participated in heterosexual activity will know how a member of their sex is *supposed* to act in such a situation.

The same is true for every other human society in the world. They all have differentiated sex roles that are maintained by teaching each new generation what is "right" and "wrong" for men and for women. All human sexual behavior is based on both physiology and social conditioning, with the social conditioning usually indicating when certain physiological responses are appropriate. This conditioning is generally so effective that perfectly adequate sexual stimulation will fail to lead to a sexual response if that stimulation comes from the wrong source or under the wrong circumstances.

The importance of social cuing means that human sexual behavior can best be understood when it is seen as an acquired or learned behavior. If the sexual norms of a society are repressive, the sexuality of the members of that society will be inhibited. If social conditioning leads to the expectation that females are not interested in sex, the females will tend to fulfill or at least pretend to fulfill these expectations. The human being is not a completely flexible organism. There are certain demands about sexual activity that simply would not be acceptable from any society. However, within broad limits, the individual's adult sexual expression is more a function of societal dictates than of anything else.

PATTERNS OF SEXUAL ACTIVITY

Although only a few studies have been done on specific forms of sexual behavior, a few generalizations can be made on the basis of the available data.

Masturbation

Masturbation, or self-stimulation for the purpose of sexual gratification, is common among humans and sometimes begins before puberty. It appears to be more common among males than among females. In the United States, for example, approximately nine out of ten males have practiced masturbation, but only one-half to two-thirds of females report having masturbated. In maturity, solitary masturbation is usually replaced by sexual relations with other persons as the major form of sexual activity. It becomes a supplementary activity or one to be used when sexual activity with others is unavailable.

Contrary to past belief, masturbation is completely harmless and in fact can be quite useful in training oneself to respond sexually and to learn which particular forms of stimulation are most enjoyable. Manual stimulation of the genitalia is the most common technique of masturbation for both males and females. Insertion of an object into the vagina or insertion of the penis into objects is less common. Many females reach orgasm more quickly and easily in masturbation than in coitus. This difference is attributed to differences in the speed and intensity of stimulation.

Orgasm and ejaculation during sleep appear to be fairly common experiences. Roughly three-quarters to nine-tenths of males and about two-fifths of females report having had this experience at some time. Orgasm in sleep is most common among adolescent males and tends to disappear later in life, whereas in females it is uncommon in adolescence and gradually increases with age, reaching its maximum in the third and fourth decades of life. Orgasm in sleep usually, but not always, is accompanied by erotic dreams. So-called "wet dreams," or nocturnal emissions, in most cases seem to be unrelated to the presence or absence of other sexual activity.

Petting

Heterosexual *petting* is best defined as sexual stimulation not involving insertion of the penis into the

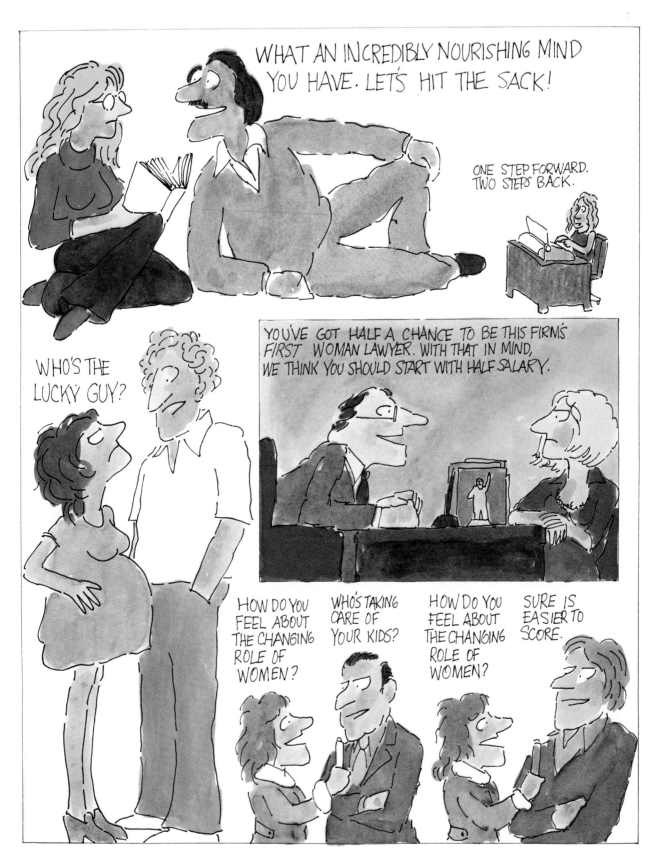

Figure 12.1 The changing nature of sex roles in America, with women seeking activities, responsibilities, and rights previously allocated only to men, has created many conflicts.

vagina. It is used in at least three ways. First, petting may be a goal in itself, a pleasurable activity that may result in orgasm. Petting of this sort often serves as a substitute for coitus between young persons wishing to avoid intercourse. Second, petting may be used by one partner to the point where coitus will be permitted. Third, when coitus has already been agreed upon or is anticipated by both individuals, petting is used as a preparation for intercourse, and in this form petting is known as *foreplay*.

In most Western societies, premarital petting tends to follow a stereotyped sequence with each new step usually initiated by the male—hugging and kissing, followed by breast and thigh caressing and proceeding to genital stimulation. Premarital petting is important as an opportunity to learn about sexual responses of the opposite sex and to obtain sexual and emotional gratification without more serious commitment. This behavior pattern seems to be a basic step toward a mature heterosexual adjustment and an integral part of courtship as a prelude to intercourse.

Petting techniques vary considerably, depending upon individual wishes and degrees of sexual sophistication. Mouth kissing is usual in Western civilization, but it is rare in some societies and absent in others. Also common is light stroking, or caressing, of various parts of the body other than the breasts or genitalia. Manual stimulation of the female breast by the male is nearly universal, and oral breast stimulation is common. In a few societies, however, this technique is regarded as too similar to infant suckling and therefore is considered inappropriate. Interestingly enough, females rarely stimulate the male breast, a potential but apparently poorly recognized source of male sexual arousal. Manual stimuation of the genitalia and adjacent skin areas is common among sexually experienced individuals.

Oral stimulation by the male of the female genitalia (*cunnilingus*) is a matter on which societies and subgroups within a given society differ markedly. In some it is common; in others it is rare or is regarded as unnatural or perverse. In the United States, such mouth-genital contact is common, oc-

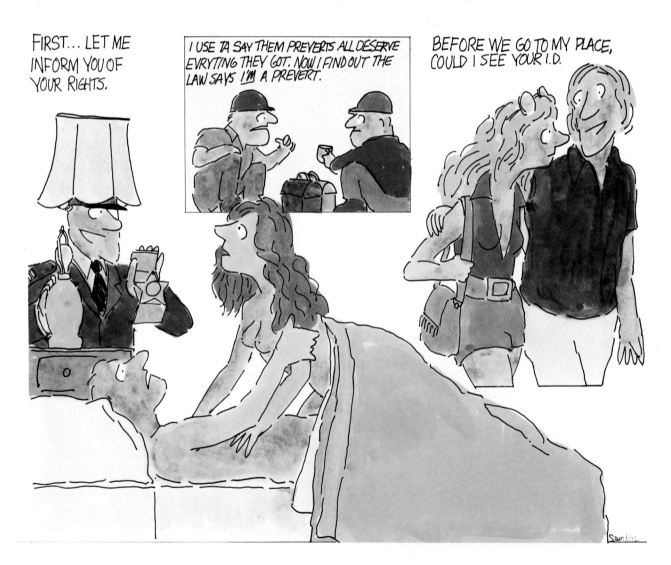

curring in more than half of marriages; however, in the criminal laws of most states, cunnilingus continues to be punishable as a felony. Oral stimulation by the female of the male genitalia (*fellatio*) is equally common in the United States. The scant anthropological data suggest that fellatio generally is more acceptable than cunnilingus. Nevertheless, it also is considered a felony along with cunnilingus in most states, usually under sodomy laws.

Coitus

In every human society, *coitus* is regarded as the ultimate and natural culmination of a full heterosexual relationship. Although coitus in marriage is universally regarded as a right, or even a duty, attitudes toward coitus under other circumstances vary greatly. For example, female *premarital coitus* is officially discouraged in many societies, yet nearly all societies permit or excuse male premarital coitus even when illegal.

Nevertheless, actual practice may vary greatly from publicly expressed attitudes. In the United States, where premarital coitus is—at least in theory—unacceptable and in most states is against the law, at least two-thirds of males and one-half of females engage in it. Males tend to have premarital coitus with more partners than do females, and with less emphasis on a total human relationship. Females generally begin coitus only after a fairly strong affectional relationship has developed. Most American females who have premarital coitus do so with males whom they hope to marry.

The social and psychological significance of premarital coitus to the individual is linked to social attitudes. In many societies, premarital coitus is expected behavior and serves a useful role in the selection of a spouse. In such societies, there seldom are negative psychological consequences. In societies that condemn the activity, there are possible negative consequences—rejection, guilt, and a greater possibility of exploitation. However, the great majority of American females who have had premarital coitus report that they do not regret it.

Even *coitus in marriage* is not wholly free of societal restrictions. In some societies, it is forbidden during menstrual flow, during part of pregnancy, or for a variable period (which can range up to many months) after childbirth. In addition, it may be forbidden before or during special ceremonies or activities.

The frequency of marital coitus varies greatly not only among societies but among individual couples within a society. During the first years of marriage between youthful partners, a couple is likely to have coitus frequently. As the male interest lessens later in life, however, male and female may seem to change places in respect to sexual drive. The wife, who in early marriage may complain of too frequent coitus, in middle age may complain it is not frequent enough.

Although age does reduce sexual activity, it need not eradicate it. If individuals are in reasonably good health and receive sexual stimulation, coitus can continue into extreme old age. In addition to its physiological benefit and its value as one of life's great pleasures, marital coitus can be an affirmation of affection and desire for each other that holds a marriage together. It is both irrational and destructive to perpetuate the notion that sexual behavior among the aged is somehow unseemly or humorous.

Extramarital coitus—that is, coitus between a married person and someone other than the spouse—often disrupts marriages and other social relationships. Some of the complications include jealousy, new emotional and social allegiances, neglect of duties, disputed paternity, and so on. Consequently, most societies either prohibit extramarital coitus or permit it only under well-defined circumstances. It may be allowed only with specified

Figure 12.2   Sex and the law. Laws regarding sex are primarily based on moral standards established in the various states in the eighteenth and nineteenth centuries. Sexual offenses range from abduction and adultery to fornication, incest, and sodomy. In most states all forms of sexual activity except face-to-face husband-wife intercourse are illegal. It is estimated that 90 percent of American adults are sex criminals under such statutes. Most sex laws are rarely enforced, although there have been a few notorious exceptions. Changes in the laws are slowly taking place, despite the protests of those who cling to the Puritan morality on which the laws were based.

persons, only during certain festivities, only with the permission of the spouse, or only where extenuating circumstances exist. Despite social disapproval and illegality, at least one-half of American husbands and one-third of American wives experience extramarital coitus at some time during their marriages. Such situations are further discussed in Chapter 15.

Postmarital coitus—occurring after a marriage has terminated but before a new one has begun—has received very little attention from students of human behavior. Restrictions tend to be minimal; even societies opposed to premarital and extramarital coitus tend to close their eyes to postmarital coitus, realizing that persons accustomed to regular coitus in marriage hardly can be expected to refrain after the marital status changes. This realization is well founded; the great majority of widowed or divorced persons continue to have coitus.

Homosexuality

Homosexuality, chiefly among males, was common in many preliterate or ancient societies. Most preliterate societies seemed to accept the homosexual activity of certain individuals but to consider them different from ordinary beings. Only a small minority of societies have treated homosexuality as normal, accepted behavior. In these societies it is recognized that homosexuality does not interfere with heterosexuality but exists in addition to it. Indeed, homosexuality and heterosexuality should not be viewed

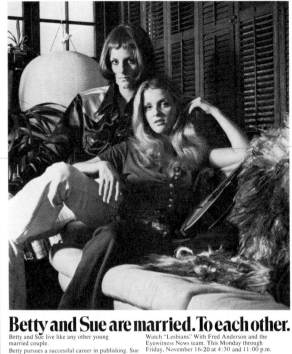

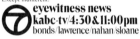

Betty and Sue are married. To each other.

Betty and Sue live like any other young married couple.
Betty pursues a successful career in publishing. Sue prefers to do the chores at home. Both will tell you they wouldn't have it any other way . . . except for one thing. Sometimes they feel very alone.
This week Eyewitness News explores the predicament of Betty, Sue and many others like them in a candid documentary entitled "Lesbians."
Hear lesbians talk openly about their philosophy and way of life. Learn about the social pressures that have forced them into hiding.

Watch "Lesbians." With Fred Anderson and the Eyewitness News team. This Monday through Friday, November 16-20 at 4:30 and 11:00 p.m.
Call the Eyewitness News team anything you like. Except indifferent.

**eyewitness news
kabc-tv/4:30 & 11:00 pm**
bonds/lawrence/nahan/sloane

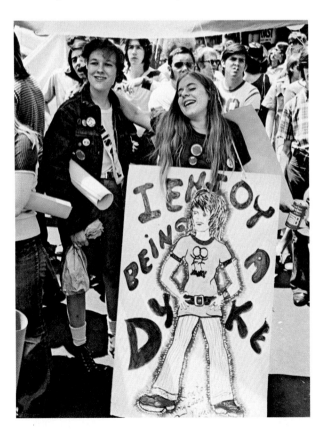

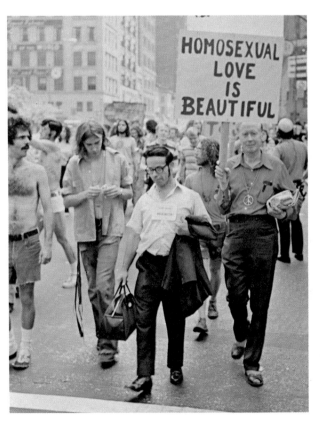

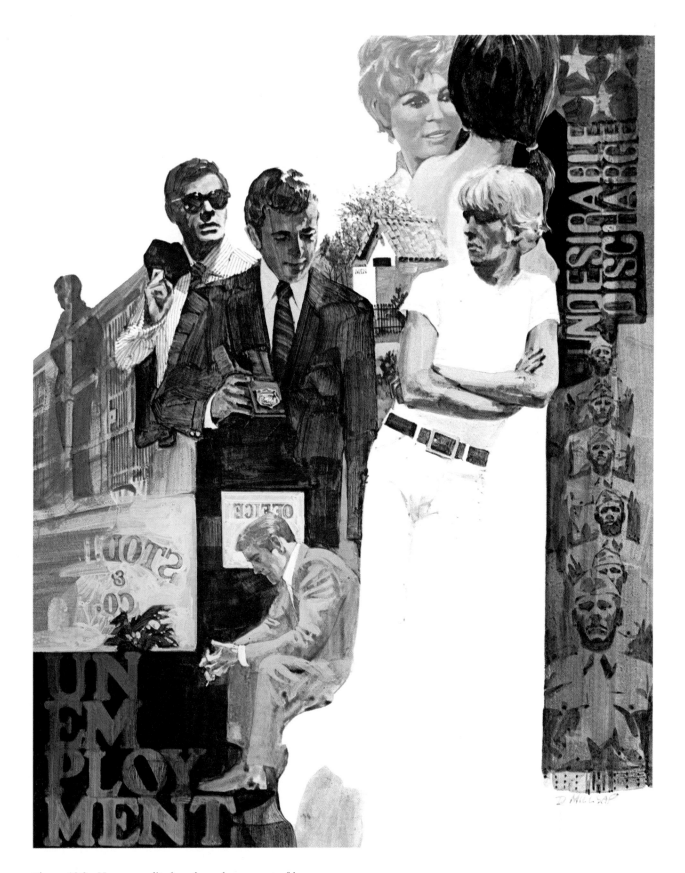

Figure 12.3 Homosexuality has always been a part of human existence. Although there seems to be a gradually increasing acceptance of the homosexual life style, there is still great pressure exerted on any individual who deviates from "the norm." This pressure is imposed in the form of job discrimination, legal restrictions, and social ostracism.

as antagonistic. Both tendencies exist to some extent in every individual, although they frequently are not expressed. Exclusively homosexual persons are uncommon, comprising about 4 percent of adult males and perhaps 2 percent of adult females in the United States.

There seems to be no one cause of homosexuality in any one individual, but there are a number of predisposing factors, none of which is a sufficient explanation by itself. In general, anything that interferes with heterosexual expression, such as being in one-sex boarding schools or prison, may predispose an individual toward homosexuality. Thus, society's own restrictions on heterosexual behavior push some individuals toward homosexuality. Incidental, temporary homosexual activity, such as that occurring during adolescent experimentation, is rather common. About one-third of American males and one-fifth of females have had such experiences.

Although extensive or even exclusive homosexual activity is a statistical deviation from the norm, it is not in itself proof of mental or emotional illness. Homosexuality is being viewed increasingly not as a disease, but as a preference. If homosexuals live in a society that condemns and punishes their behavior, they are more prone to neurosis and stress symptoms. The great majority of individuals who are chiefly or wholly homosexual cannot be identified by dress or nonsexual behavior. They lead lives that (except in the sexual sphere) are basically ordinary and normal. In the larger cities, however, some of those persons who are predominantly homosexual tend to gather together, to form homosexual organizations and a homosexual subculture. Similar tendencies to congregate for mutual support are to be found among any other minority.

There are other sexual manifestations that are statistically uncommon ("abnormal") and viewed by most societies as pathological, criminal, or both.

Figure 12.4 There are perhaps as many sexual preferences and sexual patterns as there are men and women. Persons seeking others who share similar sexual ideas often advertise in underground newspapers.

These proclivities include *sado-masochism* (sexual pleasure in giving or receiving pain or humiliation), *pedophilia* (a sexual preference for children), *fetishism* (sexual attraction to inanimate objects), and other unusual forms of sexual interest or activity. These manifestations have been the subject of much psychological study and writing.

Prostitution

Prostitution is not a particular form of sexual behavior but rather a business that caters to sexual drives. In fact, it is not easy to define a prostitute. Who should be included in such a definition? The girl who has coitus with her employer to gain promotions and salary increases? The mistress who obtains money or an apartment for her favors? The girl who insists upon gifts from her boyfriends? The gigolo? The wife who holds out for a mink coat? The fiancée who holds out for marriage? The only workable definition is an operational one: a *prostitute* is a person who, for direct and immediate payment in money or something else of value, will indiscriminately engage in sexual activity with another person, known or unknown.

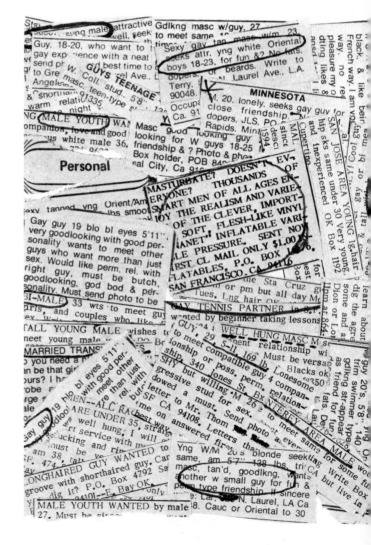

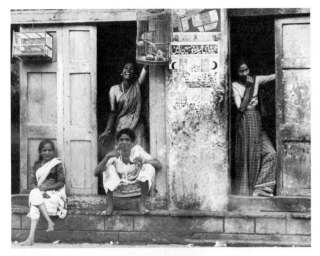

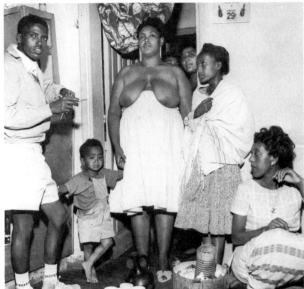

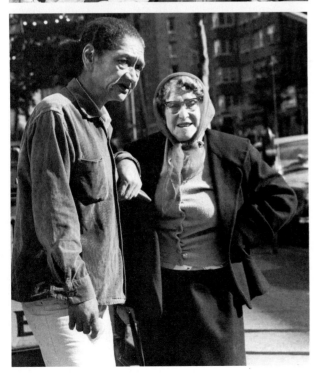

Prostitution exists in some form in almost every society. The demand is smaller in societies that are sexually more permissive, but even in such societies there are always some individuals who cannot obtain a regular sexual partner when they want one. In the United States, prostitution has become less important as premarital coitus among friends and acquaintances has increased. Brothels, or houses of prostitution, have been suppressed almost completely in most parts of the country, but the business is carried on by streetwalkers and through "call" operators (who send prostitutes to the customer in response to a phone call) and by independents operating alone or with a partner or two in the streets, hotels, apartments, or homes.

Female partners for males is the most common form of prostitution in the United States. Male prostitution for males also is relatively common. Male prostitution for females is more rare, and female prostitution for females is almost unknown.

PHYSIOLOGY OF COITUS

Until a few years ago, little more could be said about human sexual behavior than general statements of statistical frequency such as those just provided. The research of William Masters and Virginia Johnson has made possible much more specific descriptions of typical physiological and behavioral processes during coitus.

Because Masters and Johnson were the first to study genital physiological changes during sexual stimulation, they had to develop some new methods and equipment, particularly for examining the female response, which is more difficult to observe because most of it occurs internally. As the investigation proceeded, their techniques expanded to include measurement of anatomical parts during different phases of stimulation, intrauterine electrodes to measure uterine contractions, electrocardiograph tracings to monitor rate and level of car-

Figure 12.5 Prostitution. (*top*) Although prostitution is officially forbidden in India, the profession is practiced today much as it was hundreds of years ago, when it was a very respected profession. Women are born into a brothel in the same way they are born into a caste. (*center*) A second-class brothel in Addis Abbaba. In the second-class brothels most prostitutes live with their children and sometimes with their husbands. This prostitute has her small child and son with her; around her are some of the young prostitutes. (*bottom*) Prostitutes hustling on New York's Third Avenue (near the Bowery). The one on the left, who would not give her age, told the photographer, "I ain't never going to retire." It is estimated that in the United States 6 million contacts with prostitutes take place each week. If an average of seven dollars is paid for each of these encounters, the annual untaxed income from prostitution is almost 2.25 billion dollars.

diac contractions, as well as equipment to measure respiration and blood pressure. Data were collected during masturbation as well as during natural and artificial coitus. Plastic penises used for artificial coitus allowed direct observation and photography of the vagina's physiological responses.

The reaction patterns of both female and male were found to be essentially independent of the method of stimulation employed. The sexual response cycles of both women and men may be divided into four separate phases: the excitement phase, the plateau phase, the orgasmic phase, and the resolution phase. The following descriptions represent a composite of individual cycles. Individual variations are marked and usually involve duration, not intensity, of the response. The initial and final phases are of significantly longer duration than the other two.

Female Cycle

Before describing the female cycle, something must be said of the physiological equipment with which a woman is provided. The major female reproductive organs are described in Chapters 2 and 13; here the focus will be on the vagina and the external structures bordering it (see Figure 12.6).

The vagina is much more than a birth canal or a receptacle in which the male deposits sperm; it is actually a responsive muscular organ, equipped to open, receive, clasp, and rub the male organ during sexual intercourse. Ordinarily, the vagina is shaped like a flattened tube of toothpaste, about four inches long. It is lined with moist, wrinkled, elastic, skinlike mucous membrane. At the deep end of the vagina lies a firm smooth knob, the *cervix*. Encircling the vagina are the *pubococcygeus muscles*, which contract with the anal and urethral sphincters. Greater control of them can be developed by voluntary contractions that concentrate on lifting these spincters into the abdomen. Not only does control of the contraction and relaxation of these muscles increase friction during intercourse, but maintaining the tone of these muscles is believed to reduce pelvic difficulties later in life.

In virginal females, often, but certainly not always, the entrance to the vagina is narrowed by a circular fold of tissue, much like the aperture in a camera, called the *hymen*. The hymen usually has a central opening large enough to admit an examining finger or menstrual tampon. Frequently physical activity or time will obliterate the hymen, even when no intercourse has occurred. Usually with first intercourse it will stretch or even tear a little with no problem. Only occasionally will a hymen be thick or tough enough to require a doctor's help in sufficiently stretching it to accommodate the penis.

The vagina is remarkably elastic—after all, a full-sized baby can pass through it. Excessive tightness during intercourse is usually caused by an overtense condition of the encircling pubococcygeus muscles, a condition that can be overcome by learning to use these muscles properly. On the other hand, some women consider themselves "too large" or "too wide open." Usually this condition follows childbirth and can be corrected by exercises to restore normal muscle tone and use, or if necessary, by surgery.

Covering the vaginal opening are two soft, sensitive, wrinkled flaps of skin called *labia minora*, or smaller lips. Covering the labia minora are two broad, less sensitive hair-covered folds of skin called *labia majora*. Just above the vaginal opening, between the labia, lies the *urethra*, the opening from the urinary bladder. Half an inch or more above the urethra lies a sensitive organ the size of a pea, the *clitoris*. The clitoris is usually partly hooded by a flap of less sensitive skin, the prepuce, formed where the labia minora join together in an arch.

The clitoris, like its male counterpart, the penis, is an erectile organ comprising a head (clitoral glans) and a stalk (clitoral shaft). A number of lubricating glands border the vaginal and urethral openings. Most of the fluid that appears at the vaginal opening as the result of sexual stimulation, whether that stimulation is a direct physical one or merely an emotional reaction, comes from the vagina itself. With the stirring of any sort of sexual feeling, the vagina of the healthy woman begins to "sweat."

All of the external organs participate in female sexual activity. The clitoris for most women may be regarded as a sort of "message center" that receives and distributes sexual sensations. Unlike its male counterpart, the penis, the clitoris has no other function or purpose—it serves only as an erotic "switch." But the most important organ of all in any sexual response resides far outside the pelvis. It is the brain, which is the ultimate control center from which the human sexual response is directed. The stages of that response follow.

EXCITEMENT PHASE   Many parts of the body in addition to the genitalia respond to sexual stimulation. *Myotonia*, an increase in muscular tension, is a generalized sexual response involving both voluntary and involuntary muscles. Coital position has a role in determining which muscle groups will exhibit this reaction during a particular sexual response cycle. Heart-rate and blood-pressure increases begin in the excitement phase, and blood accumulates in certain blood vessels, resulting in what is known as *vasocongestion*.

Vasocongestion is a primary response to sexual stimulation and is found in a number of different body parts, including the labia minora and the clitoris. It is instrumental in the development of the sex-flush, which appears late in this phase. The *sex-flush* is a superficial vasocongestive reaction that causes a temporary rash to spread from the breasts over the lower abdomen and shoulders as sexual tension increases. Vasocongestion also is responsible for the changes occurring in other sex organs during this initial phase. The breasts show both nipple erection and a slight increase in size. Expansion or swelling of the clitoral glans always accompanies the build-up of sexual tension, although it is not always observable to the unaided eye.

PLATEAU PHASE   The first part of this phase is mainly a continuation of reactions that originated during the preceding one. If effective sexual stimulation is maintained, myotonia and vasocongestion will increase, the sex-flush will spread, and breast expansion will continue. The clitoral glans and shaft withdraw. The more effective the stimulation, the more marked this withdrawal will be.

The expansion that affected the inner two-thirds of the vagina during the excitement phase now extends to the outer one-third. This tissue, even more than the inner area, becomes grossly engorged with venous blood. Both the outer third of the vagina and the labia minora are involved in this major vasocongestive reaction. These anatomical parts respond during orgasm and therefore are called the *orgasmic platform*.

Although the uterus shows partial elevation during the excitement phase, it now attains complete elevation and moves backward toward the spine. It remains in that position until the onset of the resolution phase. The physiological reaction that leads to uterine elevation is unknown. As sexual tensions increase and orgasm becomes imminent, further increases in respiration, heartbeat, and blood pressure are seen.

ORGASMIC PHASE   Immediately before orgasm the physiological responses described for earlier phases are at their most intense level. The breasts are enlarged, with nipples erect. Sex-flush and vasocongestion are widespread. The clitoris is completely withdrawn. The vagina is lubricated and extended, with the orgasmic platform well developed. The uterus is elevated. Only myotonic tension will become even more intense with orgasm.

The physiological onset of orgasm is indicated by contractions in certain organs. The orgasmic platform is first. It displays a long contraction, lasting from two to four seconds, and then a series of shorter contractions less than a second apart. The factors that initiate this response have not been identified. They may be neural, hormonal, or muscular, or some combination of factors. The platform contractions are accompanied by uterine contrac-

tions of a less definite pattern and often by contractions of the external rectal sphincter. The frequency of these rectal contractions usually is a function of the intensity of the particular orgasmic response. No particular reaction has been observed in the breasts or the clitoris during orgasm. As indicated in Figure 12.8, unlike men, many women have the ability to experience multiple orgasms in a relatively short period of time.

Both women and physicans have long believed that orgasm resulting from vaginal stimulation (as in normal intercourse) is physiologically distinct from that resulting from clitoral stimulation alone (as in masturbation or manual stimulation by a partner). Freudian theory supported this view and maintained that, in normal sexual development,

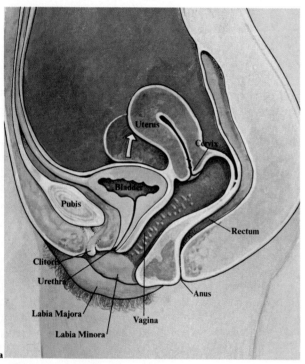

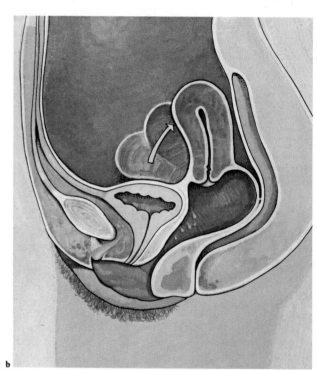

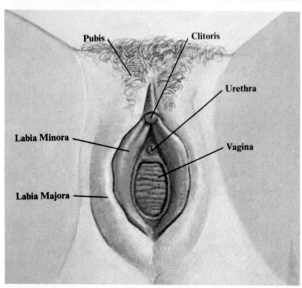

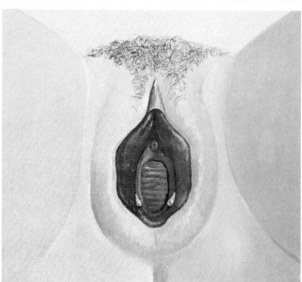

women move from clitoral response to vaginal response. Masters and Johnson's data refute this view. They found that the physiological and anatomical responses from any form of stimulation were essentially the same.

This does not mean, however, that the psychological responses from the different forms of stimulation are indistinguishable. Sexually experienced individuals know that the psychological effects of an orgasm are mainly a function of the context in which the orgasm occurs. This important new concept, the context of orgasm, is just beginning to be studied by sexologists. More knowledge about the effects of the setting in which sexual behavior occurs is essential in understanding the interaction between physiological and psychological factors.

Figure 12.6   Changes in external and internal female genitalia during the stages of sexual excitement. (a) Excitement stage: (*top*) The uterus and cervix pull away from the vagina; the vagina begins to lubricate; the inner two-thirds of the vagina lengthen and distend. (*bottom*) The clitoris increases in length; the labia majora spread flat; the labia minora increase in size. (b) Plateau stage: (*top*) The uterus is now fully elevated; the cervical end of the vagina expands; labia minora increase in size and turn bright red. (*bottom*) Clitoris retracts under hood and is tender; Bartholin glands secrete lubricant. (c) Orgasm state: (*top*) The uterus undergoes contractions similar to labor; there are strong contractions of the orgasmic platform; the male's ejaculated semen forms a pool at the cervical end of the vagina. (*bottom*) In some women the opening of the urethra dilates during orgasm. (d) Resolution stage: (*top*) The uterus and vagina return to normal; the cervix drops down into the seminal pool. The clitoris and labia slowly return to normal size and position.

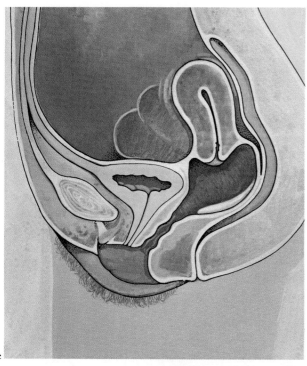

c

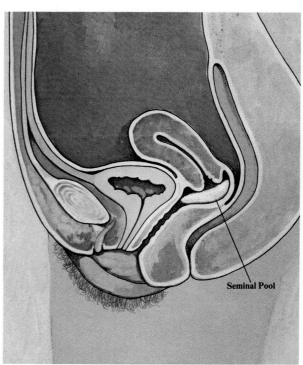

d

Seminal Pool

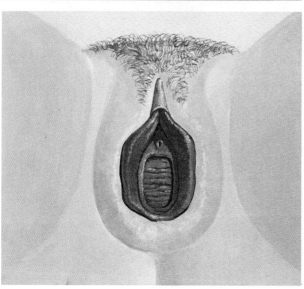

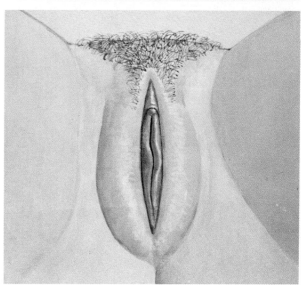

RESOLUTION PHASE This phase is characterized by return to the normal, or precoital, condition. The return is fairly rapid if orgasm has occurred. The average time is about five to ten minutes. Myotonia, sex-flush, and the orgasmic platform subside quickly. The clitoris regains normal size and position. Changes resulting from vasocongestion disappear throughout the body. This process is much slower if plateau levels of tension were reached but orgasm did not occur. In this case, thirty minutes or more may be required. Complete resolution does not occur between cycles if more than one orgasm is attained over a relatively short period.

Again, it should be stressed that the cycle described here is what Masters and Johnson see as an average cycle. Many elements may be different or missing in any particular normal cycle, but this composite picture is representative of the more than 10,000 cycles they observed.

One of the principal findings of these studies was the great extent to which a woman's entire body is involved in her response to effective sexual stimulation. Myotonia, vasocongestion, sex-flush,

and other specific reactions were observed in numerous parts of the body. Temporary loss of sharpness of vision also often accompanied orgasm, as did the appearance of perspiration. The importance of these peripheral states in the subjective experience of orgasm is unexplored.

The newly found properties of the clitoris are important to understand. The clitoris is the focal point of sensual response in the woman's pelvic area. Its unique and only known function is that of receiving, responding to, and transmitting neural messages of sexual stimulation. Its ability to respond to stimulation received at other genital points exposes the fallacy involved in typical marriage-manual instructions to maintain direct clitoral stimulation throughout coitus. This contact is both difficult and unnecessary, as the clitoris will react to the sensory input of other areas, such as the vagina. In most cases, this secondary stimulation is sufficient to cause orgasm. No correlation between intensity of orgasm and clitoral size or positioning was observed.

Another fallacy is the common belief that coitus

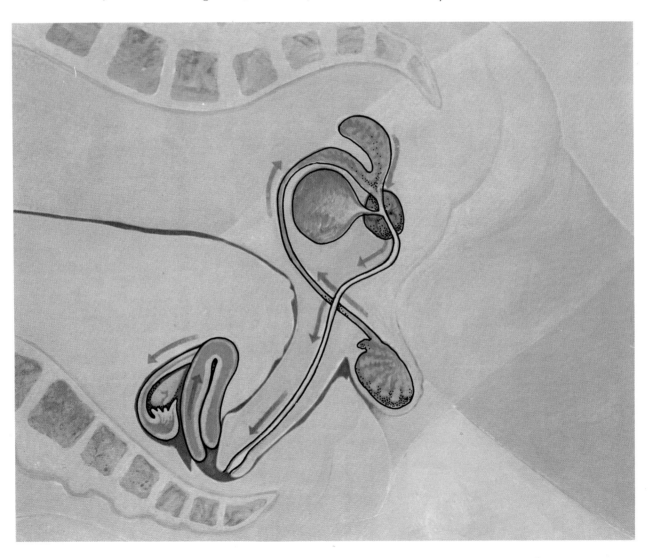

during menstruation causes physical distress to the woman. About 10 percent of the women who were menstruating regularly during their involvement with the research objected to sexual activity during menstruation on religious or aesthetic grounds. About 40 percent expressed no particular like or dislike for sexual activity during menstruation. Approximately 50 percent voiced a desire for sexual activity during the menses. Of particular interest were the 10 percent who reported frequent use of masturbation to relieve discomfort accompanying the onset of menstruation (during sexual excitement the uterus contracts, thus expelling blood clots that may contribute to cramps).

Male Cycle

A remarkable finding of the Masters and Johnson studies was the existence of numerous similarities between male and female sexual-response patterns. The similarities are much more pronounced than the differences, as is apparent in the description of the male cycle.

EXCITEMENT PHASE As in the woman, many parts of the male body besides the genital organs respond to sexual stimulation. Breast enlargement is not part of the male cycle, although the nipples may become erect. When nipple erection does occur, it usually begins late in this phase. Other extragenital responses include increased heart rate and blood pressure. Elevated tension (myotonia) in both voluntary and involuntary muscles appear early in this phase.

Early genital reactions are most visible. The penis becomes erect because of massive vasocongestion in three cavernous blood vessels that run the length of the organ. Some myotonia also is involved. Unlike female vasocongestion, mainly arterial blood is collected in the penis. Vasocongestion

Figure 12.7 (*left*) Sexual intercourse. During ejaculation the seminal fluid follows the path indicated by the arrows, and the sperm are deposited at the cervical end of the vagina.

Figure 12.8 (*right*) Masters and Johnson's phase graphs. (*top*) The man's rise in sexual tension is shown diagrammatically. Once orgasm is achieved there is a refractory period before he can have another orgasm. (*bottom*) A woman can experience one orgasm and soon after experience another (line A). If she fails to experience orgasm, however, her resolution phase is longer (line B). Line C shows a rare kind of prolonged orgasmic experience known as *status orgasmus.*

and thickening of the scrotal skin are involved in the elevation of the scrotal sac. Elevation of the testicles, on the other hand, is accomplished through shortening of the spermatic cord by an involuntary contraction of the muscles near the cord. This response begins in the excitement phase but is not completed until the plateau phase.

In some men a clear lubricating fluid may appear in droplets at the urethral outlet during all phases up to orgasm. This fluid often contains thousands of viable spermatozoa that are perfectly capable of causing conception, which is why withdrawal of the penis before ejaculation is one of the least reliable means of contraception.

PLATEAU PHASE The penis, which became fully erect during the excitement phase, will show a slight increase in circumference during this second phase. This late development is restricted to its head, or glans penis. As the testicles rise, an increase in their size becomes apparent. Testes show about a 50 percent size increase, and if plateau levels of sexual tension are prolonged without orgasm, up to 100 percent increase may occur. Like penile erection,

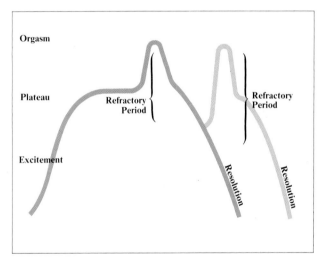

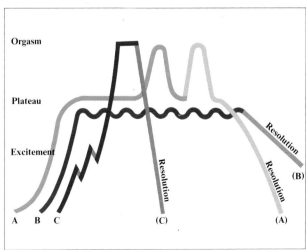

continued testicular size increase is a vast vaso-congestive response.

The approach of orgasm occasionally is accompanied by a sex-flush similar to that observed in women. In men, it usually covers the chest, neck, face, forehead, and sometimes shoulders and thighs. Impending ejaculation also is signaled by increased heart rate, breathing rate, blood pressure, and myotonia.

ORGASMIC PHASE   Although ejaculation and orgasm usually are considered as two parts of a single occurrence, they are separable. Orgasm without ejaculation—that is, without the expulsion of seminal fluids—can occur and is experienced frequently by prepubertal boys.

With the exception of fluid discharge, the physiological responses that form the basis for the male and female experience of orgasm are quite similar. Both involve the loss of general muscular control as well as massive contractions in the genital area, including the anal sphincter. The contractions of the orgasmic platform in the female and of the penile urethra in the male occur at intervals of 0.8 seconds during part of the orgasmic experience. Heart rate, breathing, and blood pressure are at their highest during orgasm in both sexes.

The contractions of reproductive accessory organs (prostate, seminal vesicles, ejaculatory duct) and the resulting seminal emission distinguish the male response from the female response. The total body response described for women also occurs in men, with myotonia and vasocongestion observable throughout the body. Just as women can voluntarily contract certain of their muscles to enhance sexual enjoyment, some men learn to heighten the intensity of orgasm by voluntarily contracting the muscles of the buttocks, abdomen, and anus before and during orgasm.

RESOLUTION PHASE   Following orgasm, the return to the unstimulated state usually is quite rapid. The sex-flush fades, and perspiration sometimes appears. Detumescence (loss of swelling) of the penis occurs with the loss of vasocongestion. This loss also leads to the descent of the testes into the relaxed scrotum. A general decrease of muscle tension then appears, usually no more than five minutes after the beginning of this phase. Nipples that showed erection in the excitement phase display no additional reactions during plateau or orgasmic phases and may require as much as an hour to return to their normal position.

Myths about the male sexual response are even more numerous than those about the female, perhaps because the external genitalia of men make their major reactions visible and consequently more a topic of discussion than the invisible and little-

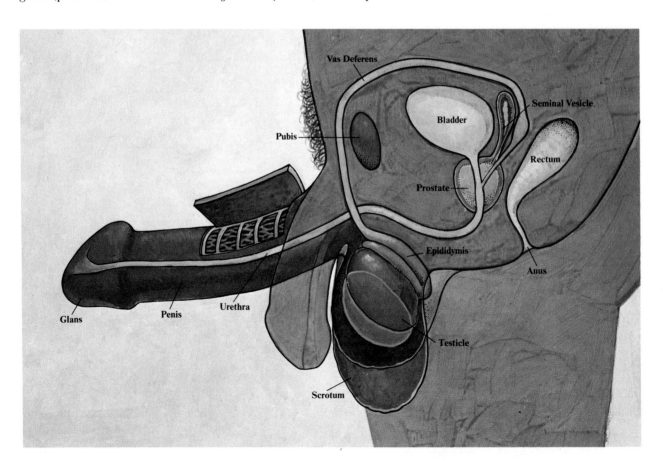

known female response. Part of Masters and Johnson's research was an investigation of the validity of popular beliefs about the male sexual response.

Contrary to popular belief, circumcision (the surgical removal of the foreskin from the tip of the penis) has no apparent influence on sexual behavior. A comparison of circumcised and uncircumcised subjects revealed no differences in degree of ejaculatory control, tendency toward impotence, or sensitivity of the penis. Another fallacy was uncovered when a study of men of all ages showed that, although some difficulty in achieving erection may appear with age, impotence is in no sense an inevitable result of aging. Furthermore, this type of impotence is a reversible condition.

It has long been believed that the larger a man's penis, the better his sexual performance and the satisfaction of his partner. Masters and Johnson's data revealed no such correlations. Their study also failed to support the belief that the large penis expands more than the small penis when erect. The small penis usually doubles its length during full erection; the large one increases to one and a half times its flaccid length, with lengths being more comparable after erection. Therefore, penis size is not a significant factor in either the man's or the woman's sexual response, particularly because the vagina accommodates to any size penis.

Sex Differences

Although there are many parallels between the sexual responses of men and women to erotic stimulation, there also are some significant differences. Men usually are more easily aroused, for example, and can engage in satisfactory coitus more rapidly than women. The female usually requires more psychological and physical stimulation before her responses begin and before she can achieve orgasm. Men also depend less upon ideal circumstances for intercourse—the proper setting, romantic circumstances, absence of distractions, and so on. A man usually can have only one orgasm until a certain period of time has elapsed, while most women are capable of several consecutive orgasms. At least some of these differences are likely to reflect psychosocial aspects of sexual behavior.

The differences between male and female responses, however, are not as great as those between different individuals. Thus there are a few women who respond very rapidly and some men who respond very slowly. An individual's response may also vary greatly from one time to another. Sickness, fatigue, preoccupation with other matters, and emotional problems all may diminish one's sexual response.

Sexual Techniques

Many young men and women become concerned with sexual techniques. Marriage manuals, photos, and films may prove of some help, and the medical profession may have to be consulted in extreme cases (frigidity, premature ejaculation, impotence), although physicians by and large do not make good sex counselors. Masters and Johnson's studies of human sexual inadequacies have shown that most cases of sexual malfunction are a result of associating unpleasant experiences with sexual behavior—incidents of societal conditioning gone awry. Most of these malfunctions can be corrected through reconditioning.

But given a normal sexual response, what becomes important in a sexual relationship is the sense of giving satisfaction to one's partner as well as to oneself. If coitus communicates a true feeling and concern for one's partner, and if one truly tries to please the other while enjoying one's own response, the relationship will probably be more satisfactory than if one thinks in terms of "personal performance." Knowledge of the physiology and psychology of both female and male sexual responses is also helpful in achieving satisfaction for both individuals.

Figure 12.9   Vasocongestion in the penis. Erection of the penis is the most obvious vasocongestive reaction.

THE SEXUAL REVOLUTION

"There is no sexual revolution, no runaway sexual permissiveness. . . . There is no generation gap of significance in sexual standards between this generation and the last." This familiar statement was made by the noted sociologist Dr. Ira L. Reiss. For those who mistakenly define the "sexual revolution" solely in terms of an increase in numbers of unmarrieds · engaging in premarital coitus or in numbers of partners encountered in experimentation, Dr. Reiss' statement of a decade ago is no longer true. This interpretation is one that many people give the term "sexual revolution," and the illusion of its validity continues to be reinforced and perpetuated through mass media.

But outside of this unfortunate and inaccurate interpretation, Dr. Reiss' statement is as valid today as it was a decade ago when written. Saying that American society is experiencing a "revolution" suggests that the motivation for premarital coital activity has changed and that something qualitatively new is occurring. This assumption has no supportive data. In fact, there is ample evidence that little change has taken place in cultural attitudes concerning premarital sexual behavior; that is, people are doing "it" now for the same reasons they were doing "it" decades ago.

Norms or value systems in all societies are undergoing evolutionary change and American society is no exception. For some fifty years in America there has been a gradual release of constraints on female sex behavior. Unlike the male, who experiences orgasm whenever he ejaculates, the female has the biological capacity for separating orgasm from

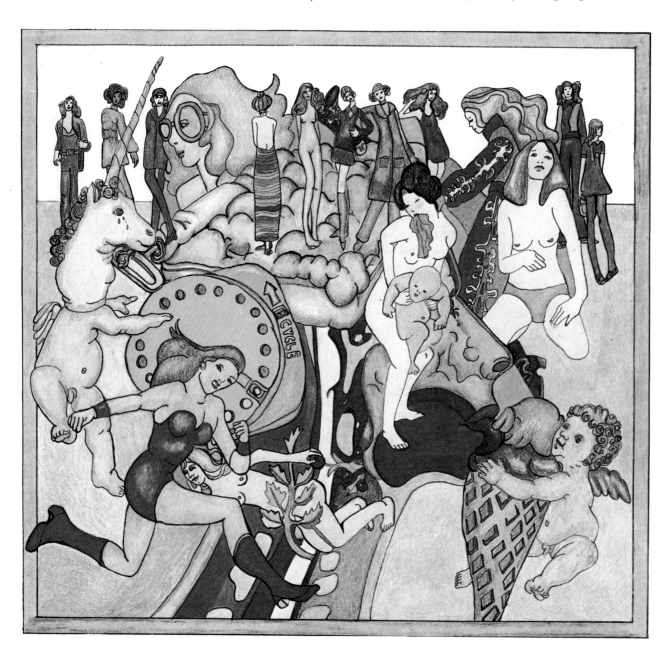

reproduction, and it is for this reason societies have been more active in suppressing female sexuality and charging her with the responsibility of supporting the cultural norms. One noted sociologist points out that female pleasure, so far as reproduction is concerned, is extremely expendable and that cultures can turn it on or off without affecting their reproductive histories in the least.

The implications of this apparent social evolution are vast indeed, but it is at least premature to conclude that release of constraints on females regarding sexual behavior will in any way change the motivational system underlying this behavior. Changes are generally viewed by most societies as social problems, not as social opportunities. To view the release of sexual constraints on women as a social opportunity would require drastic changes in the American cultural belief system.

In reality, the only change this evolutionary process has brought about is the attitude toward a female's behavior. Whereas half a century ago she was culturally forbidden to engage in premarital sexual activity, she may now do so if she likes her partner. The essence of a true sexual "revolution" would mean the separation of sexual activity from emotional commitment for women, or, in the oppo-site direction, engaging in intercourse only as part of a total interpersonal love relationship for both sexes. Such fragmentation or a similar radical break from current sexual practice has yet to occur.

There can be no question that today there are greater opportunities for men and women to express themselves sexually. But what does this opportunity mean in terms of changing the cultural norms? One writer stated the case well when he said that in the midst of all the change, young people continue to be taught pretty much what previous generations were taught about sex: that boys are usually more interested in sex than are girls; that masturbation is something that one should not do or keep a secret; that there are good girls and bad girls and you marry one and not the other.

The sexual "revolution" is a myth of the media, but society's attitudes are changing, very slowly and very cautiously. For the first time in the history of mankind the Western cultures of the twentieth century have the opportunity to make those changes on the basis of fairly sound knowledge about human sexuality. They can chose either to use this knowledge or to ignore it. If they chose to use it properly, the result will be a more satisfying, pleasurable, and fulfilling existence for everyone.

Figure 12.10 The "sexual revolution."

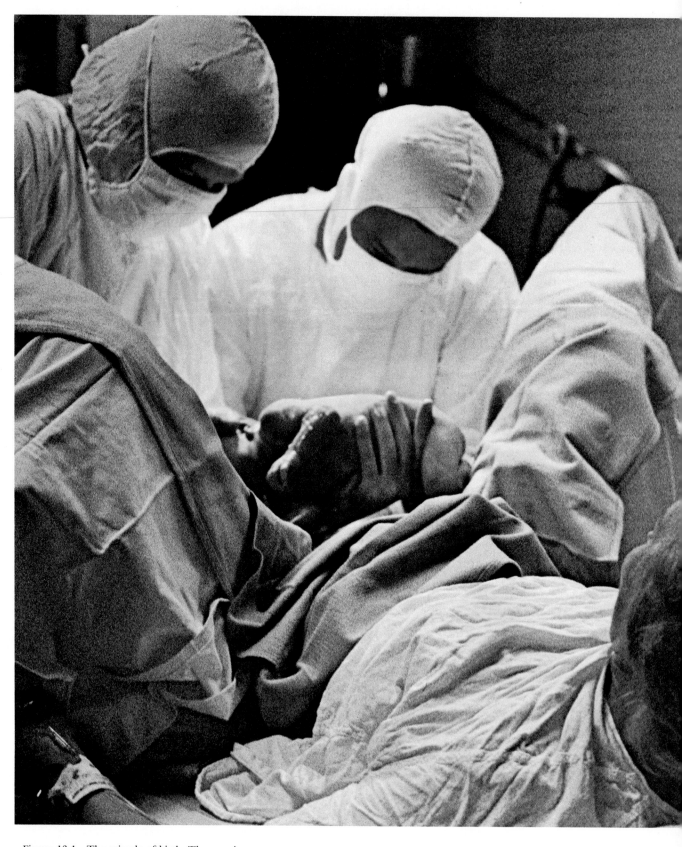

Figure 13.1   The miracle of birth. The man in green
on the right is the father.

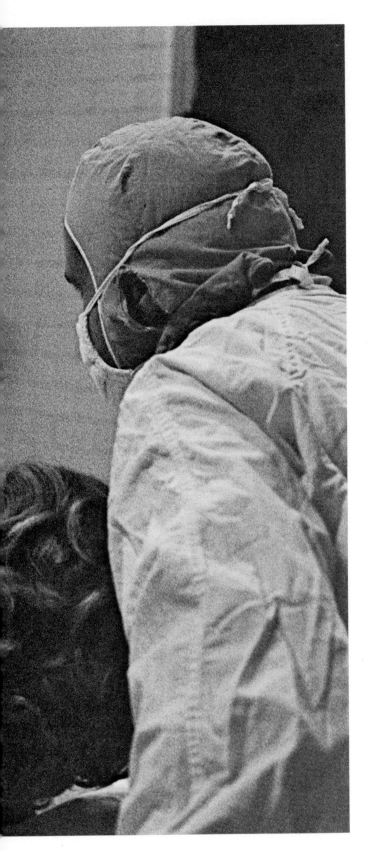

13

Perpetuation of the human species is insured by the instinctual drives that motivate individuals toward sexual union and by the extreme pleasure both sexes can experience when performing the sexual act. Yet with this great pleasure comes responsibility for the consequences of that act—the possible creation of human life and the contribution of another individual to the human population.

To take advantage of their birthright of sexual enjoyment and at the same time to assume their share of responsibility in reproductive control, every man and woman should thoroughly understand the reproductive process and how to enhance or inhibit it.

The male and female reproductive systems were described briefly in Chapter 2, and their role in sexual responsiveness was delineated in Chapter 12. Here emphasis will be on the processes that make possible the production and union of sex cells, or gametes, and the growth and birth of an individual resulting from that union. Because the essential reproductive event takes place within the female body, it is the woman's system that will be the primary focus of this chapter, but obviously the male plays a necessary role.

THE MALE CONTRIBUTION
Unlike women, who are born with a full set of egg cells already in their ovaries, men are not born with

Reproduction and Birth Control

spermatozoa. Instead their testes contain a number of undifferentiated cells, some of which are called spermatogonia. Through a long process called *spermatogenesis* (it may take as long as seventy-five days), the spermatogonia undergo various stages of development, finally becoming *spermatozoa*, the male sex cells capable of fertilizing an ovum. A normal man's testes produce about 200 million mature sperm each day. Spermatogenesis is a continuous process that can last to old age (see Figure 13.2).

The prostate, the seminal vesicles, and the bulbourethral glands constitute the accessory reproductive glands in the male. They secrete and store the *seminal fluid*, which transports the spermatozoa. Mature sperm are stored in the epididymis prior to traveling through the coiled *vas deferens* in preparation for ejaculation.

The ejaculatory process occurs in two stages. The first consists of contraction of the accessory organs (the entire male genital tract, including epididymis, vas deferens, and seminal vesicles) and the subsequent delivery of seminal fluid from the various fluid-producing organs into the urethra up to the external urethral sphincter. The second stage involves relaxation of the sphincter and the resulting expulsion of *semen* (sperm and fluid) through the penile urethra, aided by muscular contractions of the penis and urethral bulb.

Human sperm are tiny, tadpolelike cells with oval heads and long, thin tails. Several hundred million of these sperm are contained in the fluid of a single ejaculation. Such an enormous number of sperm are produced because only a small percentage of them can survive within the woman's body and actually find their way from the vagina through the cervix and uterus to the Fallopian tube, where fertilization (the union of sperm and egg to form a zygote) occurs. Many sperm are ordinarily necessary to surround the egg and break down its outer coating so that one of their number can penetrate the egg's membrane and unite with the ovum. Before discussing how the zygote develops into a living being, however, the preparation of the egg and of the environment in which a fertilized egg can develop must be explained.

THE FEMALE SYSTEM

The woman's reproductive organs were described to some extent in Chapters 2 and 12. This section will be devoted to the internal structures of reproduction (the uterus, Fallopian tubes, and ovaries).

The Uterus

The pelvis resembles a basket forming the bottom of a woman's torso. It contains all the internal reproductive organs. The sides of the basket are of bone; the bottom is of muscle with three openings

Spermatozoa

Castoff Cytoplasm

Spermatids

Spermatogonium

Primary Spermatocyte   **Secondary Spermatocytes**

Figure 13.2   Spermatogenesis.

Figure 13.3   (*right*) Monthly changes in the uterine wall. On the fifth day after menstruation (early proliferative phase), the denuded surface is fed by short basal arteries. During the proliferative phase, estrogen causes glands and arteries to proliferate, and the uterine wall thickens. After ovulation during the secretory phase, the lining swells as arteries corkscrew to the surface and the glands begin to secrete mucus. At the premenstrual phase (if fertilization has not occurred), the spiral arteries constrict, causing the surface layers to disrupt in preparation for the sloughing off of the menstrual blood.

through it: the urethra, the vagina, and the rectum. The *uterus*, or womb as it is sometimes called, is a small, pear-shaped organ that rests on its small end (the cervix) in the center of the pelvis.

The uterus has only one function: to house a growing baby from shortly after conception until it is ready to be born. During nine months of pregnancy this miraculous little organ grows from the size of a small pear into a huge muscular bag filling the entire abdomen, a bag that holds not only a seven-pound baby but a quart of water and a one-pound placenta besides.

The uterus is not a sex gland and takes little part in a woman's sexual response. Removing it does not make a woman fat or bring on the menopause, as many people seem to believe. This fact should be clearly understood by every woman who

must part with her uterus through gynecological surgery (hysterectomy) because of uterine disease. As long as the ovaries remain, the monthly ebb and flow of ovarian hormones and corresponding feelings will go right on until the normal time for menopause. Actually, a woman's sexual response may be enhanced after a hysterectomy if her uterus was tender or painful.

What ceases when the uterus is removed is *menstruation*. Menstrual blood comes only from the uterus. For thirty to forty years of a woman's life, the menstrual cycle prepares and renovates her reproductive system. Each month in "regular," nonpregnant women the lining of the uterus—the endometrium—thickens, grows, and undergoes vascular and glandular changes under the influence of various hormones preparing it to nourish a ferti-

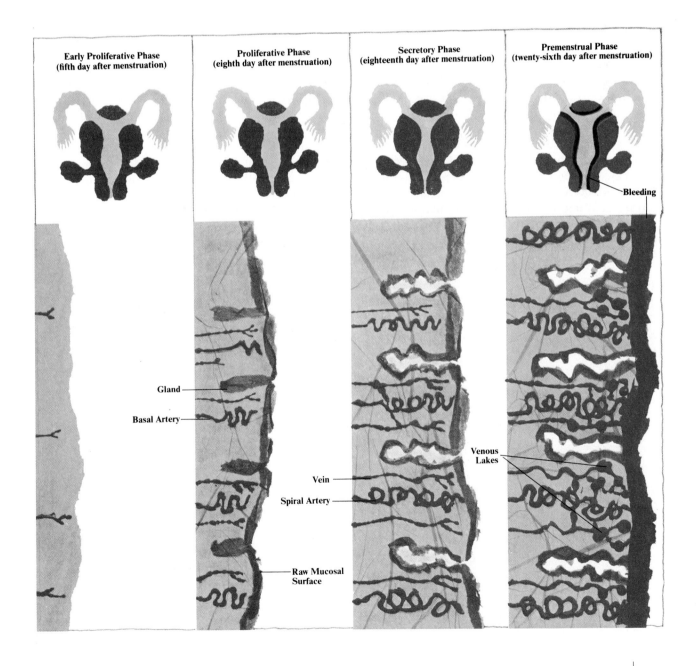

Early Proliferative Phase
(fifth day after menstruation)

Proliferative Phase
(eighth day after menstruation)

Secretory Phase
(eighteenth day after menstruation)

Premenstrual Phase
(twenty-sixth day after menstruation)

Bleeding

Gland

Basal Artery

Venous Lakes

Vein

Spiral Artery

Raw Mucosal Surface

lized ovum (see Figure 13.3). If pregnancy has not occurred, the whole lining of the uterus sloughs away monthly in the bloody discharge called menstruation, named for the Latin word *mensis*, meaning month. Whenever pregnancy does occur, of course, this lining remains to nourish the growing fetus. Menstruation is the only instance in nature where a loss of blood does not signify injury but is instead a sign of good health.

The onset of menstruation (*menarche*—pronounced men-ar-key) is variable, but it usually occurs between the ages of ten and sixteen (see Figure 13.4). In unusual cases it has been reported to begin as early as two and as late as twenty years of age. Many factors, including climate, heredity, health status, and personal hygiene appear to influence the age of menarche.

The average menstrual cycle lasts from twenty-seven to thirty days in most women. Cycles that are completely irregular or bleeding that occurs at intervals of less than eighteen or more than forty-two days should be considered abnormal, and usually ovulation does not occur. Menstrual flow generally lasts three to six days. Most women are aware of bodily changes immediately preceding their "period." They feel slightly swollen or bloated, their breasts become sore or full, and they may have backache, leg pains, or feelings of depression or lethargy. In some women, premenstrual tension may be severe enough to alter personality and behavior. It is important for these women and those in contact with them to realize the normal cyclic character of these disturbances, which last but a few days.

The Fallopian Tubes

The *Fallopian tubes*, or *oviducts*, are tiny, muscular tunnels, the setting for the drama of "Sperm Meets Egg." The soft tubes resembles miniature saxophones, attached by their small ends to either side of the uterus. They are connecting canals between the ovaries and the uterus, serving as a passageway and a meeting ground for the sperm and the egg. In order for an egg cell to develop into a baby, it must ripen first in the ovary inside what is known as a *Graafian follicle*. When the follicle is ripe, it comes up under the cover of the ovary, thins the cover into a blister, and finally the mature egg pops free from the ovary. This process is called *ovulation*. Usually only one ovary releases an egg each month.

The whole process is rather remarkable. Apparently the many-fingered fringe on the open end of the tube searches around for the ripened egg and guides it into the mouth of the tube. The tube is lined with tiny waving cilia, like miniature blades of grass, all pointing toward the uterus. These cilia gradually propel the egg toward the middle of the tube, where, if all conditions are favorable, it will meet some tiny male sperm, one of which may penetrate it. If the egg is not fertilized, it dies within a few hours and is sloughed off. But if it is fertilized, the egg moves along the tube, an ever-multiplying mass of cells, drops into the uterus, and plants itself in the lining of that organ. There it will grow to be first an embryo, then a fetus, and, finally, a baby.

The tubes become diseased or inflamed with a severity out of all proportion to their small size. Inflammation in the tubes (salpingitis) may leave scars and constrictions that prevent egg cells from passing through, making pregnancy difficult to achieve. Occasionally the tubes are only partially blocked, and the smaller male sperm cells can wriggle past the constriction, but then the much larger egg cell cannot get down to the uterus. In this case pregnancy in the tube may result. This situation is rare but always serious, for pregnancy in the tube is very difficult to detect. Eventually the tube ruptures, and immediate surgery is necessary to stop internal hemorrhage.

Figure 13.4   The decline in the age of menarche (onset of menstruation) in various European countries and the United States in the last century. (After Tanner, 1968.)

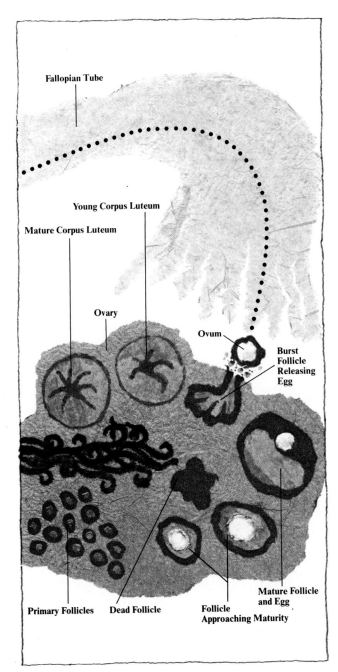

Fallopian Tube

Young Corpus Luteum

Mature Corpus Luteum

Ovary

Ovum

Burst Follicle Releasing Egg

Primary Follicles   **Dead Follicle**   **Follicle Approaching Maturity**

Mature Follicle and Egg

Figure 13.5   Oogenesis and ovulation.

The Ovaries

The *ovaries* are the true sex glands of women. Each ovary is about the size and shape of a flattened, lumpy olive and lies close to the open end of its corresponding Fallopian tube. Each month one or the other ovary will usually produce an egg on a day that is somewhere near the midpoint between menstrual periods. Many women can tell when ovulation occurs by the way they feel. The pelvis feels heavy, or there is a slight soreness on one side or the other or even a little pain that may last for a couple of days. Just why the follicle ruptures and discharges the egg at this point is not clear, but hormones are involved.

Besides making ovulation possible, the ovaries have another purpose of extreme importance to every woman. They act as endocrine glands, producing the body chemicals (ovarian hormones) that regulate the menstrual cycle, and, in fact, they influence to a great extent the general emotional attitude of a woman. Nervousness and tension before a period and relaxation afterward often parallel the ebb and flow of these ovarian hormones. The principal hormone is *estrogen*, produced mainly by certain cells of the Graafian follicle. Estrogen is responsible for the development of female characteristics as a girl matures into adulthood. This hormone declines at the menopause, though fortunately the female characteristics and sex interest remain. The other main ovarian hormone is *progesterone*, which—together with more estrogen—is produced by the *corpus luteum*, a structure evolved from the residual material of the follicle after release of the mature egg (see Figures 13.5 and 13.7).

If one ovary has to be removed or ceases functioning, the other supplies enough hormone for the body. Menstrual rhythm and ovulation remain undisturbed and childbearing may go on. But if both ovaries are removed or cease functioning, menstruation ceases.

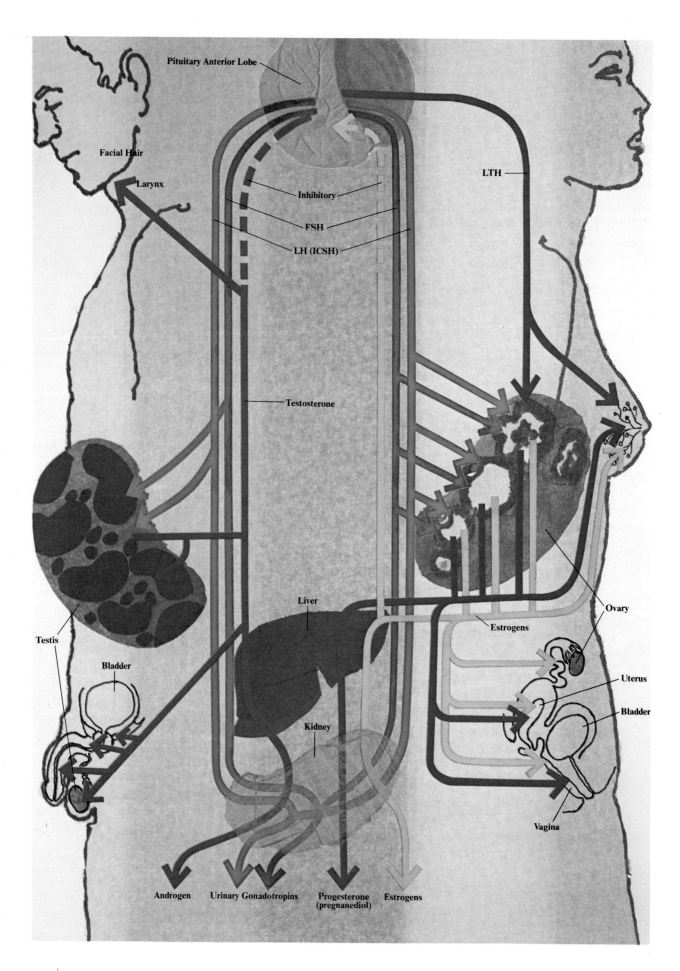

Pituitary Anterior Lobe

Facial Hair

Larynx

LTH

Inhibitory

FSH

LH (ICSH)

Testosterone

Liver

Ovary

Estrogens

Testis

Uterus

Bladder

Bladder

Kidney

Vagina

Androgen   Urinary Gonadotropins   Progesterone   Estrogens
                                     (pregnanediol)

If ovarian hormones become deficient or out of balance in relation to each other, a disturbance in menstruation often follows. In such cases menstruation may be either too scant or too excessive, and it may stop altogether for a few months. Any such menstrual disturbance demands immediate gynecological attention. Often the hormone disturbance can be corrected with artificial hormone preparations, or at least an artificial balance can be achieved until the natural balance returns.

Problems of Menstruation

Approximately 50 percent of women are slowed down or incapacitated in some degree by menstrual pain (*dysmenorrhea*). Menstrual cramps are caused by painful contractions of the uterus. There are two principal types of menstrual pain. In the primary type there is no structural disease, but the pelvic nerves are overly sensitive. The uterus normally contracts during menstrual flow, but if the nerves are too sensitive, it overcontracts in a spasm.

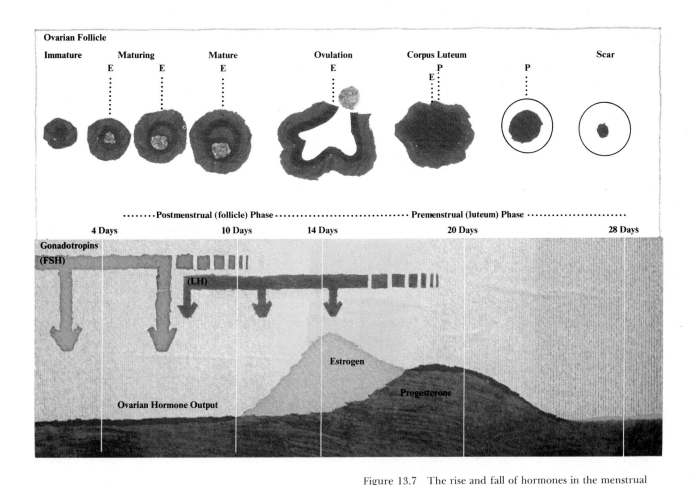

Figure 13.7 The rise and fall of hormones in the menstrual cycle. The ovarian follicle emits estrogen until the ovum is released, at which time the follicle becomes the corpus luteum and secretes both estrogen and progesterone. The gonadotropins—follicle-stimulating hormone (FSH) and leutenizing hormone (LH)—are emitted by the pituitary in the first part of the cycle.

Figure 13.6 Sex hormones. The primary gonadal hormones, testosterone and estrogen, cause maturation of the sex organs and the appearance of secondary sex characteristics associated with puberty—in males, the voice deepens and facial and pubic hair appear; in females, breasts develop, the hips become rounded, and pubic hair appears. The level of these hormones is controlled by the anterior lobe of the pituitary gland through a feedback mechanism using ICSH (LH) and FSH. The hormones are then metabolized by the liver and excreted through the kidneys. Additional female hormones include progesterone, which affects the uterine lining and breasts, and LTH, which stimulates the mammary glands to produce milk.

The second type of menstrual pain is called *organic* or *secondary dysmenorrhea*. It is caused by underlying disease or disorder of the uterus, tubes, or ovaries. Correction of the underlying disorder is, of course, necessary before one can obtain relief.

A number of studies have demonstrated that menstrual cramps tend to be more frequent and severe in underexercised women. Exercise is often successful in relieving menstrual pain. Mild work such as walking, bicycle riding, and relaxed swimming coupled with bending, stretching, relaxing movements, especially those movements including the abdominal, hip, and low back muscles, seem most useful.

Feminine Hygiene

The healthy vagina secretes sufficient fluid to keep it moist. Used-up cells are always being shed from the lining of the vagina, and these cells mixed with fluid produce a thick, white, nonirritating secretion. This secretion is clean, healthy, and odorless unless it is allowed to collect in the folds of the skin surrounding the vaginal opening. Careful bathing of this area will prevent unpleasant odor from developing, as odor usually comes from the labia and outer folds rather than the vagina itself.

When this vaginal secretion becomes excessive enough to stain clothing, or if it is yellow, irritating, watery, bloody, or smelly, then it is called a vaginal discharge, or *leukorrhea*. This type of discharge may mean infection in some part of the genital tract. There also are normal causes for increased vaginal secretion, however. Sexual tension, emotional stress, and even the sequential type of birth control pills may cause enough vaginal wetness to stain clothing. Nevertheless, heavier discharge may mean infection and should not be neglected. It is a warning signal that should bring one to a physician for examination without delay.

Although douching seems to be a popular practice among many American women, it is not necessary for good health. The normal vaginal environment is acid, which keeps it clear of undesirable bacteria. On the other hand, douching does no par-

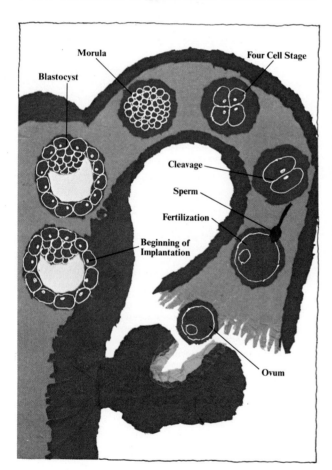

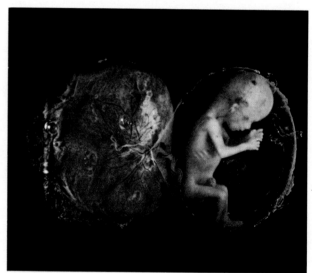

Figure 13.8   (*left*) The egg, or ovum, is released from the ovary at the time of ovulation. It begins its journey through the Fallopian tube where it is fertilized by the male sperm. The zygote immediately begins the process of cell division and within seven or eight days it is securely implanted in the uterus where it continues to develop for the duration of its prenatal life. (*above*) At four months the fetus is approximately six inches long and weighs about four ounces. (From Rugh and Shettles, *From Conception to Birth*, New York: Harper & Row, 1971).

ticular harm, provided a mild acid solution is used. Alkaline or commercial chemical douches may neutralize the protective acids so that harmful bacteria can multiply.

PRENATAL DEVELOPMENT

Assuming that ovulation has occurred and that enough sperm have been deposited in the vagina and have been swept or propelled up through the uterus to the appropriate tube at just the right time, fertilization may occur. The zygote travels down the remainder of the Fallopian tube into the uterus, a journey that takes about three days. During this journey the zygote undergoes rapid cell division. After floating free in the uterus for three or four days, the cluster of cells burrows down into the endometrium (the lining of the uterine wall) in a process called *implantation*.

Within two or three days after implantation, miraculous changes occur in the endometrium around the growing organism. Specialized cells from the maternal uterus and the now-forming embryo begin to differentiate into the *placenta*, the structure that will absorb life-giving nutrients from the mother and carry them to the developing organism for approximately the next nine months.

At the time of implantation actual pregnancy can be said to have begun. Soon thereafter physiological changes occur in the mother that can be detected by pregnancy tests. What happens during the rest of the course of the pregnancy is one of the truly amazing phenomena of life. What starts out as one cell, a speck barely visible to the human eye, in a very short time grows into a complete human being, equipped with miniature versions of all the necessary internal organs and external characteristics that not only make it human, but also a particular individual. Table 13.1 provides a synopsis of the changes that take place each month in the embryo and (after three months) the fetus.

Table 13.1 Milestones of Prenatal Development

PERIOD	*Development*
First two weeks	Zygote goes through multiple cell divisions. It attaches itself to the uterine wall, becoming an embryo, a fishlike organism floating in a fluid-filled sac.
Fourth week	Primitive heart begins beating and rudimentary organs are formed; the organism is still nonhuman in appearance.
Third month	Embryo becomes a fetus; it has a definite human appearance and is already quite active; amost all internal and external physical equipment is well developed.
Fourth month	Growth of lower body parts accelerates; most bone models formed; mother feels "quickening."
Fifth month	Fetus sleeps and wakes; it has a characteristic "lie"; it is capable of extrauterine life, except that it cannot maintain respiration.
Sixth month	Eyes (fully formed) open; eye movements occur; grasp reflex present.
Seventh month	Fetus can survive outside uterus in a highly sheltered environment.
Eighth and ninth months	Fat forms over the body, and the finishing touches are put on the organs and functional capacities.

Source: CRM Books. *Study Guide to Developmental Psychology Today.* Del Mar, Calif.: CRM Books, 1971.

Throughout its prenatal life, the developing organism is enclosed in a fluid-filled sac (the amnion), which primarily provides protection, and is attached to the placenta via the umbilical cord. As an *embryo*, the organism is less than an inch long and looks something like a curved fish. After three months it is called a *fetus* and looks distinctly human, having developed arms and legs with perfectly shaped fingers and toes. By the end of the third month, although it is only about three inches long

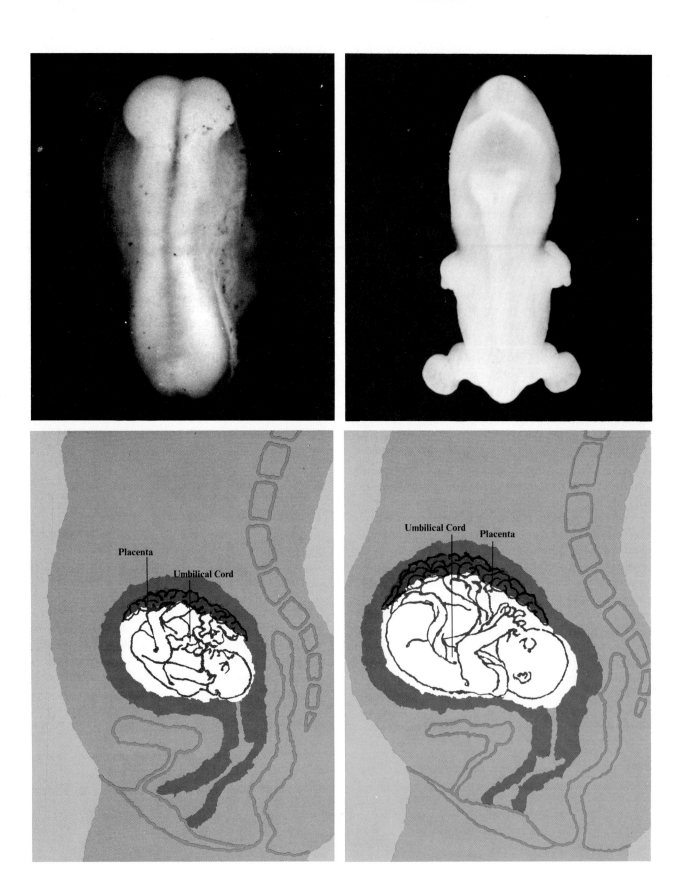

and weighs a mere ounce, the fetus can perform such actions as kicking its legs, closing its fingers, turning its head, and opening and closing its mouth. Also by this time most of its internal organs are formed and able to function, so that the remainder of the prenatal period can be spent in the process of growth and in putting the finishing touches on the organism's functional capacities.

At birth the average full-term infant weighs anywhere from five to twelve pounds and may be from seventeen to twenty-two inches long. The average length of pregnancy is 280 days, but babies born as early as 180 days or as late as 334 days after conception may be able to survive.

PREGNANCY

Under ordinary circumstances the pregnant woman is able to do almost all the things she normally enjoys, whether it be playing, working, or making love. Of course, in addition to building up her own health, strength, and energy she must fulfill the extra requirements of a growing baby, who for nine months depends on her for all body-building materials. Nevertheless, the mother cannot "eat for two" unless she is not concerned about her own and her baby's food requirements or does not want a shapely figure after the baby is born.

The medical supervision of pregnancy—helping to build health and strength, insuring that the baby's requirements are met, and watching for any complications—is called *prenatal care* and requires visits to the doctor at regular intervals. A woman in pregnancy should think of herself as an athlete in training, building up her body to the highest level of physical fitness, so that the childbirth that lies ahead will be a joy and not an ordeal. With such a plan of living and with the medical skills that are now available, she may emerge from childbirth healthier than before and with her body both strong and shapely.

Early Changes in Pregnancy

Usually the first indication of pregnancy is that an expected menstrual period does not occur. There may be a continued feeling that menstruation is about to begin but "can't quite get started." Congested and tender breasts, increased irritability, heaviness in the pelvis, and sometimes a little nausea at mealtime may or may not be noticed.

About three weeks after the missed period, an experienced doctor, by pelvic examination, can usually be fairly certain of the existence of pregnancy. Pelvic tissues are all slightly softened, the vaginal opening becomes slightly purplish in appearance, and the uterus begins to enlarge. This examination is gentle and never in any way disturbs the pregnancy.

With some women it may be impossible for the doctor to be sure for several more weeks. In such cases, pregnancy can be confirmed or ruled out within three hours with about 95 percent accuracy by examination of a urine sample for the presence of certain hormones.

Visits to the Doctor

The ideal time for the first prenatal visit to the physician is *before* pregnancy. A woman should be in the best possible general health before starting pregnancy, and for this reason it is wise for her to have a general physical examination that is thorough enough to answer the question: "Shall I have a baby now?"

If the complete examination has not been done before the start of pregnancy, it should be accomplished during the early months. Conditions that might result in complications of pregnancy, obstructed labor, or difficult delivery can then be discovered and corrected before they cause trouble. The individual plan of prenatal care will be based on the results of this examination. Needs for special exercise or special diet can be determined at this time.

Figure 13.9 (*top left*) Human embryo at twenty-nine days. At one month the embryo is only one-fifth of an inch long. (*top right*) At forty days the human embryo, shown here from the back, exhibits a well-defined spinal cord, rudimentary brain, and paddlelike arms and legs. (*bottom left*) By the end of the fifth month the fetus is about one foot long and weighs about a pound. (*bottom right*) During the final period of prenatal development, the finishing touches are put on the organs and functional capacities of the organism.

Regular medical consultation should be provided every three to four weeks in early pregnancy and more often during the last two months, even when pregnancy is normal. Sometimes if minor illness or infections that might affect the pregnancy are being treated, more frequent visits are necessary. Blood pressure, weight changes, and urinalyses are important in detecting early signs of possible serious complications.

Blood Examinations

Sometime during early pregnancy a sample of blood will be taken and a series of tests performed. Hemoglobin and red-cell counts indicate accurately the richness of blood or the possible presence of anemia. The white-cell count may reveal or rule out hidden infection or other underlying disorders. A blood test for syphilis is required by law.

The Rh test is always done for expectant mothers. Much needless worry has resulted from misunderstanding of this protective test. Briefly, some people have Rh negative blood and others (five times as many) are Rh positive. If the mother is Rh negative with an Rh positive husband, a common combination, it may affect the developing fetus. This problem is caused when Rh antigens (substances that stimulate production of antibodies) inherited from the father are present in the fetal blood, while absent in the mother's blood. Antigenic red blood cells pass into the maternal blood from the fetus during delivery, resulting in the production of anti-Rh substances in the mother's blood. These anti-Rh substances may then cross the placental barrier in subsequent children and destroy the fetal red cells, requiring a blood transfusion at birth. Sometimes the fetus may be so severely af-

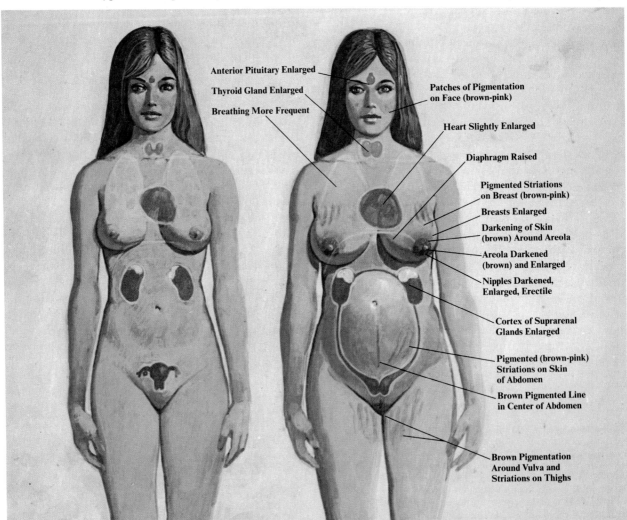

Anterior Pituitary Enlarged

Thyroid Gland Enlarged

Breathing More Frequent

Patches of Pigmentation on Face (brown-pink)

Heart Slightly Enlarged

Diaphragm Raised

Pigmented Striations on Breast (brown-pink)

Breasts Enlarged

Darkening of Skin (brown) Around Areola

Areola Darkened (brown) and Enlarged

Nipples Darkened, Enlarged, Erectile

Cortex of Suprarenal Glands Enlarged

Pigmented (brown-pink) Striations on Skin of Abdomen

Brown Pigmented Line in Center of Abdomen

Brown Pigmentation Around Vulva and Striations on Thighs

Figure 13.10 Physiological changes during pregnancy. The body is shown at conception and at thirty weeks.

fected as to require intrauterine transfusion. But under some circumstances pregnancies with an Rh incompatibility are normal and the infant is not affected.

The present treatment is to immunize all Rh negative mothers who are carrying Rh positive babies as soon as the fetus' blood type is known. This shot then blocks and covers all the antigens that may have reached the maternal circulation and prevents her immune system from "seeing" the antigen and thus from making antibodies to it. (For a further discussion of immunity, see Chapter 22.)

Discomforts of Pregnancy

One of the common discomforts of early pregnancy is "morning sickness," so called because it appears most often soon after awakening, when the stomach is empty. This type of nausea may reappear late in the morning and late in the afternoon, each time the stomach again gets empty. The exact chemical disturbance that underlies this nausea is not clearly understood. However, it is most common and more severe among "high strung" women, especially if they are distraught with anxiety and worry. Nausea usually disappears by itself around the time of the third missed period. Small, frequent meals coupled with use of antinausea medication will usually bring relief.

"Heartburn," or acid indigestion, is a common problem in the later months of pregnancy, but relief is usually easily obtained with an antacid tablet. Hemorrhoids, which are merely varicose veins of the rectum, also often occur into the later months when the baby's head presses down in the pelvis. Hemorrhoids frequently disappear without treatment after delivery.

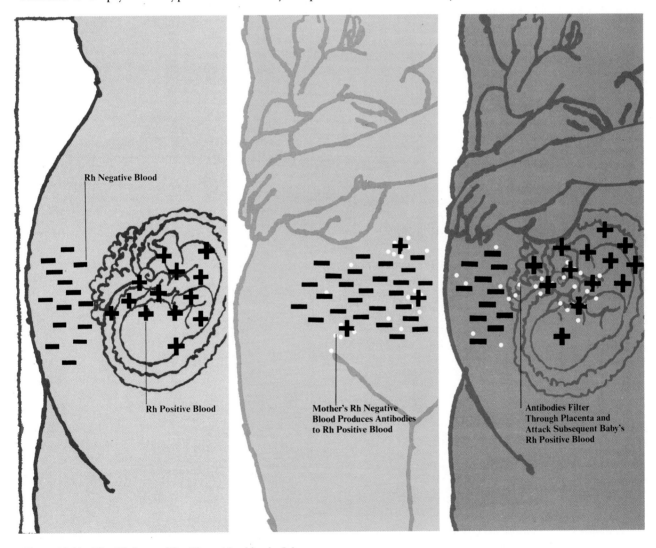

Figure 13.11 The Rh factor. The Rh positive blood of the baby may get into the mother's bloodstream at the time of birth. Her body acts by creating antibodies that may attack any subsequent Rh positive children, destroying their red blood cells. The Rh factor is only one of many blood factors by which human blood can be typed.

Many pregnant women worry about varicose veins. If the problem produces no discomfort, it may be disregarded because it will, for the most part, disappear after delivery. If the legs ache, an elastic bandage or elastic stockings will help. Elevating the lower legs on pillows each afternoon will keep them more comfortable. Pains in the tender ligaments that support the uterus also can be relaxed by elevating one's lower legs. This discomfort is common between the fourth and the seventh months.

Miscarriage

In one pregnancy out of eight, *miscarriage* (spontaneous abortion) is inevitable because either the developing organism was not implanted correctly or the egg or sperm was defective to begin with. Nature then simply gets rid of something that has no ability to survive. Bleeding and cramps continue until the uterus expels the defective fertilized ovum. When properly managed, a miscarriage is no more serious than a delivery. Future chances for childbearing are not impaired.

Automobile trips do not cause miscarriages, nor do falls, or emotional shocks. On the other hand, miscarriages may be related to general glandular or body disorders, which is one of the reasons for having a good medical examination before starting a pregnancy.

These remarks generally do not apply, however, to the rather rare problem of habitual abortion, in which a woman suffers one miscarriage after another. This discouraging condition requires the most skilled and specialized medical investigation and treatment.

There is occasional confusion of terminology regarding abortion and miscarriage. Physicians use the word "abortion" to describe the end of any pregnancy before the fetus is advanced enough to survive outside the mother's body, irrespective of whether the end of the pregnancy comes about spontaneously (miscarriage) or through external intervention.

LABOR AND BIRTH

During the last month or two of pregnancy a woman may notice her uterus contracting at irregular intervals. These contractions usually are not painful, but occasionally they are. Nervous tension alone may cause these "false labor" contractions to become painful. True labor contractions usually feel like menstrual cramps, as they both represent contractions of the uterus. A contraction may be

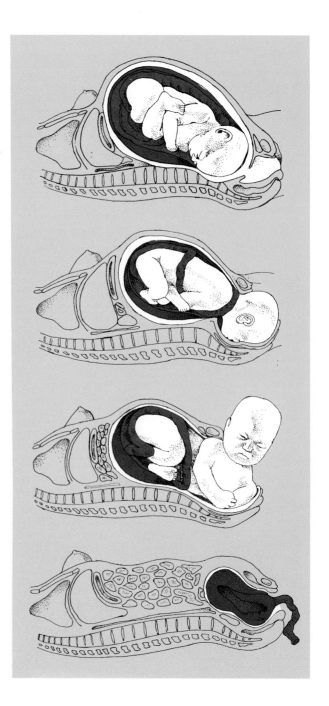

Figure 13.12 Stages of childbirth, shown both diagrammatically and in a sequence of photographs. The baby's head lies close to the cervix, which becomes fully dilated. Strong uterine contractions begin to force the head into the birth canal (vagina). After the head is born, the shoulders rotate in the birth canal and the rest of the body is expelled. In the last stage of delivery, the placenta and umbilical cord (sometimes called "afterbirth") are expelled. Note that in top middle photograph an episiotomy is being performed.

felt as only a tightness in the back. Frequently a small amount of vaginal bleeding is noticed a day or two before the onset of labor.

Sometimes, near the end of pregnancy, clear fluid will drain spontaneously from the vagina, which means that the amniotic sac, or bag of waters, has broken, and labor is likely to start shortly. Contrary to some popular opinion, early rupture of the bag of waters (dry labor) does not mean that labor will be difficult or prolonged; in fact, it is likely to be faster and easier. Rupture of the amniotic membrane itself is normal and painless. True labor contractions usually start at intervals of fifteen to twenty minutes and gradually become more fre-

quent. In some cases, however, labor sets in abruptly with contractions coming every three to five minutes.

Every woman probably has some degree of apprehension as she approaches childbirth itself. To obtain the peace of mind that is necessary to make the birth of her baby the rich and deeply satisfying experience it should be, the pregnant woman should try to obtain as much information as she can about the birth process.

First, she must understand what happens during the contractions of labor; that each contraction of the uterus brings the baby just a little closer to birth; that her own body relaxation can lessen the

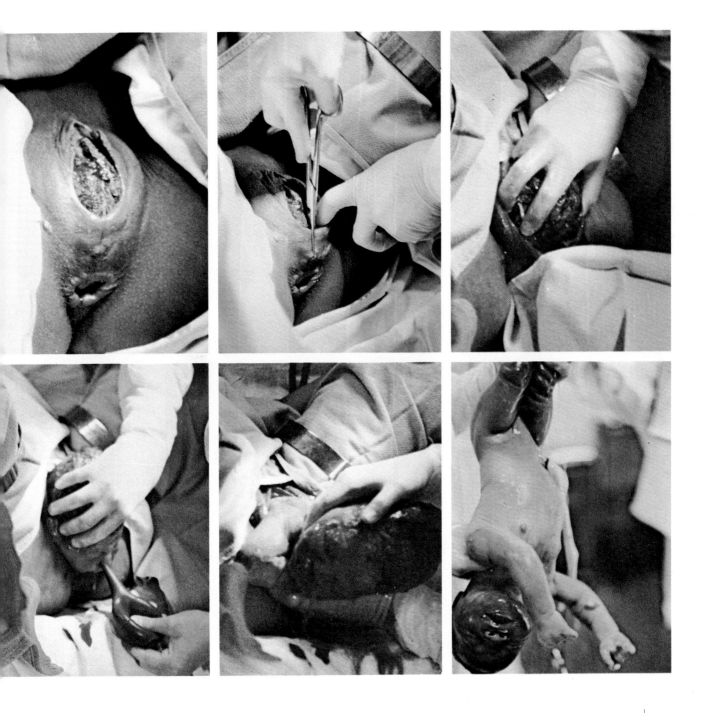

discomfort of strong contractions. She must have confidence in herself and in her ability to have a baby naturally. She must have confidence in her doctor and in his ability to make her labor comfortable. She must realize that for every possible complication, there is a method of treatment that will make it safe for her.

For example, sometimes during the course of labor it may become necessary to do a Caesarean operation (also called a Caesarean section), but this operation is now a safe one even late in labor. Instead of being delivered through the birth canal, the baby is removed through incisions in the abdomen and uterus. This operation is sometimes required when the mother has a pelvic opening so small in relation to the infant's head that normal delivery might be dangerous both to her and to her child. Caesarean section also is used in cases of malpresentation, placenta previa (the placenta is situated over the cervix, making a normal birth impossible and causing massive blood loss with the onset of labor), and previous section (because of

the danger of uterine rupture at the site of the previous incision).

In order to understand what happens during a labor contraction, one should try to visualize the uterus as a big muscular bag that is upside down with its open end emptying into the vagina. At first this opening is almost closed by an elastic ring, the cervix. Every time the walls of the bag contract, the baby's head is pressed very firmly against the cervix, and the opening dilates a little more. Finally, the elastic cervix opens wide enough for the baby's head to pass through into the vagina. Only now can the mother herself aid in expelling the baby. She then almost automatically bears down with her abdominal muscles during each contraction, very much as she would in expelling a bowel movement.

The dilating contractions of labor may be painful, and in fact, they are often called "labor pains." But it is equally true that medication usually can be used to relieve most of the pain and to make labor reasonably comfortable. Nevertheless, medication must be used with caution because overdosage

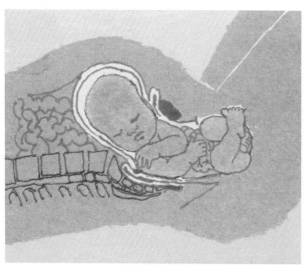

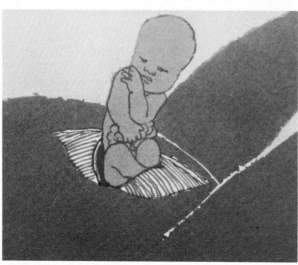

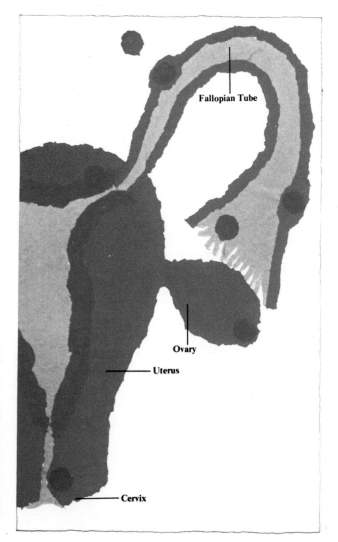

Fallopian Tube

Ovary

Uterus

Cervix

could slow down labor or affect the baby. The more one learns to relax the entire body during each contraction, the less pain there will be and the easier it will be for medications to completely relieve it.

When the baby's head is through the cervix and in the vagina, the woman feels a compulsion to bear down and expel the baby through the vaginal opening. This process goes on even under gas anesthesia. First the crown of the baby's head appears, and then gradually, with succeeding contractions, the head normally slides out face down. Once the head is out, the body usually follows easily because the head is largest in diameter. At this point the umbilical cord is tied and severed, and the newly breathing, loudly crying baby is welcomed to the world. Soon afterward the uterus contracts down into a large ball, expelling the placenta.

It is common practice to have the mother lightly asleep during the delivery. The process of labor goes on under light anesthesia just as if the mother were awake. It also is common practice to aid the birth with low forceps. This practice should not be confused with the popular conception of an "instrument delivery." Usually a surgical incision called an *episiotomy* is used to prevent undue stretching or tearing of the tissues around the vaginal opening. This incision is repaired with sutures, leaving the opening about the same as it was before pregnancy.

Many women have a strong desire to stay awake during delivery, both for the rich experience of childbirth itself and to hear their baby's first cry. This desire may be met by using low spinal anesthesia. Usually, with spinal, or "saddle," anesthesia, comfort is complete and the experience of having a baby is a happy and exciting one. At any time during labor or delivery, however, it may be necessary to abandon the method being used and switch to another.

Some women have been able to have their babies without any medication for pain relief, usually adopting one of the "natural" methods of delivery. These methods involve rather intensive education and training to prepare the mother for delivery so she will not require an anesthetic. Early in the course of training she is taught how to avoid fear and tension so she will feel less pain during labor.

INFERTILITY

In the United States today, approximately one married couple out of ten tries to have children without success. Adoption can be a solution to the problem for some. Fortunately, in recent years advances have been made in the methods of overcoming infertility, and now it is possible for many of these formerly sterile couples to have children. There are many causes of sterility, and a number of ingenious tests and procedures must be carried out by a physician before all possible causes have been identified and corrected. Often a complete investigation with appropriate treatment will last for eighteen months. Couples who start a sterility study should be prepared to go through the entire program. Those who see one doctor after another for superficial examinations rarely achieve success.

Male Infertility

In one-third or more of sterile matings, the husband has an anatomical or physiological defect that is either wholly or partially responsible for the barren marriage. It should be noted that there is no relation between a man's erotic sexual adequacy and his true fertility.

The test for fertility in males involves thorough microscopic study of a semen specimen to ascertain the degree of male fertility. Just as a low red blood count indicates anemia, so a low sperm count indicates low male fertility. A normal semen ejaculate should measure from three to eight cubic centimeters with 50 million to 100 million live and swimming spermatozoa per cubic centimeter. If defi-

Figure 13.13 (*top left*) Breech presentation occurs in approximately 3 to 4 percent of all deliveries. (*bottom left*) Caesarean sections are performed in cases in which the mother's pelvic structure is too small to admit the baby's head, when the baby's head is unusually large due to an abnormality, or in emergency situations in which a rapid delivery is imperative.

Figure 13.14 (*right*) Ectopic pregnancies are those that occur outside of the uterus, such as in the Fallopian tubes or in the abdominal cavity.

ciency is found, a thorough study is usually carried out by a physician competent in this field. Often when the cause of male sterility is found, hormone treatment is instrumental to restore fertility.

Female Infertility

Female infertility may be caused by some simple and minor condition that is easily found and corrected, but sometimes there are complicated problems in diagnosis. Frequently a series of special tests are required. Because general bodily disorders, glandular disorders, and a host of conditions outside the pelvis can underlie female sterility, more than pelvic tests must be carried out. A Rubin's test (running gas under measured pressure through the Fallopian tubes) will determine whether they are open or closed. If the tubes are blocked, an x-ray picture will show the location of the block after some iodized material has been injected into the uterus and tubes.

A Huhner test may be performed on mucus obtained from the cervix at ovulation time (as indi- cated by a rise in basal temperature) several hours after intercourse. Microscopic study of the mucus will show whether the sperm cells are still alive and whether they are able to pass into the uterus. Sometimes a small sample of the lining of the uterus will be taken in order to determine if it is favorable for nourishing a fertilized ovum. Some women's vaginas seem to contain an unknown factor that kills sperm.

THE MENOPAUSE

Menopause is the cessation of menstruation and of cyclic reproductive activity that occurs eventually in every woman. The average age of occurrence is forty-eight but it can begin earlier than forty or later than fifty-five. Menstrual periods usually falter for a few months and then cease altogether, and a woman is said to have gone through the menopause, or "change of life." This change is also sometimes known as the *climacteric*, the time that marks the end of her reproductive period.

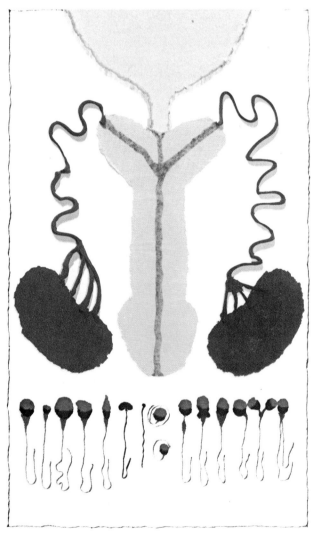

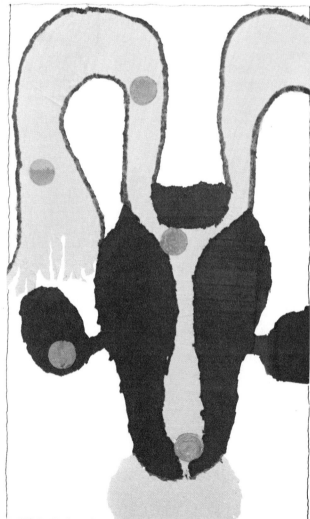

What actually has happened is that her ovaries, after thirty or forty years of activity, have finally lost their ability to produce mature eggs. Moreover, they also have lost much of their ability to produce the feminizing hormones so important in maintaining a woman's physiological state. The menopausal woman may welcome her loss of fertility, but the reduced production of feminizing hormones can create other problems.

It is not true that sex interest and sex activity always decline naturally after menopause. In fact, many menopausal and postmenopausal women, no longer concerned about becoming pregnant, actually feel more sexual desire and satisfaction, especially if their estrogen levels are maintained with hormone replacement.

Some menopausal women tend to put on weight, but this gain is primarily because they eat more and exercise less. It is not true that menopausal women become masculine, nor do they ever become psychotic from the climacteric. About 50 percent of women, when deprived of their natural estrogen supply, will experience "hot flashes" for a few months and sometimes for years. Hot flashes have two causes, hormone deficiency and emotional tension. Sometimes it is difficult to separate these two contributory causes.

Subtle and undesirable body changes may occur at menopause as the result of ovarian hormone deficiency. The skin may gradually become drier and more wrinkled. The vagina tends to become drier and its lining thinner and much more tender. The vagina also may shrink to a smaller size so that in some women intercourse becomes painful. Later, with more severe estrogen deficiency, blood vessels may harden and bones may lose calcium and become more brittle.

Fortunately, all these unpleasant symptoms and undesirable effects can be prevented. Even after these changes have occurred, they can be reversed

The Worst Thing about Middle Age	
Losing Your Husband	52%
Getting Older	18%
Cancer	16%
Children Leaving Home	9%
Menopause	4%
Change in Sexual Feelings and Behavior	1%
What I Dislike Most about Being Middle-Aged	
Getting Older	35%
Lack of Energy	21%
Poor Health or Illness	15%
Feeling Useless	2%
None of These	27%
The Best Thing about the Menopause	
Not Having to Worry about Getting Pregnant	30%
Not Having to Bother with Menstruation	44%
Better Relationship with Husband	11%
Greater Enjoyment of Sex Life	3%
None of These	12%
The Worst Thing about the Menopause	
Not Knowing What to Expect	26%
The Discomfort and Pain	19%
Sign of Getting Older	17%
Loss of Enjoyment in Sexual Relations	4%
Not Being Able to Have More Children	4%
None of These	30%
How Menopause Affects a Woman's Appearance	
Negative Changes	50%
No Effect	43%
Positive Changes	1%
No Response	6%
How Menopause Affects a Woman's Physical and Emotional Health	
Negative Changes	32%
No Effect	58%
Positive Change or Improvement	10%
How Menopause Affects a Woman's Sexual Relations	
Sexual Relations Become More Important	18%
No Effect	65%
Sexual Relations Become Less Important	17%

Figure 13.15 Infertility. (*left*) Male infertility may result from inability of the testes to produce sperm or from the production of too many malformed sperm such as those shown here in comparison to a normal sperm (first one in line). (*right*) Female infertility may result from lack of ovulation, blocked Fallopian tubes, failure of the eggs to implant in the uterine wall, or a cervical mucus that is impenetrable or that is spermicidal.

Figure 13.16 Women's views and general attitudes toward menopause. (After Neugarten, 1969.)

to a great extent. Medical science has developed effective hormone-replacement programs for estrogen deficiency. Where failing ovarian hormones cause definitely identifiable problems, they can be replaced by a "pill a day," and the body hardly knows the difference.

Men may experience a gradual reduction in sexual demand as they age, but they do not go through a true climacteric and remain fertile sometimes into the eighth decade. Hormones for men do not seem to retard the effects of aging as estrogens do for deficient women.

BIRTH CONTROL

The whole process of human reproduction is a remarkable sequence of events. But men and women do not always want a child to be conceived when they mate, and obviously coitus is pleasurable and an expression of love as well as a reproductive act. The earth would undoubtedly be completely overpopulated by now if every mating produced offspring. Even primitive peoples have recognized this fact, and throughout history both sexes have tried to find ways to prevent conception.

The wives of North African desert tribesmen mixed gunpowder solution and foam from a camel's mouth, then drank the potion. Egyptian women inserted crocodile dung into the vagina or used tampons made from lint soaked in fermented acacia juice. The Chinese fried quicksilver in oil and drank it or swallowed fourteen live tadpoles three days after menstruation. Byzantine women of the sixth century attached a tube containing cat liver to their left foot. Obviously, the unwanted child was as much concern to the ancients as to modern man. More successful and more sanitary methods of conception control are now available, based on a better knowledge of how conception and pregnancy occur. There are a number of contraceptive methods widely used in the world today.

Condoms

Condoms are thin rubber sheaths worn over the penis to capture and hold the seminal fluid so sperm will not be deposited in the vagina, thus preventing conception. The condom, properly used, also aids in preventing the transmission of venereal disease.

There are several objections to the condom. It must be applied prior to intercourse. If it is placed on the penis between sexual foreplay and coitus, it may affect both partners' desire. The man may lose his erection. In older men, it frequently reduces sensation so much that ejaculation becomes difficult or impossible. The woman may not have as much sensation or may not be able to feel her partner ejaculate. One of the biggest disadvantages of the condom as a contraceptive, however, is the carelessness in its use, so that it may come off the penis, allowing sperm to enter the vagina. Also, pregnancies have resulted from premature ejaculation before the condom was put on.

Many couples still find the condom a satisfactory form of contraception. It is highly portable, simple, and requires no medical consultation or prescription. Because more than half of first coital experiences of many college women, as indicated by one study, involved no contraception, and because the major reason given was "not prepared," the condom would seem a good alternative. Workers in planned parenthood have long advocated the carrying of condoms not only by sexually active (or about to be) young men but by young women in this category as well.

The average pregnancy rate when condoms are used is 15 per 100 woman-years; that is, 15 pregnancies will occur each year for every 100 couples who use the condom as the sole method of protection. Individuals, however, can reduce this risk substantially by exercising utmost care in the use of the condom.

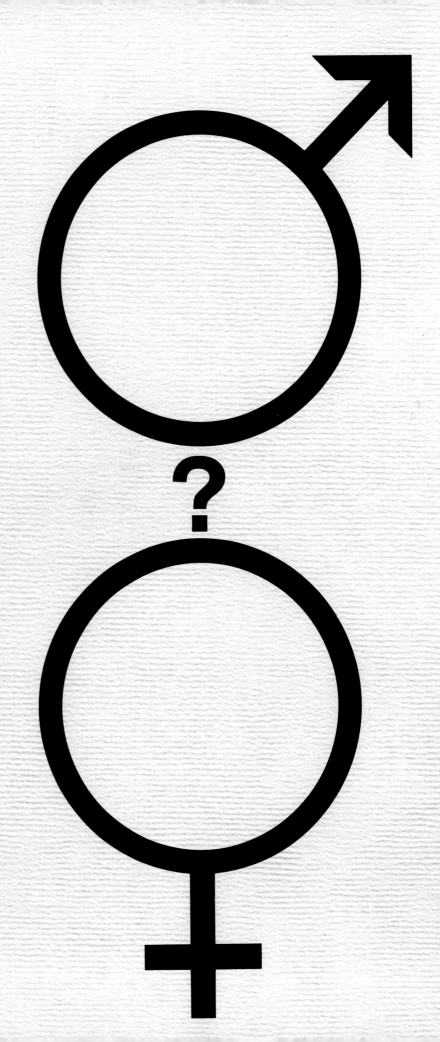

by
David M. Rorvik
with
Landrum B. Shettles, M.D.

Sitting in his office, Dr. Landrum B. Shettles recalls the night in the early 1960s when he made the discovery that may help millions select the sex of their offspring. After examining more than 500 sperm specimens, he is convinced that small, round-headed sperm carry the male-producing Y chromosomes and that a larger, oval-shaped type carry the female-producing X chromosomes. He noticed that in most cases the round sperm far outnumbered the oval-shaped sperm.

Dr. Shettles failed to find anyone who produced only the female-producing sperm, but he did encounter some men whose specimens contained almost nothing but the male-producing variety.

Dr. Shettles stresses, however, the rarity of cases in which the husband produces sperm that is predominantly of one type. And even in cases in which a man may produce unusually more sperm of one type than the other, he can still produce offspring of both sexes, provided he follows certain procedures.

Not everybody has agreed with his findings, and he does not claim scientific infallibility. But he does stand on his record, on observations he has made in the laboratory, and, most important, on his results to date. Other researchers have provided some impressive corroboration of Dr. Shettles' work.

As soon as he had made his initial discovery, Dr. Shettles had only one thing in mind: to find some means of exploiting his new knowledge to help parents choose the sex of their children. Since there definitely seemed to be a difference in the overall size of the two types of sperm, he reasoned, there must be other differences as well. Perhaps, one type was stronger than the other or faster—or both. Perhaps one type could survive longer in a certain environment than the other. There were all sorts of intriguing possibilities that could lead to a means of selecting sex—simply by interfering, even slightly, with the environment in which the sperm seek out the egg.

In terms of longevity, resistance to disease and stress, and adaptability to environment, it has long been conceded, at least by scientists, that the male is the weaker of the two sexes. This fact now appears to be borne out even at the most elemental level; the male-producing sperm (androsperm) begin with a substantial head start (perhaps a two-to-one margin) but end up only slightly ahead of the female-producing sperm (gynosperm) in the number of babies born each year.

Adapted from Rorvik, D. M., and L. B. Shettles, ''You Can Choose Your Baby's Sex,'' *Look* (April 21, 1970), pp. 88–98. Excerpted from *Your Baby's Sex: Now You Can Choose.* New York: Dodd, Mead, 1971.

What accounts for the greater slaughter of androsperm within the womb? To find out, Dr. Shettles began studying the environment that exists inside the vagina and uterus at the time of conception. He took transparent capillary tubes and filled them with cervical and vaginal secretions. Then he turned millions of sperm loose at the opening of the tubes and watched their activity through his microscope.

When the secretions in the tubes were more acidic than alkaline, the gynosperm seemed to prevail. But when the tubes were filled with cervical mucus removed from a woman very close to the time of ovulation, the smaller androsperm were clear-cut winners every time. Why?

Acid inhibits both gynosperm and androsperm, but because the gynosperm is larger than the androsperm, it seems to be protected from the acid for longer periods.

Alkaline secretions are kind to both types of sperm and generally enhance the chances for fertilization. But in the absence of hostile acids, the androsperm have the advantage due to the speed and agility that their small heads and long tails give them.

The environment within the vagina is generally acidic; the environment within the cervix and uterus is generally alkaline. Also, the closer a woman gets to ovulation the more alkaline her cervical secretions become.

Dr. Shettles' findings suggested that intercourse at or very close to the time of ovulation, when the secretions are most alkaline, would very likely result in male offspring. Intercourse two or three days before the time of ovulation, on the other hand, when an acid environment still prevails, would be likely to yield female offspring. The gynosperm can survive two or three days, while the androsperm rarely last longer than twenty-four hours.

Female orgasm helps provide additional alkaline secretions. Of course, many women never experience orgasm. These women should not think that their chances to conceive boys are diminished, because there are other ways of increasing the alkalinity that favors male offspring. Another point—abstaining from intercourse until at least a week after the conclusion of menstruation—is more significant, for this puts coitus very close to the time of ovulation in most women.

To further investigate the association between time of intercourse and gender of offspring, Dr. Shettles sifted through the data on artificial insemination. Doctors special-

izing in artificial insemination try to pinpoint the time of ovulation in their patients so that fertilization can be achieved on the first try. It occurred to Dr. Shettles that an unintended side effect of this practice ought to be an abundance of male offspring. In a series of several thousand births achieved by artificial insemination, he found that the sex ratio was 160 males for every 100 females. In another series, 76 percent were boys, and 24 percent were girls!

Dr. Shettles also noted in the course of his early research that low sperm count seems to be associated with a preponderance of female offspring; high sperm count with a greater number of male offspring. This suggested that building up the sperm count through abstinence might be another way of increasing chances of begetting male offspring.

As a result of these findings, Dr. Shettles has formulated two procedures—one to be used if a female child is desired, the other if a male is wanted. These procedures can be used in the home without prior semen analysis.

The procedure for female offspring:
1. Intercourse should cease two or three days before ovulation. Timing is the most important factor.
2. Intercourse should be immediately preceded, on each occasion, by an acidic douche consisting of two tablespoons of white vinegar to a quart of water. The timing might be enough to ensure female offspring, but the douche makes success all the more likely, since the acid environment immobilizes the androsperm.
3. If the wife normally has orgasm, she should try to avoid it. Orgasm increases the flow of alkaline secretions, and these could neutralize or weaken the acid environment that enhances the chances of the gynosperm.
4. The face-to-face, or "missionary," position should be assumed during intercourse. Dr. Shettles believes that this makes it less likely that sperm will be deposited directly at the cervix, where they might escape the acid environment of the vagina.
5. Shallow penetration by the male at the time of male orgasm is recommended. Again, this helps make certain that the sperm are exposed to the acid in the vagina and must swim through it to get to the cervix.
6. No abstinence from intercourse is necessary, until after the final intercourse two

or three days before ovulation. A low sperm count increases the possibility of female offspring, so frequent intercourse, prior to the final try two or three days before ovulation, cannot hurt and may actually help. This may be why Dr. Shettles says that "having girls is more fun."

The procedure for male offspring:
1. Intercourse should be timed as close to the moment of ovulation as possible. (A doctor can help set up a procedure for determining time of ovulation as indicated by changes in the female basal temperature.)
2. Intercourse should be immediately preceded, on each occasion, by a baking-soda douche, consisting of two tablespoons of baking soda to a quart of water. The solution should be permitted to stand for fifteen minutes before use. This allows the soda to become completely dissolved.
3. Female orgasm is not necessary but is desirable. If a woman normally has orgasm, her husband should time his to coincide with hers or let her experience orgasm first.
4. Vaginal penetration from the rear is the recommended position. This, Dr. Shettles says, helps ensure deposition of sperm at the entrance of the womb. This is desirable because the secretions within the cervix and womb will be highly alkaline, more so even than in the vagina, in spite of the alkaline douche, and an alkaline environment is most favorable to androsperm.
5. Deep penetration at the moment of male orgasm will help ensure deposition of sperm close to the cervix.
6. Prior abstinence is necessary; intercourse should be avoided completely from the beginning of the monthly cycle until the day of ovulation. This helps ensure maximum sperm count, a factor favoring androsperm.

Dr. Shettles does not guarantee that these procedures will be successful on every occasion. But, in his words, "The procedures are safe and simple. There's nothing distasteful about them, nothing any religious body has objected to. They can be carried out in the home, and they are entirely harmless. Clinical results show at least 80 percent success. And I believe that if the couple is conscientious with the douche and the timing, they can achieve success 85 to 90 percent of the time."

Coitus Interruptus

Coitus interruptus is the oldest of the useful methods of contraception. It involves having the male withdraw his penis from the vagina prior to ejaculation. Several problems arise with this method, however. Although there may be several hundred million sperm in one ejaculation, only one with the help of a few others is necessary for fertilization. A few sperm are usually present in the lubricating fluids emitted from the penis during sexual excitement, prior to ejaculation. Moreover, the male must have a great deal of willpower to use this method satisfactorily. The penis must be completely withdrawn, not only from the vagina but from the external genitalia as well. It is a little-known fact that pregnancy may occur from ejaculation into or on the labia. Because the female may gain satisfaction from the males's ejaculation against the clitoris, this practice is common. Withdrawal does not guarantee avoidance of pregnancy: the average pregnancy rate is 16 per 100 woman-years.

Rhythm Method

The principle utilized in the rhythm method is to avoid coitus during the time when the woman may be ovulating. As a practical method of contraception, several difficulties are encountered. Despite extensive research, there is no way at present to determine with any precision when ovulation is about to occur. One way a woman may try to pinpoint the time of ovulation is to chart her body temperature daily: Ovulation is followed by a slight temperature elevation that lasts until the start of the next menstrual cycle. But although this temperature change is a fairly good index that ovulation has occurred, only pregnancy is truly a proof of ovulation.

Even though a woman with a twenty-eight-day cycle usually ovulates on the fourteenth day, a considerable margin of safety must be allowed. At the very minimum, intercourse should be avoided from the eleventh to the eighteenth day of each cycle. But even a week's abstinence is no insurance, for sperm may survive for several days, or perhaps even longer, inside the female genital tract. Pregnancies have occurred after a single coitus seven days prior to apparent ovulation (as indicated by body temperature). If ovulation is early or late, the risks of pregnancy are greatly compounded. The average pregnancy rate for couples using the rhythm method is between 14 and 16 per 100 woman-years.

Spermicides and Diaphragms

Vaginal spermicides are nonprescription foams, creams, or synthetic gels that are inserted in the vagina against the cervix with a plastic applicator. They act by destroying sperm without harming the delicate vaginal lining. One application is recommended before each intercourse. The average pregnancy rate with this method is between 20 and 22 per 100 woman-years.

The newer foams are potentially far more effective than the overall failure rate would indicate, again, because of poor procedures in its use. It may be applied too long prior to coitus. It may be applied too close to the vaginal opening instead of deeply and against the cervix. It may be applied too late and after coitus. It may have been applied once and expected to last through repeated coitus. Or, the couple may have exhausted their supply and/or decided to "take a chance." All of these errors affect the failure rate. Like the condom, vaginal foam is especially useful for inexperienced, unmarried individuals who require a portable, simple, inexpensive, nonmedical method.

The diaphragm is a shallow rubber cup, the rim of which is a circular metal spring covered with fine latex rubber. The spring can be bent so the entire diaphragm can be compressed and easily

Figure 13.17 Comparison chart of various methods of birth control.

	STERILIZATION	THE PILL	INTRAUTERINE DEVICE (IUD)	DIAPHRAGM WITH CHEMICAL
How it works	Permanently blocks egg or sperm passages	Prevents ovulation	Uncertain: may stop implantation of egg	Barrier to sperm
Possible side effects	Psychological only	Initial weight gain and nausea; long-term effects not known	Initial discomfort and irregular bleeding; long-term effects not known	Chemical may cause irritation
Physician's assistance required	Operation performed by physician	Must be prescribed by doctor; periodic checkups required	Must be inserted by doctor; periodic checkups required	Must be fitted by physician
Cost	Vasectomy: $100 to $250; salpingectomy $200 to $300	Approximately $2.50 per month	From $15 to $75	From $15 to $25
Average pregnancy rate per 100 woman years	0.003	3–4 (minidose) 1–2 (sequential) 0–1 (combination)	3–4	10–12

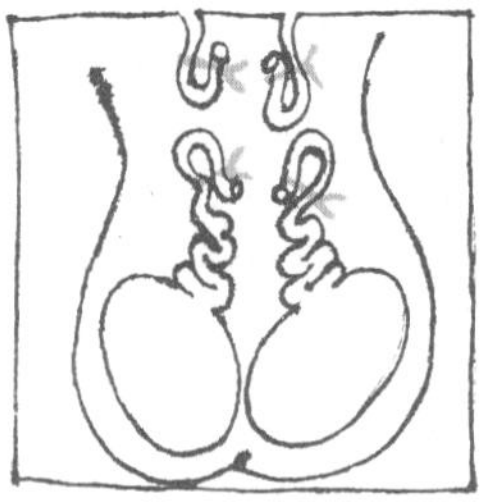

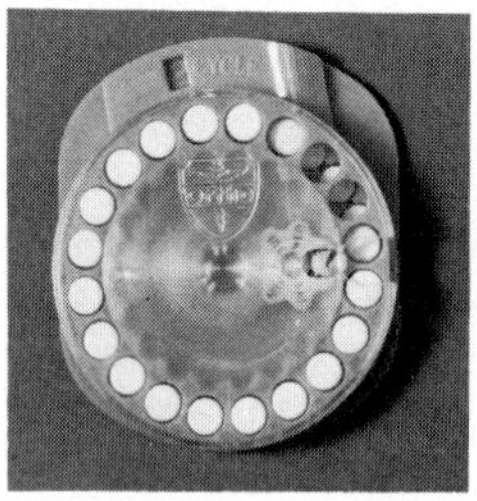

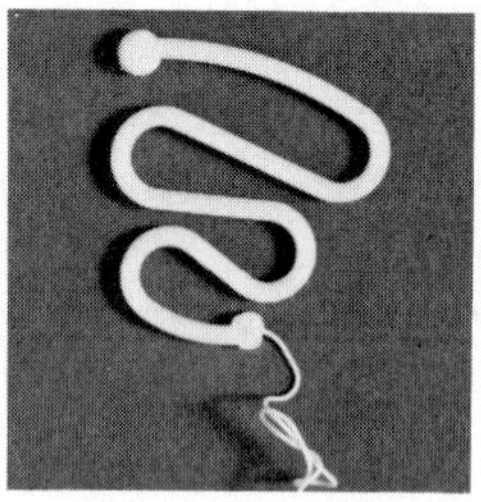

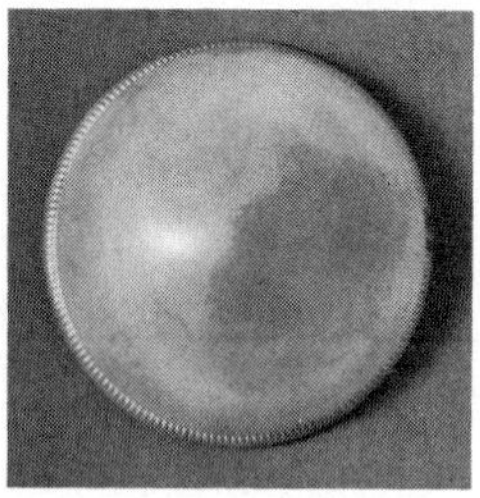

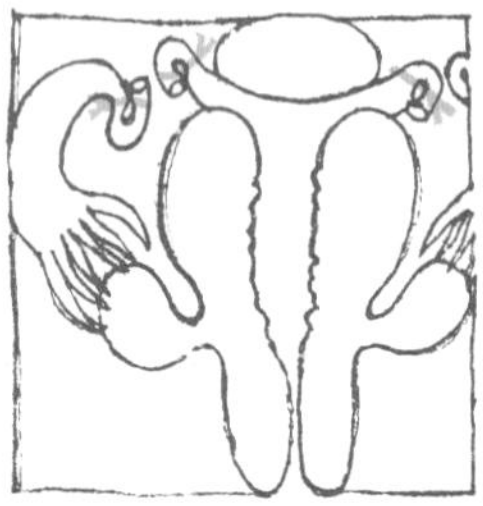

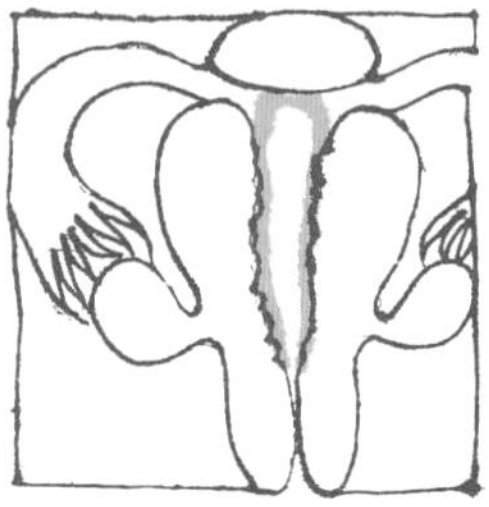

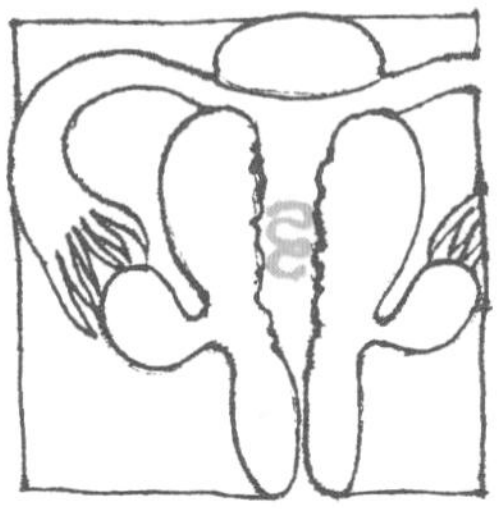

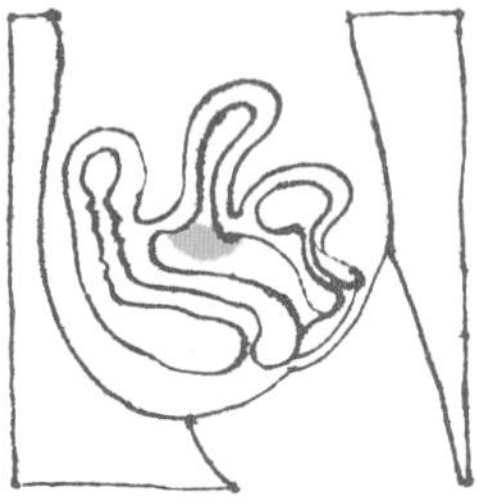

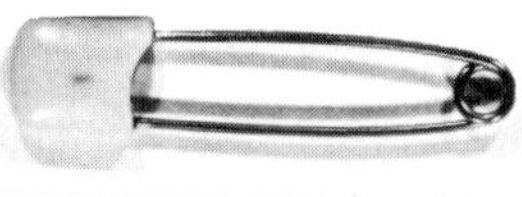

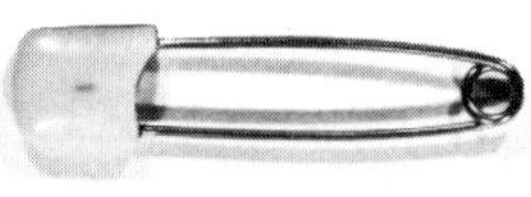

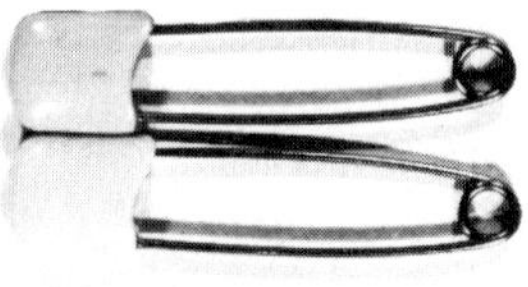

RHYTHM	CONDOM	WITHDRAWAL	FOAMS AND JELLIES	DOUCHE
Abstinence during fertile period	Prevents sperm from entering vagina	Ejaculation occurs outside the vagina	Barrier to sperm; spermicidal	Rinses sperm from vagina
Psychological only	Loss of sensation	Psychological only	May cause irritation	None
Possibly for consultation	None	None	None	None
Approximately $10 for calculator and $4.50 for basal thermometer	Approximately 3 for $.75	None	$1 to $3 per month	Approximately $2.50
14–16	15	16	20–22	36–40

passed into the vagina. It is then released in the upper and larger portion of the vagina where it covers the cervix completely.

Because the dimension of the vagina from the area behind the cervix to the pubic bone varies from woman to woman, diaphragms are available in specific sizes. This distance may be measured by a physician and the proper size prescribed. To increase the effectiveness of the diaphragm, it should be covered with a spermicidal jelly or cream. When the diaphragm is inserted properly, it will completely cover the cervix and cause no discomfort. A properly fitted diaphragm will not be noticed by the male partner. It should be inserted prior to intercourse and, preferably, be removed six to eight hours later, usually the next morning.

The pregnancy rate with use of a diaphragm is 10 to 12 per 100 woman-years. Improper insertion and forgetfulness probably account for most pregnancies with this method as well as with some other methods.

Intrauterine Devices

The methods described thus far prevent the sperm from reaching the ovum. Intrauterine devices (IUDs) utilize a different principle, although the precise mechanism of action is still unknown. Present evidence suggests that the IUD produces an inflammatory exudate that interferes with specific endometrial cell enzymes, thus preventing implantation of the egg.

IUDs are made of soft, flexible plastic, molded into various sizes and shapes. They are inserted into the uterus where they remain indefinitely. The device should be sterile and should be inserted by a physician. Insertion of IUDs may cause more discomfort in women who have not borne children than in women who have.

The IUD is useful for women who find other methods too messy or demanding or are not motivated enough to use them. Because it is long-lasting and need not be put in place every time before intercourse, it may prove especially practical for those with low motivation for taking pills. In addition, the IUD may be used by women who are unable to use the Pill because of persistent recurrent side effects.

About 20 percent of IUDs must be removed because of persistent bleeding or cramps. Another major disadvantage of the IUD is the high "fallout" rate. Occasionally the device may drop out and the loss go unnoticed by the wearer. Although expulsions usually occur during the first few months after insertion, there is a continuing, although low, incidence of recurring loss. This is particularly true of women who have had many babies and in whom the cavity of the uterus is large.

The intrauterine device should not be used if a woman has large tumors of the uterus, has had irregular or unexplained bleeding, has congenital abnormalities of the uterus, or has an infection of the cervix or vagina.

The most common major complication of the IUD is unwanted pregnancy. Effectiveness may be correlated with size of the device—the larger the device, the fewer the pregnancies. When pregnancies do occur, the incidence of abortions and pregnancies outside the uterus is higher than expected. If pregnancy is suspected, the device should be removed because of the high abortion rate with devices in place. In some instances, the IUD has been placed into a uterus already containing an unknown—or known—pregnancy. Abortion usually results and may be followed by infection, inflammation of the membrane lining the abdomen (peritonitis), and eventual sterility.

As shown in Figure 13.17, IUDs are about four times as effective as either diaphragm or condom, and about as effective as minidose oral contraceptives, but still not so effective as the sequential orals or the combination pill. New IUDs presently being tested have a pregnancy rate near zero with fewer side effects than present types.

Oral Contraceptives

In 1956 oral contraceptives were used in the first human field trials. Four years later the Food and Drug Administration approved them for use with a doctor's prescription. Since that time well over 10 million prescriptions for them have been written in the United States alone. Through the years, investigation has shown that ovulation can be effectively prevented with much smaller doses of hormones than were originally used, which is fortunate because side effects are directly related to the amount of hormone in the pill.

The Pill introduces into the body some synthetic equivalents of the natural sex hormones in such a way that the hormone cycle leading to ovulation is tampered with and ovulation is prevented. Most brands on the market today are "combination" pills; that is, each tablet contains both progestin (a synthetic progesterone derivative) and estrogen. A few brands are "sequentials," in which the first fourteen to sixteen pills contain only estrogen while the last five or six pills contain a combination of progestin and estrogen.

A major flaw in the Pill is the fact that it is to be taken daily with no omissions for three weeks and then omitted for seven days while the female menstruates. If the user forgets three or more pills, and sometimes even two or one, the contraceptive effect may be lost for the month, and pregnancy may occur.

Several attempts have been made to simplify the regimen by having the user take a pill daily. Already on the market are brands that contain an estrogen and a progestin for twenty-one days, with seven additional inert pills as "duds" or "placebos" to be taken during menstruation.

Another regimen presently being tested is a graded sequential method. This system simulates to a certain extent the gradually increasing level of estrogen after menstruation and before ovulation and then the second surge of estrogen and progestin after ovulation. This regimen also does away with having to remember when to start and stop pills and provides a more physiological method of hormone replacement.

During the last half of 1967 and early 1968, several pills with lower hormone levels were made available in an effort to reduce side effects. These pills contain only 1 mg. of progestin (as compared to 2.0 or 2.5 mg. in the prior preparations) and only .05 mg. of estrogen (half the former dosage). These doses are just as effective in conception control as the higher doses; however, because of the low amount of estrogen in these pills, breakthrough bleeding is more common. Patients taking the lower-dose pills frequently may have to double the dose until the endometrium adapts to this estrogen level.

The present formulations of the Pill still depend heavily upon estrogen. This hormone has been implicated in a possible side effect of current oral contraceptives—an increased incidence of diseases involving blood clots in the veins. These clots may impair the circulation of the legs and could cause death if they travel to lungs, heart, or brain. The danger of this complication, though, is twenty times less that the risk of similar complications during or following normal pregnancy. Hormones in the pill also are believed in rare instances to elevate the blood pressure of susceptible women and possibly to alter the metabolism of fats in the body.

Surgical Sterilization

In the past, numerous men and women have accepted surgical sterilization as a method of conception control. However, it has never been a widely popular procedure because of the permanent effect. In the female, the standard technique of dividing or tying off the Fallopian tubes is usually but not always reversible. The same problem exists in the male when the vas deferens is tied, a procedure known as *vasectomy*. Although the surgical procedure in the male is a minor one and may be performed in the office of a urologist, operation on the Fallopian tubes, called *tubal ligation*, still is a major abdominal procedure requiring hospitalization. A new technique, *laparoscopy*, is now being used to divide the tubes with a small electrode. This method requires a small incision in the abdomen and forty-eight hours of hospitalization.

For individuals who are certain that they no longer wish to conceive, voluntary sterilization provides the closest to ideal alternative available today. It is virtually 100 percent effective (failures are due to improper technique or failure to use alternate contraception for six weeks following vasectomy), painless, and has no side effects. Although the popularity of vasectomy is growing dramatically, especially among educated professional families,

many men still do not accept it because their masculine self-identities include their ability to conceive. They fear what they refer to as "loss of manhood." Dispelling this fear is yet another challenge to community education.

Abortion

Abortion is the most widely practiced method of birth control in the world today. To a physician, abortion means ending a pregnancy before the fetus can survive on its own.

Though vigorously opposed by some in the United States, the right of a woman to refuse to bear an unwanted child is a principle that seems to be gaining ground. Many states have recently legalized early abortion with minimal medical restrictions. As a result, abortion is increasingly becoming a medical concern of doctor and patient, rather than a crime against the state. Therapeutic abortion during the first twelve weeks of pregnancy is a relatively safe procedure when conducted by a qualified physician, but does require hospitalization in most states.

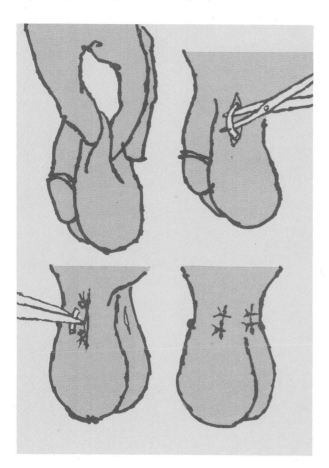

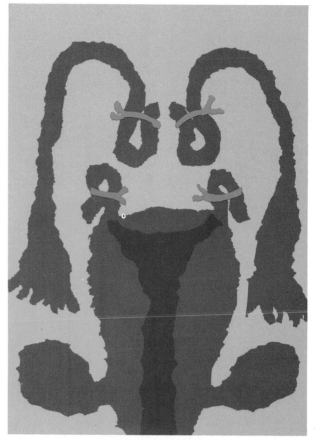

Figure 13.18 Sterilization. (*left*) How a vasectomy is performed. (*right*) The process of tubal ligation.

Methods used to about the twelfth week of pregnancy

Dilatation and Curretage (D and C) and Suction Curretage

With appropriate instruments the cervix (opening into the uterus) is dilated (stretched) large enough to accommodate forceps, curette (scraper) or suction curette (scraper connected to vacuum pump). The fetus, amnion, and placenta are suctioned or scraped from the uterine cavity. The procedure takes from fifteen to thirty minutes and rarely requires more than a twenty-four-hour stay in the hospital. Discharge is either that evening or the following morning.

Methods used between the twelfth and nineteenth weeks of pregnancy

Hysterotomy (This procedure is similar to a Caesarean Section)

An incision is made through the lower abdomen into the uterine cavity; the fetus and sac are then removed. The length of the hospital stay depends on the nature of recovery—usually five days.

(There is no removal of uterus, tubes, or ovaries. Pregnancies can occur again.)

Saline Induction

A small area of the abdomen is numbed with a local anesthetic such as novocaine. After numbing, a needle is introduced into the amniotic sac, which contains the fetus. Some fluid is withdrawn and a special salt solution is injected. After twenty-four to forty-eight hours the uterus begins to contract. After a variable amount of time the uterus will expel the fetus and placenta. A follow-up curettement (D and C) may be required to remove dead tissue that might cause infection.

Oral Means

Ergot compounds: can cause fatal kidney damage

Quinine sulphate: can cause deformities in fetus or death to mother

Estrogen and castor oil are both useless.

Nothing that is swallowed can cause abortion without also causing death or severe disability to the mother.

Solids Inserted into Uterus

Knitting Needles	Catheters
Coat Hangers	Gauze (packing)
Slippery Elm Bark	Artist Paintbrushes
Chopsticks	Curtain Rods
Ballpoint Pen	Telephone Wire

With all of the above there is the subsequent danger of perforation of uterus and bladder and death from infection or hemorrhage.

Fluids Inserted into Uterus

Soap Suds	Lye
Alcohol	Lysol
Potassium Permanganate	Pine Oil

Administration of any of the above can result in severe burning of tissues, hemorrhage, shock, and death.

Air Pumped into Uterus

Sudden violent death from gas emboli in the bloodstream.

Injections into Uterine Wall

Ergot

Pitocin

Sodium Pentothal

Other Means:

Vacuum cleaner connected to uterus—not to be confused with vacuum aspiration—is fatal almost immediately: extracts uterus from pelvic cavity.

Physical exertion such as lifting heavy objects, running, etc., is useless.

Falling down stairs: severe injury to mother with abortion rarely resulting.

Figure 13.19 Abortion methods. Butcher abortions are deadly. Only doctors or other specially trained personnel can safely use one of the four methods of abortion—all other methods can cause death but rarely induce abortion.

Prior to the twelfth week of pregnancy, gynecologists interrupt pregnancy by an operative procedure known as a "D and C"—dilatation of the cervix and curettage (or scraping out) of the uterine cavity. During the last few years most abortions have been done by dilating the cervix and then aspirating the uterine contents with a vacuum suction apparatus.

Nonmedical abortions have been produced by a variety of techniques, but all employ the insertion of a foreign object into the uterus—rubber catheters, soap solutions, irritating pastes, and various chemicals. Although these agents initiate contractions of the uterus and the expulsion of part of the products of conception, the uterus is usually never completely emptied and therefore infection is common. Soap solutions and pastes may cause immediate death if particles enter the venous circulation and travel to the lung or brain. The mortality rate from therapeutic abortion ranges from 10 to 20 deaths per 100,000. The mortality rate from criminal abortion ranges from an estimated 100 to 250 deaths per 100,000.

After the twelfth week of pregnancy medical abortion is done either by a miniature Caesarean section, requiring an abdominal incision, or by the insertion of a salt solution into the uterus via a catheter placed through the abdominal wall. The latter procedure is called "salting out," the former a hysterotomy.

Future Methods of Contraception

LONG-ACTING INJECTIONS   Extensive research has been done in the development of injectable and long-acting agents for suppression of ovulation. Such an injection must be given within twenty-four hours before menstruation or on the eighth day following the onset of menstruation. Clinical investigations by various groups throughout the United States have indicated an efficacy approaching 100 percent.

The side effects of the injection are about the same as with the Pill.

The monthly injection of estrogen and progestin works in the same way as the Pill; that is, by inhibiting ovulation. Some irregularity of cycles has been reported because of the long action of both hormones, and more than the usual incidence of breakthrough bleeding has been observed. Even longer-acting injections that would prevent ovulation for a year or more after a series of shots are under investigation.

POSTCOITAL PILLS   Extensive research in the development of a postcoital, or "morning after," pill is now under way. The reason is obvious: it may be used to protect a woman who has forgotten to take her conventional pill or might be used by women who have neglected conception control completely. If a pill were available that could be taken safely and effectively before the first missed menstrual period, it would have definite advantages over other methods. Because the woman would not know whether an egg had been fertilized, the pill could be taken with less guilt than would be involved with a pill that caused an abortion. Strictly speaking, however, postcoital pills, too, are abortional devices. One pill currently under investigation is thought either to produce contractions of the uterus that prevent the egg from implanting or to speed the egg along in the tubes so that it reaches the uterus prematurely.

A major approach to population control may come from the investigation of a new group of compounds known as *prostaglandins*, naturally occurring substances found in most body tissues. When prostaglandins are given at any stage of pregnancy, the pregnant uterus will respond by contracting. One study revealed that menstrual flow could be induced with the intravaginal application of prostaglandin tablets. Thus far, this method has proved effective for birth control. It is therefore possible that in the future prostaglandins may provide "contraception" that can be self-administered only when a woman becomes pregnant. If the menstrual period is delayed for seven to ten days, this compound could be used to initiate bleeding and thus cast off the early implanted egg. Such a method has obvious advantages over the Pill.

MALE CONTRACEPTIVES Progress in developing shots and pills to control male fertility has lagged behind developments for the female. Social influences are in part responsible for this lag. On the other hand, the slow pace of research in the male also may be due to the fact that investigators have found it difficult to separate sperm production from the process of male hormone formation. In any case there is little evidence of vast success in contraception when the method involves responsible male behavior.

Many contraceptive chemicals previously tested in women have the property of diminishing or halting normal production of sperm. Some compounds even destroy the potency of sperm. The problem with such compounds, however, is that they also cause certain unwanted side effects. For example, one preparation effective in preventing the normal development of sperm cells contains the female hormone estrogen, which tends to feminize some men, causing growth of breast tissue and reducing sex drive. Another compound that lowers sperm counts without feminizing effects is presently unusable because it causes other side effects if the user drinks even small amounts of alcohol.

The psychological and physiological factors involved in the development of a chemical or hormonal agent for male contraception are so complex that researchers in this field are not optimistic about an early breakthrough. Eventually science may be able to inactivate sperm without affecting the hormonal milieu or the masculinity of the male. At the moment, though, such attempts have not yet reached the stage of clinical investigation.

Dr. Alan Guttmacher, president of Planned Parenthood-World Population, has commented, "Even though the progress made in the past decade has been magnificent, the prospects for the next five years are even more exciting." The need is urgent. Investigators are at work. Progress in the field of contraception is inevitable. It is also inevitable that as new forms of fertility control are developed, new problems will emerge, with important implications for the social, moral, and psychological problems that already exist with the Pill.

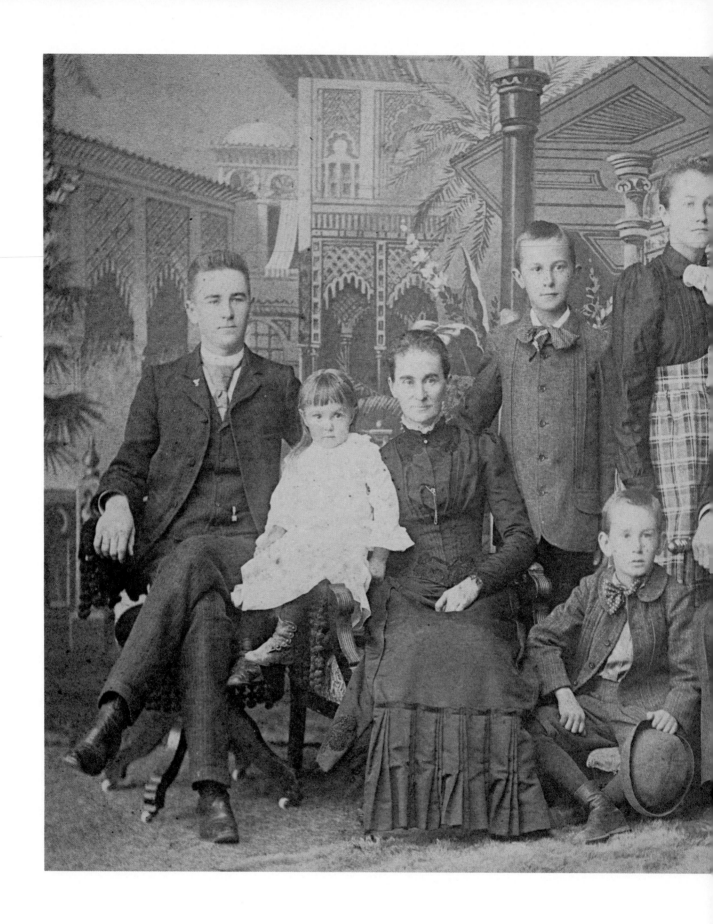

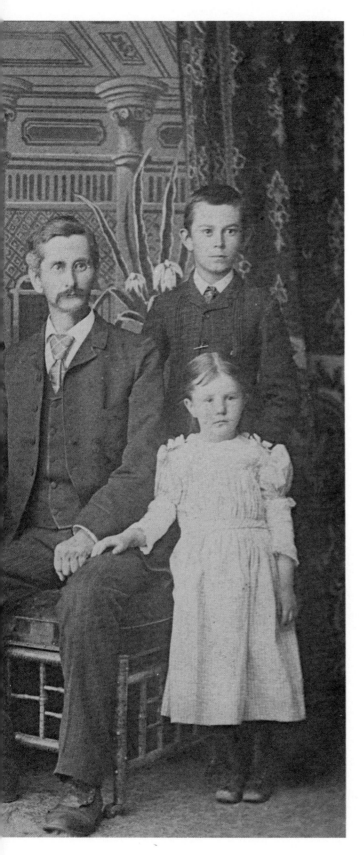

14

By the time a child is born, much of what it will be for the rest of its life has already been determined. The combination of the materials that the fertilized egg receives from the mother and father at the time of conception initiates a chain of biochemical and biological events that establishes the human nature of the future child, its appearance, whether it will be relatively healthy or seriously handicapped, and a number of physical and mental traits that will characterize it as an individual. In some cases, however, the developing fetus may be altered by environmental hazards, such as radiation, drugs used by the mother, or such maternal diseases as rubella and syphilis. But also much of what a person will be during his or her life is determined after birth, depending on the environmental conditions under which postnatal development takes place and on how the individual utilizes his genetic and environmental potentials. The question, still unresolved, is not *whether* but *how much* one human being depends on each of these determining factors—inheritance, prenatal development, and postnatal development.

Within the same family, brothers and sisters may share a number of physical and mental similarities, such as the color of hair or eyes or a talent for music, but also will display differences that may reflect the hereditary history of the mother or the father. Some of their traits may be linked with an ancestor even though the parent may not evidence it. Obvious or subtle, healthy or defective, one trait can be passed on generation after generation in the

Heredity and Health

form of *genes*. *Genetics* is the science that studies the transmission of hereditary factors and the way by which they express themselves during the development and life of an individual. One of the marvels of life is that the basic genetic laws apply equally well to a microbe, a plant, an animal, or a human being.

The more complex the living organism, the more difficult it is to discern the relationships between its observable features and the corresponding units of inheritance, the genes. The feature or features that are manifested, or *phenotype*, often are many steps removed from the inherited package of instructions, the *genotype*. One phenotypic trait may express the instructions from many genes, and conversely one gene's action may spread out to influence a number of phenotypic features (see Figure 14.1). Whether and how genotypes get expressed also is a function of the environment, internal as well as external. The phenotype represents the ultimate expression of the interplay between genotype and environment.

Even in a relatively healthy environment, to be healthy a body requires in the first place a "healthy" set of instructions handed over from the parents (genotype), a "healthy" way to transmit them from generation to generation of cells within the individual, and a "healthy" machinery to read the instructions and act upon them without mistakes. If the message from the genes is defective to begin with, becomes somewhat garbled on the way, or gets misinterpreted, life may indeed become very difficult.

THE TOOLS OF INHERITANCE

The biological directions for man's hereditary characteristics are locked in double-stranded coils of chemicals that are passed on through the parents' gametes, the egg and the sperm. These gigantic molecules, called deoxyribonucleic acid, or DNA, determine the "code of life" for an individual, as well as for his or her descendents. They lay down the rules for the body's manufacture of the vital substances called *proteins*—including enzymes, hormones, antibodies, and structural proteins—

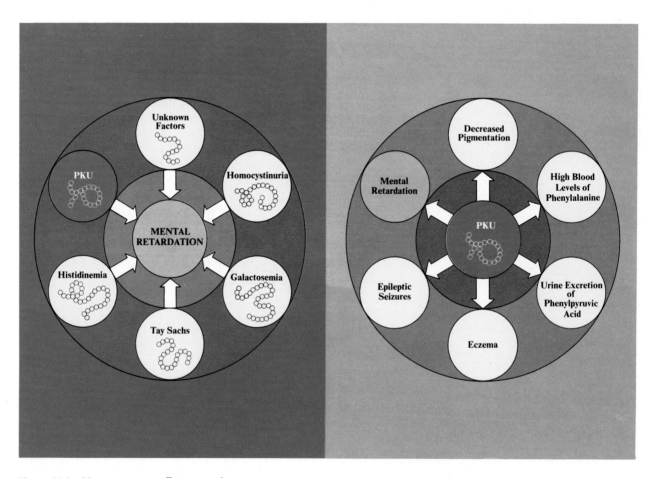

Figure 14.1 Many genes can affect one trait or phenotype (mental retardation); one gene or genotype (such as PKU) can affect many different traits.

which can make more molecules of DNA when needed, run the body's chemistry in general, and give an individual his characteristic shape and identity.

Each cell of a person, whether it be found in the skin or bloodstream or liver or brain, contains the same DNA molecules, that is, all the genetic instructions that the zygote contained in the first place. Not all these instructions are utilized all the time or by all the cells of the body, however. As the fertilized egg divides more and more extensively and the embryo grows and develops, certain cells begin to utilize selected sets of instructions within the overall common genetic endowment and therefore to acquire specialized phenotypic properties that will distinguish them from other groups of cells using different selections. This process is called *differentiation*, through which skin and blood and liver and brain cells acquire their own distinctive phenotypic features even though they all have the same *potential* abilities, that is, the same genotype.

DNA and the Genetic Code

The Nobel prize-winning work of Drs. James Watson and Francis Crick and the efforts of many other researchers have made clear some of the workings of the DNA molecule. DNA is composed of many building blocks, just as proteins are; the DNA building blocks, or nucleotides, are, however, very different from the protein building blocks, or amino acids. *Nucleotides* are made up of three different types of chemicals—*sugars*, *phosphates*, and most importantly, *bases* (see Figure 14.2). The nucleotides are chemically linked to one another to form long strands, and two such strands are entwined to form the "double-stranded helix," or coil, of DNA. The complete DNA molecule resembles, in effect, a twisted ladder in which the sugar and phosphate groupings link together in each strand to form the supports, while bases from one strand cling to those of the other to form the rungs, as is shown in Figure 14.2.

DNA molecules may be hundreds of thousands of nucleotides long, yet they contain by and large only four kinds of nucleotides because only four bases are used in their make-up. The four bases are: cytosine (C), guanine (G), thymine (T), and adenine (A). Moreover, as Watson and Crick have proved, the bases are limited in the way they cling together to form the rungs across the two opposing strands. For example, A always pairs with T, and G always pairs with C.

The nucleotides are the basic compounds, the letters of a molecular language known as the *genetic code*. Within each DNA strand, every group of three consecutive bases codes for a specific piece of genetic information, or codon (see Figure 14.2). They represent the words of the genetic alphabet. A few hundred codons, sequentially following one another along the DNA chain, constitute the gene—the genetic message unit or sentence. A DNA molecule contains several hundred genes. The genes may be thought of as forming "chapters" in the genetic language within the "volume" of the whole DNA molecule. Structural and molecular properties of the DNA make it easy to understand how it can exercise its two basic genetic functions: self-duplication to provide new generations of cells with the same genetic "library," and the imparting of instructions for the cell machinery to act on.

When a cell is preparing to divide, the two entwined strands of the DNA unzip from each other. New individual nucleotides from the cytoplasm progressively arrange themselves along each strand and faithfully reproduce its complementary sequence through the specific A-to-T and G-to-C base-pairing (see Figure 14.2). At the end of this process of *replication*, two identical double-stranded

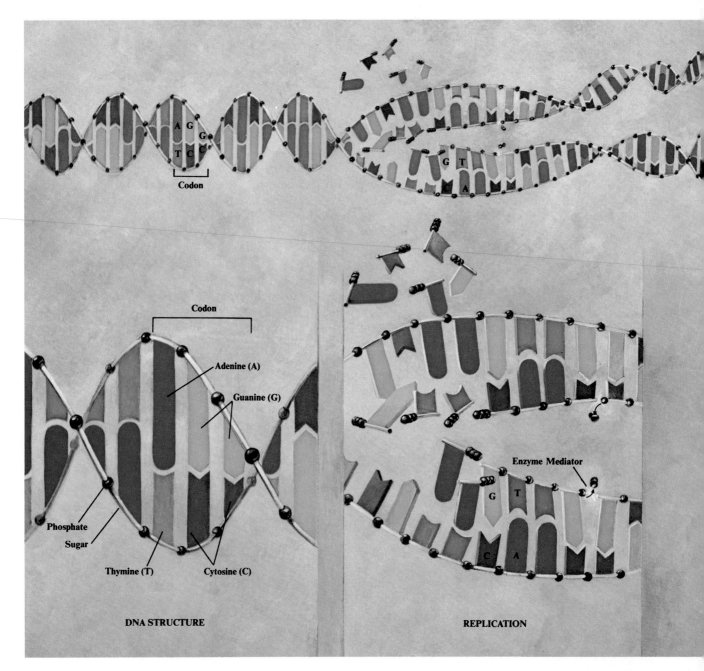

Labels in figure:

Codon

DNA STRUCTURE

Codon
Adenine (A)
Guanine (G)
Phosphate
Sugar
Thymine (T)
Cytosine (C)

REPLICATION

Enzyme Mediator

Figure 14.2   The structure of DNA. The DNA molecule, which takes the form of a double helix, is made up of sugars and phosphates to form the molecule's supports and of bases (cytosine, guanine, thymine, and adenine) to form its rungs. Any group of three base pairs is called a *codon*.

During the process of *replication*, which occurs each time a cell divides, the DNA molecule splits along its rungs and each half of the ladder builds a new half (with the help of enzyme mediators) by adding on new components from the cytoplasm in exactly the same order as they were in the original strand.

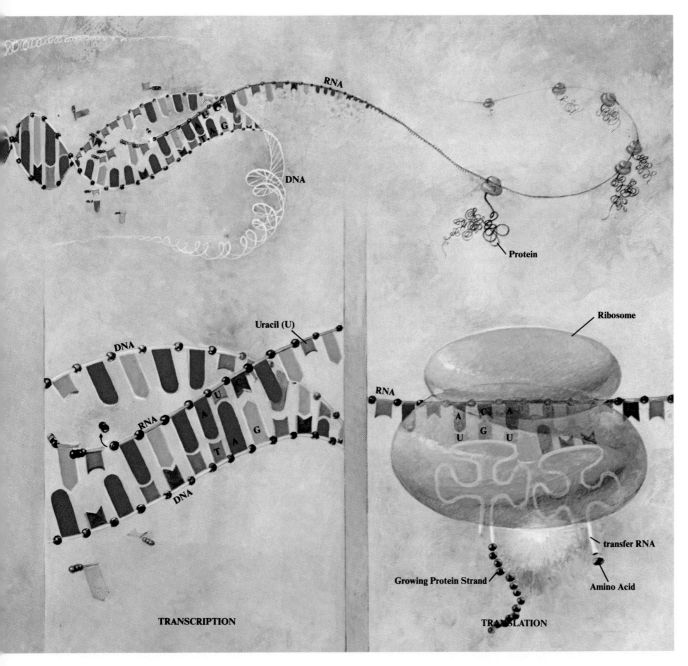

TRANSCRIPTION

TRANSLATION

Figure 14.3 The process of transcription. The sequence of nucleotide bases (A, C, T, G) on a strand of DNA forms a template for the formation of a complementary strand of messenger RNA (with bases A, C, U, G). The messenger RNA forms a negative print of the DNA (which is located only in the nucleus) and proceeds to carry its message outside the nucleus.

Figure 14.4 The process of translation. The messenger RNA carries its message from the DNA outside the nucleus to the ribosomes, where, with the help of transfer RNA, it lines up a set of amino acids to form protein molecules. Thus the DNA in the nucleus, through a series of processes, ultimately controls the production of the proteins used in so many important ways by the body.

DNA molecules have become available, each one to eventually go with one of two daughter cells.

Because the copy DNA is identical to the original DNA, both good and bad genes will be faithfully reproduced, and the daughter cells will "inherit" the whole genotype of the parent cell. However, it is possible for the replication process itself to go awry and for an error to be made that results in an "altered" copy; radiation, certain drugs, and toxic chemicals are known to favor such *genetic mutations*. As a consequence, one of the daughter cells acquires a new genotype, becomes a *mutant* cell, and, unless the mutation is lethal, passes on the new genotype to its own cell progeny.

The read-out of genetic instructions by the cell machinery starts with the process of *transcription*, which is similar to the process of replication. The transcripts are not identical to the DNA portions on which they are made; chemically, they are known as *ribonucleic acid* or RNA molecules, also constituted by chains of nucleotides using somewhat different sugars and one different base. Nevertheless, the RNA molecules faithfully reflect the nucleotide sequence encoded in their DNA "templates" and can therefore act as accurate messengers of the corresponding portions of the genetic code.

RNA molecules are, in turn, used as templates for the process of *translation* that takes place at the protein assembly line of the cell, the *ribosomes*. In the ribosomes individual amino acids are positioned in the correct sequence against the messenger RNA by other, smaller RNA molecules, and then linked with one another by appropriate enzymes to form the specific amino-acid chains characteristic of each body protein (see Figure 14.4).

In this way, through the transcription and translation processes, each group of three consecutive bases in one DNA strand—that is, each codon— ultimately codes for one given amino acid, and the codon sequence of one gene dictates the amino acid sequence of its corresponding amino-acid chain. The alteration of even one codon in the DNA may result in a different amino acid being injected in the protein chain or even in the interruption of the build-up of the chain and the failure to manufacture the corresponding protein.

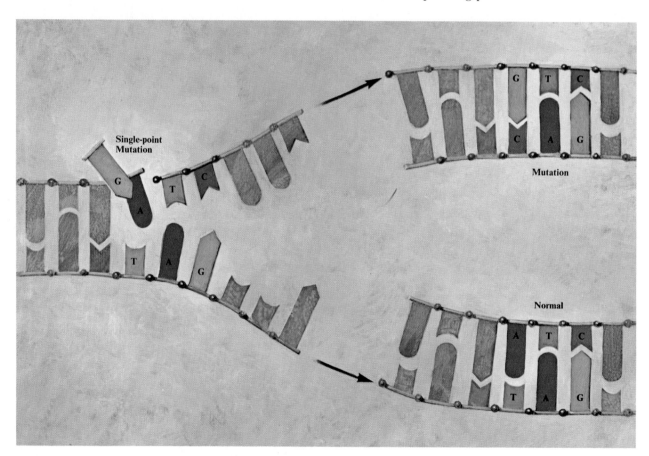

Figure 14.5 Genetic mutation. There are several ways that errors can occur during DNA replication. For example, the positions of one or more bases may be switched, causing altered copies to be formed. These altered molecules will then transmit the mutation to later generations.

Genetic Machinery of the Cell

In the human cell, as in most plant and animal cells, the DNA is concentrated within the nucleus and packaged in highly organized structures known as *chromosomes*. Each human chromosome contains a large number of genes, linearly arrayed as DNA. Except for the sex cells (eggs and sperm), all cells of the human body (somatic cells) as well as the zygote contain *two* copies of each chromosome, one derived from each parent. There are twenty-three pairs of chromosomes in the human cells. Of these, twenty-two pairs are known as *autosomes*, while the remaining pair comprises the *sex chromosomes*, XX for the female and XY for the male. In each pair of corresponding chromosomes (except the XY pair) the various genes of one chromosome have their individual counterparts in the other. These paired genes are called *alleles*.

The sex cells, or gametes, have only half the chromosome number of the somatic cells, or twenty-three instead of a total of forty-six. When egg and sperm fuse together, the newly formed zygote acquires the chromosomes from both paren-

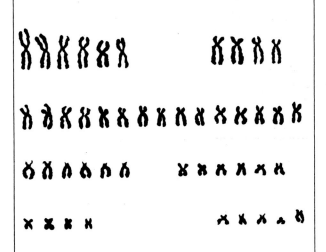

Figure 14.6 A chart of the twenty-three pairs of human chromosomes. The last chromosomes in the second and fourth rows are the sex chromosomes, which determine that this particular individual is a male.

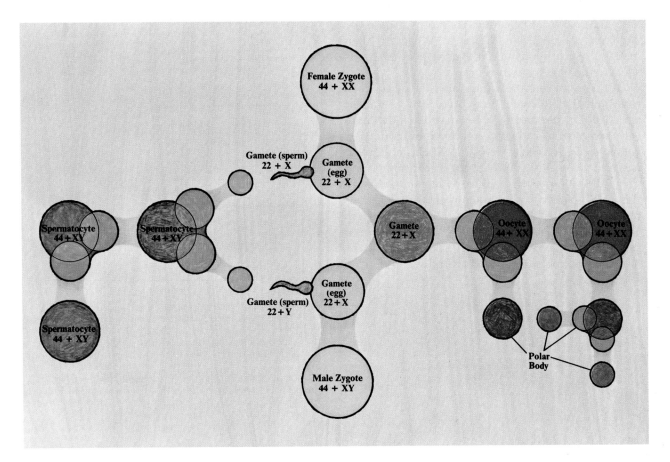

Figure 14.7 Chromosomal transmission in gametogenesis and fertilization.

tal gametes, and the full number is restored. The complete human being that will evolve from it will therefore draw on the genetic characteristics of each parent. In this way, every human being receives one allele of each pair of alleles from his father and the other from his mother.

If an individual carries two identical alleles in a given pair, he is said to be *homozygous* for that gene. When the two alleles differ from each other, he is said to be *heterozygous*. A person may be homozygous for some genes and heterozygous for others. Homo- and heterozygosity are *genotypic* qualities. Their *phenotypic* expression depends on the "products" of the similar or dissimilar alleles and when they differ, whether only one or both will be expressed in some way.

It has long been known, for example, that individuals belong to one of several different blood groups, depending on certain substances present on the surface of their red blood cells. A major blood-group classification is ABO. Individuals with the A or the B substance on their red blood cells will belong to the A or, respectively, the B groups; individuals with neither will belong to the O group, and those with both to the AB group. These are *phenotypic* classifications, however. What are their genetic constitutions—their genotypes—with respect to the blood-group genes?

It turns out that the same gene is involved in all cases and that this gene may occur in three allelic varieties: G_A, G_B, and G_O. Homozygous individuals will each have two identical alleles: their genotypes will be $G_A G_A$, or $G_B G_B$, or $G_O G_O$. Their gene products will be exclusively A, or B, or O (none), and they will belong to the A, B, or O blood groups. In this case, genotypic and phenotypic classifications match each other. Heterozygous individuals such as $G_A G_O$ or $G_B G_O$, however, will still show the A or B substance respectively on their red blood cells. What has happened is that the product of allele A

Population	O	A	B	AB
United States Whites	45%	41%	10%	4%
United States Negroes	47	28	20	5
African Pygmies	31	30	29	10
African Bushmen	56	34	8	2
Australian Aborigines	34	66	0	0
Pure Peruvian Indians	100	0	0	0
Tuamotuans of Polynesia	48	52	0	0

Parents' Phenotypes		Phenotypes of Children Possible	Phenotypes of Children Not Possible
A	A	A, O	AB, B
A	B	A, B, AB, O	
A	AB	A, B, AB	O
A	O	A, O	AB, B
B	B	B, O	A, AB
B	AB	A, B, AB	O
B	O	B, O	A, AB
AB	AB	A, B, AB	O
AB	O	A, B	O, AB
O	O	O	A, B, AB

O = O/O	A = A/A or A/O	B = B/B or O/B
		AB = A/B

Figure 14.8   ABO blood groups. (*above top*) Distribution of ABO blood types among various human populations. (*above bottom*) Blood-type inheritance. By looking at your blood type in the middle column, you can determine what types your parents may and cannot have. (*right*) How to use the table, taking the first line as an example. If the parents are phenotypically type A, their alleles must be either A/A or A/O genotypically. All the possible combinations are worked out, showing that offspring of parents who are A phenotypically can produce only children that are A or O phenotypically.

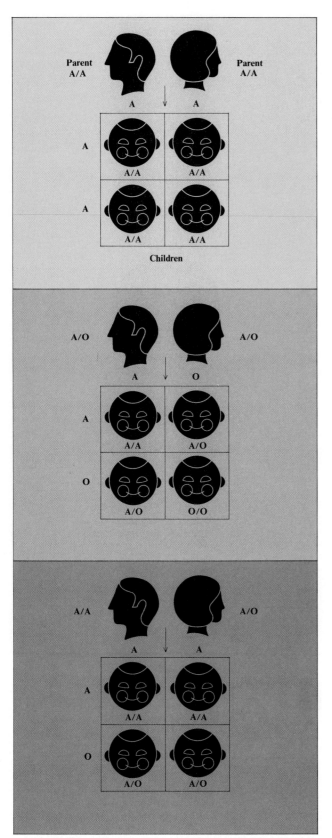

or B dominates over that of allele O and therefore is called *dominant*, while the gene that is not expressed is called *recessive*. Finally, individuals who are heterozygous with the genotype $G_A G_B$ display the products of both alleles (the A and B substances) and belong to the fourth blood group, AB. Their alleles G_A and G_B are neither dominant nor recessive relative to each other; this type of relationship—some kind of peaceful coexistence—is referred to as *codominance*.

There are many such examples of allelic relationships among genetically controlled human characteristics, both normal and abnormal. For example, some children in a family can taste a chemical called phenylthiocarbamide (PTC), while others cannot. If the child has two similar PTC-taster alleles (designated T), that is, a TT genotype, he can taste the chemical; if he has two other alleles "t" (tt genotype), he cannot. And if the individual has a Tt genotype, he can also taste PTC, indicating that the T allele is a dominant one.

Some human traits are under the control of a small number of genes, and the total genetic basis of their determination is obvious. Among these characteristics are eye color and blood groups. More complex traits (involving such things as behavioral patterns and intelligence) are *polygenic*; that is, they are influenced by many genes. These traits are not all-or-nothing in their expression, but vary continuously over a spectrum of possibilities. Furthermore, most genes contribute to a *range of potential* for a given trait, with the individual's actual state being determined by past and present experiences or environments.

MECHANISMS OF INHERITANCE

Once a zygote is formed by the fusion of egg and sperm, the parental heredity is firmly locked-in in its forty-six chromosomes. Except for somatic mutations, this heredity will be faithfully transmitted

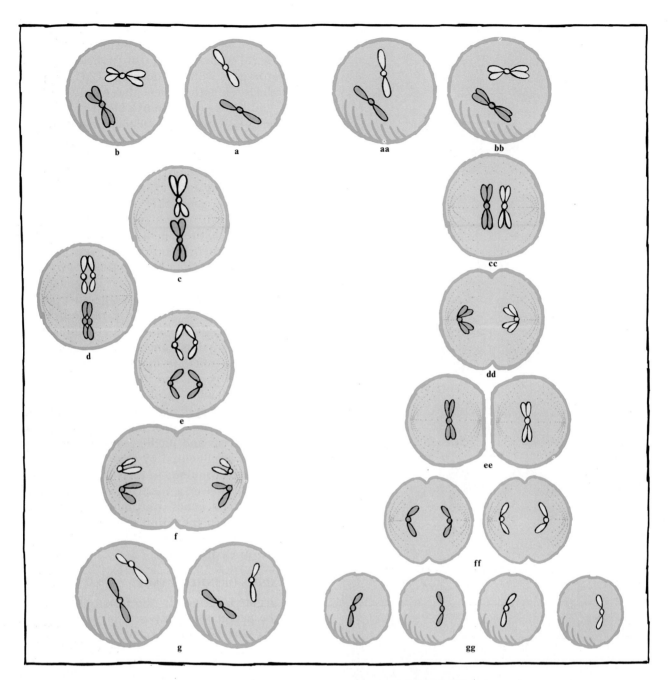

Figure 14.9 (*above left*) A schematic presentation of mitosis. (a) The chromosomes first materialize in the cell and (b) duplicate at all points but the centromere. (c, d) They line up along the equatorial plane, and (e, f) one member of each pair is pulled toward the opposite pole. (g) When the cell splits, two daughter cells, each exactly like the parent, result.

Figure 14.10 (*above right*) The process of meiosis. (aa) As in mitosis, the chromosomes appear and (bb) duplicate. (cc) They then line up in two parallel planes, and (dd) half of the chromosomes are pulled to each pole. (ee) The cell divides and (ff) quickly divides again, without the chromosomes doubling, resulting in (gg) four daughter cells—each with half the chromosomes of the parent. The drawings along the bottom illustrate the process of crossing over that occurs during meiosis. The two homologous chromosomes lie side by side, and corresponding breaks occur in each chromosome. The fragments are interchanged, resulting in two chromosomes with new alleles.

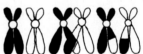

Figure 14.11 (*right*) Independent segregation. The process of reshuffling of genetic material during meiosis can be compared to the shuffling of a deck of cards. Taking only six cards as an example, suppose the red cards represent maternal chromosomes and the black cards paternal chromosomes and that cards of the same value represent homologous chromosomes. The eight sets show all the possible combinations of these chromosomes. The number of possible arrangements of such pairs in a full deck of cards would be 2^{26}. Man has forty-six chromosomes and thus may produce 2^{23} different kinds of sperm—more than 8 million possible combinations.

to *any new cell* within the growing or the adult organism by the process known as *mitosis*. Mitosis is the means by which the genetic material of the chromosomes is identically duplicated and equally distributed to the nuclei of two daughter cells (see Figure 14.9).

Quite different is the process by which gamete cells are produced to be used for the transmission of heredity from one person to his progeny. This process is called *meiosis*. In the meiotic process, genes need not remain locked within their original chromosomes but can combine across homologous pairs, that is, between corresponding paternal and maternal chromosomes within the germ cell. This exchange occurs through the mechanism of *crossing over*, where two homologous chromosomes adhere to each other at various points down their length, then break at homologous points and exchange corresponding segments (see Figure 14.10). Homologous chromosomes then segregate into two groups, each containing half the number of chromosomes as the original germ cell; this process is the meiotic *reduction*, by which the gametes end up

with half the normal number of chromosomes. During the segregation, furthermore, paternal and maternal chromosomes distribute themselves randomly between the two groups, that is, *segregate independently* from their parental origin and from one another. Lastly, each group completes chromosomal duplication and splits once again, each final set still comprising half of the original chromosome number (see Figure 14.10).

Thus, the meiotic process has not merely resulted in the generation of sex cells: Gene recombination (crossing over) and chromosome independent assortment have reshuffled paternal and maternal genes as in a deck of cards. Each gamete produced may now have quite a different gene composition, even though they all have the same number of genes located in the same sequence on the same number of chromosomes. Independent assortment alone, applied to the twenty-three chromosomes, permits the generation of more than 8 million kinds of gametes as long as the individual is heterozygous for at least one pair of alleles in each chromosome (a practical certainty). If heterozygosity

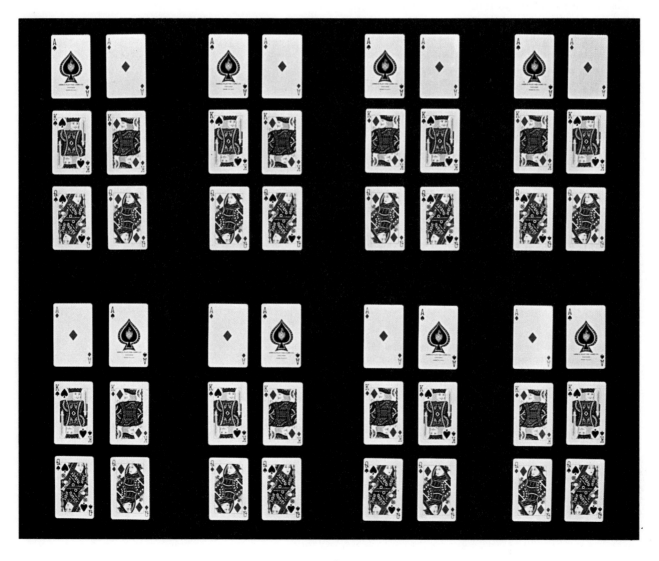

extends beyond one allele pair, and crossing over breaks up the original combinations and recombines maternal and paternal genes into new chromosomes, the potential number of different gametes that one person can produce becomes an astronomical figure. Even if individuals had lives as long as that of the earth and had a litter of children every year, the chance for two children to receive the same genotype would still be practically zero.

When the male and female gametes join together, a new game is started. The new human being will unquestionably receive, for all gene pairs, one allele from his father and one from his mother. What cannot be generally predicted, because of the gene reshuffling occurring during meiosis, is the grandparental origin of these alleles or the specific combination in which various genes are received from each grandparent.

If one focuses on a single gene pair, it is easy to see that each gamete will have an equal chance to contain one or the other and, thus, to pass it on to the next generation. This idea, as well as the whole concept of the cellular mechanism for heredity, was in fact demonstrated more than one hundred years ago by the work of the Austrian monk Gregor Mendel, using the common garden pea plant. Mendel grew various pure strains of pea plants, differing from one another by clearly recognizable traits (flower color, stem length, seed shape, and so on). He then crossed one strain with another and observed what happened to those traits in the progeny and in subsequent generations obtained by further cross-fertilization.

Mendel noted that certain traits, characteristic of one generation, disappeared in the next but could reappear in later generations—the basis for the concepts of dominance and recessiveness. He also was able to determine the genetic rules that underlie the transmission of single, clear-cut hereditary traits (see Figure 14.12). The same mathematical rules hold true for humans as well as for peas, and for genetic defects as well as for normal traits.

HEREDITY VERSUS ENVIRONMENT

Although it has been realized that heredity and environment both contribute to human characteristics, questions still remain as to the extent of genetic influence over many characteristics. One question still to be answered is: How wide is the *range of potential* that genes can provide for a given trait? A partial answer to this question lies in studies of identical twins. Because identical twins develop from the same egg, their genetic endowments are the same. Therefore, any differences between them must result from environmental influences.

Schizophrenia

One twin study has shown that if one individual of an identical twin pair exhibits schizophrenia, there is a 60 percent chance that the other individual also will be schizophrenic. At first consideration, the data seem to indicate a genetic basis to the psychosis, but this interpretation is not justifiable in light of

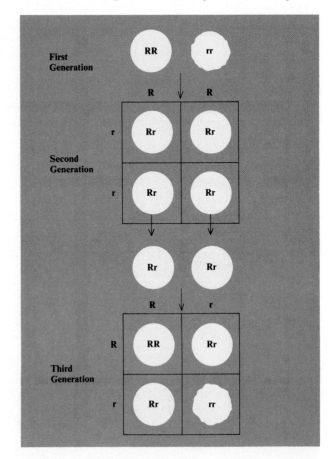

Figure 14.12 Mendel's pea experiments. Mendel found that if he crossed two homozygote pea plants, one with smooth peas and the other with wrinkled ones, their progeny would all be smooth. If, however, he crossed the second-generation peas with one another, three-fourths of the progeny were smooth and one-fourth wrinkled. From such experiments Mendel worked out the basic laws of transmittal of hereditary traits and calculated what matings would provide what types of offspring and their approximate proportions.

the 40 percent who do not share their twin's psychosis. The fact that in 40 percent of such cases only one member of the twin pair is schizophrenic indicates that if there is a genetic basis to the disease it does not exert an overwhelming influence.

Although this study of identical twins shows the existence of environmental influences in schizophrenia, a question still remains as to the possibility of genetic influences. Insight into this possibility has been obtained from studies of fraternal twins (twins developing from two different eggs and therefore having different genetic constitutions). Because such twins enter a family at the same time, it would be expected that the environment is similar for both individuals. Studies of nonidentical twins indicate that if schizophrenia occurs in one member of a twin pair, there is approximately a 10 percent chance that the other twin will also be afflicted. This lower frequency of co-occurrence suggests a genetic basis of the disease.

Again, however, there are difficulties in interpreting the data. For example, it may not be correct to assume that the environments of nonidentical twin pairs are as "similar" as those of identical twins. Because fraternal twins differ in physical and mental traits to a greater extent than identical twins, their interactions with their environment also can be expected to differ to a greater degree. Investigations have indicated, however, that schizophrenia often co-occurs in identical twins even when they are separated early in life. Although this study tends to lend strength to the argument for a genetic origin of the disease, it has been based on only a small number of identical twins reared apart and cannot be considered to be conclusive.

Intelligence

The problems involved in the study of schizophrenia are indicative of the difficulties encountered in all studies of complex human traits. Perhaps the most controversial area of dispute between proponents of genetic and environmental determinants of human existence lies in the analysis of the basis of human intelligence. Difficulties in resolving this dispute begin with the problem of establishing a measuring device for intellectual capabilities. At present the primary means available are the so-called intelligence or IQ tests.

The major difficulty in assessing the results of IQ tests is that a given examination can only be designed to test the *relative* intellectual capabilities of peoples of a similar environmental or cultural background. If significant differences in social and historical backgrounds exist between two groups, it is difficult, if not impossible, to compare results of IQ examinations.

Recently, an educational psychologist, Arthur R. Jensen, has suggested that differences in intelligence between black and white Americans as measured by IQ reflect a difference in innate intellectual capabilities of the two ethnic groups. Although it is true that black Americans tend to score lower on IQ examinations, the question remains as to whether the differences reflect innate capabilities or effects of social and cultural differences between the two groups.

One of the major arguments that Jensen cites in support of his theories is that differences in IQ persist even between blacks and whites of the same socioeconomic class. This interpretation can be questioned, however, when one considers the social deprivation (such as inferior education) that almost all blacks in America, regardless of socioeconomic class, have had to face. The dispute over the relative IQ scoring ability of blacks and whites in the United States is far from resolved, and most responsible researchers would agree that there is a significant possibility that either or both genetic and environmental causes could be at the base of the differences in measured IQ.

GENE ABNORMALITIES

It has already been mentioned that, through an error in the replication process or because of damage by radiation or certain chemicals, an even minute portion of the DNA of a cell may be altered. If that portion is part of a gene, the alteration may constitute a *gene mutation*. Mutation is the source, for better or for worse, of new allelic variants.

A large number of physiological defects due to gametic mutations (those affecting germ cells) are known, the most easily identifiable being what are called *inborn errors of metabolism*, that is, defects in certain enzymes or other proteins. Such errors occur because the immediate consequence of a gene defect is the alteration of the amino-acid chain whose production is directed by that gene, resulting in the inability of the body to produce a specific protein in its normal form. If the affected protein is an enzyme or a hormone, it will lead to problems in a certain aspect of metabolism. Some 1,500 such inborn errors are known. In most cases they are recognized as due to single gene mutations, and in a few cases it is known which protein has been affected. Most of them involve a recessive allele, spread by heterozygous carriers and often brought together through intermarriage between members of genetically closely knit groups.

Sickle Cell Anemia

Of all the body proteins, the hemoglobin of red blood cells is among the most important to the survival of a human being, for it transports oxygen to the body's cells and then helps dispose of their waste carbon dioxide. There are now about eighty known hemoglobin abnormalities resulting from some flaw in a gene involved in the manufacture of this vital protein. One of the best-known abnormalities is sickle cell anemia, an affliction that probably originated in Africa an unknown number of generations in the past. About 8 to 10 percent of North America's 20 million Negroes carry one such gene,

while in about 1 percent of them both alleles are of the "sickle" type.

Sickle cell anemia gets part of its name from the fact that the blood cells of afflicted individuals take on a sickle or crescent shape and clog up the fine capillaries of the circulatory system, cutting off the oxygen supply to nearby tissue and causing tissue damage as well as severe pain (see Figure 14.13). The disease also is complicated by the activities of the spleen, which quickly destroys the abnormal blood cells before the patient can manufacture new ones to replace them. Severe anemia results—hence the rest of the name. Typical symptoms are weakness, general lassitude, poor physical development, rheumatism, pneumonia, kidney failure, and enlargement of the spleen. The fate of a person suffering from sickle cell anemia or its complications is extremely unpleasant. Death often occurs before the age of forty.

The actual sickle cell anemia *disease* occurs only in the homozygous individual. He has inherited two defective alleles—one from each parent—that direct the manufacture of the abnormal hemoglobin molecule. Because the defective instructions are the only genetic message provided to the body, abnormal hemoglobin only is produced. On the other hand, a child who inherits only one sickle cell gene has the other allele to direct the making of normal hemoglobin, which gives him an approximately fifty-fifty mixture of the two types of hemo-

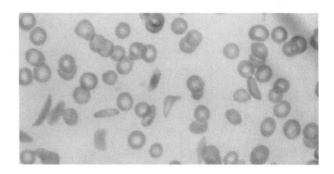

Figure 14.13   The characteristic form taken by red blood cells in the individual who has sickle cell anemia.

Figure 14.14   How phenylalanine in milk is normally metabolized, compared with what occurs in phenylketonuria.

globin in his blood. Thus, the "sickle cell" allele behaves as a *codominant* one relative to the normal allele, rather than as a recessive gene. A child with one sickle cell gene is said to carry the sickle cell "trait" and can lead a relatively normal life, but he has one serious disadvantage: if he goes to high altitudes where the oxygen in the air is thin, he can become seriously ill or die. On the other hand, the single gene has a side advantage in that it seems to protect the carrier against malaria in areas where the disease is prevalent, such as the tropics.

Phenylketonuria (PKU)

An increasing number of inherited disorders are being linked to mutant genes causing a vital enzyme to be produced in an abnormal form or not to be produced at all. One of the best known is phenylketonuria, or PKU. Its chief symptom is progressive, severe, and irreversible mental retardation, leaving most victims with an average IQ of about 50. Other accompanying symptoms are epilepticlike seizures and abnormal brain-wave patterns, a decrease in the normal pigmentation of

hair, eyes, and skin, and skin disorders such as eczema. PKU is a recessive disorder, only occurring when both parents have transmitted the aberrant gene. It is found about once in every 10,000 births.

PKU patients lack an enzyme called *phenylalaninehydroxylase*, normally located in the liver and beginning to function after birth. This enzyme converts phenylalanine—an essential dietary amino acid (one that the human body cannot manufacture)—into another amino acid called tyrosine. Tyrosine is not an essential amino acid and, like phenylalanine, is partly utilized to build body proteins; a small amount of tyrosine, however, is converted to important body substances such as the pigment melanin, the hormones and neurotransmitters adrenalin and noradrenalin, and the thyroid hormone thyroxin. Heterozygous individuals, carrying only one PKU allele, manufacture only about half the normal amounts of the phenylalanine-hydroxylase enzyme—thanks to the other, normal, allele—but that appears adequate under normal circumstances and no disease is suffered.

In the PKU patient, the lack of the enzyme is

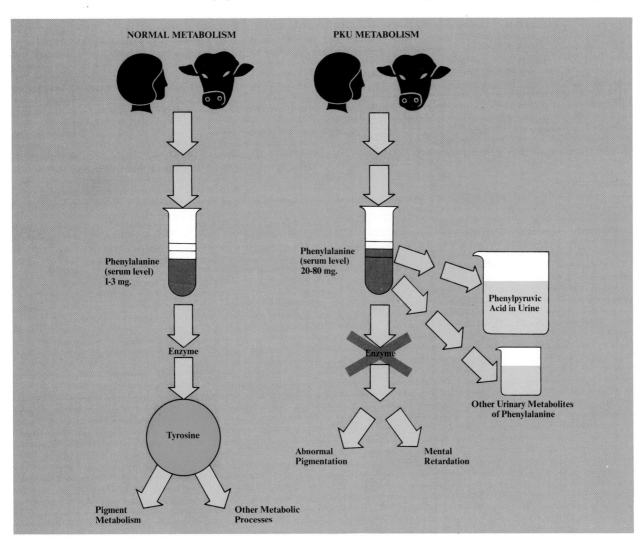

NORMAL METABOLISM

PKU METABOLISM

Phenylalanine
(serum level)
1-3 mg.

Enzyme

Tyrosine

Pigment
Metabolism

Other Metabolic
Processes

Phenylalanine
(serum level)
20-80 mg.

Enzyme

Phenylpyruvic
Acid in Urine

Other Urinary Metabolites
of Phenylalanine

Abnormal
Pigmentation

Mental
Retardation

complete. When an enzyme is missing, the outcome could be a build-up of the unprocessed substrate, a deficiency of the expected product, or both. The latter does not seem to be important in PKU, because tyrosine (the product) also is acquired from the diet and can be manufactured by the body. The levels of phenylalanine in the blood and the urine of the patient do, however, build up massively (up to twenty times normal) and so do the levels of abnormal and characteristic degradation products—from one of which (phenylketone) the disease derives its name.

Phenylalanine-low diets developed for PKU patients seem to prevent or slow down the course of the disease, provided that an afflicted child begins the diet at a very early age. Completely eliminating phenylalanine from the diet is not suitable because it is a necessary amino acid required for protein synthesis. The diet of the PKU child must therefore provide enough phenylalanine for this purpose without interfering with other bodily processes.

To detect a PKU child as soon after birth as possible, a diagnostic test developed by Dr. Robert Guthrie in 1960 has been made mandatory in many states for all newborn infants. Hospitals in all fifty states now have the facilities for the test. All it requires from the newborn child is a single drop of blood from its heel. One of the consequences of this massive testing program has been to show the disease to be twice as prevalent as previously believed. Much more important, many children have been saved from their fate and permitted to lead a life with normal or near-normal intelligence.

Sphingolipidoses

An important group of genetically caused metabolic errors is that of *sphingolipidoses*, where the genetic defect prevents normal metabolism of certain fatty substances (sphingolipids) and leads to their accumulation, or the accumulation of their abnormal products, in various body tissues, including the brain. Among these genetic disorders are Fabry's, Niemann-Pick, and Gaucher's diseases and, most prominent, *Tay-Sachs disease*, all caused by recessive genes. Tay-Sachs is a sublethal, most horrendous disease, causing mental degeneration and idiocy, blindness, convulsions or paralysis, wasting away of the child, and inevitably, death before the age of seven years. The cause of it all is the absence of an enzyme called Hex A.

As with a number of other defective genes, the Tay-Sachs allele is largely restricted to a well-defined segment of the human population—Jews whose ancestors lived in a small area on the Russian-Polish border and whose subsequent migrations have spread the gene in many countries. Of those persons affected by Tay-Sachs disease, 99 percent are people of Jewish Ashkenazic (East European) ancestry. In the United States, this ancestry is involved in more than 90 percent of all American Jews, and each year between 100 and 200 children are born with the disease.

The enzyme involved, Hex A, can now be readily tested and measured in the blood. Tay-Sachs carriers, having only one normal allele, have about half the normal level of enzyme in their blood and can, therefore, be easily detected. Programs are now under way for extensive screening of such carriers, to warn them and counsel them about their genetic heritage.

Drug Abnormalities

Although most inborn errors of metabolism become apparent in young children when the body is not able to handle naturally occurring substances, others are revealed by drugs or other materials that adults deliberately add to their own personal environment. For this reason, some physicians argue that modern medicine is working against itself in some respects; drugs intended to cure a certain illness may prove to be dangerous when taken by individuals whose genetic machinery is ill-equipped to handle them.

For example, it is now known that the anesthetic succinyl choline should not be taken by people who lack an enzyme that would ordinarily metabolize the drug and safely remove it from the bloodstream in a short time. If they do take the drug, they will experience prolonged anesthesia and become endangered.

The antituberculosis drug Isoniazid also is dangerous to some people. In fact, about half the people in the United States may carry a genetic defect that prevents them from producing the enzyme necessary for the quick breakdown of the drug, bringing on a wide variety of deleterious side effects. The hereditary basis of these abnormal reactions is suggested by the fact that the ratio of "slow metabolizers" to "fast metabolizers" varies from country to country. In South America slow metabolizers make up about one-third of the population, while only one-twentieth of Eskimos cannot tolerate the drug.

Since physicians first became aware of these drug abnormalities, the new field of *pharmacogenetics* has developed. It aims at identifying genetic drug abnormalities when they occur and then devises tests to spot defects before a patient takes a potentially harmful drug. Workers in pharmacogenetics expect that a better understanding of the genetic and chemical bases of adverse drug reactions will mean that more good drugs will get to more people. At the present time, a basically good drug can be kept off the market if it shows adverse side effects in even a small number of people. If it can be proved that the side effects are due to some genetic flaw, pharmacogeneticists maintain, there is really no good reason to prevent a much larger number of people from using a drug that could save them from death.

Sex-Linked Gene Mutations

Of the twenty-three pairs of human chromosomes, one pair (the *sex chromosomes*) is special compared to the other twenty-two (the somatic chromosomes, or autosomes). In the female, the sex-chromosome pair comprises two homologous chromosomes, XX. The male, however, has only one X chromosome, and its "homologous" equivalent is represented by an altogether different chromosome, Y. When the XY male germ cells go through meiosis, gametes are produced that have either the X or the Y sex chromosome only; female gametes, on the other hand, are only of the X type. Fertilization of an X-containing egg by an X-containing sperm will produce an individual with an XX sex-chromosome pair, that is, a female, while fertilization by a Y-containing sperm will lead to the birth of an XY, hence male, child. Each man receives his Y chromosome from his father and can only pass it on to his sons and receives his X chromosome from the mother and only passes it on to his daughters. Every woman, on the other hand, receives one X chromosome from each parent and can pass either one to her children, whatever their sex.

Besides their role in sex determination, X chromosomes carry a large number of genes, known as sex-linked genes, and their mode of transmission is called sex-linked inheritance. Female cells have two alleles of all X-linked genes and can be either homozygous or heterozygous for them. Male cells, having only one X chromosome, are called *hemizygous* for X-linked alleles. A *recessive* X-linked gene would therefore be free to express itself in the male even though it would not do so in presence of its dominant allele in a heterozygous female.

The gene abnormalities discussed thus far were "autosomal" defects, that is, they involved alleles located on autosomes (somatic chromosomes) and could occur equally in male and female individuals. There are a number of sex-linked gene abnormalities that, because of the peculiarity of the sex chromosomes and the sex-linked inheritance, deserve a separate look. One must be aware, however, that the occurrence of an inheritable sex-linked *disease* could also be due to an autosomal gene defect whose phenotypic expression differs in the two sexes.

One of the most famous inherited diseases is the bleeder disease, or *hemophilia*. Injury or physical stress results in excessive bleeding, usually because of deficiencies in certain blood components necessary for effective and rapid blood clotting. In classical hemophilia, or hemophilia A, the defective gene is an X-linked, recessive allele (h) unable to direct adequate synthesis of a protein, the "anti-hemophilic globulin." A male bearing the h gene on his X chromosome cannot have a normal allele counterpart H (because he has no second X) and will therefore always show the disease. Moreover, because the aberrant gene is linked to X, he cannot breed a male child bearing it and no male child of his will be diseased unless it inherits the gene from the mother. He will, however, transmit the gene to all of his daughters. A woman bearing the h gene on only one X chromosome will not show the disease because of the dominant H allele present on her other X. She will transmit the aberrant gene to half of her progeny, whether male or female, and therefore half of her male children may be hemophiliacs and half of her daughters hemophilia-carriers. Homozygous recessive females (hh) are extremely rare. Thus, by and large, hemophilia will skip a generation, a man with the disease transmitting the gene to a daughter (no disease) and through her to some of his grandsons (diseased).

Other X-linked, recessive gene defects are involved in red-green *color-blindness* (actually, a group of diseases). If a color-blind man marries a normal woman, all children will appear normal. If a color-blind woman (hence homozygous for the recessive gene) mates with a normal man, all sons will be color-blind and all daughters will be phenotypically normal and yet carriers for the color-blindness gene. A color-blind female child can be born only of a color-blind father and either a color-blind or a carrier mother.

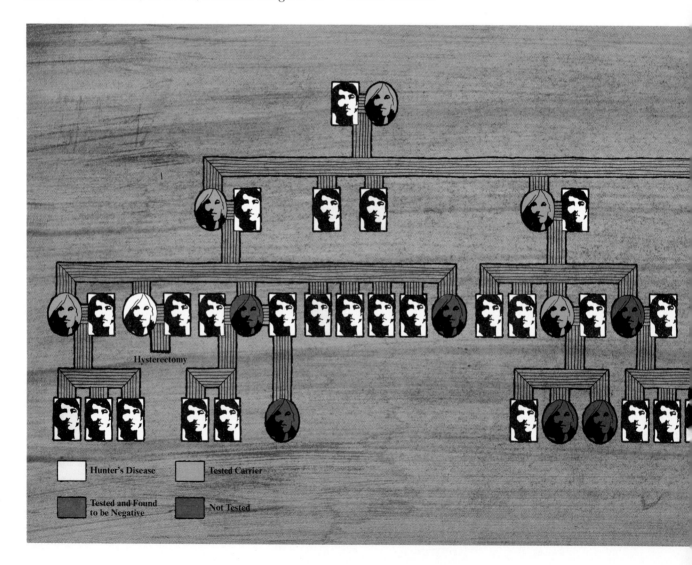

Many other traits are known, or strongly suspected, to be controlled by X-linked alleles. Such is one type of muscular dystrophy, two types of diabetes insipidus (one due to the deficiency of the pituitary hormone ADH), hypogamma globulinemia, a still poorly understood inability of the body to adequately produce gamma globulins (including the immunity proteins), and so on.

CHROMOSOME ABNORMALITIES

Gene mutations lead to gene abnormalities, that is, a change in the *quality* of the genetic material. But the *quantity* of genetic material and the way by which it is *arranged* also are important for well-balanced functioning of the cells and a harmonious development of the human body. Developmental or functional disorders, therefore, also can be due to *chromosome abnormalities*, be they in their number, their integrity, or the gene distribution within them. They, too, are genetic disorders, may involve somatic cells and be transmitted to subsequent cell progenies, or may involve germ cells and be passed on from one individual to the next generation through his or her gametes. Chromosome abnormalities are sometimes referred to as "chromosomal mutations."

Normal mitosis during development of a human being from the fertilized egg produces only cells with a full and correct number of chromosomes. For various reasons, including environmental factors such as radiation or drugs, the duplication of chromosomes during mitosis may occasionally go wrong and affect the *number* or the *content* of the two sets of chromosomes that will constitute the genetic material of the two daughter cells. After replication, two sister chromosomes may fail to move to opposite poles (a phenomenon called *nondisjunction*), causing one daughter cell to have forty-six plus one, or forty-seven, chromosomes and the other forty-six minus one, or forty-five chromosomes. The atypical chromosome numbers could then be perpetuated through cell proliferation by correct mitotic processes.

Another potential mechanism for chromosomal abnormalities is chromosome *breakage*, where a fragment may be split off a chromosome and get lost or

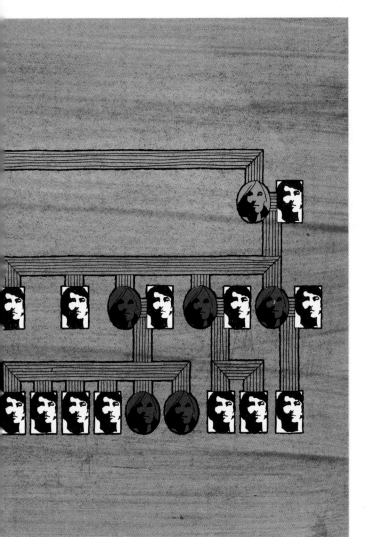

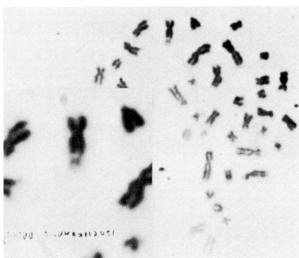

Figure 14.16   Chromosomal breakage. Such breakage may be due to any one of a number of factors. Some of the factors that have been implicated in such abnormalities are ingestion of drugs, including caffeine and aspirin, and radiation.

Figure 14.15   Hunter's disease, one of six known hereditary disorders in which complex sugar molecules (mucopolysaccharides) accumulate for lack of their degrading enzyme. In Hunter's, the missing enzyme is an X-linked recessive gene. The disease involves enlargement of the liver, coarse and deformed bones and joints, slowly progressive mental retardation, and excessive levels of mucopolysaccharides in the urine. Note that all carriers are female and that all diseased individuals are male.

fuse to another one; again, the defect may persist through the cell progeny. Chromosome abnormalities passed on through a gamete to a new individual are often lethal; if the zygote survives, the new human being will, to one degree or another, develop defectively.

In *Down's syndrome*, also known as mongolism, one normal gamete has fused with an abnormal one containing an extra chromosome, so that the affected person has forty-seven instead of forty-six chromosomes in his or her cells. The chromosome with an extra copy (called *trisomic* because there are now three of them) is, in this case, a small one known as number 21. Because of its presence, the individual is born with physical abnormalities of the face, tongue, eyelids (the name comes from the slanted-eyed or mongoloid appearance), and other parts of the body (for example, the heart) and is physically and mentally retarded. As with many other chromosomal abnormalities, "mongoloid" children are more likely to be produced by mothers over forty than by younger mothers. The number of previous pregnancies or the age of the father do not appear to be relevant. The age of the mother is believed to be important not because of her physical condition during pregnancy but because of her greater tendency to produce "nondisjunctional" eggs and thus contribute an abnormal gamete to the new individual.

Examples of abnormal chromosome numbers also are found with respect to the sex chromosomes. In *Turner's syndrome*, the individual has only one X chromosome (often designated as XO); the genital apparatus, both internal and external, is female but the ovaries are lacking or rudimentary. The converse case of an extra X chromosome (XXX) is less common. In males, *Klinefelter's syndrome* (abnormally small testes with no mature sperm) is associated with an XXY sex-chromosome set. The syndrome appears to be the counterpart of the Turner's in the sense of the affected persons being "origin opposites." Nondisjunction with respect to the sex chromosomes, occurring in a male germ cell, could produce O and XY sperm (instead of the normal X and Y); upon fusion with normal X eggs, they would result in zygotes of the XO or

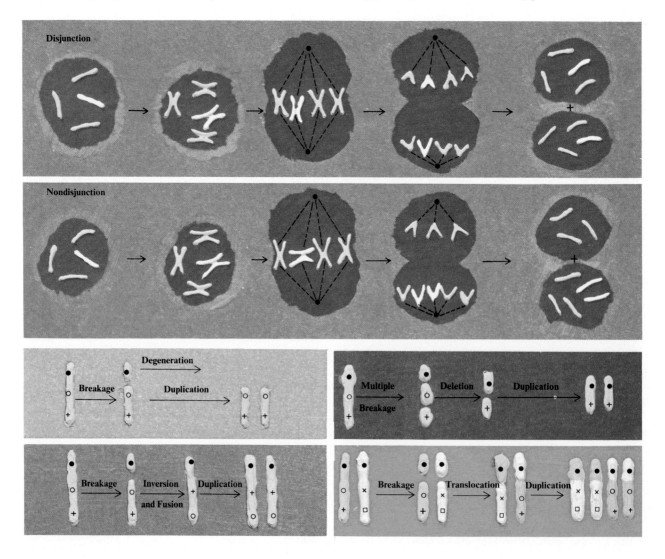

the XXY types respectively—although other mechanisms may also explain such aberrations.

Recently, much attention has been given to another sex trisomic situation, the XYY male. Individuals with an extra Y chromosome appear to be less rare than was previously thought, are taller than usual, and seem to be medically normal. However, some physicians and lawyers suspect that the XYY condition may be linked to asocial behavior and could at least in some cases be responsible for violent criminal acts. Although the point is not as yet fully established, it could cast a completely different light on future criminal trials, providing them with a medical rather than a purely social base.

CONGENITAL DEFECTS

Any defect with which a child is born is a *congenital* defect. Included in this category are, therefore, all gene or chromosome abnormalities. More restrictively, the term *congenital malformation* is applied to *phenotypic* defects present at birth, as contrasted with any that would appear only during postnatal development. Besides those derived from gene or chromosome abnormalities, many malformations could arise from *injury* to the growing embryo.

Although the fetus appears to be well protected from most of the hazards associated with life in the outside world, its proper development can be seriously altered by a great number of external factors, most of which come to it by way of the mother's bloodstream. If the mother takes even relatively harmless drugs, smokes excessively, is x-rayed, does not eat enough, or is otherwise unhealthy, the developing embryo can be killed, stunted, or severely deformed. The frequency of congenital malformations increases with the age of the mother beyond thirty-five years.

Some of the most prevalent congenital abnormalities resulting from one or more of the above factors are:

1. *Spina bifida*, a major deformity of the spinal cord that affects two in every 1,000 babies.
2. *Hydrocephalus*, or water on the brain, which often accompanies *spina bifida*. Its usually lethal course can now be temporarily diverted by shunting the excess brain fluids into the bloodstream through a system of valves.

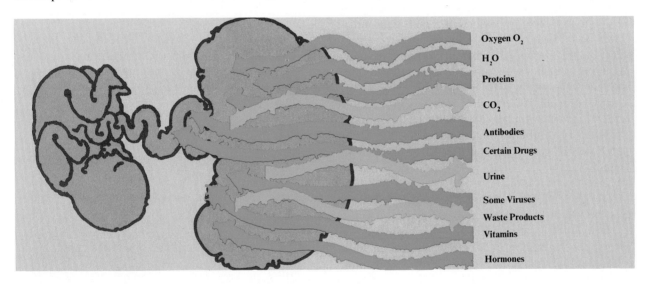

Oxygen O$_2$

H$_2$O

Proteins

CO$_2$

Antibodies

Certain Drugs

Urine

Some Viruses

Waste Products

Vitamins

Hormones

Figure 14.18   Fetal and maternal circulation, showing which substances can cross the placental barrier. A selectively porous membrane separates the two circulatory systems.

Figure 14.17   Chromosome abnormalities. Abnormalities may occur in the *quantity* of chromosomal material, such as occurs in nondisjunction, or in the *quality* of the chromosomal material, as occurs in degeneration, inversion, translocation, deletion, or other results of chromosomal breakage.

3. *Spastic cerebral palsy*, the most widely known type of congenital brain damage, which may be caused by almost any injury to the brain before or at birth.
4. *Congenital heart disease*, discussed in greater detail in Chapter 24. Such defects can often be corrected when the child is strong enough to withstand major surgery.

Lesser abnormalities such as hare lip or cleft palate also can be corrected by surgery. Congenital malformations in addition can be the consequence of imperfect attempts at abortion or injury during or before delivery.

Most physicians now believe that *timing* is the most crucial factor in determining whether or not an abnormality will appear in the fetus, and what kind it will be. Various bodily organs develop along their own special timetables, and if some outside influence disturbs that schedule, the organ will probably never be able to develop fully. For example, if development is interrupted between the seventh to the tenth week when the inner ear is being formed, the child may be born deaf.

The *thalidomide* disaster proved just how seriously bad timing and an apparently harmless drug can combine to affect the future of the developing child. The drug was prescribed as a mild tranquilizer and was taken in the first few months of pregnancy by thousands of pregnant women in Germany and elsewhere. As a result, more than 8,000 children were born with *phocomelia*, a condition marked by stunted arms and legs but little other physical deformation. This tragedy has led many doctors to recommend that mothers abstain from taking *any* drugs during the first three months of pregnancy, when the embryo is especially prone to congenital malformations.

Rubella, or German measles, is another frightening example of how important timing can be in the development of deformities in the embryo. Although the disease is relatively harmless in children, its occurrence in women during the first three months of pregnancy can be disastrous to the unborn child. In the last great rubella epidemic in the United States during the early 1960s, about 20,000 children born to mothers who had rubella were afflicted with a pathetic number of congenital deformities, including blindness, deafness, imbecility or mental retardation, and limb abnormalities. About 30,000 were lost by spontaneous abortions or stillbirths. A similar outbreak is expected some time in the early 1970s, although a new antirubella vaccine should reduce the impact of the coming epidemic.

Syphilis in the mother can cause abortions and stillbirths, as well as blindness, deafness, and other defects in newborn children. But because the disease can now be detected by a blood test during pregnancy and can be treated with penicillin, few babies should be affected. Blindness may also occur from a gonorrhea-infected mother, a serious danger given the current epidemic rise of this disease (see Chapter 22).

There also is growing evidence that such commonly accepted drugs as alcohol and tobacco can

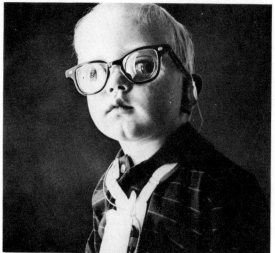

The mother got over her rubella in three days. Unfortunately, her unborn child didn't.

To pregnant mothers, rubella (German measles) means a few days in bed, a sore throat, a runny nose, temperature, and a rash.

But if they're in their first month when they catch it, there's a 40% chance that to their unborn babies it can mean deafness, or a heart condition, or brain damage, or cataracts which cause at least partial blindness.

Only last year, an immunization against rubella became available. But when a pregnant mother gets immunized, the prevention may be as harmful to her baby as the disease.

So if unborn babies are going to be protected, it will have to be by inoculating the kids who infect the mothers who in turn infect the fetuses.

And it will have to be done now. You see, rubella epidemics break out every six to nine years. The last outbreak was in 1964. Which means the next one is due any day now.

In the last epidemic, 20,000 babies were deprived of a normal childhood—and 30,000 more deprived of any childhood at all—because no immunization existed.

It would be unforgivable if the same thing happened again because an immunization existed and nobody used it.

 Metropolitan Life
We sell life insurance.
But our business is life.

For a free booklet about immunization, write One Madison Avenue, N.Y., N.Y. 10010.

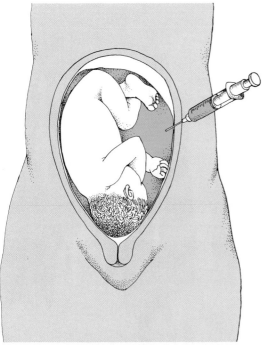

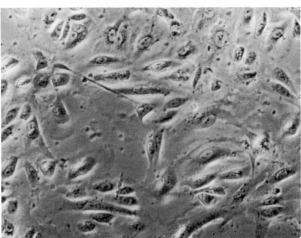

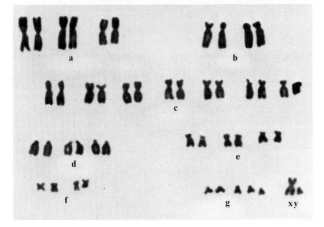

Figure 14.19 Amniocentesis. (*top*) How the culture cells are taken. (*center*) What the culture cells look like. They are examined for evidence of any chromosomal abnormalities such as Down's syndrome (*bottom*), in which there is an extra chromosome in the twenty-first pair (g).

impair fetal growth when a pregnant woman smokes or drinks to excess. In addition, hundreds of studies conducted in several underdeveloped nations show that if pregnant women are on diets inadequate in protein, the child can be born mentally retarded and will probably remain so for the rest of its life.

GENETIC COUNSELING

As man's understanding of genetic diseases grows, more approaches toward the *treatment* of the diseased persons become accessible. Besides attempting to relieve the symptoms from which they suffer, science has learned to provide a missing hormone—as in diabetes—or to reduce the abnormal levels of toxic substances—as in PKU. Perhaps in the future science will find ways to provide an enzyme for which the genetic instructions are missing. Better still, the enormous progress that the science of genetics has made over the last two decades suggests that man may be at the threshold of a new era of *genetic engineering* when it will become possible to provide the genetically abnormal person with the very gene that is missing or replace one that is defective.

The most critical question in such approaches is the identification of the affected individual at a sufficiently early time when irreversible damage to the developing body, and particularly the developing brain, has not yet set in. For a growing number of genetic disorders it is now possible to apply *diagnostic tests* directly to the developing fetus as early as the first few weeks or months of life. Through the technique known as *amniocentesis*, a few cells derived from the fetus are removed from the amniotic fluid that surrounds it; the cells are grown in *tissue culture*—that is, in a vessel outside the organism—for an appropriate period of time and then examined. For Tay-Sachs disease, the Hex A enzyme can be measured to determine whether the

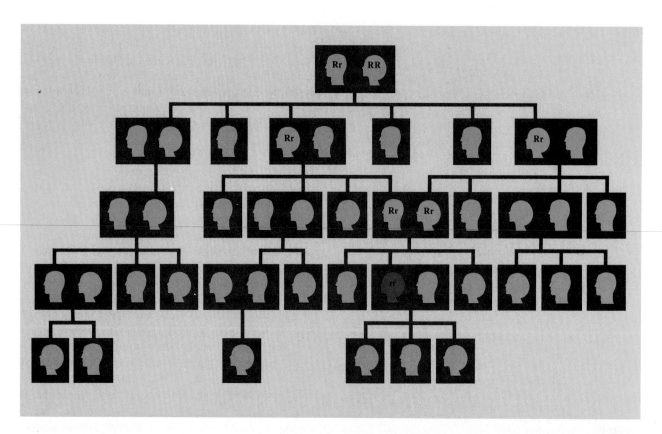

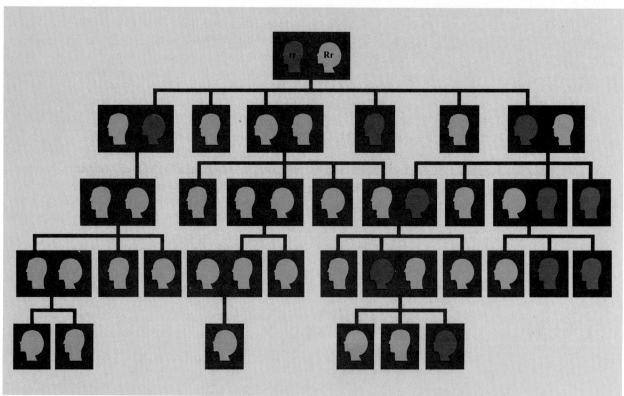

Figure 14.20 A typical family pattern of a recessive trait (*top*) and a dominant trait (*bottom*). The orange represents appearance of the dominant trait, magenta, the recessive trait.

child will be genetically normal, have the disease, or be a carrier of the abnormal gene. The sex of the unborn child can be established by measuring the amount of sex chromatin (or Barr chromatin), an easily stainable substance detectable in female but not male cells and probably related to the X chromosomes; sex diagnosis may be particularly important in such sex-linked genetic diseases as hemophilia. A chromosome count and examination will provide information for a diagnosis of such chromosomal abnormalities as Down's syndrome.

Whenever there is an indication that the unborn child may carry a genetic disease—based on occurrence of the disease in family members, identified carrier parents, advanced age of the mother, and so on—the availability of such diagnostic tests will be invaluable. If the fetus is not affected, the parents will have a greater peace of mind about the forthcoming birth than was ever before possible. If the test shows the developing baby to be affected, and a reasonable treatment is available, it will be possible to start the treatment at an effectively early date. As a last resort, the positive diagnosis will suggest the advisability of a therapeutic abortion.

As for all diseases, however, the best treatment remains *prevention*. In the case of gene abnormalities, prevention means identifying the presence of the aberrant gene in the parents and avoiding the conception of a new diseased human being. Identification of possible genetic problems and giving advice based on that identification is the role of *genetic counseling*. Because many genetic diseases are due to recessive alleles, both prospective parents must be carriers for the future child to be affected. Thus, early recognition of carrier individuals is usually the first, often still difficult, step. No doubts are left when a previous child has already been born diseased, or when the prospective father or mother had a diseased parent. In other cases, a detailed study of the *pedigree* (family tree) of each spouse and tests performed on selected cells may permit one to recognize them as carriers.

Armed with this information, the consulting geneticist can make an objective assessment about the future child. He can only do so, however, in terms of *probability*. Science has learned, for example, that matings of two recessive heterozygous individuals would result, *on the average*, in one normal, two carriers, and one diseased child for every four children born. But chance has no memory. These same probabilities apply to every single new birth, irrespective of what happens with previous ones. Thus, even for two carrier parents the chances are always 25 percent to have an affected baby and 75 percent not to. In most such cases, the prospective parents may still choose to go ahead and rely on subsequent diagnostic tests on the fetus for a decision on whether to terminate or complete the pregnancy.

Although congenital defects of one kind or another, or for any one of the causes just discussed, still occur with an approximate frequency of one every hundred births, one must wonder at the progress that modern health science has achieved already. Just a few years ago, physicians could only shake their heads at genetic or environmentally caused abnormalities. They could label them but they could do little to treat the children. Now medicine is knocking on biological doors that are opening to a new understanding of what has gone wrong at the level of molecules and cells. With such previously untreatable diseases as sickle cell anemia and PKU, the doors have opened to new methods of treatment, new hope.

These discoveries have put the genetic counselor on an entirely different level of sophistication. It may be that in a decade or two, he will have moved even further ahead. From his present options of suggesting abortion or discouraging parents with certain genetic flaws from having children, he may have become capable of prescribing a program based on some new conquest of the molecular medicine that has evolved from a closer look at the double-stranded coil of a chemical called DNA.

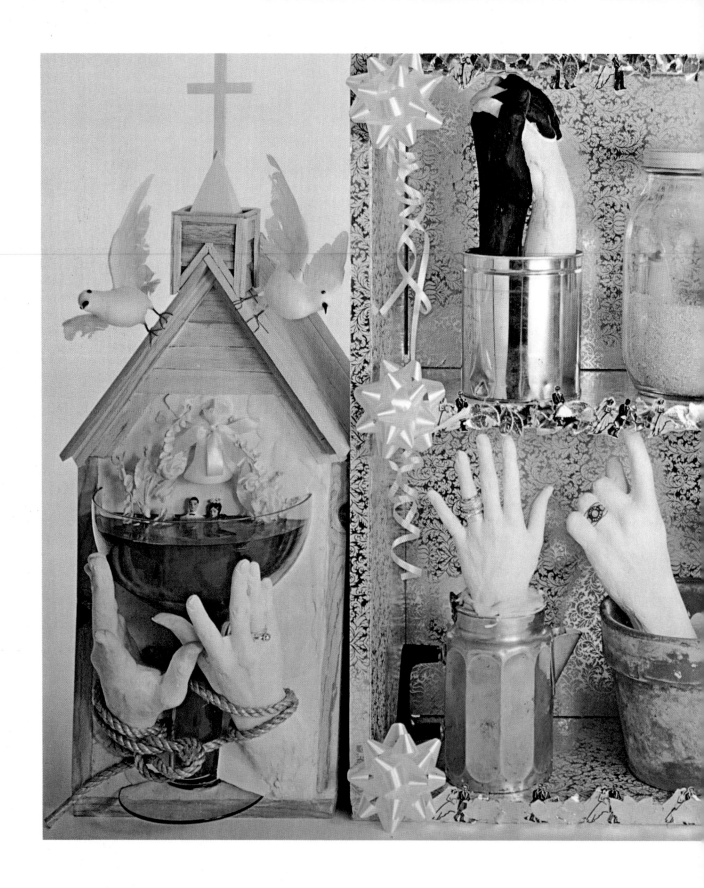

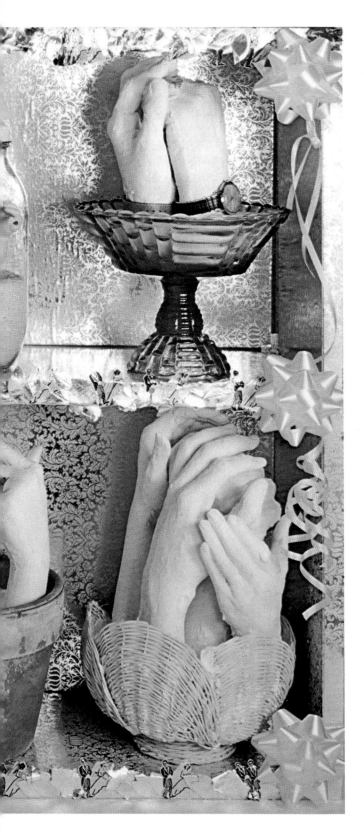

15

More than a century ago the Swiss historian and ethnologist J. J. Bachofen postulated that early man lived in small packs, ignorant of marriage and indulging in beastlike sexual promiscuity. He could hardly have suggested anything more revolting, or more fascinating, to the puritanical and prurient sensibility of his time. Anthropologists based whole theories of the family and of society on his notion. As the Victorian fog dissipated, however, evidence began to show that among the hundreds of primitive peoples still on earth—many of whom live much like early man—not a single one was without *some form of marriage* and some limitations on the sexual freedom of the married. Marriage, it appeared, was a genuine human universal.

Nevertheless, Bachofen's myth died hard, because it appealed to a longing, deep in everyone, for total freedom to do whatever one wants. And recently, it has sprung up from its own ashes in the form of a startling new notion: Even if there never was a time when marriage did not exist, there soon will be. Lately, the air has been filled with such prophecies of the decline and impending fall of marriage. Some of the prophets are grieved at this prospect and warn that hedonism and easy divorce are eroding the foundations of family life. Others rejoice at the thought of the death of marriage, saying that marriage is obsolete and that any sensible person can live and love better without it.

Marriage in American Society

But are there, in fact, any real indications of a mass revolt against traditional marriage? There certainly seem to be. For one thing, in 1969 there were 660,000 divorces in America—an all-time record—and the divorce rate seems certain to achieve new highs in the next few years. For another thing, marital infidelity seems to have increased markedly since Alfred Kinsey's first surveys of a generation ago and is now tried, sooner or later, by some 60 percent of married men and 30 to 35 percent of married women in the United States. But in what is much more of a departure from the past, infidelity is now tacitly accepted by a fair number of the spouses of the unfaithful. For some couples it has become a shared hobby; mate-swapping and group-sex parties now involve thousands of middle-class marriages.

Yet another indication of change is a sharp increase not only in the number of young men and women who, dispensing with legalities, live together unwed but also in the kind of people who are doing so; although common-law marriage has long been popular among the poor, in the past few years it has become widespread—and often esteemed—within the middle class. Furthermore, the strive to abandon the "double standard" of the sexes and to reach a real, effective equality for man and woman is bound to reshape the rules, attitudes, and content of legalized or unlegalized marriages.

An even more radical attack on the American marriage system is the effort of people in hundreds of communes around the country to construct "families," or group marriages, in which the adults own everything in common, often consider that they all belong to one another, and play mix and match sexually. A quite different but equally radical break with tradition is being made by a rapidly growing percentage of America's male and female homosexuals, who nowadays feel freer than ever to avoid "cover" marriages and to live openly as homo-sexuals. Their lead is almost certain to be followed by countless others within the next decade or so as American society grows ever more tolerant of personal choice in sexual matters.

Nevertheless, reports of the death of marriage are, to paraphrase Mark Twain, greatly exaggerated. Most human beings regard whatever they grew up with as right and good and see nearly every change in human behavior as a decline in standards and a fall from grace. But change often means adaptation and evolution. The many signs of contemporary revolt against marriage have been viewed as symptoms of a fatal disease, but they may, instead, be signs of a change from an obsolescent form of marriage—patriarchal monogamy—into new forms better suited to present needs.

CHANGING PERSPECTIVES

Marriage as a social structure is exceedingly plastic, being shaped by the interplay of culture and of human needs into hundreds of different forms. In societies where women could do valuable productive work, it often made sense for a man to acquire more than one wife; where women were idle or relatively unproductive—and, hence, a burden—monogamy was more likely to be the pattern. When women had means of their own or could easily fall back upon relatives, divorce was apt to be easy; where they were wholly dependent on their husbands, it was generally difficult. Under marginal and primitive living conditions, men kept their women in useful subjugation; in wealthier and more leisured societies, women often managed to acquire a degree of independence and power.

For a long while, the only acceptable form of marriage in America was a lifelong one-to-one union, sexually faithful, all but indissoluble, productive of goods and children, and strongly husband-dominated. It was a thoroughly functional mechanism during the eighteenth and much of the nine-

Figure 15.1 The roles of husband and wife in a marriage vary from culture to culture. In some societies the social roles are interchangeable; in others, the woman's role is a clearly defined subservient one. In some cultures the roles in marriage are defined in terms of more than just husband and wife and involve all the members of the extended family group.

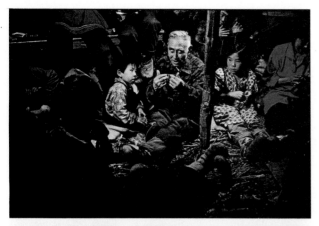

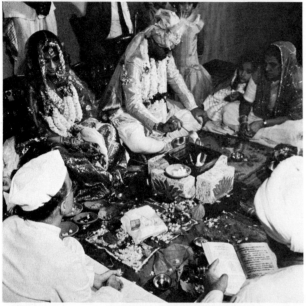

teenth centuries, when men were struggling to secure the land and needed women who would clothe and feed them, produce and rear children to help them, and obey their orders without question for an entire lifetime. It was functional, too, for the women of that time who, uneducated, unfit for other kinds of work, and endowed by the law with almost no legal or property rights, needed men who would support them, give them social status, and be their guides and protectors for life.

But as time passed, men had less and less need for their women to produce goods and their children to help on the farm; more and more, women were educated, had time to spare, made their way into the job market—and realized that they no longer had to cling to their men for life. As patriarchalism lost its usefulness, women began to want and demand contraceptives, the vote, and respect; men, finding the world growing ever more impersonal and cold, began to want wives who were warm, understanding, companionable, and sexy.

Yet, strangely enough, as all these things were happening, marriage not only did not lose ground but grew more popular, and today, when it is under full-scale attack on most fronts, it is more widespread than ever. Indeed, a considerably larger percentage of the adult population was married in 1970 than was the case in 1890; the marriage rate, though still below the level of the 1940s, has been climbing steadily since 1963.

The explanation of this paradox is that as marriage was losing its former uses, it was gaining new ones. The changes that were robbing marriage of practical and life-affirming values were turning America into a mechanized urban society in which people felt like numbers, not individuals, in which they had many neighbors but few friends, and in which their lives were controlled by remote governments, huge companies, and insensate computers. Alone and powerless, how were they to find inti-

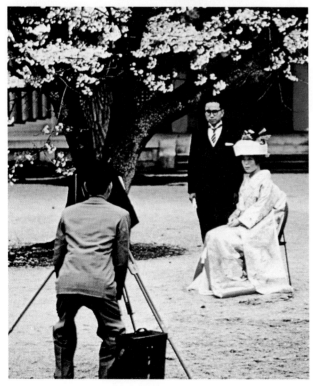

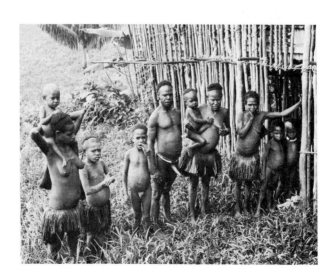

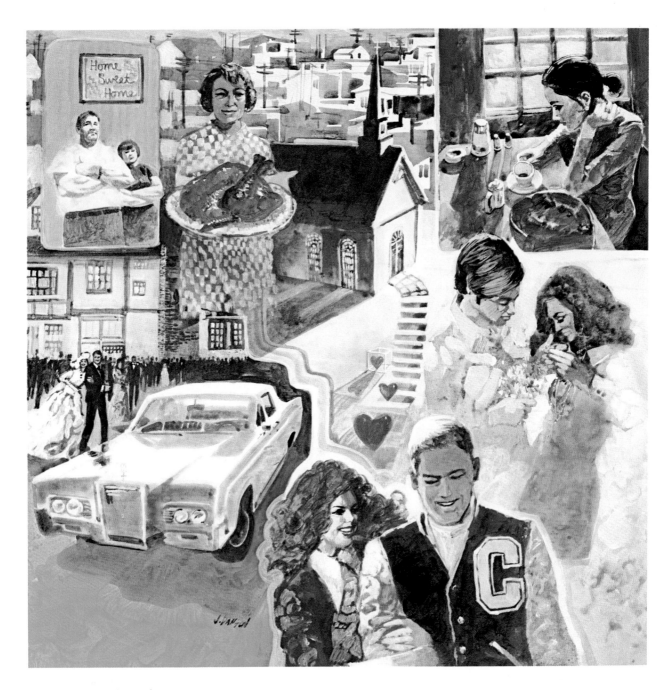

Figure 15.2 American culture puts many pressures on young men and women to get married. Some of these pressures are subtle, such as the wording of advertising. Others are more obvious, such as parental urgings.

macy and warmth, sympathy and loyalty, enduring friendship and a feeling of personal importance? Why, obviously, through loving and marrying. Marriage is a microcosm, a world within which one seeks to correct the shortcomings of the macrocosm around him.

The model of marriage that served the old purposes excellently serves the new ones poorly. But most of the contemporary assaults upon it are not efforts to destroy it; they are efforts to modify and remold it. Only traditional patriarchal marriage is dying, while everywhere marriage is being reborn in a variety of new forms.

DIVORCE

Far from being a wasting illness, divorce is a healthful adaptation, enabling monogamy to survive in a time when patriarchal powers, privileges, and marital systems have become unworkable; far from being a radical change in the institution of marriage, divorce is a relatively minor modification of it and thoroughly supportive of most of its conventions.

Not that it seemed so at first. When divorce was introduced to Christian Europe, it appeared an extreme and rather sinful measure to most people; even among the wealthy—the only people who could afford it—it remained for centuries quite rare and thoroughly scandalous. In 1816, president Timothy Dwight of Yale thundered against the "alarming and terrible" divorce rate in Connecticut—a rate of about 1 percent. But as women began achieving a certain degree of emancipation during the nineteenth century, and as the purposes of marriage changed, divorce laws were liberalized and the rate began climbing. Between 1870 and 1905, both the United States population and the divorce rate more than doubled; since then, the divorce rate has increased more than four times.

And not only for the reasons already noted but for yet another: the increase in longevity. When people married in their late twenties and marriage was likely to end in death by the time the last child was leaving home, divorce seemed not only wrong, but hardly worth the trouble; this was especially true where the only defect in a marriage was boredom. Today, however, when people marry earlier and have finished raising their children with half of their adult lives still ahead of them, boredom seems a good reason for getting divorced. Half of all divorces occur after eight years of marriage and a quarter of them after fifteen—most of them being the result not of bad initial choices but of disparity or dullness that has grown with time.

Divorced people, however, are seeking not to escape from marriage for the rest of their lives but to exchange unhappy or boring marriages for satisfying ones. Whatever bitter things they say at the time of divorce, the vast majority do remarry, most of their second marriages lasting the rest of their lives; even those whose second marriages fail are likely to divorce and remarry and, that failing,

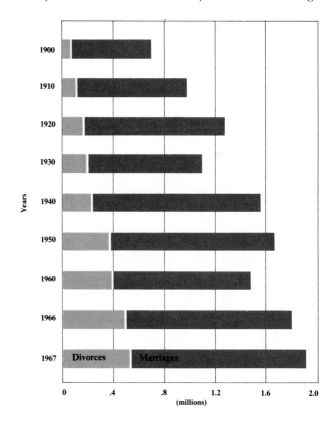

Figure 15.3 Marriages and divorces in the United States, 1900–1967.

marry yet again. Divorcing people are actually marrying people, and divorce is not a negation of marriage but a workable cross between traditional monogamy and multiple marriage; sociologists have even referred to it as "serial polygamy."

Despite its costs and hardships, divorce is thus a compromise between the monogamous ideal and the realities of present-day life. To judge from the statistics, it is becoming more useful and more socially acceptable every year. Although the divorce rate leveled off for a dozen years or so after the postwar surge of 1946, it has been climbing steadily since 1962, and the rate for the entire nation now stands at nearly *one for every three marriages*. In some areas, it is even higher. In California, where a new ultraliberal law went into effect in 1970, nearly two of every three marriages end in divorce—a fact that astonishes people in other areas of the country but that Californians themselves already accept with equanimity. They still approve of, and very much enjoy, being married; they have simply gone further than the rest of the country in using divorce to keep monogamy workable in today's world.

INFIDELITY

Seen in the same light, marital infidelity also is a frequently useful modification of the marriage contract rather than a repudiation of it. It violates the conventional moral code to a greater degree than does divorce but, as practiced in America, is only a limited departure from the monogamous pattern. Unfaithful Americans, by and large, neither have extramarital love affairs that last for many years nor do they engage in a continuous series of minor liaisons; rather, their infidelity consists of relatively brief and widely scattered episodes, so that in the course of a married lifetime, they spend many more years being faithful than being unfaithful. Furthermore, American infidelity, unlike its European counterparts, has no recognized status as part of the marital system; except in a few circles, it remains impermissible, hidden, and isolated from the other aspects of one's life.

This impermissibility is not true at all levels of American society, however: Upper-class men—and to some extent, women—have long regarded the discreet love affair as an essential complement to

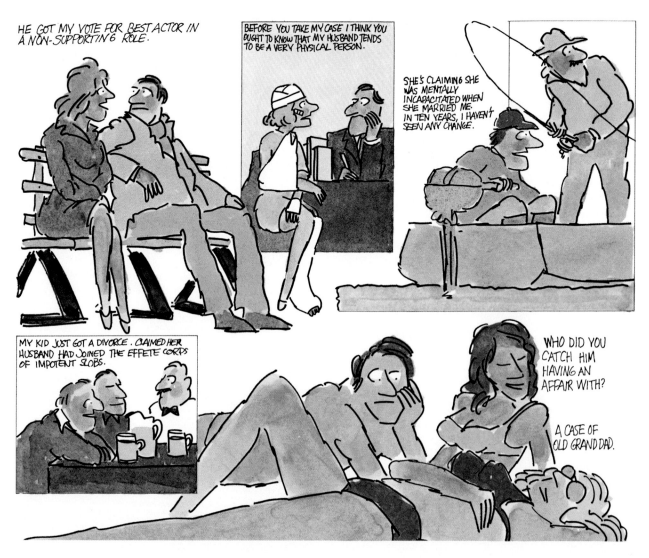

marriage, and lower-class husbands have always considered an extracurricular roll in the hay important to a married man's peace of mind. Indeed, few societies have ever tried to make both husband and wife sexually faithful over a lifetime; the totally monogamous ideal is statistically an abnormality. Professors Clellan Ford and Frank Beach state in *Patterns of Sexual Behavior* that less than 16 percent of 185 societies studied by anthropologists had formal restrictions to a single mate—and, of these, less than one-third wholly disapproved of both premarital and extramarital relationships.

America's middle-class, puritanical society, however, has long held that infidelity of any sort is impossible if one truly loves one's mate and is happily married, that any deviation from fidelity stems from an evil or neurotic character, and that it inevitably damages both the sinner and the sinned-against. This credo drew support from earlier generations of psychotherapists, for almost all the adulterers they treated were neurotic, unhappily married, or out of sorts with life in general. But it is just such people who seek psychotherapy; they are hardly a fair sample. Recently, sex researchers have examined the unfaithful more representatively and have come up with quite different findings. They agree in general that:

1. Many of the unfaithful—perhaps even a majority—are not seriously dissatisfied with their marriages or their mates and a fair number are more or less happily married.
2. Only about one-third—perhaps even fewer—appear to seek extramarital sex for neurotic motives; the rest do so for nonpathological reasons.
3. Many of the unfaithful—perhaps even a majority—do not feel that they, their mates, or their marriages have been harmed; in one sample, one-tenth said that their marriages had been helped or made more tolerable by their infidelity.

It is still true that many a "deceived" husband or wife, learning about his or her mate's infidelity,

Figure 15.4 Some of the grounds for divorce in the various states, in addition to those depicted here, are mental cruelty, pregnancy at the time of marriage, drug addiction, bigamy, and fraudulent contract. Divorce laws vary greatly from state to state.

feels humiliated, betrayed, and unloved and is filled with rage and the desire for revenge; it is still true, too, that infidelity is a cause in perhaps one-third of all divorces. But more often than not, deceived spouses never know of their mates' infidelity nor are their marriages perceptibly harmed by it. (The chance of harm, moreover, would be still smaller if the element of "deceit" were gone.)

The bulk of present-day infidelity remains hidden beneath the disguise of conventional marital behavior. But a minority of unfettered husbands and wives openly grant each other the right to outside relationships, limiting that right to certain occasions and certain kinds of involvement in order to keep the marital relationship all-important and unimpaired. A few couples, for instance, take separate vacations or allow each other one night out alone per week, it being understood that their extramarital involvements are to be confined to those times. Similar freedoms have been urged by radical marriage reformers for decades but have never really caught on, and probably never will, for one simple reason: What is out of sight is not necessarily out of mind. What husband can feel sure, despite his wife's promises, that she might not find some other man who will make her dreams come true? What wife can feel sure that her husband will not fall in love with some woman he is supposed to be having only a friendly tumble with?

COMARITAL SEX

It is another matter when husband and wife go together in search of extramarital frolic and do their thing with other people, in full view of each other, where it is visibly and safely devoid of romantic feeling. This lack of emotional involvement is the very essence of marital swinging, or, as it is sometimes called, comarital sex. Whether it consists of a quiet mate exchange between two couples, a small sociable group-sex party, or a large orgiastic rum-

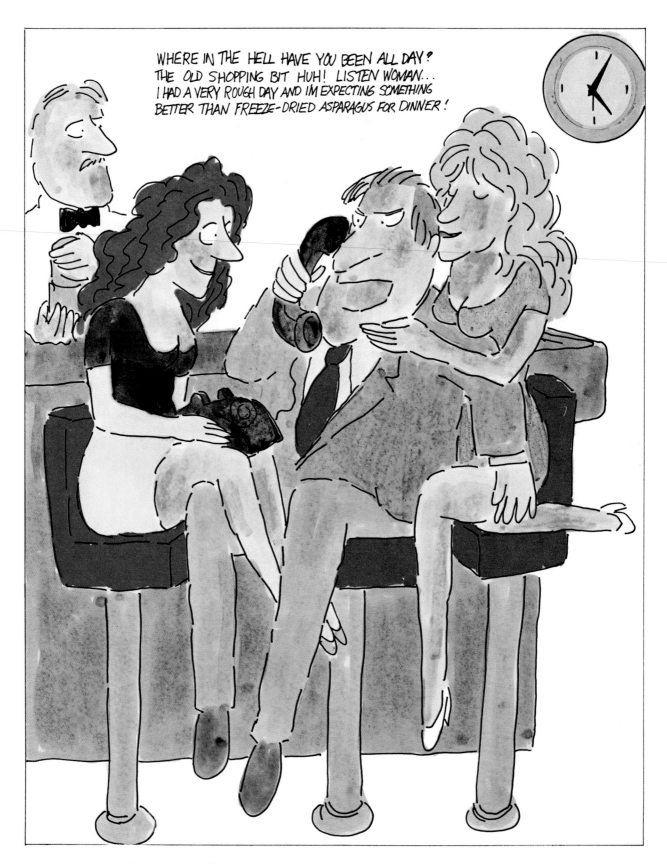

Figure 15.5   The double standard is still ever-present
in American marriages.

pus, the premise is the same: As long as the extra-marital sex is open, shared, and purely recreational, it is not considered divisive of marriage.

The very exhibitionism of marital swinging enforces its most important ground rule—the tacit understanding that participants will not indulge in emotional involvements with fellow swingers, no matter what physical acts they perform together. According to several researchers, this proves that married swingers value their marriages: They want sexual fun and stimulation but nothing that would jeopardize their marital relationships. As sociologists Duane Denfeld and Michael Gordon of the University of Connecticut write, marital swingers "favor monogamy and want to maintain it" and do their swinging "in order to support and improve their marriages."

To the outsider, this must sound very odd, not to say outlandish. How could anyone hope to preserve the warmth and intimacy of marriage by performing the most private and personal sexual acts with other people in front of his own mate or watching his mate do so with others?

Such a question implies that sex is integrally interwoven with the rest of one's feelings about the mate; swingers, however, maintain that sex can be detached and enjoyed apart from those romantic feelings, without changing them in any way. Marital swinging is supposed to involve only this one segment of the marital relationship and during only a few hours of any week or month; all else is meant to remain intact, monogamous, and conventional.

Experts maintain that some people swing out of neurotic needs; others have sexual problems in their marriages that do not arise in casual sex relationships; still others are bored and in need of new stimuli; and still others need the ego lift of many conquests. But the average swinger, whatever his or her motive, normal or pathological, is apt to believe that he loves his spouse, that he has a good marriage, and that detaching sex—and sex alone—from

marital restrictions not only will do the marriage no harm but will rid it of any aura of confinement or entrapment.

NONLEGAL MARRIAGES

There seems to be a far broader and more thorough rejection of marriage on the part of those men and women who choose to live together unwed. Informal, nonlegal unions have long been widespread among poor blacks, largely for economic reasons, but the present wave of such unions among middle-class whites has an ideological basis, for most of those who choose this arrangement consider themselves to have a more honest and vital relationship than conventional marriage.

For example, in one such arrangement, the woman shunned traditional marriage because she hated homemaking, was career oriented, and feared that if she became a legal wife, she would automatically be committed to traditional female roles and to dependency. Hence, she and her boyfriend rejected marriage and chose an arrangement without legal obligations, without a head of the household, and without a primary money earner or homemaker, though she, as it happens, does do 90 percent of the cooking. Both believe that their freedom from legal ties and their constant need to rechoose each other make for a more exciting, real, and growing relationship.

A fair number of the avant-garde and many of the young have begun to find this not only a fashionably rebellious but thoroughly congenial attitude toward marriage; in particular, couples are living together on many a college campus, often openly, risking punishment by college authorities (but finding the risk smaller every day) and bucking their parents' strenuous disapproval (but getting their glum acceptance more and more often).

When one examines the situation closely, however, it becomes clear that most of these couples live together in close, warm, committed, and monogamous fashion, much like married people: they keep house together (although often dividing their roles in untraditional ways), and neither is free to have sex with anyone else, date anyone else, or find anyone else intriguing. Anthropologists Margaret Mead and Ashley Montagu, sociologist John Gagnon, and other close observers of the youth scene feel that living together, whatever its defects, is actually an apprentice marriage and not a true rebellion against marriage at all.

Dr. Mead in fact suggested in 1966 that laws be revised so that there would be two kinds of marital status: "individual marriage," a legal but easily dissolved form for young people who are unready for parenthood or full commitment to each other but who want to live together with social acceptance; and "parental marriage," a union involving all the legal commitments and responsibilities—and difficulties of dissolution—of marriage as it is presently known. Her suggestion aroused a great deal of public debate. The middle-aged, for the most part, condemned her proposal as being an attack upon and a debasement of marriage, while the young replied that the whole idea was unnecessary. The young were right: They were already creating their own new marital folkway in the form of close, serious-but-informal unions that achieve all the goals of individual marriage except its legality and acceptance by the middle-aged. Thinking themselves rebels against marriage, they have only created a new form of marriage closely resembling the very thing Dr. Mead had suggested.

GROUP MARRIAGE

If these modifications of monogamy are not quite as alarming or as revolutionary as they seem to be, one contemporary experiment in marriage is a genuine and total break with Western tradition. This approach is group marriage—a catchall term

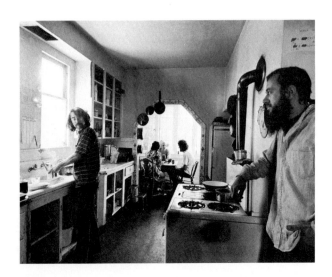

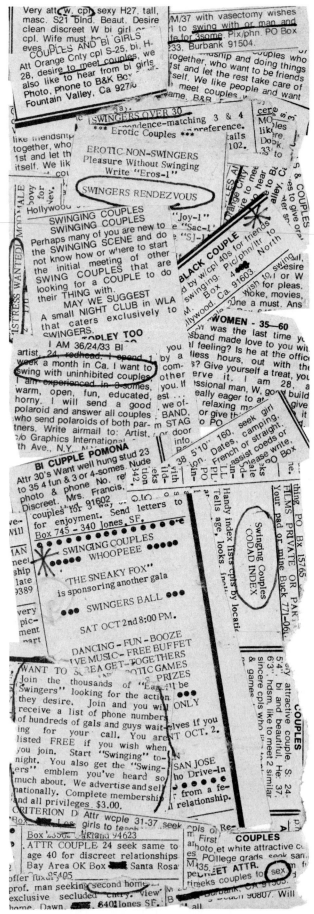

applied to a wide variety of polygamous experiments in which small groups of adult males and females, and their children, live together under one roof or in a closeknit settlement, calling themselves a family, tribe, commune, or, more grandly, intentional community and considering themselves all married to one another.

As the term intentional community indicates, these are experiments not merely in marriage but in the building of a new type of society. They are utopian minisocieties existing within, but almost wholly opposed to, the mores and values of present-day American society.

A few of these associations are located in cities and have members who appear conventional and hold regular jobs; some, both urban and rural, consist largely of dropouts, acid heads, panhandlers, and petty thieves; but most are rural communities, have hippie-looking members, and aim at a self-sufficient farming-and-handicraft way of life. A few communes are politically conservative, some are in the middle, and most are pacifist, anarchist, and/or New Leftist. Nearly all, whatever their national political bent, are islands of primitive communism in which everything is collectively owned and all members work for the common good.

Their communism extends to—or perhaps really begins with—sexual collectivism. Though some communes consist of married couples who are conventionally faithful, many are built around some kind of group sexual sharing. In some, couples are paired off but occasionally sleep with other members of the group; in others, pairing off is actively discouraged and the members drift around sexually from one partner to another—a night here, a night there, as they wish.

Group marriage has captured the imagination of many thousands of college students in the past few years through its idealistic and romantic portrayal in three novels widely read by the young—

Robert Heinlein's *Stranger in a Strange Land* and Robert Rimmer's *The Harrad Experiment* and *Proposition 31*. The underground press, too, has paid a good deal of sympathetic attention—and the establishment press a good deal of hostile attention—to communes.

All this attention sometimes gives one the feeling that group marriage is sweeping the country; but, based on even the most exaggerated figures—estimates of the number of communes vary from a few hundred to 12,000—and counting a generous average of twenty people per commune, no more than 250,000 adults—approximately one-tenth of 1 percent of the United States population—are presently involved in group marriages. And even these figures seem high.

Nevertheless, group marriage offers solutions to a number of the nagging problems and discontents of modern monogamy. Collective parenthood—every parent being partly responsible for every child in the group—not only provides a warm and enveloping atmosphere for children but removes some of the pressures from individual parents; moreover, it minimizes the disruptive effects of divorce on the child's world. Sexual sharing is an answer to boredom and solves the problem of infidelity, or seeks to, by declaring extramarital experiences acceptable and admirable. It avoids the success-status-possession syndrome of middle-class family life by turning toward simplicity, communal ownership, and communal goals.

Finally, it avoids the loneliness and confinement of monogamy by creating something comparable to what anthropologists call the extended family, a larger grouping of related people living together. (There is a difference, of course; in group marriage, the extended family is not composed of blood relatives.) Even when sexual switching is not the focus, there is a warm feeling of being affectionally connected to everyone else.

Figure 15.6   Alternatives to marriage. (*left*) A commune in Berkeley, California. (*right*) "Swinging" has become a way of life for many couples, who often join clubs or advertise in search of like-minded individuals.

There is, however, a negative side: This drastic reformulation of marriage makes for new problems, some of them more severe than the ones it has solved. Psychologist Albert Ellis has enumerated several categories of serious difficulties with group marriage, including the near impossibility of finding four or more adults who can live harmoniously and lovingly together, the stubborn intrusion of jealousy and love conflicts, and the innumerable difficulties of coordinating many lives.

Other writers, including those who have sampled communal life, also talk about the problems of leadership (most communes have few rules to start with; those that survive for any time do so by becoming almost conventional and traditional) and the difficulties in communal work sharing (there are always some members who are slovenly and lazy and others who are neat and hard-working, the latter either having to expel the former or give up and let the commune slowly die).

A more serious defect is that most group marriages, being based upon a simple semiprimitive agrarian life, reintroduce old-style patriarchalism, because such a life puts a premium on masculine muscle power and endurance and leaves the classic domestic and subservient roles to women. Even a most sympathetic observer, psychiatrist Joseph Downing, writes, "In the tribal families, while both sexes work, women are generally in a service role . . . Male dominance is held desirable by both sexes."

Most serious of all are the emotional limitations of group marriage. Its ideal is sexual freedom and universal love, but the group marriages that most nearly achieve this ideal have the least cohesiveness and the shallowest interpersonal involvements; people come and go, and there is really no marriage at all but only a continuously changing and highly unstable encounter group. The longer-lasting and more cohesive group marriages are, in fact, those in which, as Dr. Downing reports, the initial sexual spree "generally gives way to the quiet, semipermanent, monogamous relationship characteristic of many in our general society."

Not surprisingly, therefore, Dr. Ellis finds that most group marriages are unstable and last only several months to a few years; and sociologist Lewis Yablonsky, who has visited and lived in a number of communes, says that they are often idealistic but rarely successful or enduring. Over and above their specific difficulties, they are utopian—they seek to construct a new society from whole cloth. But all utopias thus far have failed; human behavior is so incredibly complex that every totally new order, no matter how well planned, generates innumerable unforeseen problems.

THE FUTURE OF MARRIAGE

All in all, then, the evidence is overwhelming that old-fashioned marriage is not dying and that nearly all of what passes for rebellion against it is a series of patchwork modifications enabling marriage to serve the needs of modern man without being unduly costly or painful.

Although this is the present situation, is it possible to extrapolate it into the future? Will marriage continue to exist in some recognizable form?

It is clear that, in the future, people are going to have an even greater need than they now do for love relationships that offer intimacy, warmth, companionship, and a reasonable degree of reliability. Such relationships need not, of course, be heterosexual. With the increasing tolerance of sexual diversity, it seems likely that many homosexual men and women will find it publicly acceptable to live together in quasimarital alliances.

The great majority of men and women, however, will continue to find heterosexual love the preferred form, for a variety of biological and psychological reasons. But need heterosexual love be embodied within marriage? If the world is already badly overpopulated and daily getting worse, why add to its burden—and if one does not intend to have children, why seek to enclose love within a legal cage? Formal promises to love are promises no one can keep, for love is not an act of will, and legal bonds have no power to keep love alive when it is dying.

Such reasoning—more cogent today than ever, due to the climate of sexual permissiveness and to the twin technical advances of the Pill and the IUD—lies behind the growth of unwed unions. From all indications, however, such unions will not replace marriage as an institution but only precede it in the life of the individual.

It seems probable that more and more young people will live together unwed for a time and then marry each other or break up and make another similar alliance, and another, until one of them turns into a formal, legal marriage. In fifty years, perhaps less, America may come close to the Scandinavian pattern, in which a great many couples live together prior to marriage. It may be, moreover, that the spread of this practice will decrease the divorce rate among the young (50 percent of teen-age marriages end in divorce), for many of the mistakes that are recognized too late and are undone in divorce court will be recognized and undone outside the legal system with less social and emotional damage than divorce involves.

If, therefore, marriage continues to be important, what form will it take? The only truly revolutionary innovation is group marriage—and, as has been seen, it poses innumerable and possibly insuperable practical and emotional difficulties. A marriage of one man and one woman involves only one interrelationship, yet everyone knows how difficult it is to find that one right fit and to keep it in working order. But add one more person, making the smallest possible group marriage, and there are three relationships (A-B, B-C, and A-C); add a fourth to make two couples and there are six relationships; add enough to make a typical group marriage of fifteen persons and there are 105 relationships involved.

This is an abstract way of saying that human beings are all very different and that finding a satisfying and workable love relationship is not easy, even for a twosome, and is impossibly difficult for aggregations of a dozen or so. It might prove less difficult, a generation hence, for children brought up in group-marriage communes. Such children would not have known the close, intense, parent-child relationships of monogamous marriage and could more easily spread their affections thinly and undemandingly among many. But this is mere conjecture, for no communal-marriage experiment in America has lasted long enough for there to be noticeable results, except the famous Oneida Community in Upstate New York; it endured from 1848 to 1879, and then died, its offspring vanishing back into the surrounding ocean of monogamy.

Those group marriages that do endure in the future will probably be dedicated to a rural and semiprimitive agrarian life style. Urban communes may last for some years but with an ever-changing membership and a lack of inner familial identity; in the city, one's work life lies outside the group, and with only emotional ties to hold the group together, any dissension or conflict will result in a turnover of membership. But although agrarian communes may have a sounder foundation, they can never become a mass movement; there is simply no way for the land to support well over 200 million people with the low-efficiency productive methods of a century or two ago.

Agrarian communes not only cannot become a mass movement in the future but will not even have much chance of surviving as islands in a sea of modern industrialism. For semiprimitive agrarianism is so marginal, so backbreaking, and so tedious a way of life that it is unlikely to hold most of its converts against the competing attractions of conventional civilization. Even Dr. Downing, for all his enthusiasm about the "Society of Awakening," as he calls the tribal family living, predicts that for the foreseeable future, only a small minority will be attracted to it and that most of them will return to more normal surroundings and relationships after a matter of weeks or months.

Thus, monogamy will prevail; on this, nearly all experts agree. But it will almost certainly continue to change in the same general direction in which it has been changing for the past few generations: namely, toward a redefinition of the special roles played by husband and wife, so as to achieve a more equal distribution of the rights, privileges, and life expectations of man and woman.

THE WOMAN'S ROLE

The marriage of today has come a long way from patriarchy toward the goal of equality. The prevalent marital style has been termed companionship marriage by a generation of sociologists; in contrast to nineteenth-century marriage, it is relatively egalitarian and intimate, husband and wife being intellectually and emotionally close, sexually compatible, and nearly equal in personal power and in the quantity and quality of the labor each contributes to the marriage.

From an absolute point of view, however, it still is contaminated by patriarchalism. Although each partner votes, most husbands (and wives) still think that men understand politics better; although each may have had similar schooling and believes both sexes to be intellectually equal, most husbands and wives still act as if men were innately better equipped to handle money, drive the car, fill out tax returns, and replace fuses. There may be something close to equality in their homemaking, but nearly always it is his career that counts, not hers.

If his company wants to move him to another city, she quits her job and looks for another in their new location; and when they want to have children, it is seldom questioned that he will continue to work while she will stay home.

In practice, then, with the advent of the first child there is a considerable shift back toward traditional role assignments: The husband stops waxing the floors and washing dishes, begins to speak with greater authority about how their money is to be spent, tells his wife (rather than consults her) when he would like to work late or take a business trip, gives (or withholds) his approval of her suggestions for parties, vacations, and child discipline. The more he takes on the airs of his father, the more she learns to connive and manipulate like her mother. Feeling trapped and discriminated against, resenting the men of the world, she thinks she makes an exception of her husband, but in the hidden recesses of her mind he is one with the others. Bearing the burden of being a man in the world, and resenting the easy life of women, he thinks he makes an exception of his wife but deep down classifies her with the rest.

These are the reasons why a great many women yearn for change; these are the problems the majority of women's liberation members are actively attacking. A handful of radicals in the movement think that the answer is the total elimination of marriage, that real freedom for women will come about only through the abolition of legal bonds to men and the establishment of governmentally operated nurseries to rid women once and for all of domestic entrapment. But most women in the movement, and nearly all those outside it, have no sympathy with antimarriage extremists; they very much want to keep marriage alive but are seeking to push toward completion the evolutionary trends that have been under way so long.

Concretely, women want their husbands to treat them as equals; they want male participation in domestic duties; they want help with child-rearing; they want day-care centers and other agencies to free them to work at least part-time while their children are small, so that they will not have to give up their careers and slide into the imprisonment of domesticity. They want an equal voice in all the decisions made in the home—including job decisions that affect married life; they want their husbands to respect them, not indulge them; they want, in short, to be treated as if they were their husbands' best friends—which, in fact, they are, or should be.

Further progress in this direction is bound to be made, if only as a continuation of the developments in marriage over the past century and a quarter. The key question is: How far can marriage evolve in this direction without making excessive demands upon both partners? Can most husbands and wives have full-time, uninterrupted careers, share all the chores and obligations of homemaking and parenthood, and still find time for the essential business of love and companionship?

From the time of the early suffragettes, there have been women with the drive and talent to be full-time doctors, lawyers, retailers, and the like and at the same time to run homes and raise children with the help of housekeepers, nannies, and thoughtful husbands. But judging from these current examples, it is unlikely that this pattern will prevail in the future, for it would take more energy, money, and good luck than the great majority of women possess and more skilled helpers than the country could possibly provide. But what if child care were more efficiently handled in state-run centers, which would make the totally egalitarian marriage much more feasible? The question then becomes: How many middle-class American women would really prefer full-time work to something less demanding that would give them more time with their children? Women's liberation leaders are largely middle-to-upper-echelon professionals, and

it is no wonder they think every wife would be better off working full-time, but the truth is that most of the world's work is dull and wearisome rather than exhilarating and inspiring.

Married women *are* working more outside the home all the time—in 1970, more than one-half of all mothers whose children were in school held jobs—but the middle-class women among them pick and choose things they like to do rather than *have* to do for a living; moreover, many work part-time until their children have grown old enough to make mothering a minor assignment. Accordingly, they make much less money than their husbands, rarely ever rise to any high positions in their fields, and, to some extent, play certain traditionally female roles within marriage. It is a compromise, and, like all compromises, it delights no one—but serves nearly everyone better than more clear-cut and idealistic solutions.

Though the growth of egalitarianism will not solve all the problems of marriage, it may help to solve the problems of a *bad* marriage. With the increasing independence of women, fewer wives will feel compelled to remain confined within unhappy or unrewarding marriages. Divorce, therefore, can be expected to continue to increase, despite the offsetting effect of extramarital liaisons. Extrapolating the rising divorce rate, it can conservatively be expected that within another generation, one-half or more of all persons who marry will be divorced at least once. But even if divorce were to become an almost universal experience, it would not be the *antithesis* of marriage but only a part of the marital experience; most people will, as always, spend their adult lives married—not continuously, in a single marriage, but segmentally, in two or more marriages. For all the dislocations and pain these divorces cause, the sum total of emotional satisfaction in the lives of the divorced and remarried may well be greater than their great-grandparents were able to achieve.

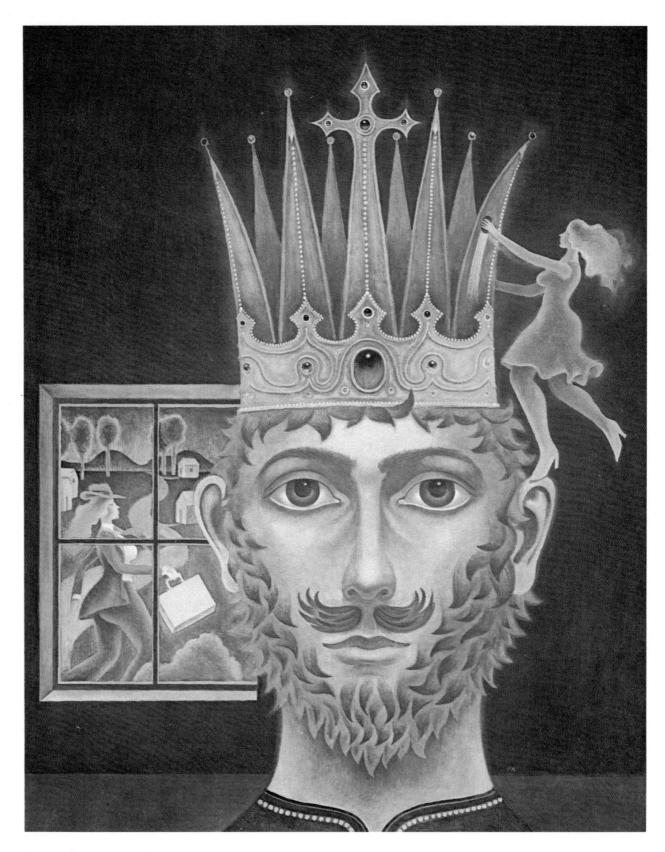

Figure 15.7   Woman's role in marriage.

Marital infidelity, because it also relieves some of the pressures and discontents of unsuccessful or boring marriages—and does so in most cases without breaking up the existing home—will remain an alternative to divorce and will probably continue to increase, all the more so as women come to share more fully the traditional male privileges. Within another generation, based on present trends, four of five husbands and two of three wives whose marriages last more than several years will have at least a few extramarital involvements.

Overt permissiveness, particularly in the form of marital swinging, though it may be more widely tried than it is now, will not predominate; most of those who test it out will do so only briefly rather than permanently adopting it as a way of life. Swinging has a number of built-in difficulties, the first and most important of which is that the avoidance of all emotional involvement—the keystone of swinging—is exceedingly hard to achieve. Jealousy is a frequent and severely disruptive problem. And not only jealously but sexual competitiveness: Men often have potency problems while being watched by other men or after seeing other men outperform them. In addition, the whole thing is truly workable only for the young and attractive.

There will be wider and freer variations in marital styles—America is a pluralistic nation, growing more tolerant of diversity all the time—but throughout all the styles of marriage in the future will run the predominant motif that has been implicit in the evolution of marriage for a century and a quarter and that will finally come to full flowering in a generation or so: the marriage of the future will be a heterosexual friendship, a free and unconstrained union of a man and a woman who are companions, partners, comrades, and sexual lovers.

There will still be a certain degree of specialization within marriage, but by and large, the daily business of living together—the talk, the meals, the going out to work and coming home again, the spending of money, the lovemaking, the caring for the children, even the indulgence or nonindulgence in outside affairs—will be governed by this fundamental relationship rather than by the lord-and-servant relationship of patriarchal marriage. Like all friendships, it will exist only as long as it is valid; it will rarely last a lifetime, yet each marriage, while it does last, will meet the needs of the men and women of the future as no earlier form of marriage could have.

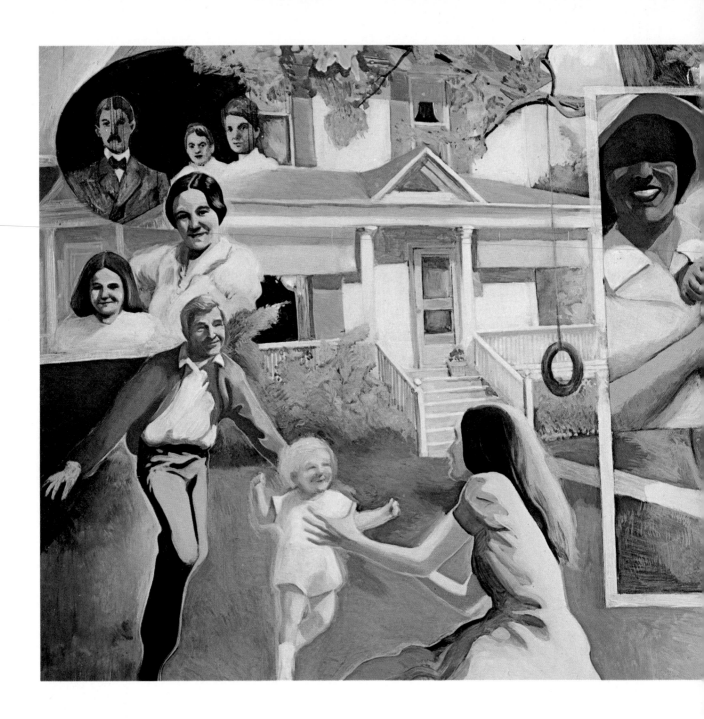

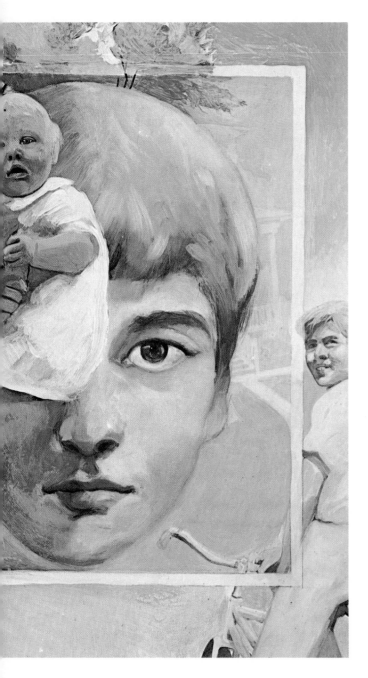

16

Although children are not essential to a marriage, parenthood is an expected part of most man-woman unions. Children can bring moments of true joy to their parents, who may feel a sense of creative accomplishment in guiding and helping a child grow into a well-functioning, mature adult. At best, though, the pleasures of child-rearing are bittersweet. Children bring difficulties, conflict, quarrels, sickness, and responsibilities, and their arrival always alters the relationship between partners. If the couple allows relations with their children to take precedence over their marriage, trouble is inevitable.

Taking such factors into consideration, many couples today are beginning to reject the parenthood role. In the past, society expected all married couples capable of having children to have them, but social expectations are changing. Cognizant of the population problem, many groups are encouraging couples to limit the size of their families or to have one child of their own but to adopt others.

The desire to be a parent is socially learned—it is not a universally sought-after role. In fact, many persons who yield to various pressures and bear children should definitely *not* be parents, simply because they do not have the time, desire, or ability to react to a child as another human being worthy of respect or to help him become a mature, fully functioning adult.

TO HAVE OR NOT TO HAVE

In the past, it was to people's economic advantage to have children—sons could become hands on the farm or apprentices in a trade; daughters could relieve some of the drudgery of the mother's house-

Parenthood

work and marry men who could provide additional help and income to the family.

Today, despite greater knowledge of birth control and availability of birth-control methods, people still have children, but the reasons are much more diverse. Studies on why people have children have uncovered many of the motives, yet the reason least mentioned by parents is a love for children. There are many *wrong* reasons for couples to decide to have children; a few of them are:

1. To try to bring stability to a shaky marriage.
2. To provide objects for exercising dominance.
3. To give the parents "immortality."
4. To substitute a love object for love missing between man and wife.
5. To maintain family traditions.
6. To "even up" the number of children of each sex in the family or to provide playmates for an only child.
7. To prove that the man is virile and that the wife is a woman.
8. To keep the wife "out of circulation."
9. To give the bored wife something to do.
10. To project part of themselves—a chance to raise a copy of themselves that will have "the things they never had" and achieve the goals they never reached.
11. To exercise the only "self-expression" left accessible in a deprived socioeconomic condition—a self-perpetuating situation.
12. To provide their parents with grandchildren.
13. To provide themselves with security in old age.

When any of these reasons is a couple's predominant (conscious or unconscious) motivation, having children will be a mistake. It is the couple primarily motivated to enjoy and respect another human being that is most likely to be successful.

Unwed Mothers

Although unwed motherhood does not carry the stigma it did in the days of Hawthorne's *The Scarlet Letter*, it still presents a number of social and psychological problems to the woman involved—and to her child. Finding herself pregnant, a woman may be pressured by social convention or other people or her own principles or whims to carry through and give birth to a child.

Unwed mothers do not fall into any one stereotyped category of social class, race, age, or personality type. Most have a love relationship or close friendship with the child's father and more than half eventually marry.

Some psychologists contend that unwed mothers are nearly always emotionally immature, frustrated, unsure of themselves, or unable to form satisfactory interpersonal relationships. These psychologists point out that such women often bear children in an effort to prove their identity and personal worth or to get the father to marry them.

No matter what motivates the unwed mother to have a child, her task as a parent is made difficult by having to be both father and mother to the child while having to support it and having to cope with negative social attitudes. If she has become a mother for neurotic reasons, she is more than likely to have ambivalent feelings toward the child, a situation that will further complicate her problems and that will have negative effects on the child's psychological development.

Effects of Children on Marriage

Children cannot help but change the structure of a marriage, sometimes for the better, sometimes for the worse. If the mother works, she must usually leave her job, at least while the child is an infant. The husband and wife come to live in two separate worlds—he, the world of his job, she, the world of diapers, vacuum cleaners, and baby food. Many husbands complain that their wives become duller, less fun once they've become housewife-mothers, while women complain that their husbands do not take enough interest in their activities and in the children.

Figure 16.1   Childbirth rates per 1,000 women (ages 15–44) since 1910. Note the drop in the rate since 1960.

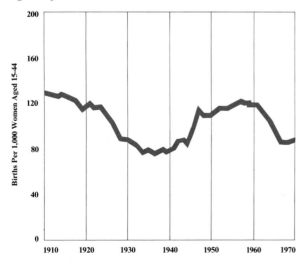

The further the husband and wife drift apart, the more tension they feel, and the more flare-ups are caused by "little" problems. The couple who can overcome these pitfalls by maintaining mutual as well as separate interests and who can share in the "drudgery" part of caring for a home and children are more likely not only to have a happier marriage but to raise happier, healthier children.

THE PARENTS' ROLE

Child psychiatrist J. Louise Despert has pointed out that this is an age of conscientious parents—mothers and fathers exert themselves with zeal for their children's sake. They attend lectures, read books, absorb magazine articles, and yet they feel even more perplexed and anxious at the tasks of parenthood. The more they read and hear about theories of child-rearing, the more confused they become, for, as was described in Chapter 4, there are many conflicting theories of child development, and most stress the crucial importance of the parental role.

As a result, a large number of parents have become overly concerned over every event in their child's life, continually asking themselves if being too strict or too permissive in a certain situation will cause a trauma that will permanently "warp" their child's personality. Some parents choose to be consistently "strict"—sheltering the child from any contact with the "bad" parts of life by limiting his activities. Others are permissive, giving the child anything he wants, giving in during all conflicts, so that the child never gets the proper guidance, never develops a good sense of right and wrong, and never learns self-control. Still other parents arbitrarily mix permissive and strict actions, often in the same situation, thus giving the child a feeling of helplessness—he never knows what response to expect from his actions.

Because a parent is the most important teacher a child will ever have, it is important for all parents

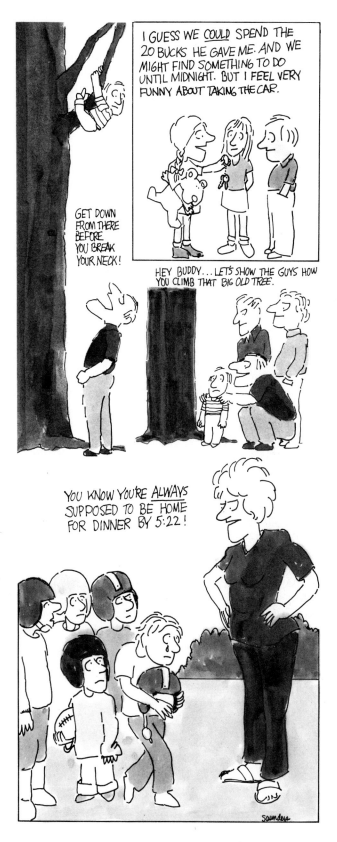

Figure 16.2 Differences in parental styles. Permissive parents run homes that are unstructured—the children are allowed to do whatever they want. Some parents are inconsistent, being strict sometimes, permissive other times, even in similar situations. Strict parents establish thousands of ironclad rules, weighing the child down.

to consider their various roles in the child's life and to understand themselves and what the child means to them. Perhaps the most difficult part of being a parent is in recognizing the child as a distinct and separate entity. The child must be thought of as a separate human being with individual thoughts and needs at every stage.

Role in Emotional Development

Several theories of child development were outlined in Chapter 4. They suggested that children pass through various stages on the road to adulthood and that the way a parent reacts to a particular stage has a great deal to do with how successful the child will be in coping with events at that stage.

Whatever theory they tend to favor, psychologists have determined that the first five years are most important for emotional development. The family is the child's emotional school, where his needs are either satisfied or denied. The infant has physical needs (food, clothing, shelter, protection) and sociocultural needs (learning of communication, social control, basic skills, awareness of self in relation to others). Most important perhaps is his need for love, for if denied this response by his parents or parent substitutes, he will be handicapped in his emotional development.

Children strive for a uniqueness of personality. They want to be "special" and they want their parents to treat them differently from other siblings, and they do not want to be forced into roles that are inconsistent with their self-image (boys reject "sissy" things, for example). Nevertheless, children are also conformists in wanting "what the other kids have."

As sociologist Clifford Kirkpatrick has indicated, children can be thought of as organisms striving for control of environment, for freedom, and for self-realization. Parents can either help or hinder these natural tendencies. One way in which a par-

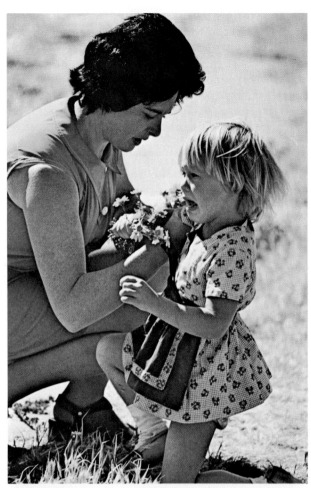

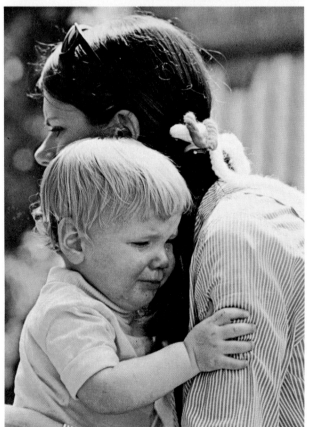

Figure 16.3   A primary function of parenthood is to satisfy the child's emotional needs and to give emotional support.

ent hinders the child's strivings is to exploit the child for the parent's own purposes, such as dominating the child for pleasure in the authoritarian role or making excessive demands for satisfaction of parental pride. Parents also can interfere in the child's development by imposing their own personal prejudices with no explanation but "mother knows best." But parents can *help* their child's natural development by leading, guiding, and providing models for healthy ways of dealing with emotions.

Role in Social Development

Parents usually do not deliberately set out to indoctrinate their children with the sorts of attitudes toward the world that the parents would like the children to have; yet, for all practical purposes, indoctrination is precisely what does take place in most families. Most adults cannot recall having their fathers and mothers tell them to which political party they ought to belong, but social scientists know from hundreds of studies that almost everyone votes the way his parents do. How does this type of indoctrination take place? Part of attitude learning takes place through imitation.

A child tends to emulate or imitate those adults who occupy large chunks of his awareness. Parents are important for several reasons. First, and perhaps foremost, they are important because they loom so large in a child's world, because they are the adults with whom the child has greatest contact. But it also is true that parents are important because they have the power to reward and punish a child's responses; they exhibit or withhold love and warmth in response to the child's first independent actions. Although much attitude learning occurs at the overt level ("Big boys don't cry"; "Little girls don't say things like that"), much of it is covert and hidden. Parents tend to show interest in (and hence reward) their children when they echo the parents' attitudes; on the other hand, parents tend to be dis-

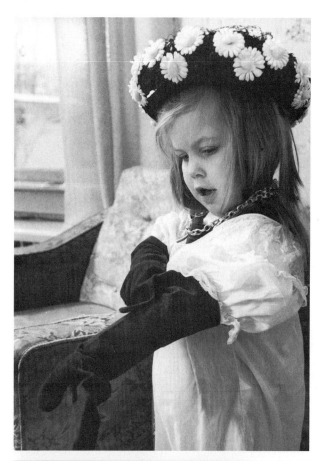

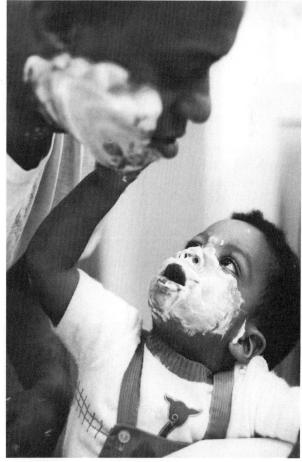

Figure 16.4 The parents serve as sex-role models for their children.

interested, bored, or even hostile when the child expresses some opinion that the parents do not share. The parents are not likely to see this type of response on their part as being a definite program by which they are inculcating their own values, but the result is the same as if it were planned.

Parents also "indoctrinate" their children, partly unconsciously, in their proper sex roles. Before the child even learns there are two sexes, parents begin helping their children to acquire the proper sex preference and to learn the associated behaviors, attitudes, and feelings that fit each role. These sex roles are, of course, inevitably interwoven with the status society attaches to each role. In general, the male role (with its freedom, authority, and power) is preferred by both sexes while they are growing up. Because sexual behavior is patterned after adult performance, the model provided for the child to study is exceptionally important, as is the quality and stability of the relationship between husband and wife. The wife-husband relationship is always the first model a child perceives, hence this relationship establishes his response to sex.

Socioeconomic or class-related behavior is another way in which parents, often unwittingly, act as models for their children to imitate or reject. Children whose parents went to college are most likely also to go to college. Parents who could not escape a life of poverty may pass on a resigned, despondent, or rebellious approach to life, or generate in the child an antisocial set of values.

Role in Intellectual Development

As with emotional development, the crucial period in the child's intellectual development is the first five years. Benjamin S. Bloom, a psychologist from the University of Chicago, believes that about half of a person's intellectual capacity has developed by the time he is four, about three-fourths by the time he is eight, and the remainder by age seventeen. What is missed in the preschool years may be diffi-

cult to make up in later years, as has been suggested in studies of children in deprived areas who usually receive no intellectual stimulation until entering school at age six or later. Many middle- and upper-class parents also may have actually hindered their children's intellectual development by following the advice of child psychologists who recommend that children be kept away from learning materials until they are old enough for school and that children be encouraged to spend all their time playing.

Psychologists have finally realized that not only *should* preschoolers learn, but in infancy they actually *love* to learn—they do not need to be conditioned to do so. They have found that children have an innate drive for curiosity and a need for competence. As mentioned in Chapter 4, Robert White has theorized that the drive for competence and mastery is essential to the individual's development, because the child must learn to function in the world and to take care of himself. This theory fits in quite well with Jean Piaget's idea that the more stimulation the child is given, the more he will be able to cope with new stimuli as he grows older, thus contributing further to his sense of competence and his self-esteem.

Many experimenters have supported the idea that children will learn for the pleasure of learning—that is, to satisfy the needs of their curiosity. They need no other reward. It is when they are forced to learn and are threatened with punishment for failure that learning becomes a chore.

The best home environment for intellectual development is one in which parents are warm and loving, take time to explain their actions, let the children participate in decisions, try to answer questions, and are concerned with their child's development of competence. In such homes, researchers have found, children experienced an average IQ increase of about eight points over a three-year period. In homes where parents are

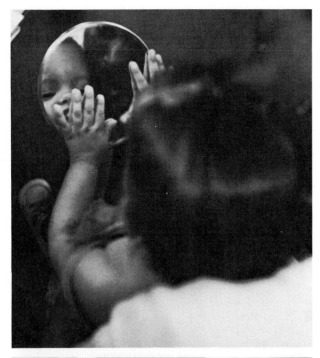

neglectful, hostile, or restrictive toward children, IQ actually decreased over this time.

Writer Joan Beck, who has done considerable research in this area, has made a few general suggestions as to how parents can promote intellectual development, particularly in the preschooler:

1. It helps for the parent to explain the whys behind the rules he sets up and decisions he enforces on his child. These explanations can serve as a teaching device so the child can learn to evaluate alternatives.
2. Even a two-year-old can be given more opportunities to make choices in his life: Does he want to wear the red shirt or the green shirt? Would he rather have peas or carrots? Does he want to do a puzzle or hear a story?
3. The parent should emphasize what the child has done right, rather than scolding him for what he does wrong. Many a youngster has had his ability to learn stifled because he spends his energy worrying, trying to keep out of trouble, and avoiding mistakes.
4. The parent should encourage the child to try—failure is not a crime. If the child does fail, the parent should try to make him understand what went wrong and how it could be prevented.
5. The parent can serve as the child's teacher by example, by creating a stimulating environment, by talking to the child, by listening to him seriously, by introducing him to interesting things, by taking advantage of everyday happenings and transforming them into learning experiences.

The role of early learning in all of a person's later life is coming to be seen as more and more important. In this area, as in the area of emotional development, the parent can either do a significant disservice to his child or provide him with a foundation for which he can always be thankful.

PARENT-CHILD INTERACTION

The ultimate goal of the parent should be to help his children to become self-regulating, mature individuals. A real child cannot be separated into segments and labeled the emotionally developing

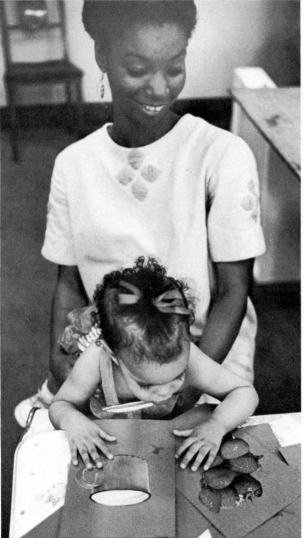

Figure 16.5   Intellectual stimulation in infancy. In this study, culturally deprived infants are engaged in activities designed to enhance their cognitive and intellectual functioning.

child, the socially developing child, and the intellectually developing child. He must be treated as a whole individual, in which all these aspects are interacting, conflicting, growing. In addition to the child's development, the parent must also take into account his *own* needs and interests—he cannot spend all his time following the child around, nor would that be desirable.

Discipline

In trying to take both his and the child's interests into account, the parent must develop a few rules to govern his relationship with his children; such rules generally fall under the heading of discipline. Dr. Fitzhugh Dodson, a child psychologist, has come up with the following methods of discipline, all designed to help the child develop self-regulation while at the same time minimizing parent-child conflict:

1. Parents should control the child's environment to minimize the need for discipline, especially with young children. For example, a mother who tries to handle a toddler or preschooler in a house that is full of things he must not touch and that has little in the way of play equipment geared to his level will probably have to contend with needless discipline problems.

2. Parents should give a child freedom to explore his environment and to assume the degree of self-regulation suitable to his stage of development so that he builds a positive self-concept. As soon as the child can feed or dress himself or turn on his own bath water, he should be allowed to do so. It is certainly faster to do these things for a small child than to let him do them, but it is much more beneficial if he does them himself.

3. It is important for parents to make the distinction between feelings and actions—a child can learn to control his actions; he cannot learn to control his feelings. He cannot help being angry sometimes, but he can refrain from hitting or kicking—he can learn to control his actions in response to that anger. To be psychologically healthy, children should learn that feelings are rational and may be expressed in actions that do not bring dire consequences.

4. It is important for parents to set firm limits to the actions of their child, so that he knows what he is permitted and not permitted to do. These limits

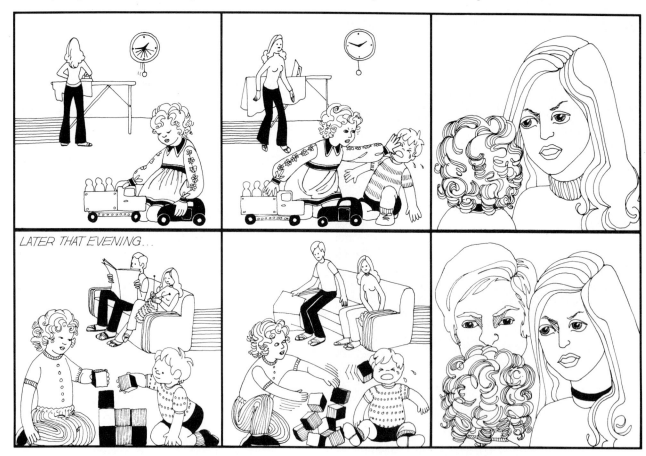

Figure 16.6   Parents often reinforce bad behavior in their children by ignoring them (not rewarding them) when they are good and by punishing them (giving them attention) when they are bad.

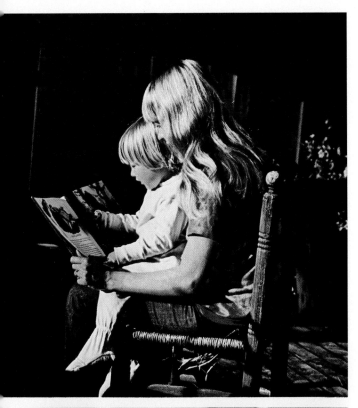

should be reasonable, consistent, and suited to the child's stage of development. In addition, parents should be able to justify these limits to themselves and explain them to their children.

5. Children's feelings not only need to be talked about; they must be understood and sympathized with. When children are afraid, helpless, angry, or hurt, they want their parents to understand. A parent may make a superficial show of understanding by simply saying, "I know just how you feel," but that will not necessarily convince a child. A better way for the parent to show the child he understands is to put the child's feelings into his own words and reflect them back to the child as in a mirror.

No-Lose Method

It is inevitable that conflicts will arise between parent and child. Often parents resolve conflict so that someone wins and someone loses. If the parent wins, he pays a high price for victory: The child has little or no motivation to carry out the solution, because he had no voice in making the decision. If he cannot get out of it, he goes through the motions, barely doing what is required and nothing more. In addition, this method of resolving conflict causes the child to resent the parent and offers no opportunity for the child to gain self-discipline.

If the child wins, on the other hand, he will never acquire inner controls on his impulses. He will therefore become self-centered, demanding, and often unmanageable. Such children frequently have great difficulties with their peers: they are so accustomed to getting their way with their parents that they assume they should get their way in other situations as well. These children also have difficulties in adjusting to school rules and regulations.

In the "no-lose" method of resolving conflict, when a parent and child encounter a conflict situation, the parent asks the child to join him in a joint search for some solution *acceptable to both*. Both

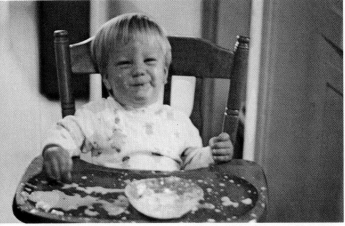

Figure 16.7 (*top*) A child's parent is his first and most important teacher.

Figure 16.8 (*bottom*) A child should be allowed to try to do things for himself, even when he has not completely mastered the task.

child and parent offer possible solutions to the problem and then evaluate the proposed solutions. Eventually they decide on a final solution acceptable to both, so neither party "loses." An example of this sort of solution is illustrated in Figure 16.10.

The "no-lose" method of resolving conflicts has several psychological advantages for both parents and children. The child is motivated to carry out the solution because he has participated in the decision-making process and because the decision has not been imposed upon him by his parents. The technique also should improve family harmony, for when both parent and child can agree on a solution, resentment and hostility typically do not arise. Another advantage of this method is that it helps to develop the child's thinking processes. Because it is a problem-solving process, the "no-lose" method often gets beyond the superficial problem to the real problem that underlies it. Thus the chances for a genuine solution are greatly increased.

Adolescence

Adolescence, particularly, is a potential period of explosive conflict between parent and child. In adolescence more than ever a child needs parents who know who they are, what they stand for, and what their values are, not only to serve as examples to emulate or reject but to represent stability in a world that has suddenly become complex and full of choices for the adolescent. He encounters major conflicts—his aspirations versus doubts of being able to achieve them, his longing for independence versus his need for dependence, his exaggerated image of his parents versus the realization that they are humans who can make mistakes. The adolescent's life is further complicated by increased sexual needs, his interest in the other sex, and his need to establish new intimacies outside the family.

The goal of the parent during this time should be to strengthen and confirm the child in his development without making him feel dependent.

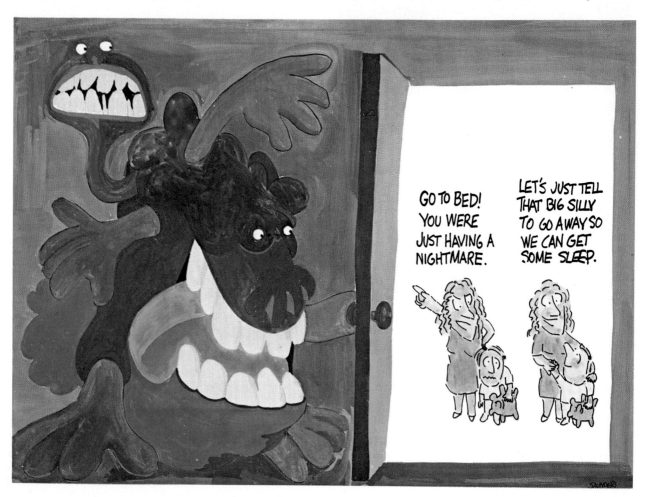

Figure 16.9 The reflection of feelings technique. The parent tries to understand the child's fears and problems and to let the child know he understands.

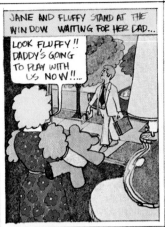

JANE AND FLUFFY STAND AT THE WINDOW WAITING FOR HER DAD...

LOOK FLUFFY!! DADDY'S GOING TO PLAY WITH US NOW!!...

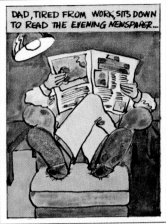

DAD, TIRED FROM WORK, SITS DOWN TO READ THE EVENING NEWSPAPER...

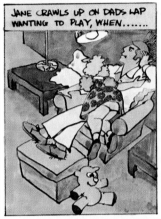

JANE CRAWLS UP ON DADS LAP WANTING TO PLAY, WHEN.......

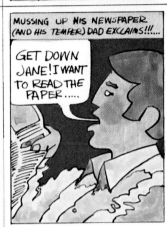

MUSSING UP HIS NEWSPAPER (AND HIS TEMPER) DAD EXCLAIMS!!!...

GET DOWN JANE! I WANT TO READ THE PAPER.....

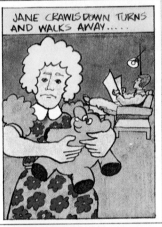

JANE CRAWLS DOWN TURNS AND WALKS AWAY.....

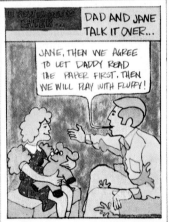

A FEW MINUTES LATER... DAD AND JANE TALK IT OVER...

JANE, THEN WE AGREE TO LET DADDY READ THE PAPER FIRST, THEN WE WILL PLAY WITH FLUFFY!

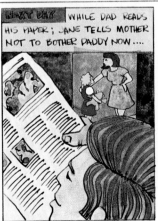

NEXT DAY WHILE DAD READS HIS PAPER; JANE TELLS MOTHER NOT TO BOTHER DADDY NOW.....

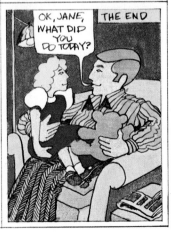

OK, JANE, WHAT DID YOU DO TODAY? THE END

Parents who either attempt to retain total control or totally abdicate involvement may actually retard the adolescent's growth.

Adolescence is, of all the later stages of development, the one that can most readily permit profound and benign transformations of personality. A challenging, responsive, and confirming environment can enable an adolescent to undo vast damage done in earlier childhood, to heal the wounds from parental inconsistency, ignorance, or neglect, and to move beyond these handicaps to a responsible and satisfying maturity. Adolescence can provide a second chance—the opportunity to move away from the malignancies of family pathology, social disorganization, and cultural deprivation in order to pursue the goals of becoming independent, self-directing, tolerant, humane, and ethical.

SOCIAL-CLASS DIFFERENCES

The values, child-rearing methods, and life styles of families in the various classes differ, as do their religious affiliations, the number of children the mother bears, the financial security of the family, the schools the child attends, and the associates he encounters. What adults consider desirable, probable, and possible in life determine the qualities that are instilled in their children. Certain qualities of children are emphasized in particular social classes and others in different social classes. For example, lower-class parents generally value overt conformity to the prescriptions and proscriptions of society, while middle-class parents stress the development of self-direction in children. These lessons are often taught casually and with little pressure in the middle classes but intensely and under close guard in lower classes.

Middle-class parents tend to stress independent action and personal responsibility well before adolescence, and they are likely to give reasons why they want the child to do something and why they punish him. Lower-class parents, on the other

Figure 16.10 The no-lose method of parent-child interaction. Jean wanted her Daddy to play with her immediately after he arrived home from work every night. Daddy, however, generally felt tired from driving the crowded freeways after work and needed relaxation. Jean would frequently climb on his lap, muss the paper, and persistently interrupt him with coaxing and begging. He was dissatisfied with disappointing the child if he refused to play, but he felt resentful if he gave in. He stated the conflict to Jean and suggested they try to find a solution agreeable to both. In just a few minutes they agreed on a solution: Daddy promised to play with Jean provided she waited until he had finished reading the paper. They both kept to their agreement, and later Jean told her mother, "Now don't you interrupt Daddy during his rest period." (After Gordon, 1970.)

hand, begin independence training later and are less likely to provide an explicit rationale for rules they enforce. Lower-class parents tend to value obedience and are inclined to obtain it through coercion—physical punishment is used much more in the lower class than in other social strata.

But although there are general patterns of child-rearing on these different social levels, there are wide variations within each level. A lower-class parent may well provide stimulation and begin independence training at an early age; and there are plenty of middle-class parents who exercise coercive control over children they won't allow to grow up. Class does not define what kind of a parent one will be—it merely provides a background against which children are raised and, therefore, exerts an influence on what a person expects parenthood to be like.

Nevertheless, there are groups of people who may find it impossible to provide for even the basic physical needs of their children, much less for emotional, social, or intellectual needs. Economic disadvantage is one such situation, ranging from the extreme poverty of some American families to the daily uncertainty of many others. Social disadvantage is another. In a society like America where racial discrimination—imposed on more than 20 million citizens—has been as rigid a principle of segregation as caste or class discriminations are in other societies, one must face up to the existence of parents who never have the opportunity or the freedom to provide appropriate care for their children—and of children suffering the consequences.

Insufficient nourishment, inadequate physical environment, the time and energy erosion of parents trapped in poverty or segregated in a ghetto, the frequent absence of one or the other parent, and indifferent or prejudiced teachers who discourage any spark of intellectual ambition may be more crippling to the developing child than a severe disease would be to an adult.

The disadvantage of so many in one society cannot help but be damaging to all the others as well. Individual parents must do the best they can to help their children's development, but there are great limitations to what disadvantaged parents can accomplish, given their social context. It is a critical part of every parent's responsibility to play an effective and constructive role in minimizing those restrictive social conditions both for his own family and for the families of others.

A CHANGING SOCIETY

Physical, emotional, and social development are so interrelated that it is tempting to always treat them together. This approach may be appropriate in a slowly evolving social framework in which the parents' world is mirrored in the world of their children when they grow up, but it is no longer accurate when the social context in which their children will live is quite different from the one in which they were brought up.

The separation of social development from the physical and emotional can be pertinent to many situations. A child raised in a rural subculture, for example, will have to undergo a different type of social development when he moves to an urban environment. Similarly, a child growing up in a deprived situation—of poverty, racial segregation,

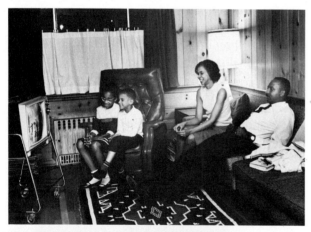

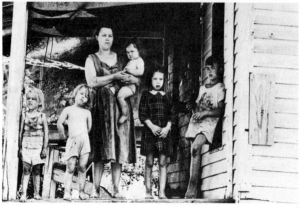

Figure 16.11   Social-class differences in child-rearing. Middle-class parents tend to be more strict but they give reasons for their rules. Lower-class parents tend to run their homes more loosely but are more physical in their disciplining if the children break any of the few rules they do make.

WANTED:

A Dr. Spock for Black Mothers

by
Joanne Dann

The middle-class white mother consults her pediatrician, a Bank Street-trained nursery school teacher, or a child psychologist when her child throws tantrums. She consults Spock when her child wets his bed. And she rushes to a psychiatrist when she finds traces of marijuana in her teen-ager's desk drawer.

The urban black mother has few of these resources, and she isn't sure she would use them if she could.

"I put my faith in me," a twenty-five-year-old mother of four said. "I'm all there is to put it in."

"Dr. Spock? He's for rich kids. How can he help my children? He doesn't know my child," said another.

The middle-class white mother tends to accept norms and generalizations about child-rearing, but not the black mother. "Nobody knows my child as well as I do," is a frequent refrain. In their eyes, the generalizations that they reject fit white kids, not their kids growing up in crowded city blocks.

Sensitive, caring deeply about her children, the black mother looks to her family, not to outsiders, for the advice every mother needs—on feeding a newborn, temper tantrums, toilet training, discipline, loneliness. She consults her own mother, grandmother, aunt, or sister when she's in doubt.

Dr. James Comer, a black psychiatrist and associate professor at the Yale Child Study Center, praises the black mother's independent approach. "White mothers," he says, "tend to go too much by the book. Plain common sense is important."

He praises, too, the independence of the black youngster who fixes his own breakfast, stays home alone after school until his mother gets home from work, knows how to take care of himself. This, Dr. Comer maintains, is preferable to the middle-class white situation where overprotection can crush independence.

But the large black family whose emotional support helped nourish this independence has almost disappeared, especially in the cities. Black mobility and the working grandmother have transformed it into a nuclear family of parents and child—very often just one parent, the mother, and several children. This leaves the mother, and the low-income mother in particular, stranded. She has no one and no place—or knows of none—to turn for advice.

Little written material on child-rearing is available to or directed toward the black mother. The New York City Baby Book, distributed at health stations, was prepared for the low-income mother. It's a laudable attempt, but its heavy blocks of type tend to discourage women who may not have finished high school. There's a gap, too, in books for the educated parent.

At this stage in black history, it may be that what is needed is a black Dr. Spock. Many black behavioral scientists are convinced that black parents face child-rearing problems different from those of white parents.

The black middle class, for instance, differs from its white counterpart in that it believes in strict discipline. Spanking and scolding are taken more for granted.

"We don't tolerate sassiness or horsing around," one mother told me.

"You never see a black child having a tantrum in a supermarket the way a white child does," said another. "If he has a tantrum at home, I hit him."

Dr. Comer sees nothing wrong with firmness. "There must be a proper balance of course, but in too many white families, parents share their kids' rebellion. There's no reason to play out anti-authority feelings through your own children."

He worries about the black parent who tries too hard to train his child to conform. The chief concern of the intellectual black mother—or father—today, says Dr. Comer, is how much acceptance of the black-white situation to teach young children.

"There are still parents who teach conformity and acceptance. But there are many more who don't," Dr. Comer reports. "You must help a child develop ways to survive, but you mustn't hurt his sense of self."

He told me an anecdote of his own childhood. "I'd gotten a scolding for clowning in class. When my mother heard about it, she was angry. I said Mary and Johnny had done it, too. My mother's answer was, 'Mary and Johnny are white. They can get away with it. Besides—if they jumped out of the window, would you?' "

Today, it's not enough to say that Mary and Johnny are white and can get away with it. "The black parent," says Dr. Comer, "must add, 'That's not the way it should be.' You must not allow a child's sense of self to be damaged."

Some mothers still discipline, often harshly, to protect their children from what they see as a hostile world. Dr. Leonette Vanderhost, a consulting psychologist to Haryou-Act Headstart, explains that this stems from long experience that the placid black child was safe in a white world and the self-assertive one in danger.

These protective controls extend into late adolescence. One mother recently complained that she had trouble getting her nineteen-year-old son home by nine o'clock each night. She imposed this curfew because the police in her neighborhood interrogate boys out on the streets at night. The fact that white mothers relinquish this kind of control by the mid-teens was news to her.

Dr. Comer advised the mother to talk to her son in terms of consequences. "You have to get it across," he said, "that the boy is in real danger of being arrested as a suspect or getting a police record. The parent must point out that this is unfair. And then the boy must be allowed to make his own decision."

The trick, he says, is to help the black youngster establish internal controls and still be self-assertive without jeopardizing his long-range goals. "It's difficult in this society," he adds, "where what a black kid does in third grade can be held against him for life."

Fatherless homes also concern black psychiatrists and psychologists. But, according to Dr. Vanderhost, a more sophisticated awareness of the importance of men as role models is developing. "Mothers have become very sensitive about how their lovers or friends treat their children," she says. When several generations of a family still live together, uncles or brothers-in-law can provide a masculine model for a boy to pattern himself after if his father is no longer living at home.

But if the father has gotten into trouble and has deserted the family, the mother is often overly concerned lest her son follow his father's pattern. She must be counseled to provide her son with a healthy picture of manhood through her own relationships with and attitude toward men, says Dr. Comer. "She shouldn't crush his masculinity by criticizing all men."

Dr. Comer worries about the overwhelmed mother, the mother of six, for instance, with no husband, no steady job. She gives her children independence enough, but not the right kind. This kind of freedom creates "little men and women on the sur-

face, who are still children underneath."

He told of a fourteen-year-old girl whose mother had, in effect, abdicated her role. The teen-ager was responsible for feeding the younger children. She had to stay home from school when one of them was sick or if her mother was away. So much responsibility at too early an age forced the girl into erratic behavior. She would go out on nightclub dates with older men on weekends. Other times she would just curl up on her bed sucking her thumb.

Her mother had to be told that despite her daughter's bravado and capabilities, she was really anxious and afraid, Dr. Comer said, and needed more mothering.

This kind of advice is not available to the majority of black mothers. Sometimes, just because the black mother has always been so independent, it is too late when she realizes she needs help. One mother who had had no place to turn for advice when her obstreperous son was young ended up by taking him to Children's Court in an effort to stop his chronic truancy. Another woman put her daughter in a detention home "to find herself," because she could not control her.

As a rule it's the schools that reach parents. They call them in to discuss truancy or bad behavior or learning problems. But they rarely offer parents a chance to discuss the "normal" developmental problems all children have.

There are exceptions. A guidance counselor who works in low-income communities on Long Island has experimented with holding discussion groups on such subjects as why children disobey, how to prevent failure, how to encourage youngsters to assume responsibility. She found that the black mothers who attended were "almost too trusting. They have a great willingness to change and learn," she reports.

But too often, the black mother is afraid to reach out lest she be "rejected or condescended to," says one black psychologist. "For all her independence, she worries whether she'll be criticized for the way she is raising her child."

This is a problem she never faced when supported by yesterday's large family. "So much had to do with survival," says one black researcher, "that how other people thought children should be brought up didn't matter. Just hunger, shelter, health."

While the urban white mother usually does not lack for help or advice, the urban black mother may have only the clinic. This is usually unsatisfactory, at least as a source of child-guidance information. ("Have you ever waited all day in a clinic holding a cranky baby?")

And today, more and more black mothers wonder if the advice dispensed by a white doctor really applies to them and their children. One woman had several sessions with a white psychiatrist when her husband was committed to a mental hospital. "I felt the

psychiatrist, being white, wasn't aware of black needs," she said. "He told me I would marry again. I know there aren't that many black men around who are going to take care of me and my children."

The day-care and preschool movements may turn out to be the way to reach both black parent and child. Dr. Comer is cautiously optimistic about this, but he warns, "If government sees day care merely as a way to get mothers into jobs and off welfare, neither parents nor children will be aided."

Under the Haryou-Act Family Day Care plan (where "provider" mothers take children into their homes so "career" mothers can work) group discussion of child-development problems is part of the program. Early childhood education specialist, Mrs. Evelyn Silverman, has led such groups for nearly a year.

At a recent meeting a mother told of her difficulty in leaving her crying five-year-old that morning: "I told him he was going to school and I was going to work. But when he kept crying, I told him to shut up. Then I lied to him. I said I'd pick him up at lunchtime."

Mothers often feel guilty when they go to work, Mrs. Silverman responded. She suggested the mother "just once" bring her child to see where she worked. It might reassure him.

She urges mothers to let their children experiment. A two-year-old should have the opportunity to feed himself. Many mothers pointed out they didn't have time. "Give him a chance to be on his own, to be independent," Mrs. Silverman repeated. Bedwetting, discipline, and school problems are the biggest worries. "Mothers have become more concerned and aware now," she says.

If children skip a day at school, Headstart mothers are visited at home by community workers. Many of these mothers are so isolated in the loneliness of the cities that they cannot even give the name of someone to turn to in case of emergency. If problems are complex, they are referred to a psychologist. Perhaps once a year mothers ask for a group discussion on common problems.

Yet Headstart and some 150 publicly supported day-care centers reach only a relative handful of parents and children. What about the rest?

Half-sheepishly Dr. Comer wonders if television may prove to be the black Dr. Spock. He suggests the same skillful approach used on "Sesame Street" for children might be used for parents.

In finding ways to help mothers help their children, the greatest resource in the long run will be the tremendous strength and resilience of the black mother. Society must make sure, however, that this basic strength isn't tested beyond endurance. Dr. Comer puts it simply: "People shouldn't have to climb Pike's Peak every day just to get by."

or social isolation—will have to reorient himself if he is to ever counteract the "depriving" conditions. In both these situations, individual values and vocational models are different in the new and the old contexts, and a time of adjustment is necessary. The same holds true when a rapidly evolving society challenges the old traditional values, and in so doing creates disaffection between generations.

This is a time of transition, and America is a society of accelerating change. The values and models to which yesterday's adult was geared may not hold for the world in which tomorrow's adults will live. This is where the "*no-lose*" method expands to acquire the value of a general principle applicable to all interhuman problems. Solutions, not only to conflict situations but to unclear ones as well, can be sought together by child and parent,

student and teacher, young and old, black and white. A no-lose approach will reduce confrontation and disaffection but, more important still, will bring together different values, different perspectives, and different talents toward the solution of common problems. Until everyone learns to interact in this way, parents will continue to produce winners and losers, with the negative features of both and the unresolved frustration of all.

WHAT MAKES A GOOD PARENT?

A few things can be said about what constitutes a good parent. Basically, he is one who respects the child as a separate, unique human being and who also provides for the psychological and biological needs of the child. He is honest in his interaction with his child and admits to his mistakes. He is

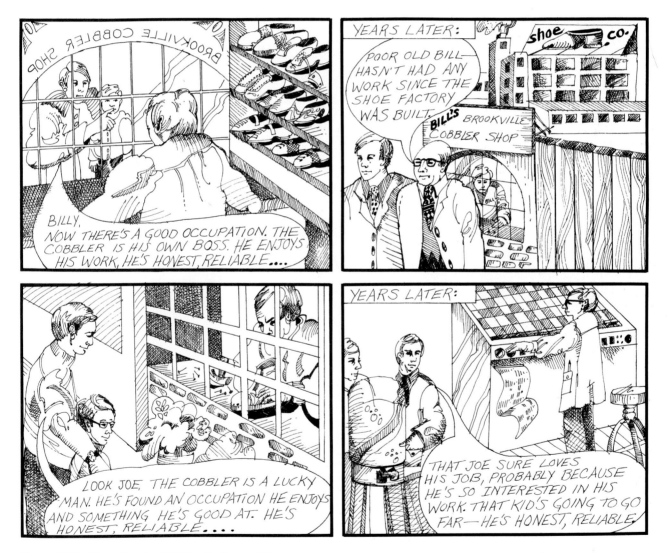

Figure 16.12 Preparing the child for the future. The parent should emphasize concepts rather than concretes so that the child will be able to cope in a variety of situations.

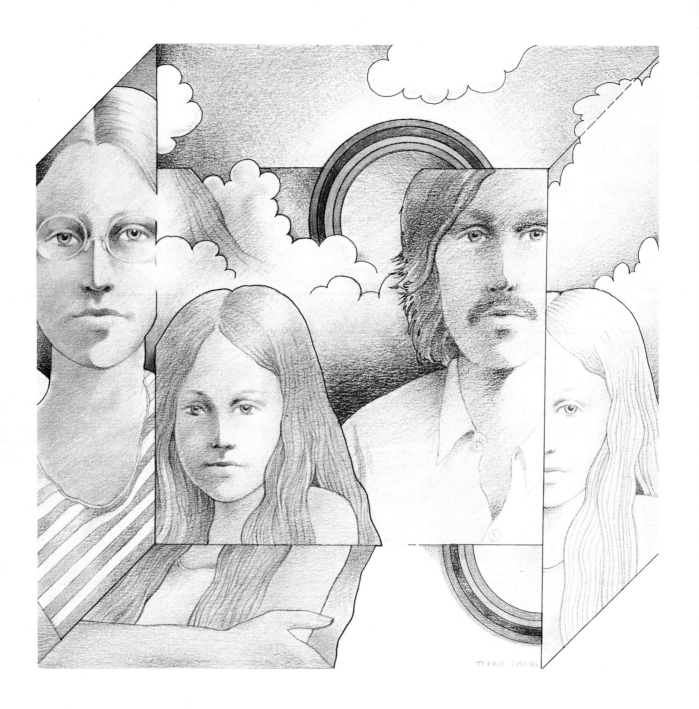

careful in choosing the few essential rules he sets for his child and is consistent in enforcing them. And he provides the child with emotional security, sympathy, and understanding.

These are simply guidelines for the adult once he has become a parent. Perhaps even more critical is the evaluation of needs and goals that a couple hopes to satisfy by deciding to have children. A child need never be a "mistake." There are adequate birth-control methods to allow each individual to decide whether parenthood is a part of his requirement for a full and satisfying life. Once parenthood is decided upon, the responsibilities accompanying it must be accepted. Whether a child is one's own or adopted is of little importance in the role of parenthood; more and more couples are having one child and adopting others. When the goals of parenthood are defined, and the couple mature enough to make a decision to become parents, the experience can be a rewarding one.

Parenthood may seem at times to be an awesome responsibility and, in a sense, it is, but it is also an unparalleled opportunity to express one's humaneness, to be fulfilled, and to contribute constructively to the world. Although study and understanding of the rudiments of child development and parenthood are undoubtedly helpful, the day-to-day business of being a good parent involves rather relaxed living and family relationships. Even the best parents make mistakes, but children are actually quite resilient. No child is ruined by occasional parental mistakes, rather the quality of parent-child relationships over the long haul is most responsible for successful child-rearing.

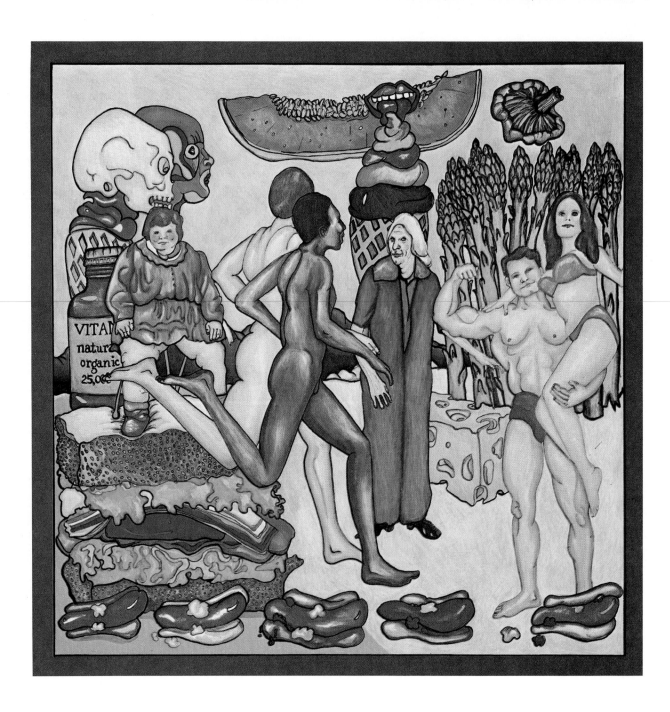

V PERSONAL HEALTH CARE

In many respects, the health of individuals and groups results from forces of culture and environment over which they have little control. Whether one is nurtured in a warm and loving family or a cold and aloof one, whether or not he grows up in the midst of polluted air, whether he is tempted by drugs in a neighborhood saturated with drug abuse or in a community offering better alternatives, these and countless other influences determine to a large extent who he will be and what opportunities for health he will have. ¶ Despite the influences that limit alternatives, however, the basis of choices leading to optimum health is, obviously, education —knowing the facts. Man does make himself. In making "right choices" about what he eats, the amount and kind of physical activity he will do, the amount of rest he gets, and the way in which he takes care of the external parts of his body, he both facilitates his own survival and frees himself from unnecessary disability and suffering. ¶ Personal health care is an area open to quackery, old wives' tales, advertising boasts, and advice from friends, family, and pseudoexperts. Can people have naturally "soft" teeth? Are "organic" foods better for people than processed foods? Will bowling every night keep one physically fit? Do contact lenses really help people or are they only good for cosmetic purposes? Do mouthwashes really destroy bad breath? Do dreams happen only in a split second before awakening? Can rock music harm hearing? Will eating red beets cure anemia? Does vitamin C cure the common cold? These are the kinds of questions people ask about their health every day. The purpose of the chapters in this unit is to provide some of the knowledge for evaluating the statements and claims made daily about nutrition, physical fitness, and care of eyes, ears, teeth, skin, and hair.

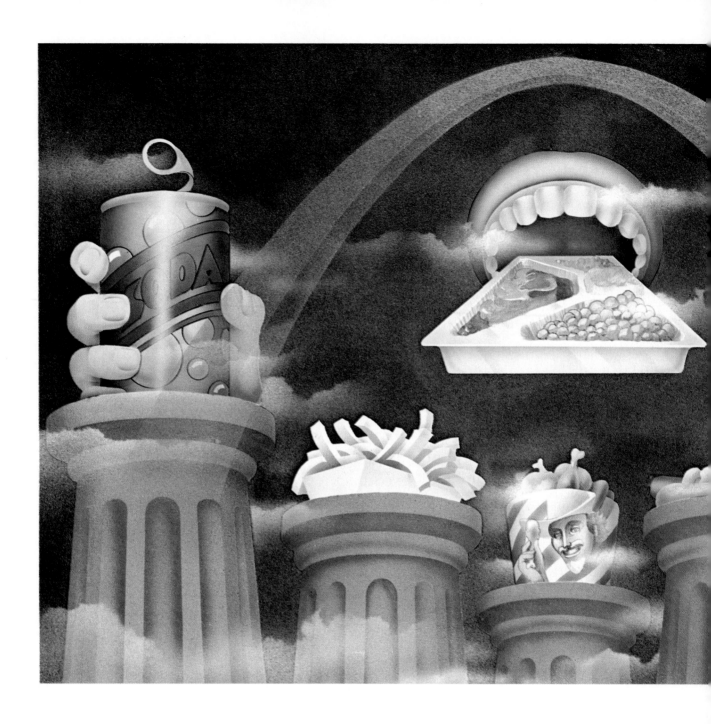

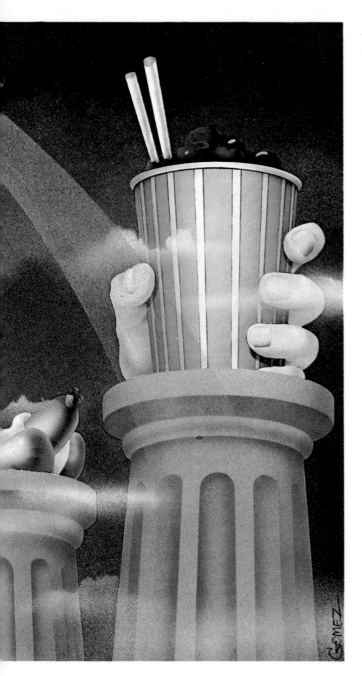

17

The bulging bellies of starving children have appeared on the front pages of newspapers with increasing frequency in the past few years. One can recall the agonizing reports of the thousands of people—men, women, and children—who starved to death during the Biafran war, or the pictures more recently of thousands upon thousands of people in Pakistan who are dying from the lack of food.

Starvation is the illness caused by extreme malnutrition. Nutrition, the relation of the health of an organism to its food requirements, has become an increasingly important subject as people become more and more aware of the dangers of overpopulation.

All living things—humans, animals, plants, even cells—have certain well-defined nutritional requirements. Although nutritional requirements vary from species to species—in fact, from individual to individual—a number of different chemical substances are needed in varying proportions by all organisms. They are usually divided into five main categories, according to their chemical or functional properties: carbohydrates, fats, amino acids (protein), vitamins, and minerals. Some of these substances, or *nutrients*, must be received from outside because the organism is unable to manufacture them (*essential* nutrients); others can be produced by the body provided adequate source material is taken in.

NUTRITION AND SOCIETY

Problems occur for an organism when the delicate metabolic balance is upset by an excess or deficien-

Nutrition

cy of one or more nutrients. The starving millions of the world suffer and die prematurely because their diets do not provide adequate amounts or the right kind of protein, lack carbohydrates, or are deficient in essential vitamins or minerals. Even in a well-developed country such as the United States, where hunger and starvation are not a major problem, deficiencies are not uncommon. A common form of malnutrition in Western countries is the overconsumption of food, which can create such serious health problems as obesity and heart disease and contribute to the development of certain forms of diabetes.

Using current analytical techniques, it is relatively easy to calculate the approximate amounts and proportions of fats, carbohydrates, proteins, vitamins, and minerals that should go into the "ideal" diet. Most people, however, do not read nutritional charts, nor do they know how to define nutritional requirements in terms of actual food consumed. They tend to eat what and when they like or can afford to, whether or not the meal has the right nutrients. In the United States, for instance, many students dash off to classes after a breakfast of coffee and toast or with no breakfast at all, then settle for a lunch of hamburger and french fries, snacking along the way on candy bars or soft drinks. This kind of diet can provide enough calories to give one energy to get through the day, but it is otherwise inadequate. It does not have a balance of the nutrients needed to nourish all of the body's systems. Because such diets can contribute to weight gain, they frequently are coupled with crash diets that make additional inroads into the individual's nutritional reserves. Thus poor nutrition also can exist in the midst of plenty. In contrast, in the poor areas of the United States, such as Appalachia, parts of the South, and the ghetto communities of the large cities, many people cannot afford to purchase the food necessary for a balanced diet, even if they know what such a diet is.

Figure 17.1 A nutritional calorie is the amount of heat required to raise the temperature of one kilogram of water one degree centigrade.

In many countries, eating habits are dictated by tradition, crop availability, and economics more often that on the basis of nutritional need. Cultural, social, and religious factors also affect what people eat, sometimes to the detriment of nutritional values. Although limited amounts of protein supplements are now being produced to meet the needs of protein-deficient population groups, food experts find that the exchange of old food traditions for good nutrition is not an easy step. Any food supplement must be incorporated by the people as a natural choice, otherwise it remains an experimental prop.

Thousands of myths, taboos, and fallacies stand in the way of good nutrition. The Zulus of South Africa believe that a pregnant woman has an evil influence on cows, so they forbid her to consume milk during the period when she needs it most. In many areas of India, the cow is sacred and cannot be slaughtered, even though it is an excellent source of needed protein.

Religion also influences eating habits; Orthodox Jews will eat meat that comes only from cud-chewing divided-hoof quadrupeds that must be drained of blood. Seventh-Day Adventists will not eat any meat. Some philosophical attitudes toward life in general entail unusual attitudes toward food: ascetes find a taste for good food somehow demeaning, while hedonists revel in it.

COMPONENTS OF NUTRITION

The energy supplied by food, good or bad, is measured as *calories*. Caloric content, or value, of a given food is the number of calories produced by a specified amount of it when it is eaten and "burned" by the combination of all metabolic processes in the body. Because the same number of calories are released when that food is burned outside the body under standard conditions, the caloric content of different kinds of food can be precisely measured (see Figure 17.1).

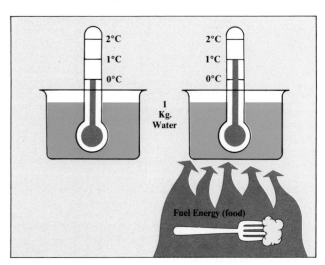

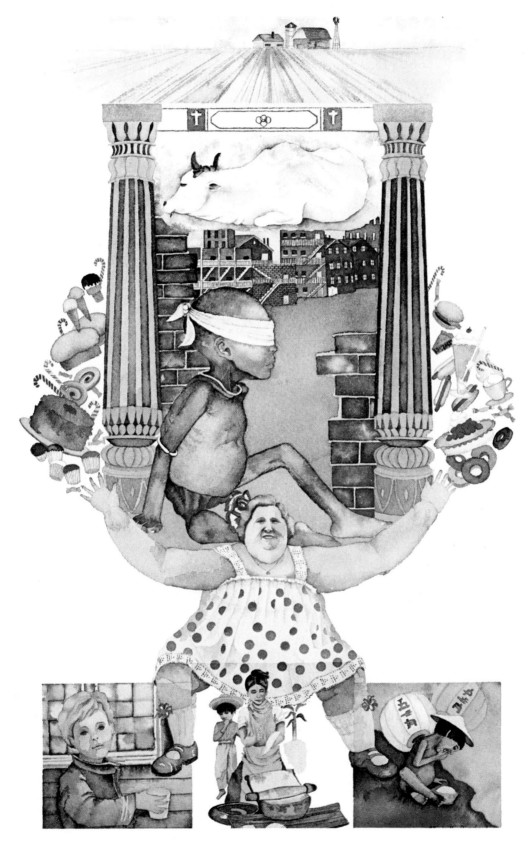

Figure 17.2   Factors related to defective nutrition. Poor nutrition can result from unavailability of necessary dietary elements, prohibitive costs of nutritional foods, lack of knowledge of good and bad foods and daily requirements, poor eating habits, tradition or religious and political beliefs that confine one to specific foods, or some combination of these factors.

Humans differ widely in their caloric requirements, depending on size, age, sex, occupation, and so on. The average middle-aged male needs about 2,600 calories a day, a woman needs about 1,900, and a twelve-to-fifteen-year-old girl or boy will require from 2,500 to 3,000, respectively. Because many more calories are required by physically active persons, however, a football player might burn as much as 3,500 to 4,500 calories a day during football season, and a long-distance runner may require more than 5,000 calories.

If an individual takes in more calories than he burns (as too many American adults do), the extra calories are converted to fat, and the person gains weight. However, if one does not take in enough calories to sustain his daily activities, his body begins to convert its own tissue into the calories it needs, and he loses weight. Reducing diets based on this principle, unless carefully balanced, often are accompanied by a lack of necessary vitamins and other essential nutrients. Such a calorie-deprived condition may result in severe malnutrition. More prevalent as the result of food unavailability, this disease is common among young children in many of the poor nations of Asia, Africa, and Latin America and is then known as *marasmus*.

Carbohydrates

Carbohydrates have a number of nutritional functions. They are involved in the composition of many important cell constituents (nucleic acids, glycoproteins, glycolipids, and so on) and can be used as substitutes (raw materials) for the biological synthesis of other types of nutrients (fats, amino acids).

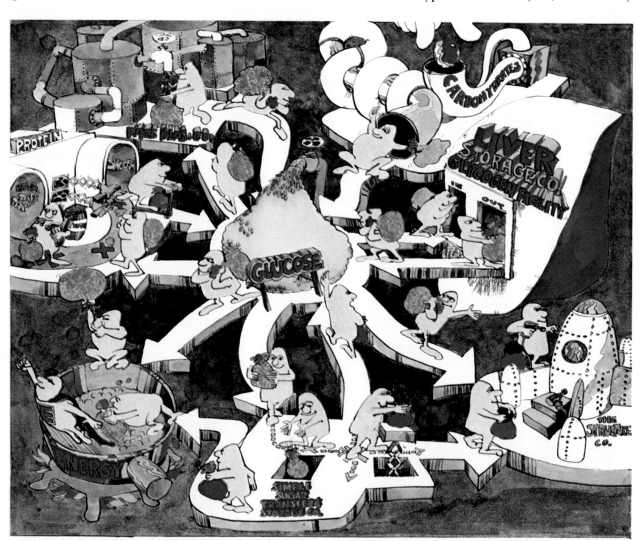

Figure 17.3   Utilization of carbohydrates by the body. Carbohydrates are broken down into glucose, which can be used directly as energy or as a building component in cells or can be converted into fats, amino acids, simple sugars, or glycogen, all of which can be reconverted to glucose if necessary.

They also are the major source of animal energy and the general chemical "currency" for transfer of energy from plants to animals. Carbohydrates contain four calories per gram. *Sugars* and *starches* are the major food sources of carbohydrates for man (cellulose is another source for many animals) and are quickly converted by the body to *glucose*, which can then be used as energy or converted into fat for future use. Glucose also may be stored in the liver as *glycogen*; the rapid release of glucose from glycogen stores helps to maintain the normal blood-sugar level and provides an instant energy resource.

Some of the most familiar sugars besides glucose are *fructose*, found naturally and predominantly in fruit; *sucrose* (table sugar) from sugar cane, sugar beets, and some fruits; *lactose* from milk; and *maltose* from malt. Starches are found in all plants, especially in the cereal grains, such as corn, rice, wheat, and oats, and in potatoes.

Fats

Fats contain even more calories than the carbohydrates—nine calories per gram. Theoretically, an individual could survive without any fats at all, because the body can make most of the fats it needs from carbohydrates. However, some fats, such as *linoleic acid*, cannot be made by the body and must be taken in with the diet if an individual is to be adequately nourished. It is now known, for instance, that a deficiency of linoleic acid can lead to skin disorders. It also may lead to the accumulation of abnormal amounts of cholesterol in the arteries.

Fats are mixtures of substances called *triglycerides*, which are composed of glycerol and fatty acids. The *saturated* fats are found primarily in meat, butterfat, and coconut oil and are solid at room temperature. *Unsaturated* fats (like, for example, linoleic acid) are most abundant in those fats or oils that are liquid at room temperature, such as the common vegetable oils, olive oil, and oils found in

fish and poultry. A saturated fat contains all of the hydrogen atoms that it can chemically accommodate, whereas an unsaturated fatty-acid molecule has bonds that are not filled with hydrogen (see Figure 17.4). Some unsaturated vegetable oils used in cooking have been chemically "hydrogenated" to the solid saturated form. As will be discussed in greater detail later in this chapter, it is now strongly suspected that an excess of saturated fats in the diet may be related to higher risks of some common kinds of heart disease.

Triglycerides are but one category of what are called *lipids*. Other important lipid categories—which the body can itself build from adequate substances—are the *phospholipids* (phosphate-containing lipids), the *glycolipids* (carbohydrate-containing lipids), and the *steroids* such as cholesterol (with an entirely different chemical structure but sharing certain properties with the other lipids), some liposoluble vitamins, and some hormones.

Proteins

Proteins are necessary structural and functional components of every living cell, tissue, organ, and organism. The oxygen-carrying activity of blood cells is based on hemoglobin, a protein; muscles contract through the involvement of two proteins, actin and myosin; and all disease-fighting antibodies are proteins, as are all enzymes, without which life could not exist. Proteins also are used as energy sources, with a caloric content similar to that of carbohydrates (four calories per gram).

All proteins are made up of long chains of small building blocks known as *amino acids*. Digestive enzymes break down other proteins in food into amino-acid fragments, which are absorbed in the bloodstream and distributed throughout the body. They are then chemically recombined into blood protein, muscle protein, eye protein, enzymes, hemoglobin, and so on.

Figure 17.4 The chemical structure of fats. Saturated fats are composed of fatty-acid chains with the maximum of hydrogen atoms. Unsaturated fats have less than the maximum hydrogen atoms, while polyunsaturated fats have the least. Polyunsaturated fats that are hydrogenated to make them solid (as in many margarines) have the maximum hydrogen atoms, as with saturated fats.

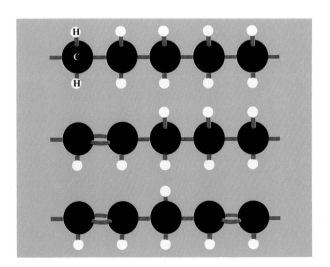

Of the twenty-odd amino acids found in foods, eight cannot be made by the adult human body and must be supplied in the diet. These eight *essential* amino acids, found to greater or lesser extent in different types of food, are: leucine, isoleucine, valine, lysine, methionine, phenylalanine, threonine, and tryptophan. Two others, arginine and histidine, also may be nutritionally necessary, particularly during development.

The best sources of all the essential amino acids are animal proteins, such as those present in meat, eggs, milk, and other dairy products. Vegetable products, which form the bulk of the diet in many underdeveloped nations, are usually low in one or more essential amino acids, although mixtures of vegetables can provide a good "balance" if chosen with care. For instance, corn contains only small amounts of lysine and tryptophan. Many other vegetables contain enough tryptophan and lysine, but lack methionine.

Nutritionists recommend that a normal adult male receive about sixty-five grams of protein a day from a variety of sources. These recommendations can be met more easily in nations where it is still possible to use lands for feeding animals to produce foodstuffs.

In most underdeveloped areas, cereal protein from corn, wheat, tapioca, or rice is the chief dietary staple. Cereals contain about 10 percent protein, but they are low in some essential amino acids found in meat, milk, eggs, or fish. If a child does not eat enough protein, he can develop a disease called *kwashiorkor*. Kwashiorkor is a Ghanaian word that is said to mean "first after second"; it is derived from the custom in Ghana of stopping breast feeding at too early an age because of the greater needs of a younger child. Once the child is deprived of the protein provided by his mother's milk, he is forced to live on a protein-low diet of gruel because he has no teeth for chewing meat. The symptoms of kwashiorkor quickly become obvious—his muscle mass wastes away (even though the weight loss may be masked by water accumulation); he becomes weak; he may have discolored hair, become extremely irritable, and show intestinal and liver damage; and his mental development may be permanently impaired. In areas where kwashiorkor is prevalent the death rate of children may be up to fifteen times greater than normal.

The problem of protein maldistribution is compounded by the world's population increase. Research scientists are attempting to reduce the protein deficit by supplementing cereal-based diets with beans, lentils, or less conventional food sources rich in vegetable protein. Some experts favor greater exploitation of the great protein resources of the sea—fish and algae. Although these research efforts have already led to the development of fish-protein concentrates—flourlike products that are designed to be mixed with other dietary staples—economic considerations often limit the use of these products where they are most needed. For example, although Peru has one of the largest fish-meal-producing industries in the world, rather than feeding its people it sells most of its fish meal to the richer nations, who use it as a feed for farm animals.

Another possible source of protein for the future is "single-cell protein" that is rich in essential amino acids and that can be produced by feeding bacteria any number of exotic diets, including petroleum and natural gas. The protein is then extracted from the bacteria and used to supplement cereals or other low-protein foods. In Central America a milk substitute called Incaparina, made of corn, sorghum, cottonseed flour, and small amounts of yeast and calcium salts, has been developed to treat and prevent kwashiorkor.

Vitamins

Unlike fats, carbohydrates, and proteins, vitamins are able to carry out their extremely important

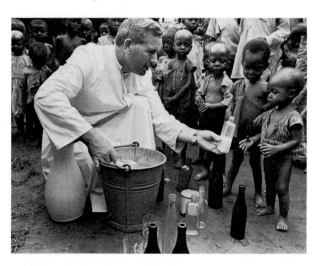

Figure 17.5   Milk is handed out to starving Biafran children, many of them suffering from the protein-deficiency disease kwashiorkor.

Table 17.1　Water-Soluble Vitamins

VITAMIN	Deficiency Syndrome		Physiological Role	Food Source	Recommended Daily Allowance*
	Disease	*Symptoms*			
C (ascorbic acid)	Scurvy	Rough, scaly skin; anemia; gum eruptions; pain in extremities; retarded healing	Collagen formation and maintenance; protects against infection	Citrus fruits, tomatoes, cabbage, broccoli, potatoes, peppers	Men:　60 Women: 55
B_1 (thiamin)	Beriberi	Numbness in toes and feet, tingling of legs; muscular weakness; cardiac abnormalities	Changes glucose into energy or fat; helps prevent nervous irritability; necessary for good appetite	Whole-grain or enriched cereals, liver, yeast, nuts, legumes, wheat germ	Men:　1.4 Women: 1.0
B_2 (riboflavin)	Ariboflavinosis	Cracking of the mouth corners; sore skin; bloodshot eyes; sensitivity to light	Transports hydrogen; is essential in the metabolism of carbohydrates, fats, and proteins; helps keep skin in healthy condition	Liver, green leafy vegetables, milk, cheese, eggs, fish, whole-grain or enriched cereals	Men:　1.6 Women: 1.5
niacin	Pellagra	Diarrhea; skin rash; mental disorders	Hydrogen transport; important to maintenance of all body tissues; energy production	Yeast, liver, wheat germ, kidneys, eggs, fish; can be synthesized from the essential amino acid tryptophan	Men:　18 Women: 13
B_6 (pyridoxine)	—	Greasy scaliness around eyes, nose, and mouth; mental depression	Essential to amino-acid and carbohydrate metabolism	Yeast, wheat bran and germ, liver, kidneys, meat, whole grains, fish, vegetables	Men:　2.0 Women: 2.0
Pantothenic acid	—	Enlargement of adrenal glands; personality changes; low blood sugar; nausea; headaches; muscle cramps	Functions in the breakdown and synthesis of carbohydrates, fats, and proteins; necessary for synthesis of some of the adrenal hormones	Liver, kidney, milk, yeast, wheat germ, whole grain cereals and breads, green vegetables	Not known
Folacin (folic acid)	—	Anemia yielding immature red blood cells; smooth, red tongue; diarrhea	Necessary for the production of RNA and DNA and normal red blood cells	Liver, nuts, green vegetables, orange juice	Men:　.04 Women: .04
B_{12} (Cyanocobalamin)	Pernicious anemia	Drop in number of red blood cells; irritability; drowsiness and depression	Necessary for production of red blood cells and normal growth	Meat, liver, eggs, milk	Men:　5.0 micrograms Women: 5.0 micrograms
Biotin	—	Scaliness of skin; pain in muscles; sensitivity to light; can possibly lead to eczema	Important in carbohydrate metabolism and fatty-acid synthesis; probably essential for biosynthesis of folic acid	Same as other B vitamins	Not known
Choline	—	None observed and identified in man	Synthesis of protein and hormones of adrenal gland; important in maintenance of normal nerve-impulse transmission	Brains, liver, yeast, wheat germ, egg yolk	Not known

*Values are given for men and women ages 18 to 22 (in milligrams unless otherwise indicated).
Source: Values are taken from *Recommended Dietary Allowances*. 7th ed. Washington, D.C.: National Academy of Sciences Publication 1694, 1968.

nutritional role in very small concentrations. More than ninety years ago scientists discovered that when rats were fed on a supposedly adequate diet of highly purified carbohydrates, fats, proteins, and minerals, they soon died. Their experiments suggested that some essential components of an adequate diet must have been missing. It was not until 1911, however, that Casimir Funk, a Polish biochemist, was able to concentrate a substance from unpolished rice that prevented beriberi. He called the substance (which was thiamin) a "vitamine" (amine of life). Since then, researchers have identified, purified, synthesized, and determined the role of a great number of chemically unrelated substances that are loosely grouped together as vitamins.

Vitamins do not usually act alone in the body but are part of enzyme systems. Other dietary components, such as minerals, may be essential parts of such enzyme systems. Vitamins are usually divided into two groups, depending on whether they dissolve in water or fat. Vitamins A, D, E, and K are fat soluble, while the remaining vitamins, including C and the large array of B-complex vitamins, are water soluble. The role each vitamin plays in the body and various vitamin deficiencies are shown in Tables 17.1 and 17.2.

Minerals

Long before nutrition reached its present level of sophistication, people who visited health resorts and spas convinced themselves that drinking "mineral waters" of the area was good for them. And in many countries, mineral waters are still consumed as avidly as soft drinks or ordinary water. Modern-day nutritionists know that the early mineral-water drinkers were theoretically correct and that certain minerals are as essential to the diet and and to good health as fats, carbohydrates, proteins, and vitamins. In many cases, the mineral elements act in conjunction with other dietary components, including the vitamins—a deficiency in one can prevent the other from being used. The minerals required by the human body, their function, and what foods provide them are given in Table 17.3.

THE WELL-BALANCED DIET

Each individual's nutritional needs are shaped by many variables, including his size, sex, age, and activities. In addition, in some instances his hereditary background may have provided him with a deficiency or surplus of enzymes, hormones, or other biological substances that prevent him from using the same nutrients in exactly the same way

Table 17.2   Fat-Soluble Vitamins

VITAMIN	Deficiency	Excess	Physiological Role	Food Source	Recommended Daily Allowance (international units)
A	Night blindness; growth decrease; eye secretions cease	Swelling of feet and ankles; weight loss; lassitude; eye hemorrhages	Maintenance of epithelial tissue; strengthens tooth enamel and favors utilization of calcium and phosphorus in bone formation	Milk and other dairy products, green vegetables, carrots, animal liver; carotene in vegetables is converted to Vitamin A in the body	Men: 5,000 Women: 5,000
D	Rickets: a softening of the bones causing bow legs or other bone deformities	Thirst, nausea, vomiting; loss of weight; calcium deposits in kidney or heart	Promotes absorption and utilization of calcium and phosphorus; essential for normal bone and tooth development	Fish oils, beef, butter, eggs, milk; produced in the skin upon exposure to ultraviolet rays in sunlight	Men: 400 Women: 400
E	Increased red cell destruction	—	May relate to oxidation and longevity, as well as a protection against red blood cell destruction	Widely distributed in foods: yellow vegetables, vegetable oils, and wheat germ	Men: 30 Women: 25
K	Poor blood clotting (hemorrhage)	Jaundice in infants	Shortens blood-clotting time	Spinach, eggs, liver, cabbage, tomatoes; produced by intestinal bacteria	Not known

Source: Values are taken from *Recommended Dietary Allowances.* 7th ed. Washington, D.C.: National Academy of Sciences Publication 1694, 1968.

Table 13.3   Minerals*

MINERAL	*Primary Function in Man*	*Food Source*	*Daily Requirement*
Calcium (Ca)	Building material of bones and teeth; regulation of body functions: heart muscle contraction, blood clotting	Dairy products, leafy vegetables, apricots	Men: .8 grams Women: .8 grams
Phosphorus (P)	Combines with calcium to give rigidity to bones and teeth; essential in cell metabolism; serves as a buffer to maintain proper acid-base balance of blood	Peas, beans, milk, liver, meat, cottage cheese, broccoli, whole grains	Men: .8 grams Women: .8 grams
Iron (Fe)	Component of the red blood cell's oxygen and carbon dioxide transport system; enzyme constituent necessary for cellular respiration	Liver, meat, shellfish, lentils, peanuts, parsley, dried fruits, eggs	Men: 10 mg. Women: 18 mg.
Iodine (I)	Essential component of the thyroid hormone, thyroxin, which controls the rate of cell oxidation	Iodized salt, seafood	Men: 140 mcg. Women: 100 mcg.
Sodium (Na)	Regulates the fluid and acid-base balance in the body	Table salt, dried apricots, beans, beets, brown sugar, raisins, spinach, yeast	Men: 10–15 grams Women: 10–15 grams
Chloride (Cl)	Associated with sodium and its functions; a component of the gastric juice hydrochloric acid; the chloride ion also functions in the starch splitting system of saliva	Same as sodium	Men: 10–15 grams Women: 10–15 grams
Potassium (K)	Component of the system that controls the acid-base and liquid balances; is probably an important enzyme-activator in the use of amino acids	Readily available in most foods	
Magnesium (Mg)	Enzyme-activator related to carbohydrate metabolism	Readily available in most foods	Men: 400 mg. Women: 350 mg.
Sulfur (S)	Component of the hormone insulin and the sulfur amino acids; builds hair, nails, skin	Nuts, dried fruits, barley and oatmeal, beans, cheese, eggs, lentils, brown sugar	?
Manganese (Mn)	Enzyme activator for systems related to carbohydrate, protein, and fat metabolism	Wheat germ, nuts, bran, green leafy vegetables, cereal grains, meat	?
Copper (Cu)	The function of copper has not been fully resolved although it is known to function in the synthesis of the red blood cell and the oxidation system of the body	Kidney, liver, beans, Brazil nuts, wholemeal flour, lentils, parsley	?
Zinc (Z)	The function is unknown although it is a component of many enzyme systems and is an essential component of the pancreatic hormone insulin	Shellfish, meat, milk, eggs	?
Cobalt (Co)	A component of the vitamin B_{12} molecule	Vitamin B_{12}	?
Fluorine (F)	Essential to normal tooth and bone development and maintenance; excesses are undesirable	Drinking water in some areas	1 part per million in drinking water

*Several trace minerals—chromium, silenium, nickel, molybdinum, vanodium, and tin—are now known to be required in very small amounts by experimental animals (studies have not been done on man). Their distribution in food varies considerably, depending in part on the composition of the soil in which plants are raised.

Source: Values are taken from *Recommended Dietary Allowances*. 7th ed. Washington, D.C.: National Academy of Sciences Publication 1694, 1968.

that someone else does. For instance, a diabetic cannot metabolize sugar properly, and other individuals may be genetically predisposed to be obese. In addition, the definition of a well-balanced diet tends to change as scientists learn more about the fundamentals of nutrition.

Nevertheless, within limitations, it is safe to say that the average American should be eating a proper balance of four different food groups: milk, and milk products; meat, eggs, beans, and protein sources; vegetables and fruits; and breads and cereals. Meals of convenience foods selected from these food groups in the right proportions will contain all the carbohydrates, fats, proteins, vitamins, and minerals needed daily.

WEIGHT CONTROL

When a person increases his caloric intake beyond his body's capacity to utilize those calories, he stores the nutrients in the form of fat as reserve against a future need. However, the maintenance of weight by diet is a complex subject because psychological and other factors play an important role in human weight control.

Every person has an ideal weight that is based upon his height, sex, and bone structure (see Table 17.4). The term "overweight" is used when an individual exceeds his ideal weight by up to 20 percent. If the individual is more than 20 percent over his ideal weight, he is categorized as being "obese." The distinction is a subtle one—an athlete may be overweight because of an excess of muscle, but an obese individual is overweight because of the excess fat his body has retained.

Obesity

More adults than children are obese; however, socioeconomic, sex, and occupational factors are far more important variables than age. It is impor-

Table 17.4 Desirable Weights for Men and Women*

GROUP	Height (with shoes on)	Small Frame	Medium Frame	Large Frame
Men (1-inch heels)	5' 2"	112–120	118–129	126–141
	5' 3"	115–123	121–133	129–144
	5' 4"	118–126	124–136	132–148
	5' 5"	121–129	127–139	135–152
	5' 6"	124–133	130–143	138–156
	5' 7"	128–137	134–147	142–161
	5' 8"	132–141	138–152	147–166
	5' 9"	136–145	142–156	151–170
	5' 10"	140–150	146–160	155–174
	5' 11"	144–154	150–165	159–179
	6' 0"	148–158	154–170	164–184
	6' 1"	152–162	158–175	168–189
	6' 2"	156–167	162–180	173–194
	6' 3"	160–171	167–185	178–199
	6' 4"	164–175	172–190	182–204
Women† (2-inch heels)	4' 10"	92–98	96–107	104–119
	4' 11"	94–101	98–110	106–122
	5' 0"	96–104	101–113	109–125
	5' 1"	99–107	104–116	112–128
	5' 2"	102–110	107–119	115–131
	5' 3"	105–113	110–122	118–134
	5' 4"	108–116	113–116	121–138
	5' 5"	111–119	116–130	125–142
	5' 6"	114–123	120–135	129–146
	5' 7"	118–127	124–139	133–150
	5' 8"	122–131	128–143	137–154
	5' 9"	126–135	132–147	141–158
	5' 10"	130–140	136–151	145–163
	5' 11"	134–144	140–155	149–168
	6' 0"	138–148	144–159	153–173

*Weight in pounds according to frame (in indoor clothing).
†For girls between 18 and 25, subtract one pound for each year under 25.
Source: Metropolitan Life Insurance Company, 1959.

tant for young adults to determine their ideal weight, based on their anatomical make-up, so that they can avoid unnecessary food intake throughout their adult lives. Poor eating and snacking habits and lack of physical activity may show little effects in adults in their early twenties, but as increased age decreases the necessary caloric intake, these same habits later may lead to obesity. Obesity brings with it many health hazards and, statistically, a shortened life span.

To assess one's body fatness, he should pinch the back of his upper arm lightly. If there is a thick fold of fat in that area he is probably too "fat." Standards of obesity have been based on this kind of measurement because this area is a subcutaneous fat deposit in most individuals. Weight charts such as Table 17.4 are valuable for a first approximation of optimum weight based only on sex, age, and height. But a person must remember the other factors that are important in determining ideal weight.

Obesity is always the result of food intake in excess of needs. In turn, this intake is sometimes due to endocrinological abnormalities or other diseases. Psychological factors also may, in some

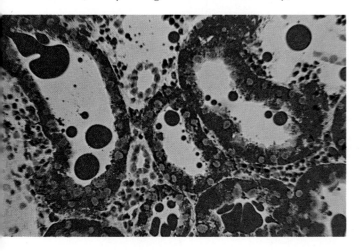

Figure 17.6 Fat cells. One theory of why many people become overweight is that overeating in childhood causes an increase in the size and number of fat cells in the body. These cells constantly crave nourishment and as the individual grows older are increasingly difficult to shed, resulting in an obesity in adulthood that it is extremely difficult to combat.

cases, be a cause of obesity. Obesity in turn causes considerable physiological and psychological stress. Before attempting to diet, a person should consult his physician. In some cases the diet is already moderate and it is more important to increase physical activity than to decrease food intake.

Dieting

Although "dieting" has great popular appeal and continuous publicity, it is essentially inadequate as an approach to weight control. To most people dieting implies going on some special eating program different from one's usual program, implying that at some future time the dieter will go off the special program and back to his usual program that resulted in the problem in the first place. What happens overwhelmingly, then, is what Jean Mayer has termed the "rhythm system of girth control"—gaining and losing periodically and a continuation of the problem. In the face of this problem the only approach that works is a permanent change in one's eating and exercise habits, with no going back. Because permanent weight control among obese persons is extremely rare, obesity is considered by many experts to be a chronic incurable disorder.

There are as many kinds of weight-loss diets as there are individuals. No one diet can be successful for everyone, no matter what the claims. Reducing diets need to be adjusted to each person and his weight problem. There are, however, inherent dangers in *every* diet. No extensive weight loss should be attempted without first having a thorough physical examination. As staid as this advice sounds, it is still the only intelligent way to approach dieting. Fad diets usually emphasize intake of one kind of nutrient and deemphasize other kinds, thus unbalancing the normal diet.

Exercise can help take off weight by burning up calories that might otherwise be stored as fat. A physician is perhaps best equipped to determine if a sudden program of exercise can be tolerated by an obese patient, but it is possible to estimate how much and what kind of exercise will burn up calories, as illustrated in Table 17.5.

Research has shown that if one is able to lose weight quickly, he also tends to put it on quickly. The slower weight is removed, the more stable and permanent the new desired weight becomes.

DIET AND HEART DISEASE

Overweight can aggravate heart disease because it places a greater strain on an organ that is already operating below peak efficiency. Furthermore, many years of scientific research and studies of various population groups indicate that diet contributes to atherosclerosis, a particular form of blood-vessel and heart disease (see Chapter 24).

In 1913 Nikolai Anichkov, a Russian pathologist,

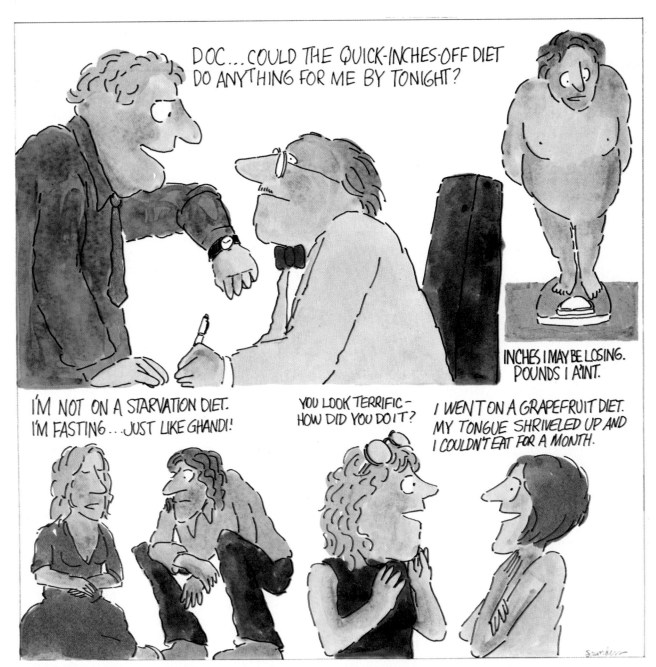

Figure 17.7 There are a number of potentially hazardous diets that rise and fall in popularity yearly in the United States. For example, high-protein, low-carbohydrate diets, such as the "Air Force" diet and the "Doctor's Quick Weight-Loss Diet," are dangerously low in necessary carbohydrates, causing excessive protein breakdown and other undesirable metabolic responses. In addition, these diets bring about water loss rather than weight loss and are usually high in fat, which may contri- bute to atherosclerosis. High-carbohydrate, low-protein diets (such as rice diets) do not supply adequate nutrition, save little in calories, and may cause the dieter to lose protein from his body, thus weakening it. Long stays on liquid or formula diets cause such side effects as constipation, diarrhea, nausea, and cramps, due to the lack of bulk. Other diets that emphasize one component of the diet and deemphasizes the others bring about similar problems.

Table 17.5 Expenditure of Calories

| FOOD | Calories | Minutes of Activity | | | | |
		Walking	Riding Bicycle	Swimming	Running	Reclining
Apple, large	101	19	12	9	5	78
Bacon, 2 strips	96	18	12	9	5	74
Banana, small	88	17	11	8	4	68
Beans, green, 1 cup	27	5	3	2	1	21
Beer, 1 glass	114	22	14	10	6	88
Bread and butter	78	15	10	7	4	60
Cake, 2 layer, 1/12	356	68	43	32	18	274
Carbonated beverage, 1 glass	106	20	13	9	5	82
Carrot, raw	42	8	5	4	2	32
Cereal, dry, 1/2 cup with milk, sugar	200	38	24	18	10	154
Cheese, cottage, 1 tbs.	27	5	3	2	1	21
Cheese, cheddar, 1 oz.	111	21	14	10	6	85
Chicken, fried, 1/2 breast	232	45	28	21	12	178
Chicken, TV dinner	542	104	66	48	28	417
Cookie, plain	15	3	2	1	1	12
Cookie, chocolate chip	51	10	6	5	3	39
Doughnut	151	29	18	13	8	116
Egg, fried	110	21	13	10	6	85
Egg, boiled	77	15	9	7	4	59
French dressing, 1 tbs.	59	11	7	5	3	45
Halibut steak, 1/4 lb.	205	39	25	18	11	158
Ham, 2 slices	167	32	20	15	9	128
Hamburger sandwich	350	67	43	31	18	269
Ice cream, 1/6 qt.	193	37	24	17	10	148
Ice cream soda	255	49	31	23	13	196
Ice milk, 1/6 qt.	144	28	18	13	7	111
Mayonnaise, 1 tbs.	92	18	11	8	5	71
Milk, 1 glass	166	32	20	15	9	128
Milk, skim, 1 glass	81	16	10	7	4	62
Milk shake	421	81	51	38	22	324
Orange, medium	68	13	8	6	4	52
Orange juice, 1 glass	120	23	15	11	6	92
Pancake with syrup	124	24	15	11	6	95
Peach, medium	46	9	6	4	2	35
Peas, green, 1/2 cup	56	11	7	5	3	43
Pie, apple, 1/6	377	73	46	34	19	290
Pizza, cheese, 1/8	180	35	22	16	9	138
Pork chop, loin	314	60	38	28	16	242
Potato chips, 1 serving	108	21	13	10	6	83
Sherbet, 1/6 qt.	177	34	22	16	9	136
Shrimp, French fried	180	35	22	16	9	138
Spaghetti, 1 serving	396	76	48	35	20	305
Steak, T-bone	235	45	29	21	12	181
Strawberry shortcake	400	77	49	36	21	308
Tuna-salad sandwich	278	53	34	25	14	214

Source: Adapted from F. Konishi, "Food Energy Equivalents of Various Activities," *Journal of the American Dietetic Association*, 46 (1965), 186.

found that rabbits fed on large amounts of cholesterol (a waxy fat derivative formed normally in the body) and animal fat developed atherosclerosis. Other researchers have since duplicated his findings in other animals. Studies on humans have shown that saturated fats will increase blood cholesterol levels, while unsaturated fats do not. In addition, people who live in countries where large amounts of saturated fats are eaten develop heart disease at a higher rate than people on low-fat diets. In sections of Finland, for instance, saturated fats make up about 22 percent of the calories in the diet and the heart-disease rate is 120 in 1,000. Americans derive about 17 percent of their calories from saturated fats and the heart-disease rate is 80 in 1,000. In Japan, however, where saturated fats make up only 3 percent of dietary calories, the heart-disease rate is only 20 in 1,000. Though the evidence is only circumstantial as yet, the significance of these findings is dramatized by the fact that heart disease killed more than 600,000 Americans last year. Of these, 165,000 victims were younger than sixty-five.

As presented in Chapter 24, there are many reasons for heart disease, including smoking, stress, inherited "defects," and lack of exercise, as well as diet. If a young adult comes from a family with a record of heart disease he should keep in close contact with a physician. His dietary pattern should be determined by his physician after a laboratory test for the various blood "lipoproteins" and cholesterol. Some individuals will need to reduce their intake of saturated fats, while for others excessive carbohydrates or calories in any form should be avoided.

NUTRITION DURING PREGNANCY

Many studies have demonstrated that if a pregnant woman lives on a seriously deficient diet, the child may mirror the deprivation after it is born or may literally starve to death while still in the womb. Dr. R. L. Naeye of the Department of Pathology at the Pennsylvania State University Medical School completed more than 1,000 autopsies of children from lower-income as well as middle- or upper-income families. ("Lower-income" means that the family could spend only 75 cents a day for food for each child.) He found that infants from the low-income families weighed from 12 percent to 15 percent less than infants from richer families. Although many of the mothers of the dead infants had received some nutritional counseling, they could not afford to follow the advice. Naeye found that not only was every vital organ severely stunted, but the cells themselves were starved, as indicated by a decrease in cytoplasm, the portion of the cell that normally contains the necessary cellular nutrients.

Other studies reviewed recently by the National Research Council (NRC) of the United States suggested that current medical practices of restricting pregnant women to a weight gain of only ten to fourteen pounds may be contributing to the relatively high infant mortality rate in the United States. (It ranks nineteenth among forty countries in infant mortality.) The NRC recommended instead an average gain of twenty-four pounds and cautioned that weight reduction programs and severe calorie restrictions should not be undertaken during pregnancy. Weight restrictions are particularly harmful to underweight women and especially to pregnant adolescents.

THE NUTRITION GAP

Even though a well-balanced diet can now be established with scientific precision, a recent federal survey showed that the American diet is worse today than it was twenty years ago. The studies stressed that obesity was certainly a major problem but that about 24 million people were not getting the right amounts of vitamins and minerals. The survey also

by James Trager

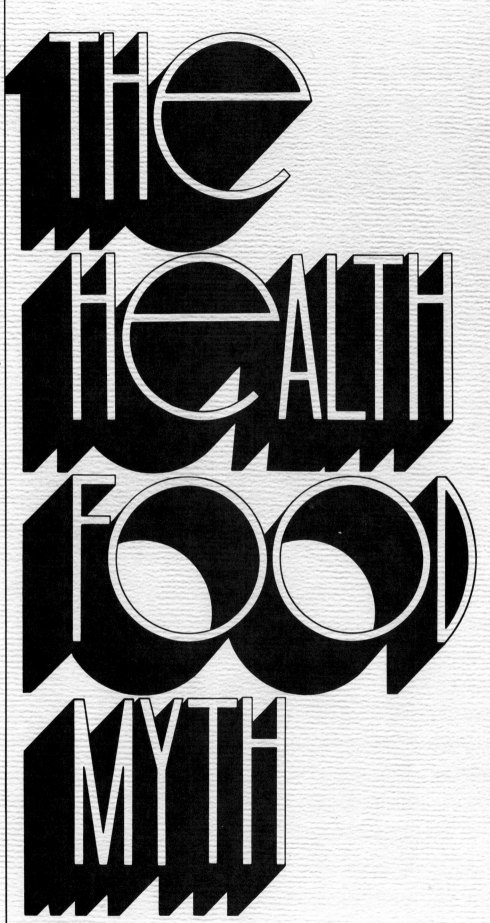

THE HEALTH FOOD MYTH

A few months ago I was in Los Angeles and was asked to dinner by people who had an imposing house high up on Angelo Drive in the Holmby Hills. It was everything a fine estate should be, with an unobtrusive swimming pool, perfect landscaping, the works—including guard dogs and a silent burglar-alarm system, reminders that the Tate-Polanski house was close by. In the valley far below glittered the phony tinsel—and the real tinsel—of Hollywood.

My host confided to me over brandy that he had bought the place back in the early 1940s from a man named Hauser. Gaylord Hauser. Perhaps I had heard of him? Suddenly a whole corny chain of B-movie optics and sound effects went off inside my head. So this was the house that blackstrap molasses built. And brewer's yeast, wheat germ, and yogurt, the "wonder foods" with which the debonair Hauser had charmed the Hollywood crowd in the 1930s and 1940s and which he touted in his 1950-1951 best seller, *Look Younger, Live Longer*. If anyone had any doubt about the money to be made in "health" foods, this house had to be convincing.

Today a new crop of millionaires is building dream houses with money generated by the "health" food mystique, the questionable notion that all men's ills are rooted in what he eats and that they can all be cured or avoided by special diets.

Medicine is still full of unanswered questions. Through the gaps in medical knowledge, the "health" food exponents rush in, advancing speculations and conjectures as unequivocal truths, offering "case histories" as evidence. No single magazine article can begin to examine all the claims, the half-truths, the theories long ago disproved, the exaggerations on which the "health" food movement is based. Nor can we analyze the movement's psychology, which appears at first as a joyful, positive glorification of nature, but soon reveals itself as a basic distrust of orthodox medicine and a dark suspicion that greedy "interests" are ruthlessly, recklessly exploiting the public.

So, let us merely look at one key idea that "health" food enthusiasts take as an article of faith. This is the myth that "organically grown" foods—fruits and vegetables fertilized with animal manure or green compost—are filled with "natural" vitamins and minerals never found in foods fertilized with inorganic nitrates, potash, and phosphates.

The only trouble with this rosy-cheeked idea is that it isn't true. According to the Department of Agriculture, "for the most part,

Adapted from Trager, J. "Exploding the Health Food Myth," *Family Circle*, (July 1971), p. 58, 84, 106.

elements essential to plant growth enter the plant in the inorganic form. If an element is originally present in the soil in some organic combination, this organic combination is broken down to an inorganic form by the microorganisms in the soil before the element enters the plant."

Agricultural Information Bulletin No. 299 is available for 15 cents from the Superintendent of Documents, U.S. Government Printing Office, Washington, D.C. 20402. It goes into great detail on the subject, but its key point is that any differences in the content of "essential elements or vitamins that have been noted . . . have been too small to be of any nutritional significance, and have been in favor of the inorganic fertilized plants as often as in favor of those grown with organic materials."

Robert Rodale, of the Rodale Press, is one who disagrees. Rodale wrote me recently that his organization's "claim that organic food is generally of superior nutritional value has long been challenged by people in the food establishment. However, the weight of evidence does indicate that the mineral composition of plants varies according to the quality of the soil in which they are grown. Vitamin content is much more difficult to influence by changing soil quality."

A mutual friend tells me that Rodale is a sincere man, a man who "really wants to help people." I have no doubt of it. Nor does anyone question that the presence of mineral elements in plants is related to the presence of mineral elements in the soil. This is why sophisticated farmers employ soil experts to treat their soils with trace elements and thus correct specific deficiencies. If you raise livestock that eat only the grass from a rather limited area of land, this can be important. But our own food comes from so many soils that nutritional deficiencies based on soil inadequacy are virtually impossible. In any event, the whole subject begs the question of whether "organic food is generally of superior nutritional value" as people like Rodale claim it is.

There are militant "health" food zealots who reject any findings of the Agriculture Department but accept, on the other hand, far-out claims that declare blackstrap molasses as a cure for anemia, arthritis, ulcers, varicose veins, and as a cancer preventive. In such ways, fortunes are made.

Desperate people will try anything, and anything includes, along with blackstrap molasses, brewer's yeast for B vitamins; rosehip or acerola-berry jam for vitamin C (as-corbic acid); wheat germ for iron, vitamin E, and the B vitamins; apple-cider vinegar for potassium; yogurt for calcium and riboflavin. Huge claims are made for these and other "health" food items, while doubters are dismissed as being members of the "medical establishment."

The militancy of the movement is deceptively wrapped in a kind of occult, spiritual fervor, an old-time religion that gets in the way of old-fashioned common sense. In this world of fouled air and water, of ugly technology, in this time of yearning for an idyllic, unspoiled past of basic simplicity, the bucolic virtues of nature do seem a kind of salvation. There may be nothing much a woman can do about some things except to write letters and join protest groups, but there is something she can do about what she feeds her family. She can feed them "pure," "natural" foods and see them glow with health. What a fine, satisfying thought that is!

Of course, she may decide that natural butter is not as healthy for her husband's heart as artificial butter made with polyunsaturated vegetable oils. She may not consider natural raw milk worth the risk of having her children come down with undulant fever, staphyloccocal food poisoning, or other diseases sometimes transmitted by unpasteurized milk. (In most places in the United States such milk is not legally obtainable.)

Going back to grandma's ways may give a woman an emotional kick; it will perhaps come as a shock that grandma's spring tonic, sassafras tea, is no longer legally available unless it is free of a liquid called safrole. Back about a dozen years or so, it was found that safrole, which occurs naturally in the bark and roots of the sassafras tree, produced cancer in the small intestines of test rats.

In short, there is nothing safe about being natural. Dr. Julius Coons, a ranking expert on poisons in natural foods, says, in fact, that "at present, the unknowns in regard to the chemical make-up and toxicology of our natural food resources seem much more extensive and numerous than those related to additives and (pesticide) residues." I introduce Dr. Coons at this point because "health" food zealots have made such a bugaboo of chemicals.

Exaggerated fears of chemicals have had unfortunate effects. Opposition to iodized table salt has made such "chemically treated" salt unavailable in some communities in the Midwest, with the result that many people may have disfiguring goiters or suffer other thyroid gland problems due to a deficiency of iodine in their diets. Opposition to fluoridation of community drinking water in many areas has meant a high rate of juvenile dental problems.

This phobia against chemicals is basic to the "organic" food fad, which opposes chemical pesticides as well as chemical fertilizers. In recent years this position has brought the "organic" food people into the camp of those who are fighting to save the environment. It has also muddied the "organic" argument.

Ecology is a magic word today. We are all against DDT, which is still used on almost 1 percent of United States food crop acreage. But the major concern about DDT and similar pesticides is with their effect on wildlife. These is little to support claims that DDT causes cancer or other diseases in humans.

Chemical fertilizers, which promote the high crop yields that keep our food prices low, do sometimes run off into waterways and promote the growth of unwanted weeds and algae. This process lowers the submerged oxygen levels in the water and jeopardizes fish life. You may elect to pay high "health" food prices as a protest against environmental decay, but have no illusions that the extra money is guarding the health of your family.

You may also elect to pay extra for fresher fruits and vegetables, or fresher eggs, than those usually offered at the supermarket. Nobody can deny that some of the efficiencies that have made American food such a bargain (no other country spends such a small part of average personal income to feed itself) have sacrificed certain taste values in our foods. Some small stores, including "health" food stores, will have tomatoes, peaches, melons, and other items that have not been picked prematurely and have not traveled far. They will taste better, but they will not be more nutritious and will not be worth premium prices on the basis of health.

Food prices are high enough these days without paying fancy prices for the dubious virtues of "health" foods and diet supplements. If you are worried about your family's health, find a good doctor. But do not confuse "health" foods with medicine. Despite their screeches against the "commercial" food interests, the "health" food people represent a commercial food interest themselves. Let them build their mansions with somebody else's food dollars.

showed that after puberty women are more apt to have inadequate diets than men, especially with regard to iron intake. Studies of underprivileged children show that in some areas between 10 percent and 25 percent are anemic. On this basis, the American Medical Association and other groups have recommended that iron should be added to flour and cereals, to bring it up from a level of 16.5 milligrams per pound to 60 milligrams per pound, a measure that has received general support. It also has been suggested that food manufacturers label their products more accurately and completely as to their nutritional content.

World Food Needs

If inadequate nutrition is a problem in the United States, it takes on catastrophic proportions in other parts of the world. In 1969, a conference of the United Nations Food and Agriculture Organization (FAO) projected world food needs to 1985, based on the expected population increase to more than 7 billion compared to the present 3 billion. Noting that about 1.5 billion of the additional people will live in the developing or underdeveloped nations, the conference participants agreed that the population explosion will require an 80 percent increase in food supplies in 1985, compared to the 1962 figure, just to keep nutrition *at its present level.*

The Green Revolution

Agricultural planners hope that the anticipated food-population crises might be at least partially averted by the growth of the so-called "Green Revolution": increased production of cereal crop sta-

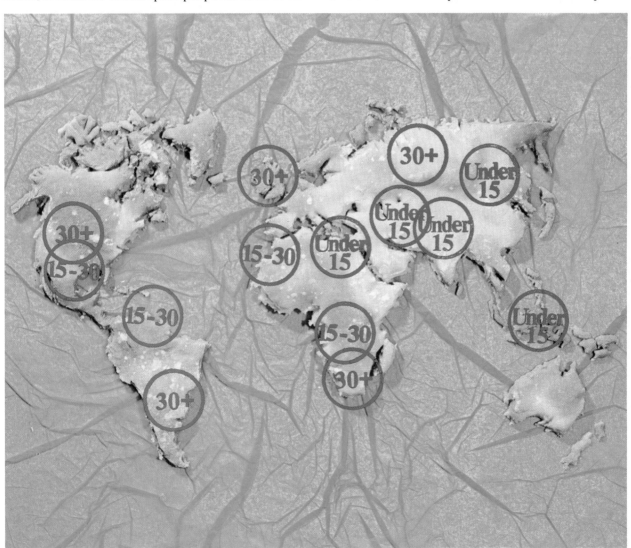

Figure 17.8 Animal protein levels in selected countries. Protein supplies the body with essential amino acids. One of the best sources of protein is the meat of animals. In countries where natural resources or tradition do not allow for even minimal consumption of meat and poultry, an adequate diet should contain alternative sources of protein, such as soybeans and cottonseed.

SATISFACTORY DIET	Milk Group	Meat Group	Fruit-Vegetable Group	Bread-Cereal Group	Calories	Protein	Fats	Calcium
Breakfast								
Oatmeal				▓	150	✕		
Milk	▓				165	✕	✕	✕ ✕ ✕
Sugar					50			
Grapefruit (½)			▓		50			
Coffee								
Lunch								
Chili beans								
a. Chili sauce			▓		190			
b. Meat		▓			250	✕ ✕ ✕	✕ ✕ ✕	
c. Beans		▓			230	✕ ✕		✕
Toast (2 slices)					110			
Broccoli spears			▓		45	✕		✕ ✕
Orange			▓		70			
Butter (4 pats)	▓				200		✕ ✕ ✕ ✕	
Milk	▓				165	✕	✕	✕ ✕ ✕
Dinner								
Cottage cheese (4 oz.)	▓				120	✕ ✕		✕ ✕ ✕
Chicken		▓			250	✕ ✕ ✕ ✕	✕ ✕	
Peas (⅔ c.)			▓		50	✕		
Carrots (⅓ c.)					20			
Baked potato			▓		90		•	
Strawberry sauce			▓		250			
Shortcake					130		✕	✕
Milk	▓				165	✕	✕	✕ ✕ ✕
Butter (2 pats)	▓				100		✕ ✕	
TOTAL					2,850 cal.	17✕ = 102 g.	15✕ = 90 g.	16✕ = 1,600 mg.
Standard for X (or X =)						6 g.	6 g.	100 mg.
Minimum daily requirement Male: 150 lbs., 69 in., 22 yrs.					2,800 cal.	60 g.		800 mg.
UNSATISFACTORY DIET	Milk Group	Meat Group	Fruit-Vegetable Group	Bread-Cereal Group	Calories	Protein	Fats	Calcium
Breakfast								
Toast (2 slices)				▓	110			
Coffee and sugar					50			
Butter (4 pats)	▓				200		✕ ✕ ✕ ✕	
Lunch								
Hot dog		▓			155	✕	✕ ✕	
Bun					125			
Potato chips (large bag)			▓		440		✕ ✕ ✕ ✕	
Coke					105			✕ ✕ ✕
Snack								
Chocolate Bar (4 oz.)					580	✕ ✕ ✕ ✕ ✕ ✕		✕ ✕
Coke					105			✕ ✕ ✕
Dinner								
Hamburger		▓			250	✕ ✕ ✕	✕ ✕ ✕	
Tomato (slice)			▓		10			
Lettuce			▓		5			
Bun					220	✕		
French fries					300		✕ ✕	
Coke					105			✕ ✕ ✕
Tapioca					545			
TOTAL					3,305 cal.	5✕ = 30 g.	21✕ = 126 g.	11✕ = 1,100 mg.
Standard for X (or X =)						6 g.	6 g.	100 mg.
Minimum daily requirement Male: 150 lbs., 69 in., 22 yrs.					2,800 cal.	60 g.		800 mg.

Figure 17.9 A comparison of a poor and a good day's dietary intake, classified by basic food groups, main dietary components, and calories. The poor diet is high in calories and missing in many nutrients. The good diet contains all the recommended daily requirements.

Phosphorus	Iron	Vitamin A	Vitamin B₁	Vitamin B₂	Niacin	Vitamin C	Vitamin D
	××		××				
×××				×××			×
						××	
		×			×		
	×××		×		××××		
×	××××		×	×	×		
	×		×	×	×		
	××	×××××	×	××	×	×××××	
			×			×××	
		×					
×××				×××			×
×××							×
	××			××	××××		
	××	×	×××	××	×××	×	
		××××××					
	×		×		××	×	
	×			×		×××××	
	×		×	×	×		
×××				×××			×
13×=1,300 mg.	19× = 19 mg.	14×=14,000 IU	12×=1.2 mg.	19×=1.9 mg.	18×=18 mg.	17×=340 mg.	4×=400 IU
100 mg.	1 mg.	1,000 IU	.1 mg.	.1 mg.	1 mg.	20 mg.	100 IU
800 mg.	10 mg.	5,000 IU	1.4 mg.	1.6 mg.	18 mg.	60 mg.	400 IU

Phosphorus	Iron	Vitamin A	Vitamin B₁	Vitamin B₂	Niacin	Vitamin C	Vitamin D
	×		×	×	×		
		×					
	×		×	×	×		
	×		×	×	×		
	××		××		××		
×××							
				××××			
×××							
	×××		×		××××		
	××		××	××	××		
	×		×	×	××××	×	
×××							
11×=1,100 mg.	11× = 11 mg.	1×=1,000 IU	9× =.9 mg	10×=1.0 mg.	15×=15 mg.	1× = 20 mg.	0×= 0 IU
100 mg.	1 mg.	1,000 IU	.1 mg.	.1 mg.	1 mg.	20 mg.	100 IU
800 mg.	10 mg.	5,000 IU	1.4 mg.	1.6 mg.	18 mg.	60 mg.	400 IU

ples by using chemical fertilizers, irrigation, and new breeds of high-yield crops. Hopefully, combination of the three approaches may make it possible to increase cereal production from the 1962 level of 230 million metric tons to the 920 million metric tons needed by 1985.

Although cereal crops are by no means the complete answer to malnutrition in underdeveloped nations, they do provide a basic protein source that can, if necessary, be supplemented with essential amino acids, such as lysine and methionine. Since the early 1960s, many underdeveloped nations previously unable to produce the cereal crops they needed began to produce bumper crops of so-called "miracle wheat" and "miracle rice." First to appear was a dwarf variety of hardy, high-yield wheat that could be produced in great abundance under a wide variety of climatic conditions. The miracle wheat was so adaptable to growing conditions in various climates that Mexico, Pakistan, India, Turkey, and Afghanistan have become prolific wheat producers, in some cases changing from wheat importers to exporters.

Miracle wheat was also the prototype of a high-yield rice developed at the International Rice Research Institute in the Philippines in the mid-1960s. It is now being produced by many previously rice-starved nations. In some quarters, the Green Revolution has been criticized because ancient techniques for distribution and marketing have not been able to keep up with the production of the new strains of wheat and rice. It also has put an economic squeeze on farmers who are still producing the older varieties of the cereal crops and who cannot compete with the new varieties. A more serious objection has been that dependence of so many millions of people on a single variety of wheat or rice could result in a famine more massive than the world has ever known if the new miracle grains should suddenly succumb to a blight that could wipe out the entire crop in a matter of a season or two. A research program is currently under way to diversify the "miracle" strains and reduce the risks of such a disaster.

Some of the criticisms may be well placed, but many agricultural researchers now believe such

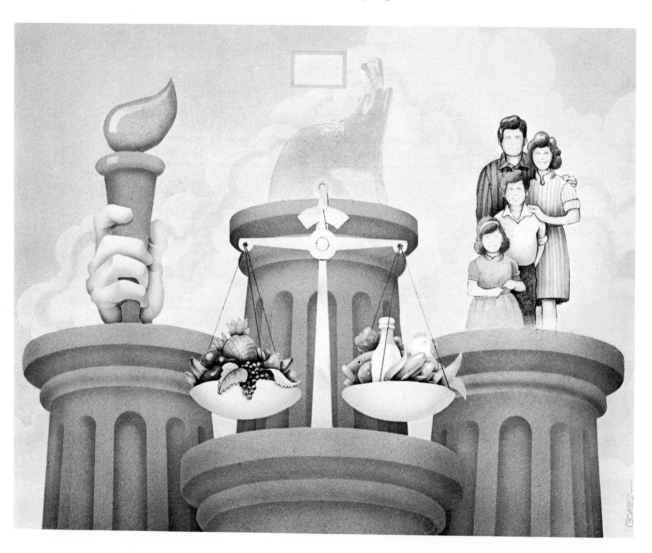

temporary economic and social disadvantages are obliterated by the immediate effects that the new cereal strains—including new varieties of corn—are now having on the world's hunger problems. They point out that because of the Green Revolution many of the underdeveloped nations are now going through a period of agricultural expansion that may have as much impact in those countries as the industrial revolution had in Europe at the turn of the century.

MISCONCEPTIONS ABOUT NUTRITION

Since the importance of vitamins for a balanced diet became known, nutritionists, drug manufacturers, and food faddists have all accepted them, but from different points of view. The drug manufacturers maintain, with good scientific certainty, that the vitamins they make in the laboratory are exactly the same as the vitamins produced in nature. However, pure-food enthusiasts and organic gardeners, among others, insist that "natural" vitamins are more nutritious than the man-made variety. There is little basis for this claim.

The "organic" food stores now sprouting up all over the country are a direct result of the nation's interest in ecology and the realization that man has disrupted the balance of his environment with a number of potentially harmful substances. Thus organic farmers grow their crops using natural fertilizers instead of chemicals, refusing to treat them with insecticides or herbicides. Their program is defensible on purely agricultural grounds, but it has its economic disadvantages because organically grown food usually costs more than mass-produced food. Organic gardening does not contribute significantly to the world's food needs, because there is not enough natural fertilizer to go around, and

chemical crop and pest control is necessary to assure the large crops that will be needed.

The outcry against food additives is another related problem, spawned in part by scientific findings that the cyclamate sugar substitutes cause cancer in animals, that a herbicide used on cranberries was found to be carcinogenic, and that the flavor-enhancer monosodium glutamate (MSG) causes brain and eye lesions in young animals if given in large amounts and a form of acute discomfort ("Chinese restaurant syndrome") in susceptible individuals. Recent findings indicate that a chemical used in certain food dyes may be carcinogenic and that sulfur dioxide, a chemical widely used in foods, may cause gene damage. Chemical contaminants of foodstuffs may be in the form of food additives designed to increase the flavor, stability, nutritional value or saleability of a food, but insecticides and herbicides also may get into crops through the soil, water, or spraying programs. Federal agencies, especially the United States Food and Drug Administration, hope to avert such potential or actual disasters by more stringent restrictions and new evaluations of food additives. It now costs from 300,000 to 1 million dollars for a manufacturer to carry out the testing program that the FDA requires for new food additives. (Such FDA activities are further discussed in Chapter 27.)

Nutrition is a science about which man knows much less than he would like. Until more is known about what actually happens with every chemical ingested by the body, controversy will continue to rage as to what is and what is not "good" for one to eat. Meanwhile, the best approach to nutrition is to eat a wide variety of foods in an effort to provide all essential nutrients as well as to avoid the possibly damaging effects of "overexposure" to any one dietary component.

Figure 17.10 Aspects of the ideal diet. Good nutrition consists of a balanced diet of all main components in adequate but not excessive amounts, of appropriate calorie intake in relation to energy expenditure, and of individual tailoring to one's age, sex, size, heredity, and activities.

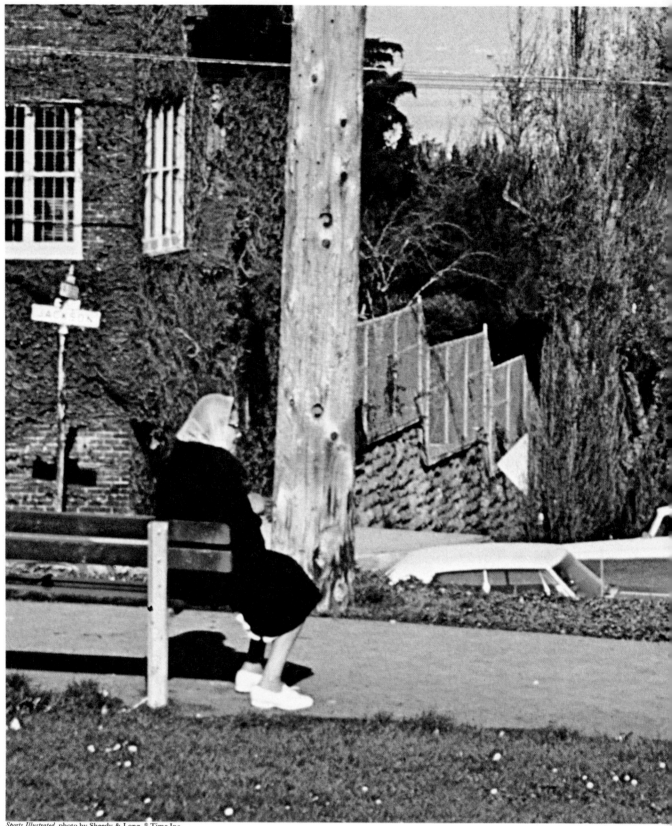

Sports Illustrated, photo by Sheedy & Long, ® Time Inc.

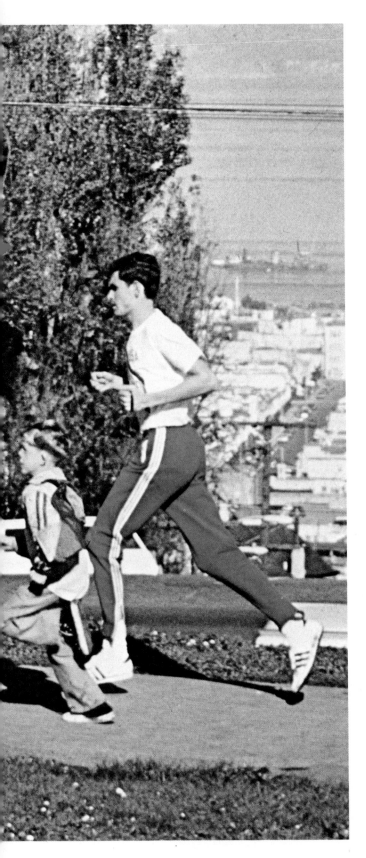

18

Hardly a day passes without someone breaking a record in one sport or another. Each generation of athletes, trained to achieve maximum performance with their bodies, minds, and emotions, runs faster, jumps higher, lifts more, and scores better than previous generations. Certainly, for their events and their eras, champions emerge as the fittest individuals in society. But they represent only a minute proportion of the population. What about the millions of people who do not participate or even aspire to set records and who rarely come close to achieving a major fraction of their own potential for physical performance? Are exercise and fitness relevant to *them*? As will be discussed in this chapter, exercise and fitness are not only relevant but important for both physical and mental health. In addition, exercise and fitness play an important role in how much and how often an individual feels fatigue and in the quality of sleep he may experience.

ROLE OF FITNESS

The record-breaking athlete, like the great painter, musician, or scientist, demonstrates how far the human species can reach. But although most people can identify with the athlete and can share the excitement of his accomplishments, few people realistically can aspire to such greatness themselves. The motivation for improved fitness often is not so much from emulation of champions but from pure self-interest.

Until recently humans could not have survived without well-developed physical abilities of the kind required to obtain food, seek shelter, and escape from danger. Modern technology and social philos-

Physical Fitness

If you're not using your body, you're not using your head.

The more we use our heads, the less we use our bodies.

And that can lead to things like fat.

And fat can lead to heart disease, diabetes, strokes, high blood pressure.

And that can lead to death.

Maybe you're taking life too easy.

Maybe you should make things a little harder on yourself.

Walk instead of taking the bus. Skip the elevator and take the stairs. Ski. Skate. Smack a handball. Jog. Dance. Do calisthenics.

Use your head.

Use your body.

We can help. For information, pick up a pencil and write to us.

The walk to the post office is a start in the right direction.

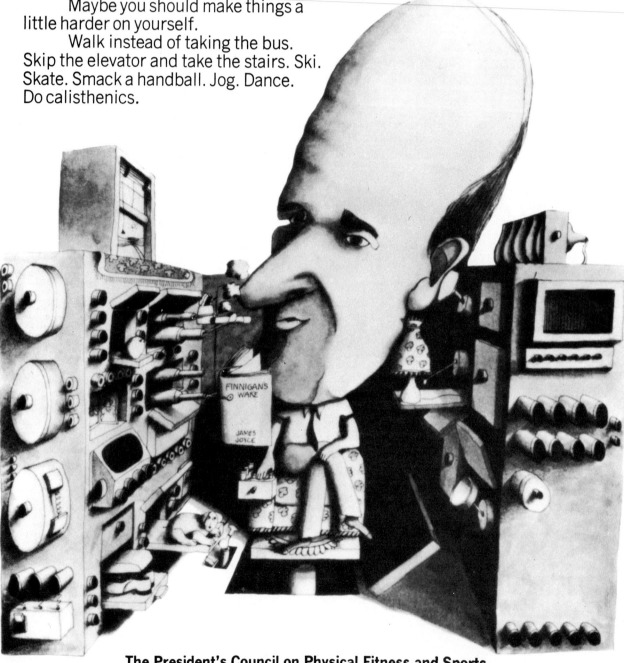

The President's Council on Physical Fitness and Sports
Washington, D.C. 20201

ophy have changed some of the physical demands for survival, so that even severely handicapped individuals often can live productively. Nevertheless, every human has a body and imprinted upon it is the need to move—a basic requirement that modern life may even intensify. The efficient fat-storage mechanism in man might have assured his survival in his history of starvation and deprivation, but in times of overnutrition and underactivity this same mechanism conspires against his health and survival. Thus, fitness must be considered relative to the time and circumstance of the human condition. There is an appropriate level of physical activity for each individual. As a minimum, this activity should be of the kind, intensity, and frequency sufficient to keep him fit for the world he now faces and will face in the future.

Physical fitness is more a means than an end, for it enables the organism to use its physical abilities to capitalize on its emotional, intellectual, and social attributes and to achieve "total fitness." The concept of total fitness implies a reasonable balance between anatomical-physiological development, performance skills for graceful, efficient movements, and the emotional and social qualities needed to guide the individual in using his attributes effectively.

The achievement of this kind of fitness is not restricted to the dedicated athlete. With a basic understanding of fitness, and a personal commitment to a physically active life style, virtually any man or woman can be fit. The tragedy is that many North Americans have simply accepted early aging and physical deterioration as their inevitable personal cost of technological progress. There are better alternatives. Understanding and action based on that understanding are essential, especially in communities where there is more reinforcement for sedentary living than for physically active living.

ELEMENTS OF FITNESS

Movement capacity involves the development of three fitness elements: strength, suppleness, and stamina.

Strength is the basic muscular force required for movement. Normally, strength is developed by overcoming resistances, such as those supplied by parts of the body in normal daily activity; by the whole body in lifting, pulling, walking, and climbing; by another person's body as in football or wrestling; or by inanimate objects like grocery bags, trash cans, books, barbells, or dumbbells.

The quickest and most direct means of improving strength is through weight training. Isometric (static) exercise that develops tension also may improve strength; however, except for special circumstances and rehabilitation purposes, resistive exercise with movement is preferred because it does not inhibit blood flow or raise blood pressure to the same extent that static exercise does. Moreover, weight training seems to bring about greater strength achievement over a wider range of movement than isometric procedures, which tend to have an effect that is limited to specific angles of application.

Suppleness, or flexibility, is the quality of muscles, bones, tendons, and ligaments that permits full range of movement in a joint. One may be supple in some joints but not in others, and there may even be large differences in the same joint on either side of the body. For example, many individuals have greater range of movement in one shoulder than the other. The ability to move one's limbs and other bendable parts effectively through the full range is maintained by periodic full-range bending and stretching movements. Immobilization or restricted movement is associated with reduced suppleness, often giving rise to postural and orthopedic problems.

Figure 18.1 An unfortunate "by-product" of the technological advances of the twentieth century has been the instigation and perpetuation of a sedentary society. Unlike their ancestors, who were forced to labor to heat their homes, collect water, gather food, and so on, most Americans get far too little exercise, so that today, although infectious diseases have been largely conquered, Americans are being killed by life styles and attitudes that admit little time for exercise.

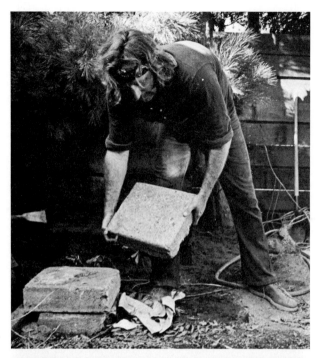

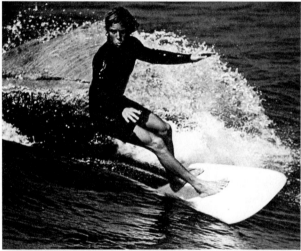

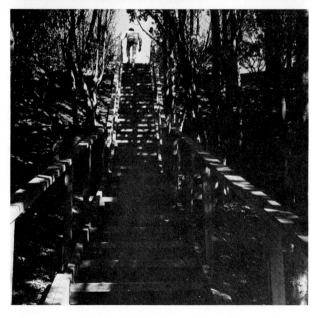

Stamina, or endurance, is the quality that enables an individual to mobilize energy to maintain movement over an extended period of time. As discussed later in this chapter, stamina is largely a matter of developing an adequate oxygen-transport system. Normally, stamina is achieved by sustained whole-body exercise, such as running, cycling, and swimming.

The fitness elements cannot be developed or maintained unless the specific exercise experience is reasonably intense and frequent. People who lead sedentary lives offer a marked contrast to those whose life styles provide activity of the kind, intensity, and frequency that are necessary for the development and maintenance of strength, suppleness, and stamina. Some of the easily identifiable effects of training are summarized in Figure 18.3.

Essentially, the trained individual is leaner, stronger for his body size, has an enhanced circulatory and energy-mobilization capacity, and recovers more quickly following exercise. The untrained individual often exhibits the physical characteristics associated with early aging. Physiological middle age for the unfit may arrive before they are chronologically twenty-one years old. At the other end of the fitness spectrum, there are vigorous "youngsters" chronologically in their sixties and beyond. There is evidence to indicate that training postpones physiological aging in adulthood and enhances strength and stamina in old age. However, a declining suppleness may be one infirmity shared by the fit and unfit senior citizen, because deterioration of joints does not appear to be reversible.

EXERCISE AND HEALTH

For centuries man has been vaguely aware that exercise and fitness are important to his well-being. Not until recently, however, has science begun to document the nature and extent of the relationship between exercise and health. Studies comparing

Figure 18.2 The three main components of fitness: (*top*) strength, as needed for lifting or carrying, (*center*) suppleness, to be able to reach and bend, and (*bottom*) stamina, such as is necessary for climbing stairs, walking long distances, and so on.

the cardiovascular systems and heart-disease experiences of sedentary and active workers within specific occupations have shown that the more active workers have less disease and lower death rates than their sedentary counterparts. If persons are compared on the basis of degree of exertion, the least active tend to have the greatest degenerative disease and death rates, with quality of health and life span increasing in direct proportion to increased physical activity (see Table 18.1).

Fascinated by this kind of evidence, two American physicians, Wilhelm Raab and Hans Kraus, reviewed the many studies on the subject, added some research of their own, and in 1961 published a book entitled *Hypokinetic Disease*, which catalogued a wide variety of human disorders that occur more often among sedentary people than among the physically active. "Hypokinetic" means insufficient movement, so these disorders are specifically linked with or complicated by too little exercise. Some of the hypokinetic disorders identified were chronic fatigue, shortness of breath, overweight, digestive upsets, headache, backache, anxiety states, muscular weakness and atrophy, musculoskeletal (muscle, bone, joint, ligament, tendon) pain and injuries, high blood pressure, atherosclerosis, coronary artery disease, and generalized, accelerated, degenerative aging.

Role of Exercise in Hypokinetic Disorders

What is the connection between lack of exercise and each of these disorders? There is no basis for the belief that exercise has value in pathological processes. Exercise does, however, provide for greater physical reserves and has value in improving body structures and functions. There seem to be a number of areas in which exercise may alleviate or prevent problems.

RELEASED TENSION   Exercise may provide the movement activity to physiologically express and release tension that accumulates when one is under stress. Primitive man survived, in part, through his "fight or flight" reactions: when danger threatened, his

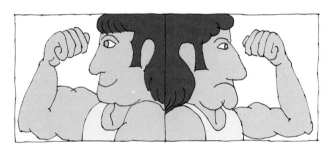

Trained State

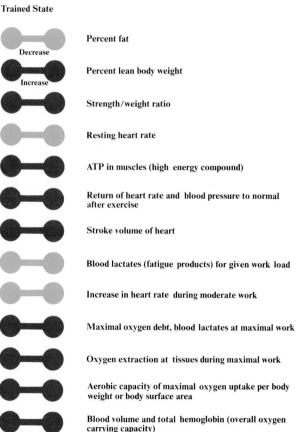

Decrease

Increase

Percent fat

Percent lean body weight

Strength/weight ratio

Resting heart rate

ATP in muscles (high energy compound)

Return of heart rate and blood pressure to normal after exercise

Stroke volume of heart

Blood lactates (fatigue products) for given work load

Increase in heart rate during moderate work

Maximal oxygen debt, blood lactates at maximal work

Oxygen extraction at tissues during maximal work

Aerobic capacity of maximal oxygen uptake per body weight or body surface area

Blood volume and total hemoglobin (overall oxygen carrying capacity)

Cardiac and skeletal muscle vascularization

Postural problems and low back pain

Table 18.1   Deaths* per 100 Men by Degree of Exertion

AGE	No Exercise	Slight Exercise	Moderate Exercise	Heavy Exercise
40–49	1.46	1.17	1.12	1.00
50–59	1.43	1.17	1.06	1.00
60–69	1.91	1.64	1.19	1.00
70–79	2.91	2.03	1.45	1.00

*From coronary heart disease.

Source: E. C. Hammond and L. Garfinkel, "Coronary Heart Disease, Stroke, and Aortic Aneurysm," *Archives of Environmental Health*, 19 (August 1969), 174. Data are based on a study of more than 1,000,000 men and women followed over a six-year period.

Figure 18.3   A summary of the physiological effects of training.

body reacted by releasing catecholamines (adrenalin and noradrenalin) into the blood. These hormones sharpened and quickened his physical responses. In modern life, environmental stress is still a very real part of human experience, though dangers seldom threaten one's life. Still, the body reacts in the same fashion as it did when threatened by wild beasts (see Chapter 3).

Primitive man was required to move, to work, to "exercise" in order to survive. Modern urban man under stress is often required to sit still and appear relaxed and calm, thereby inhibiting natural expression. Accordingly, the catecholamine-induced tense state is not resolved in activity. Unresolved stress is persistently accompanied by constricted arterioles, high blood pressure, and increased heart rate. Such unremitting stress is thought to contribute to a variety of degenerative effects, particularly in relation to the digestive and cardiovascular systems. Deliberate and appropriate exercise, then, enables modern man to release psychological tension and achieve physical relaxation.

STRENGTH AND RESISTANCE Appropriate exercise and fitness have maintenance values for a number of tissues and so survival value to the whole organism. Untrained muscles grow smaller and weaker than trained muscles. When a broken arm is immobilized in a cast for several weeks, *atrophy* begins to take place—the muscles waste away, and the bones and joints deteriorate with inactivity. Astronauts' muscles grow weak and deteriorate rapidly in weightless environments unless they exercise artificially with isometrics. Such exercise compensates for the absence of the minimal exercise involved in maintaining posture and simple movement against gravity. Sedentary man suffers the same kind of atrophy, weakness, and resulting vulnerability to injury.

SUPPORT OF DEVELOPMENTAL GROWTH Children require exercise for normal growth and development. Al-

though sedentary youngsters may survive, their muscles, bones, nervous systems, hearts, and lungs, and the functions dependent on these organs are impaired by insufficient movement. Exercise is necessary for fitness at any age, but if restrictions are imposed on it during the developmental years from birth to age twenty, a child may become permanently handicapped. The handicap may become seriously apparent only at middle age, however, Deprived of the benefits of physical fitness in the developmental years, the middle-aged man or woman frequently suffers from a variety of hypokinetic disorders such as those mentioned above. Medical treatment may provide some relief when these disorders strike, but the tragedy is that they could have been prevented or postponed by fitness in childhood and continued fitness through life.

HOW FIT IS "FIT ENOUGH"?

How fit is "fit enough"? What generalizations are justified in view of the very broad range of individual differences in goals and abilities? Ultimately each person decides these issues for himself within the framework of his perceptions, understandings, and style of living. However, research in the health sciences and understandings evolved from professional practice in medicine and physical education have pointed toward some criteria that may be helpful in personal decision making.

Fit enough to maintain orthopedic fitness—that is, to enjoy active living with minimal risk of orthopedic injury or disability—is one dimension of the "how fit" question. Men and women should have the skills and be strong and supple enough to work and play with ease and without undue fatigue. The activities to which this type of fitness may apply range from lifting babies and trash cans, or pushing vacuum cleaners and lawn mowers, to playing three hard sets of tennis or swimming half a mile.

But why not just do what one has to and wants to and let one's fitness grow and adapt accordingly?

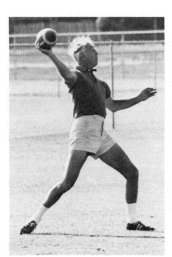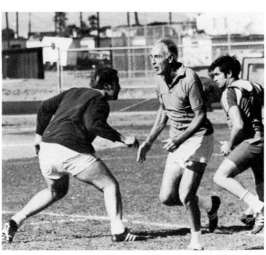

Figure 18.4 Care for one's health and physical fitness pays off in a variety of benefits as one grows older. This sixty-year-old man continues to enjoy participation in football, tennis, and other sports as one of the benefits of having kept his body in top condition.

For one thing, the body adapts to the specific demands placed on it and no more. In youth this adaptation works fairly well because of the natural resiliency of the young organism. When a younger person "overlifts" or "overexerts," he may get a few sore muscles or become fatigued, but he quickly recovers. Natural resiliency diminishes with age, however. If one does nothing more strenuous than lifting babies or pushing lawn mowers, the body adapts to those limits, and even slight exertion beyond the normal may produce injury or fatigue. Therefore, controlled extra training beyond the routine minimal daily demands is needed to maintain a safety margin for those times when an extra demand is imposed.

In developing and maintaining strength and suppleness in adults, calisthenic activity is most useful. Bending and stretching exercises (all body parts in all directions and to the limits without inordinate strain), bent-knee sit-ups, leg squats, and a wide variety of additional, controlled, no-strain movements are among the best exercises to maintain orthopedic adequacy. Once these minimal levels of muscular fitness are achieved, one might add resistive exercises such as push-ups and pull-ups or use inanimate objects such as weights, pulleys, and springs if his exercise goals go beyond minimal orthopedic safety.

Fit enough to insure against heart attack is often cited as a criterion for the "how fit" question. There is, of course, no absolute protection against heart attack, but the development of stamina (cardiovascular-respiratory endurance) appears to be one way to reduce each of the risk factors for coronary artery disease (see Chapter 24). Here is how exercise seems to work:

First, stamina training (to be described in detail later) involves continuous rhythmic cardiovascular-respiratory overload, lasting from eight minutes to an hour or longer depending on the individual's level of fitness and his fitness goals. The body responds to the demands imposed by this training by adapting; that is, it rebuilds itself in order to accommodate these training demands with less or no stress. In time the muscles involved, especially the heart muscle, develop an increased vascularization and the increased size of the capillary network offers more available routes for oxygen transport by the blood.

In the coronary system—the circulation serving the heart—such vascularization may provide valuable protection because it offers an increased blood supply capacity, making a fatal heart attack less likely. If a clot blocks a coronary vessel and causes a heart attack, there is the possibility that *collateral circulation* (by-pass blood vessels), promoted by stamina training, will allow alternate routes for blood and oxygen. Accordingly, damage is likely to be slighter and recovery quicker.

With training, the heart also becomes stronger and more efficient. An increased amount of blood is pumped on each beat, with a more complete emptying of the heart, even though the heart will not increase much in size. Cardiac output at resting is not affected because the resting heart rate be-

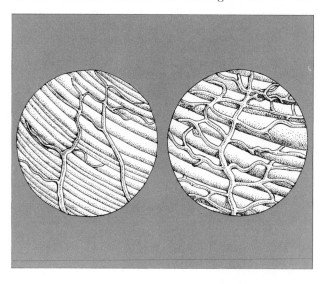

Figure 18.5 Capillarization. On the left is a drawing of an untrained muscle with relatively few capillaries. On the right is trained muscle with thicker fibers and increased number of capillaries. Studies have shown that the heart muscle in particular benefits from such training.

comes slower. Whereas the normal adult resting pulse rate is around seventy beats per minute, and eighty to ninety beats is not unusual in untrained individuals, the stamina-trained adult usually has resting pulse rates of fifty-five to sixty beats per minute. His heart beats thousands of times less per day, which appears to be beneficial in reducing the wear and tear on heart valves.

Stamina training also has been shown to improve *peripheral circulation*. It may reduce some forms of hypertension (high blood pressure), which over a period of time would seriously damage many parts of the body. Stamina training tends to relax the arterioles that work much like nozzles in controlling blood pressure and to reduce fats in the blood (cholesterol and triglycerides), which have been implicated in degenerative cardiovascular disease. The mechanism of this fat reduction is not known, but one theory holds that the fats are "used up" in exercise metabolism. Reduction in blood clotting is thought to be another benefit of stamina training.

Stamina training stresses other body systems, thereby stressing the body as a whole and in this way also contributes to the welfare of the heart. Exercise burns calories, which contributes, obviously, to weight control. In typical adult training programs occurring three days per week, partially trained participants expending energy at about 400 calories per session may undergo a weight reduction of about seventeen pounds per year as a concomitant benefit of stamina training. Rhythmic, relaxing stamina exercises tend to release muscle tension through motor expression of emotions and to reduce stress stimuli and their unnecessary burden to the heart. Finally, the entire respiratory system is employed in adapting to training. Typically the lungs increase the amount of air inspired and expired at one time (vital capacity) and the amount of air taken in over a period of time (maximum breathing capacity). Efficiency of gaseous exchange in the alveoli and the oxygen-delivery function of the blood are enhanced due to an increase in the number of red blood cells, increase in total blood volume, and better perfusion of the tissues made possible by increased capillary circulation. Togeth-

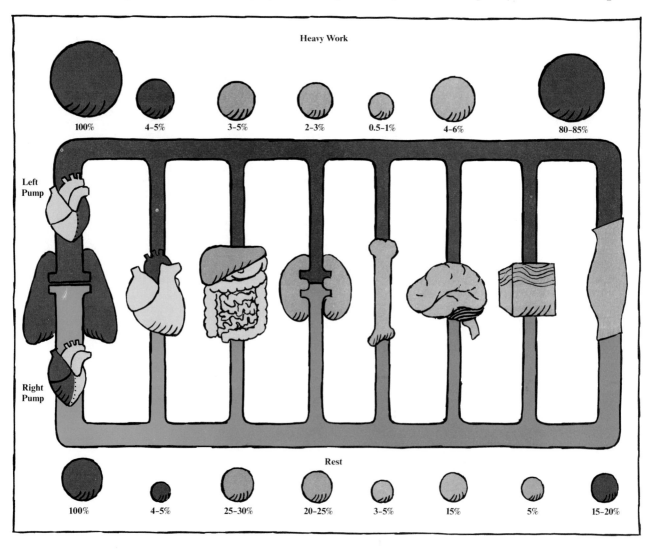

er, the adaptive effects of stamina training build and maintain the complex oxygen-transport system to protect against heart attack.

WHAT EXERCISE AND HOW MUCH?

Exactly how much and what kind of exercise is needed for fitness? Although precise answers to this question depend on individual variations in development, prior fitness, and particular goals sought, useful guidelines have been provided by fitness research and health professionals.

Because strength, suppleness, and stamina and the supporting structures and functions diminish not only with disuse but also at an accelerating rate with age (see Figure 18.7), it is important to continue to move in ways that maintain these capabilities. Resiliency and resistance to injury tend to diminish with age; therefore, exercise of an easy, flowing,

rhythmic nature is required, rather than movement demanding quick bursts of strength, speed or violent effort. Calisthenics should fully stretch the muscles and joints as gently as possible instead of applying powerful, forced stress. Sport and endurance activities in adulthood should be accompanied by a preliminary calisthenic routine to maintain reserve strength and suppleness and to avoid potential injury.

Stamina training is, of course, the most vital form of adult exercise. When properly conducted so as to be individually appropriate, such training is well within the capabilities of all normal adults regardless of age. The major concept of stamina training has been termed "aerobics" by Kenneth H. Cooper, a physician who conducted major research projects in adult fitness for the United States Air Force. *Aerobic* means "with oxygen," or, in this sense, extended exercise in which the oxygen demands of the body are being met by a sufficient delivery. Exercise in which the demand exceeds the supply and produces "oxygen debt" is termed *anaerobic*.

Oxygen is necessary for body cells to extract energy from food and store it in a special, energy-rich phosphate compound called adenosinetriphosphate, or ATP. The breakdown of ATP releases energy for the transport of substances in and out of cells, the synthesis of all the necessary biological chemicals, the complex structural organization of living matter, the maintenance of body heat, the functioning of all organs and systems of the body—including the contraction of the muscles. Truly, oxygen is the breath of life. Life's processes and extended physical work are supported aerobically.

Upon initial demand or when the activity is especially energy demanding (as in sprinting), the availability of oxygen is not sufficient for the requirement. In these instances some additional ener-

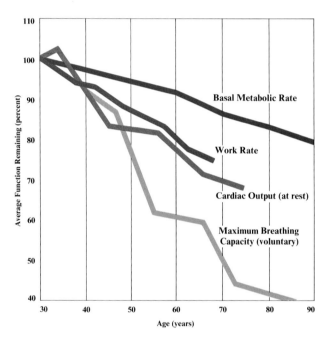

Figure 18.7 (*above*) The percentage of change with age for various physiological functions, based on 100 percent at age thirty. (After "The Physiology of Aging," by Nathan W. Shock, *Scientific American*, January 1962, p. 110. Copyright © 1962 by Scientific American, Inc. All rights reserved.)

Figure 18.6 (*left*) Comparison of cardiac output during rest and during heavy work. Cardiac output may increase as much as five times when changing from rest to strenuous exercise. The figures indicate the relative distribution of blood to the various organs during exercise (*top*) and at rest (*bottom*). Note that the blood goes primarily to the muscles during work while primarily to the digestive and excretory systems during rest. (After Astrand and Rodahl, 1970.)

gy is available anaerobically, that is, without oxygen. This energy is obtained by the splitting of sugar (glucose) and the production of lactic acid in the absence of adequate oxygen. This mechanism is a limited one that brings about the fatigue that everyone has felt at one time or another by overexerting himself. The greater one's aerobic capacity, the more intense the activity that can be supported before anaerobic processes are called upon to supply the energy needs.

Cooper's studies and others have shown that controlled aerobic exercise of sufficient duration and intensity is more comfortable, less hazardous, and produces better results than anaerobic spurts. The minimum duration of aerobic exercise for a "training effect" is about eight minutes. Less exercise than that produces little or no improvement. More exercise than that leads to greater and faster improvement.

The optimum duration for aerobic exercise training has not yet been established, but for normal individuals interested in their general fitness, fifteen to thirty minutes appears to be about right. Progress is slow with less than fifteen minutes of exercise, and more than thirty minutes yields diminishing returns. Endurance athletes in training for competition, of course, may work several hours a day to reach top performance potential.

How frequent should aerobic workouts be? Cooper, building on the work of other exercise physiologists, determined that the positive adaptive effects of an aerobic workout last about two days, after which "detraining" begins. Ideally, then, intervals between workouts should not exceed two days. Another researcher found that three-day-per-week exercise programs resulted in double the progress in a six-month period over two-day-per-week programs. Daily workouts result in the greatest progress, but four days per week appear to be a more realistic optimal frequency.

It has been difficult to determine how strenuous workouts should be to produce optimal results. The use of heart rate is common. W. D. Ross and W. R. Duncan suggest the plan shown in Table 18.2. In this plan, all rates are shown as ten-second values and maximal heart rates are from age estimates. In order to monitor the exercise heart rate, a ten-second pulse count is taken five seconds after ceasing the activity. For the first two to three months the exercise heart-rate range suggested is 65 to 80 percent of maximal. This intensity is a conservative one, determined for novices, and can easily be adjusted if it is warranted by training performance.

In general one should gradually work up to achieve the "brisk" or upper limit of the training range and should continue at this intensity for eight full minutes or longer in order to achieve a training effect. Rest intervals when needed should be somewhat less than the "easy" or lower limit of the training range. Although individual adjustments may be required, the intensity guide serves equally well for men and women.

Table 18.2   Suggested Heart Rates for Stamina Training*

AGE	Heart Rate Max.	0–2 Months Training		3–6 Months Training	
		Easy	Brisk	Easy	Brisk
15	35	23	28	25	30
25	34	22	27	24	29
35	32	21	26	22	27
40	30	20	24	21	26
45	28	19	23	20	24
50	27	18	22	19	23
55	26	17	21	18	22

*beats per ten-second interval

Source: W. D. Ross and W. R. Duncan, "Heart Rate Monitoring," *Fitness for Living* (January/February 1968), p. 52.

TOO MUCH OR TOO LITTLE

When it comes to exercise, Americans tend to do either too much or too little. A man will play football all afternoon with his boys and then get no exercise for the rest of the week. What is essential for lifetime fitness is continuous, regular exercise combining calisthenic effects with stamina training. It requires physical activity several times a week. Such a program is not compatible with sporadic exercise, fitness fads, and the like. A few words of caution about these matters are in order.

One should try to avoid *overexertion*. It does not contribute to overall fitness, because activity is reduced while one is recovering. Injuries may also result either from a mishap because of fatigue or from overworking bones, joints, or muscles. If one begins exercise training gradually and is satisfied with steady though slow progress achievable with the previously outlined principles, the likelihood of overexertion is minimized. Mistakes, however, are possible and the following signs of overexertion may be helpful:

1. Pulse rate not recovered to 120 beats per minute or lower within two minutes of stopping exercise.
2. Subjective feeling of fatigue not passed within ten minutes of stopping workout. (Proper workout should leave one relaxed, refreshed, and pleasantly exhausted rather than deeply fatigued.)
3. Lingering fatigue and difficulty in sleeping.
4. Fatigue the day following a workout.

Any combination of these signs calls for reexamination of one's fitness program and a reduction in strenuousness.

Medical clearance for beginning a fitness program is wise, especially for the inactive or those over thirty-five. A number of medical conditions are aggravated by physical exertion and should be ruled out by a medical examination before an endurance program begins. It is a good idea to plan one's tentative fitness program and present it for approval to a physician who is aware of one's physical condition and past medical history.

Recreational sports require performance that is difficult to control. Hence sports are not as useful for maintaining fitness as calisthenics and endurance training. Few sports provide the continuous rhythmic controlled overload and range of movement called for. Competition is always an invitation to overexertion. Also, most active sports have certain requirements that do not provide regular or frequent enough activity—one has to have a court, for example, or a team for many games. Sports do, however, supplement a controlled fitness program and the "fit" person is likely to enjoy many plus years of sports competence.

Fitness *gadgets and devices* may be useful but certainly are not essential. Weights, springs, and other devices for increasing resistance help build strength beyond minimal levels, but they have limited use in developing endurance. Exercise bicycles and treadmills provide for endurance training but jogging in place is just as helpful. It is to be expected that a consumer-oriented culture would develop consumer products to facilitate fitness, even though, obviously, fitness needs may be met without them.

Fitness fads are rampant, and most are harmful at worst and inadequate at best. Isometrics, which create muscle tension without movement, may build strength, especially in weak individuals. But they do not maintain or improve joint flexibility or maintain endurance. Food-for-fitness fads come and go but the only way to achieve and maintain physical fitness is through appropriate exercise and eating a balanced diet. Seconds-per-day "miracle programs" are widely advertised, but none will work because fitness training requires more time than a few seconds to produce physiological effects. Spot-reducing exercises are useless because one cannot tailor the loss or redistribution of body fat through exercise.

A LIFETIME NEED

The options for individual programs of physical fitness are virtually limitless, even within the guidelines presented in this chapter. Programs should obviously be selected and planned according to individual needs, goals, and levels of fitness. Figure 18.9 provides some basic options designed to meet most contingencies for normal adults.

Functional fitness for living that provides adequate levels of strength, suppleness, and stamina is often gained and maintained by appropriate exercise management. Moreover, the successful resolution of modern stress may be achieved in part through physical recreation. Thus, a primary health and education requisite for modern industrialized man may be the learning of recreational

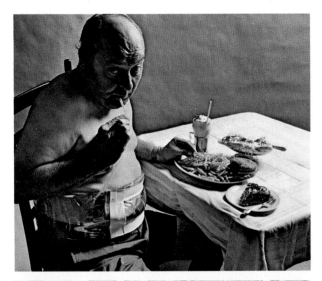

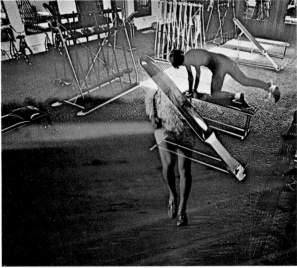

Figure 18.8 Fitness gadgets and devices only work if the individual exercises strenuously while using them. One cannot expect the gadget to automatically make one fit. Fitness devices serve primarily to provide motivation and variety in one's exercise program.

skills and the development of a life-long play attitude. It is not a matter of choosing between exercise and the activities in one's life, as those who claim that they have "no time for exercise" would like to believe. Instead, the fitness benefits of exercise increase one's capacity both to carry out and to enjoy those "other activities." The benefits are twofold. First, if physical fitness adds years to life (and there is some evidence that it does), the time invested is repaid with interest. Second, because physical fitness maintains functional capacities at a high level, health benefits are realized immediately.

There is little evidence in American culture that would lead one to believe that Americans will adopt, en masse, precise fitness programs tailored to individual needs. America's cities, neighborhoods, and predominant life styles exert immense pressures and reinforcement for sedentary living. Still, physical activity is available to those individuals who understand the advantages of appropriate exercise and who believe in its importance. Physical fitness is not a temporary or intermittent need but should continue throughout life. Its substantial benefits are enjoyed most by persons who incorporate appropriate exercise into their life styles.

FATIGUE

Fatigue is quite a complex syndrome with both mental and physical aspects that have baffled experts for years. Fatigue is generally viewed as a symptom, but that "tired feeling" is by far one of the most frequent of health complaints. Although research into the complexities of fatigue is still in its infancy, enough is known today to prevent and deal with much of the suffering and incapacity resulting from fatigue.

Fatigue may be defined as a conscious state of discomfort, accompanied by a desire for rest, a feeling of being unable to carry on, or a feeling of inadequacy to the task ahead, perhaps accompa-

Figure 18.9 (*right*) Individual exercise programs. If you cannot walk for five minutes at a brisk pace, you should begin with the RED program. If you can walk for more than five minutes but less than ten, you should begin with the third week of the RED program. If you can walk for the full ten minutes but are somewhat tired and sore, you should start the WHITE program. The BLUE program is for those who can alternately walk fifty steps and jog fifty steps for ten minutes or more without difficulty. The exercise program consists of three parts: the warm-up, which is very important; the conditioning exercises, which contribute to strength and flexibility; and circulatory activities, which improve the efficiency of the cardiovascular and respiratory systems and increase stamina. This program should be practiced daily or, at a minimum, every other day. If at any time during this program you experience nausea, trembling, extreme breathlessness, pounding in the head, or pain in the chest, stop immediately. If the symptoms persist beyond the point of temporary discomfort, check with your physician.

	Red	White	Blue
Warm-up Exercises			
1. Walk (for 2 minutes at comfortable pace)	X	X	X
2. Side Body Bend	2–5	5–10	10
3. Chest and Shoulder Stretch	2–5	5–10	10–20
4. Head Rotation	2–10	10	10
5. Forward Trunk Bend	2–10	10	10
6. Trunk Rotation	1–4	5–7	8–10
Conditioning Exercises			
1. Leg Raise and Bend	1–4	5–7	8–10
2. Knee Push-up	3–10	———	———
3. Regular Push-up	———	2–8	9+
4. Side Leg Raises	2–6	7–10	11–15
5. Head and Shoulder Curl	2–5	———	———
6. Bent Knee Sit-up	———	2–10	11–25
7. Half Knee Bends	2–5	6–9	10–15
8. Wall Press	2–4	5	5
9. Diver's Stance	Hold 5 secs.	10 secs.	15 secs.

Circulatory Activities

Week	Daily Activity		
1	Walk at brisk pace for 5 minutes, or for a shorter time if you become uncomfortably tired. Walk slowly or rest for 3 minutes. Again walk briskly for 5 minutes, or until you become uncomfortably tired.	Walk at brisk pace for 10 minutes, or for a shorter time if you become uncomfortably tired. Walk slowly or rest for 3 minutes. Again walk briskly for 10 minutes, or until you become uncomfortably tired.	Jog 40 sec. (100 yds.). Walk 1 min. (100 yds.). Repeat 9 times.
2	Same as Week 1, but increase pace as soon as you can walk 5 minutes without soreness or fatigue.	Walk at brisk pace for 15 minutes, or for a shorter time if you become uncomfortably tired. Walk slowly for 3 minutes.	Jog 1 min. (150 yds.). Walk 1 min. (100 yds.). Repeat 8 times.
3	Walk at brisk pace for 8 minutes, or for a shorter time if you become uncomfortably tired. Walk slowly or rest for 3 minutes. Again walk briskly for 8 minutes, or until you become uncomfortably tired.	Jog 10 sec. (25 yds.). Walk 1 min. (100 yds.). Repeat 12 times.	Jog 2 min. (300 yds.). Walk 1 min. (100 yds.). Repeat 6 times.
4	Same as Week 3, but increase pace as soon as you can walk 8 minutes without soreness or fatigue.	Jog 20 sec. (50 yds.). Walk 1 min. (100 yds.). Repeat 12 times.	Jog 4 min. (600 yds.). Walk 1 min. (100 yds.). Repeat 4 times.
5	*When you have completed Week 4 of the RED program, begin at Week 1 of the WHITE program.*	*When you have completed Week 4 of the WHITE program, begin at Week 1 of the BLUE program.*	Jog 6 min. (900 yds.). Walk 1 min. (100 yds.). Repeat 3 times.
6			Jog 8 min. (1200 yds.). Walk 2 min. (200 yds.). Repeat 2 times.
7			Jog 10 min. (1500 yds.). Walk 2 min. (200 yds.). Repeat 2 times.
8			Jog 12 min. (1700 yds.). Walk 2 min. (200 yds.). Repeat 2 times.

nied by a feeling of futility and a need to escape. Fatigue may be physical, mental, acute, chronic, healthy, or pathological.

Physical Fatigue

Fatigue resulting from physical activity, as described earlier in this chapter, involves a build-up of cell waste products. A healthy person feels fatigue as a natural protective mechanism to prevent injury from overexertion and underrest. It is probable that humans, along with other animals, evolved the fatigue syndrome in order to force the rest required for survival.

Normal fatigue is experienced when a healthy organism works a muscle or its whole body intensely and quickly over a prolonged period of time. At first a feeling of discomfort and weakness may be felt in the muscles, speed and precision of movement usually are impaired, and, if the work continues, the muscles may cramp or stop working.

Fatigue also may be perceived in the absence of intense or extended muscular work, such as when one engages in mild movements or holds unusual postures. Simply standing in one place for a period of time can be quite fatiguing to one who is not accustomed to it. Thus, whether one becomes fatigued by a particular activity may depend on the degree to which his body is trained to adapt to the specific activity.

A third cause of normal fatigue is lack of rest and sleep. Although the need for sleep continues to evade research, the prevailing theory holds that a complex neurochemical disorganization, or "fatigue debt," accumulates while one is awake that can be reorganized or "repaid" only when the body processes slow down during sleep.

Normal fatigue is rarely a health problem in routine day-to-day living. When one exercises strenuously, he becomes fatigued and rest restores him. When fatigue comes from unaccustomed activity, one relieves it by ceasing that activity or by repeating it during a period of training until he has adapted. And, obviously, sleep solves the problem of sleep deprivation.

Fatigue is a component of most disease processes. The body recovers more quickly from disease under conditions of rest, rather than continued exertion. Fatigue is not only a symptom of many kinds of illness but a frequent aftermath of acute diseases. Fatigue in such situations often stems from two factors: the disability, which has a metabolic basis, and the patient's depression in not being able to do as much as he wishes.

Mental Fatigue

Everyone has felt tired without having previously overexerted himself. This kind of fatigue is popularly called "mental" fatigue, but it is mental only in the sense that it is produced by intellectual activity. Among the tasks associated with normal mental fatigue are studying, reading, writing, working mathematical problems, working puzzles, and other similar activities. Mental fatigue may also be caused by anticipation of a task that one expects to cause fatigue and frustration.

Emotional disorders can cause a fatigue that is extremely resistant to intervention. For example, the *hypocondriac*, an individual inordinately preoccupied with the functions and malfunctions (real or imagined) of his body, often suffers and exhibits deep fatigue. In *neurasthenia*, another type of emotionally based fatigue, an otherwise normal individual becomes irritable, complains of oppressive fatigue, is unable to perform physical work, and may go to bed and stay there. He also may complain of headaches, backaches, muscle and joint pain, digestive upsets, blurring of vision, and loss of sex drive. When the effects are expressed more in terms of disinterest, intellectual dullness, and lack of ability to concentrate, the condition is called *psychasthenia*.

Figure 18.10 Methods of "sense relaxation." (*left*) After both backs are slapped, the couple stands back to back with eyes closed, and through movement gets to know each other's backs. (*right*) The couple sits on the floor next to one another, knee to knee. They close their eyes and take each other's hands, feeling them, exploring the backs, palms, fingers, wrists. They then explore the forearms, the elbows, the upper arm, and eventually the shoulders, moving over and around. These methods are designed to release tension and to enhance sensitivity, feeling, and awareness. (From Bernard Gunther, *Sense Relaxation.* New York: Macmillan, 1968.)

"Battle fatigue," "soldier's heart," "effort syndrome," and "anxiety neurosis" are additional labels that have been attached to fatigue impairment with presumed emotional bases. The syndrome was referred to as "irritable heart" in the Crimean War and has been studied in all American wars since the Civil War. Typically, the victim, usually under twenty-five years of age, suffers chest pain, palpitation upon physical exertion, shortness of breath, headaches, excess perspiration, and profound fatigue. Experts suggest that the cause of "effort syndrome" is a maladaptation of the victim to demands of his environment. Unable to cope with what is required or expected of him, he "adapts" by withdrawing into illness and fatigue.

Causes of Fatigue

A variety of factors have been implicated in causing fatigue. Seldom is any one of them the only cause; rather, it is a combination of one or more of the causes that results in fatigue. Among these causes are:

1. Prolongation—any task that is greatly prolonged causes physical exhaustion, boredom, or both.
2. Pacing—doing a job at a specific rate or rhythm can be fatiguing, often regardless of the length of task.
3. Unclear goals—tasks in which one does not know whether he is succeeding contribute greatly to the production of fatigue.
4. Remote goals—when one discovers that the end of the task he is to perform is far off, he may experience a letdown and the onset of fatigue.
5. Frustration—when one is constantly blocked in his attempts to achieve goals or complete projects, he is likely to experience fatigue.
6. Limiting conditions—environmental or nutritive conditions that put a limit on vital human processes, and thus limit performance, include temperature extremes, deficits of oxygen, sugar, water, or salt, and excess light or glare.
7. Too exacting demands—any situation in which the demand on specific body mechanisms is too exacting for it to act comfortably or effectively may bring on fatigue.

Overcoming Fatigue

A person may avoid or overcome fatigue by certain forms of physical and mental *stimulation*. Competition and challenge, used in business to encourage greater output, may boost activity—it is easier to complete repetitive activity if one thinks he will get a bonus or earn extra time off, for instance. And almost everyone has experienced the excitement of new stimuli, whether they are sights and sounds or brilliant ideas. Fatigue is diminished or eliminated, even though one may be physically impaired, when one has been "turned on" by a beautiful view, exciting music, or stimulating conversation. In addition, motivation and involvement in the task one must perform serve to reduce the fatigue the task is likely to cause.

Relaxation is another approach to relieving fatigue. Tension, although the individual feels it emotionally, depends largely on actual muscle tension. One may develop skill in relaxing and removing tension by observing several rules and by learning through practice a few simple relaxation techniques. For example, if sedentary activity or emotional stress has produced the tension, physical activity may express and release it—one of the benefits of exercise. Especially useful are rhythmic whole-body movements that place a gentle stretch on tense muscles. Because tension tends to center most uncomfortably in the upper body and neck, rotating the head gently, shrugging and relaxing the shoulders, and rotating the arms at the shoulders are particularly effective. Controlled breathing also facilitates relaxation and is most effective when it is deep, slow, and accompanied by relaxing movements. For example, one inhales deeply as the shoulders are raised slowly; then, as the shoulders are lowered, one exhales slowly, being conscious of "letting go"—relaxing.

Warm baths tend to relax tense muscles. Some forms of massage also are profoundly relaxing.

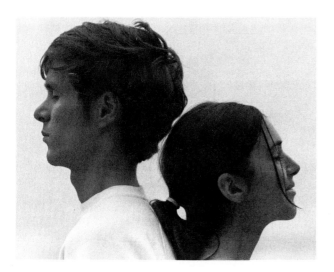

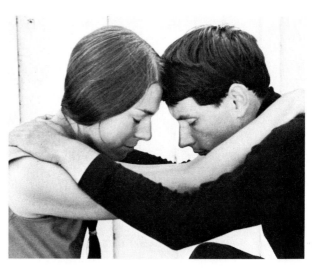

Such massage usually employs long, sweeping hand strokes with palms and fingers pressing gently over the body contours.

Drug solutions to fatigue, such as using coffee, cigarettes, or amphetamines for stimulation or alcohol or barbiturates for relaxation, carry with them complex psychological, physiological, and social implications, many of which were discussed in Unit III. Such solutions may lead to more problems than the original fatigue. Nevertheless, tranquilizers have been used with some success against fatigue, and both smoking and coffee drinking can provide a "break" that helps relieve fatigue.

SLEEP

Researchers who are concerned with understanding fatigue and how to alleviate it sooner or later turn to the study of sleep. Although physiologists can explain the function of various body processes such as breathing, digesting, and sweating, they are unable to explain fully why people should sleep and how they do so. Humans spend more than a third of their lifetimes sleeping, yet the function of sleep as a physiological process remains a mystery.

The focus of investigations on sleep is brain-wave patterns (electroencephalograms, or EEGs), which differ in waking states, sleep, and hypnosis. Sleep is now considered to be as active a state as wakefulness. Each individual appears to have a "signature EEG" during sleep that is consistent from night to night as long as the person is healthy, but it undergoes changes with age.

Instrumental analysis of sleep (by EEG as well as other recording techniques) has shown that there are two kinds of sleep. One of the two is characterized by rapid eye movements (REMs): by waking subjects when REM was observed, researchers found that it is during this period that dreaming occurs. The other type of sleep, the non-REM kind, seems to occur in four distinctive stages recurring several times each night in a pattern. Figure 18.11 outlines what happens at each stage. Prior to the first stage is a period known as the "alpha rhythm," which begins while the person is still awake but has entered a state of complete relaxation. As relaxation deepens, a neural jerk or spasm may interrupt this phase; this spasm is known as a *myoclonic jerk* and is due to a spurt of activity in the brain. The person perceives it as a "falling" feeling or a sudden jerk.

The onset of sleep occurs in the first non-REM stage and deepens through the second, third, and fourth stages, paralleled by corresponding EEG changes. In the first stage, the physiological functions are slowing down, but the person is easily awakened. In the second stage, the eyes usually roll from side to side, but sleep is deep, and if awakened, the individual has no recollection of having had any dreams. Physiological characteristics such as pulse, temperature, and blood pressure are slowed or lowered in stage three, and sleep is deep and calm. Apparently stage four is the period of deepest sleep, although of briefest duration. It is during this period that nightmares and sleepwalking are thought to occur. After stage four the sleeper ascends back through stages three and two and from there enters the REM stage, during which there is vivid dreaming about 85 percent of the time. The REM stage is followed by another cycle of deeper, then lighter sleep stages culminating in a second REM sleep period, and this cycle recurs three to four times during one night. As the night progresses, the REM periods increase in duration and their dreams become more vivid.

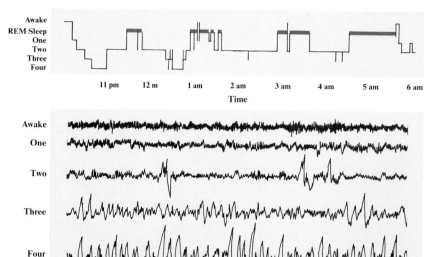

Figure 18.11 (*top line*) A record of one night's sleep. (*bottom*) EEG patterns that occur at each of the stages of sleep and during REM sleep.

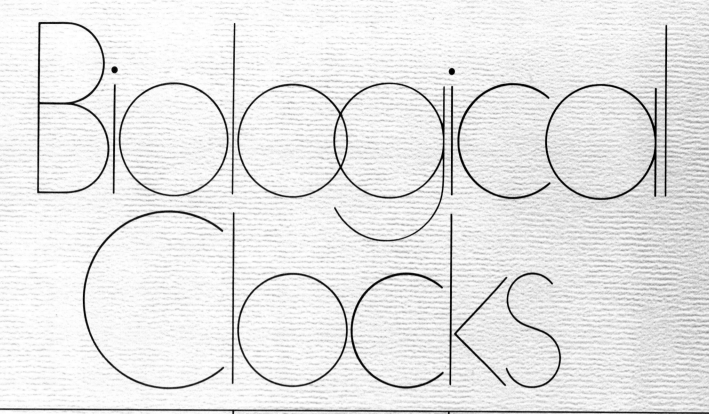

Biological Clocks

by William Barry Furlong

Until recently, man understood little of the body's time clock. He was aware of his physical and neural structure—his nerves, his muscles, the skeletal workings of his fingers and toes. But he was unaware that he was organized in time as well.

Even now, few men are aware of the arcane variety of cycles, ranging in length from microseconds to years, that influence our lives. The body temperature of every individual, for instance, varies rhythmically every day, changing as much as two degrees. So do the heartbeat, respiration, blood pressure, glandular activity, energy level, kidney secretion, and liver action. Without the rhythmic surge of activity in liver and kidney enzymes, we would be poisoned by the food we eat instead of nourished by it.

We know that man's immunity to disease changes according to a daily time clock—the hour at which an infection is incurred may have a significant effect on the intensity of illness. The response to penicillin, antihistamines, even aspirin varies according to the biological time of day at which the medicine is taken.

Man reacts mysteriously to the seasons: Eskimos suffer a winter malady called "arctic hysteria," which appears hormonal in origin. Natives of the temperate zone secrete a mysterious "summer hormone" from the thyroid that tends to reduce body heat. In fact, there is a boundless array of cycles that are important to the behavior of man and his environment.

For example, we know:

That the skin renews itself, especially between midnight and 4 a.m.

That the body's temperature is higher on the left side during sleep, is higher on the right side during wakefulness.

That we sleep in cycles of 90 minutes.

That our senses of taste, smell, and sight are at their keenest around 7 p.m. and again around 2 or 3 a.m.

That people with ulcers and certain psychoses suffer more in the spring than at any other time of year.

That our livers are early risers: They reach a peak of metabolic activity just before or just after we get up in the morning.

That epileptic seizures take place from 10 p.m. to 11 p.m. more often than at any other hour of the day.

That the male sex hormone reaches its peak activity in the early morning.

That insulin administered at 4 a.m. or 4 p.m. has a greater effect on diabetics than an identical dose given at any other time.

That an injection of house dust under an allergy patient's skin raises a greater welt after an 11 p.m. treatment than an injection at any other hour.

That we use our nostrils rhythmically and alternately: Normally we breathe mostly through one nostril while the other is engorged with tissue, then after three hours we switch and breathe predominantly through the other.

The impact of these cycles is personal and unremitting. The pace of modern life has put more stress on man's body clock than ever before. In the last few years man has become aware of the "jet-plane" syndrome. That is the way in which a person's body clock is thrown out of kilter after he passes swiftly through a number of time zones.

The traveler who takes a jet across the country, or across the oceans, frequently lands at his destination feeling irritable and out of sorts. He is terribly fatigued when the sun is at its zenith; he is terribly hungry at 3 a.m. and he cannot excrete his body wastes at the accustomed times. His judgment and alertness decline so much that the U.S. government and many large corporations suggest that their key men leave on trips twenty-four hours early so they can get a complete rest after a long jet flight. These employers feel that reducing the chance of a blunder due to the jet-plane syndrome is more valuable than the cost of a day's rest.

Many airline flight crews display a significant drop in efficiency as they try to defy their body clocks. Studies by the Aerospace Medical School of the U.S. Air Force showed that pilot-performance dropped as much as 50 percent when the pilots were asked to work against the rhythms of their body clocks.

The Russians are so sensitive to flight error due to out-of-phase schedules that they are rumored to lodge crews on the Moscow-to-Havana flight—who pass through nine time zones—at a hotel in Havana that is run on Moscow time. Reportedly, the shades are pulled to simulate midnight at three in the afternoon, and breakfast is served at 11 p.m., because that's wake-up time in Moscow.

Understanding man's biological time clock may be as important to society as to the individual. The safety of individuals within society often depends on people who work at night—police, fire, hospital personnel, even truck drivers. Yet few night-workers are selected on the basis that they are most competent during night hours. The opposite is likely to be true—so true that many night-workers are given the chance to rotate back to the day shift after a number of weeks or months. The arbitrary selection of night-workers unquestionably tends to work against safety and efficiency.

There are other times when adjusting to the biological rhythm of the individual is literally a matter of life and death. Surgery is one of them. As surgery becomes more sophisticated, it may rely more heavily on understanding the body clock. For example, should the different heartbeat rhythms of the individual be taken into account before attempting a heart transplant? What is the impact of a donor's heart—whose owner is dead but whose biological rhythm may live on in the pulsing heart—when it is asked, in a highly traumatic circumstance, to adjust to an entirely different biological rhythm?

Should the different excretory rhythms of the kidneys be matched in a kidney transplant? Chemicals are secreted by the kidneys with certain individual rhythms. It may be that the body clock of the recipient has been adjusted through a lifetime of kidney cycles to need the excretion of those chemicals at a certain hour; the question is whether the rhythm of the donor's kidney can meet that need.

Should surgery be scheduled to catch both the doctor and the patient at their physiological peaks? Why schedule surgery for early morning when the surgeon may not achieve the top of his circadian rhythm (from circa dies—"about the day"), with its peak of concentration and competence, until late evening?

Similarly, the arbitrary scheduling of surgery may catch the patient when all of his physiological systems are sinking to the nadir of his daily cycle. It seems wiser to schedule the trauma of surgery at that time when the patient's respiration, pulse, and other physiological rhythms are surging upward rather than sinking. The timing of the surgery can improve the performance of his body during and after the trauma. Ultimately it might be possible to match the body clock of the patient with that of the surgeon.

Beyond this, the mysterious workings of man's time-mechanism affect virtually every phase of modern medicine. A patient's biological rhythms create changes in his body temperature, pulse, and blood pressure. In diagnosis, a circadian rise in temperature might be mistaken for a low-grade fever, particularly if the temperature is taken regularly at the same biological time of day. Even a biopsy must be examined in the light of the time at which it was taken: Cell division reaches its peak according to individual cycles.

A perceptible change in known body rhythms can be of profound help in discerning certain illnesses. In many cancer victims, body temperature fluctuates wildly instead of in a strong daily rhythm. Laboratory studies under Dr. Franz Halberg of the University of Minnesota Medical School suggest that many cancers might be detected in their earliest stages, long before other more recognizable physical symptoms, through certain erratic cell behavior at the surface of the body. (One exception: Breast cancers maintain a daily rhythm of cell division.)

In the use of drugs, the biological time of day for treatment may be as important as the dosage. Doctor Halberg found that the death rate in mice (which have a metabolism akin to that of humans)—ranged from 5 percent to 76 percent, depending on what biological time of day an anesthetic called halothane was administered. Another test disclosed that an amphetamine administered in rats in the middle of their activity cycle killed 77.6 percent of them. But only 6 percent died if the drug was administered at the end of their activity period.

At the Children's Asthma Research Institute and Hospital in Denver, it was discovered that treatment with adrenal hormones at 1 a.m. and 7 a.m. benefited patients more than treatment at any other time. Adrenal hormones, used to relieve asthma symptoms, have an unfortunate side effect—they tend to retard growth and delay maturation. Through proper timing, they might be used to achieve the greatest medical good with the smallest side effect.

Daily rhythms change perceptibly in disturbed persons. Chronically depressed persons, for instance, adopt aberrant rhythms in their sleep—light sleep at first, hours of lying awake, with deep sleep coming in the early morning just before they get up (roughly the opposite of the normal sleep pattern)—and in the secretion of certain chemicals in their blood and urine.

These changes in emotionally disturbed patients are so great that Dr. William Bunney Jr. of the National Institute of Mental Health has begun using aberrant levels of adrenal hormones in the blood and urine to measure stress and to try to predict suicides among the disturbed.

The timing mechanism also suggests dramatic new ways to treat emotional disturbances. At the Institute of Living in Hartford, Connecticut, Dr. Charles F. Stroebel found that the most successful way to extinguish certain anxiety emotions from laboratory animals is to administer treatment at exactly the same time of day that the animal received the emotional impression.

The basic need is to determine the pattern of individual body rhythms. In the past, that has not been convenient. To make even the most primary "map" of the body's energy-cycle, a series of rectal readings of body temperature would have to be made at intervals of an hour or less. Further measurement of physiological cycles involving the heartbeat, respiration, blood pressure, and skin conductivity would demand hospitalization, a controlled environment, and medical attention for several days.

Today there are more sophisticated techniques close at hand. It is possible to design biotelemetric instruments—akin to those used on astronauts during space flights—that will relay changes in a person's body temperature, pulse, respiration, skin conductivity, and other functions to a remote computer without continually intruding on the awareness of the individual. Through such instrumentation, patterns or "maps" of an individual's body rhythms could be produced. These might become an important and permanent part of his medical record.

Through such maps, the physician of the future may discern changes in an individual's rhythms that predict disease at its earliest stages. The doctor also might use the maps to make treatment more effective by scheduling therapy for that biological time of day that is best suited for a particular patient.

Researchers are seeking ways to alter the body clock—to "set" it at will. The Russians have experimented with electrical stimulation of the brain in efforts to change certain rhythms.

At the School of Medicine in Lyon, France, investigators have used monoamine oxidase inhibitors, mood-elevating drugs sometimes prescribed for treatment of the depressed, to shift the daily activity-rest cycle in rats so that the laboratory animals need less sleep. Ultimately, they hope to extend the circadian cycles of activity-rest in humans from twenty-four hours to forty-eight hours or even seventy-two hours, thus altering the need for sleep within the cycle.

As our knowledge increases, the concept that there is a single "master clock" regulating all the body's rhythms has tended to lose favor. It seems that there are many cycles affecting many systems.

Discovering the variety of biological rhythms has taken many years and vast effort. Identifying the nature and subtle workings of the body clock promises to be difficult. But once their meanings have been discerned, many of the imperative questions of medicine and psychiatry might be answered.

Various experiments in which subjects have been kept awake for long periods show that a number of processes become distorted with lack of sleep. Perception becomes markedly abnormal. A sleep-deprived person often tells of "hearing" or "seeing" things. The subjects also become paranoid and feel that people are plotting against them.

Insomnia is the label loosely applied to inability to sleep. Judging from the magnitude of advertising for proprietary sleeping drugs and the mounting statistics on barbiturate addiction, insomnia would seem to be prevalent and growing. It is not unreasonable, however, to presume that sleeping-pill advertising in fact reinforces through suggestion both inability to sleep and drug solutions to the problem.

There are effective ways to deal with lack of sleep in one's life without worry or drugs. First, it is useful to understand that human needs for sleep vary with individuals and within individuals from time to time. By and large, one sleeps naturally when and as much as he needs to, if the environmental conditions are not too discouraging. Comfort and quiet are thought to be prerequisites for adequate sleep, but these values are relative. Individuals and cultures seem to adapt to most environmental circumstances and learn to live (or sleep) with them. For many years, for example, apartment dwellers along the route of the elevated train in New York City were jostled every twenty minutes or so by the vibration and the screeching, clanking noises of the train, yet they slept well.

When the train system was demolished, several thousand persons along the route were reported to have awakened a couple of times per hour asking, "What was that?" for several days following the demolition.

Constant, regular, or familiar noise seems generally to be less inhibiting of sleep than irregular, unfamiliar noise. As urban and suburban environments have become noisier, many people have turned to the use of "white noise" to mask out the unwanted noise during sleep. White noise is pleasant, constant, and controlled, usually similar to the sound of rushing air or a waterfall. Electric fans, room humidifiers, or other sound-making devices are sold especially for this purpose.

Exercise and sleep are closely interrelated. Sleep is facilitated by relaxation, relaxation is largely a muscular phenomenon, and exercised muscles relax more readily. Intense stress from unaccustomed exhausting exercise may disturb the homeostatic balance of the system and inhibit sleep, but regular exercise that leaves one comfortably tired facilitates normal sleep.

Both trouble in sleeping and fatigue are largely problems of one's life style. They can be affected by diet, exercise, emotional stress, and the management of living within environments often hostile to human needs. Solutions to problems of fatigue and "insomnia" can be quite complex, but they necessarily involve both individual choices in modifying behavior and the reorganization of environments to reinforce those choices.

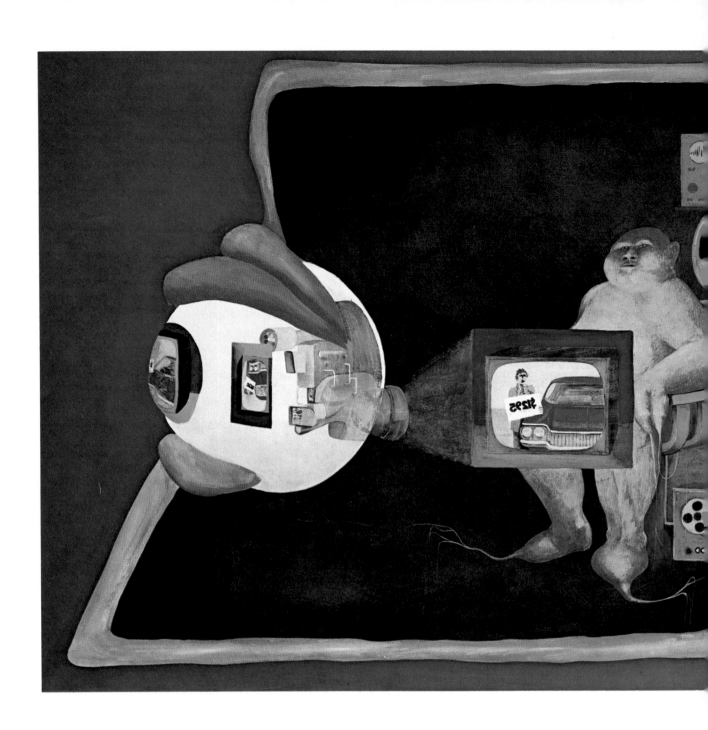

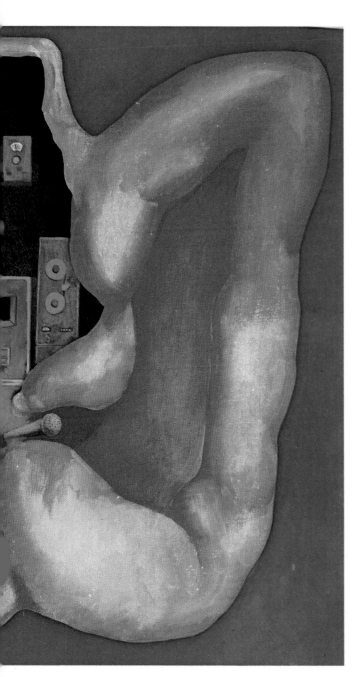

19

Man "perceives" the world largely through his senses—his eyes provide him with sight, his ears with hearing, his tongue with taste, his skin with touch, his nose with smell. If one or more of these vital receptors is disabled or malfunctioning, man can make adjustments. A deaf person sees lips that he reads; a blind man develops an acute sense of hearing and touch, which helps make up for his lack of vision; but if *all* of the senses were disabled or blocked, man would be forced to exist in a state of solitary confinement, with thought as his only release. This chapter will focus on two vital senses, the eyes and ears, as representative of the sensory system.

THE EYES

What is involved in "seeing" something? Through vision one can sense the color, the shape, the texture, the size, and the distance of an object, as well as its location in relation to other objects. The eye also can be selective—focusing on one object and blurring or blotting out others, and it can be integrative—noting objects only when they move. The eye provides the brain with all kinds of visual cues, so that the brain can construct an image of the physical world.

Structure and Function

The eye is a sphere, almost one inch in diameter, whose structure is shown in Figure 19.1. The outer layer of the eye is a white, glassy structure called

The Eyes and Ears

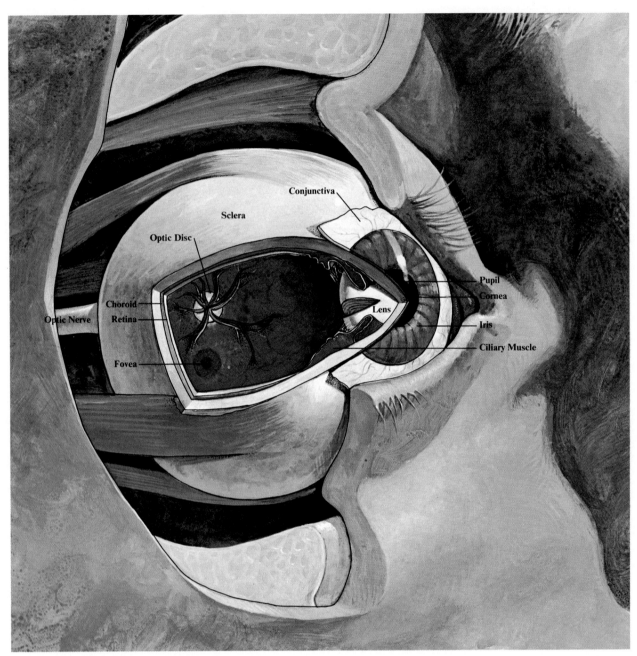

Figure 19.1 The eye. (*above*) A three-dimensional presentation. Note the thickness of the clear outer cornea. (*left*) A cross section, showing the various fluid-filled chambers of the eye.

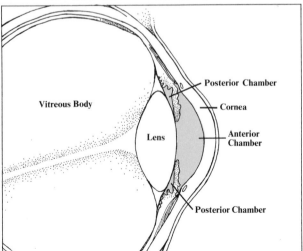

the *sclera* (the "white of the eye"), whose anterior portion is modified to provide a transparent window, or *cornea*. Inside the sclera runs a pigmented layer, the *choroid*, which contains most of the blood vessels nourishing the eye. The choroid also provides specialized structures in its anterior region. Foremost is the opaque *iris*, which contains the pigments responsible for eye color and which encircles a round aperture, or *pupil*, whose diameter contracts or expands under the action of two sets of antagonistic muscles in the iris. Posterior to the iris, the choroid thickens into the *ciliary body*, which contains the *ciliary muscles* and to which is attached a circular *lens ligament* (or zonula) holding in place the lens (see below). The entire inner face of the choroid and its derived structures is coated by the third layer of the eye, the *pigmented retina*; the portion posterior to the ciliary body has, in addition, an innermost layer known as the *neural retina*.

The *lens* is a transparent, elastic, circular, biconvex structure, suspended from the lens ligament of the ciliary body, right behind the iris and pupil. It consists of transparent fibers that increase in number as a person gets older, the newer fibers being laid down in a fashion similar to the annual deposit of rings on a tree. The shape of the lens can be altered by the contraction of the ciliary muscles transmitted to the lens margin by the lens ligament.

The lens divides the inside of the eyeball into two main fluid-filled compartments. The space between the front of the lens and the back of the cornea, the *antechamber*, or *anterior chamber*, and the space between the lens and iris, called the *posterior chamber*, are filled with a transparent fluid called the *aqueous humor*, which is continually secreted by the ciliary body. Because it is mandatory for the pressure within the anterior chamber to remain constant, comparable amounts of fluid must leak out through what is known as the *canal of Schlemm*, located laterally between the anterior margins of

sclera and choroid. When this canal gets plugged, the pressure within the anterior chamber increases, causing the condition known as glaucoma, which will be discussed later. The major portion of the eye interior, between the back of the lens and the retina, is called the *vitreous body* and is filled with a gelatinous, semisolid fluid called the *vitreous humor*.

The *neural retina* is the light-sensitive component of the eye. It is a highly complex structure comprising ten distinct layers, the major components of which are the *photoreceptor cells*, the *bipolar cells*, and the *ganglion cells*. The photoreceptor cell layer is the farthest back from the incoming light, running directly against the pigmented retina. It consists of specialized elements: the *cones* (some 7 million of them) that respond to bright light and color, and the *rods* (about 125 million) that respond to low-intensity light, such as twilight illumination. The axons of cones and rods synapse with the processes of the bipolar cells, located in a more forward layer, and the bipolar cells in turn synapse with the large, multipolar ganglion cells, whose layer is closest to the incoming light. The axons of the ganglion cells converge toward the center of the retina, cross its posterior layers, and emerge from the back of the eyeball bundled up into the *optic nerve* that connects the neural retina to the *visual portions of the brain* (see Figure 19.2).

Only a small portion of the eyeball is visible from the outside, namely the cornea with its transition into the sclera and—through the corneal window—the iris-surrounded pupil. The eye is well protected from injury by a number of structures and mechanisms: the bony walls of the *orbit* in which it is encased; the *eyelids* with their complement of eyelashes; the thin transparent membrane, or *conjunctiva*, that forms the inner surface of the eyelids and curves out to cover the exposed portions of the eye (cornea and anterior part of the sclera); the secretion from the *lacrimal* or *tear glands* (located in the upper region of the orbit), which flows over the cornea to keep it moist and clear and empties via the lacrimal sac and the naso-lacrimal duct into the nasal cavity. The eyeball can move within the orbit through the action of six ocular muscles that impart to the eye lateral, medial, upward, downward, and oblique rotations.

The eye is much more complex than a camera, but functions similarly. A beam of light enters the eye through the transparent cornea, traverses the transparent aqueous humor of the anterior chamber, passes through the hole of the pupil (whose aperture is regulated much like a camera diaphragm), and reaches the lens. It then goes through the transparent lens, where it is bent, and continues through the transparent vitreous humor and the foremost layers of the neural retina to finally focus on the photoreceptor cell layer. The photoreceptor retinal layer is analogous with the film in a camera. It receives the image and through nerve impulses conveys the visual pattern along the optic nerve to the visual centers of the brain, where the neural signals are integrated into vision.

Problems in Vision

Visual acuity is usually tested by reading letters of differing sizes on a chart. If a person has 20/20 vision, it means that he is able to see clearly at twenty feet the letters that the designer of the chart defined as normally visible at twenty feet. If one has 20/40 vision, it means that he sees well at twenty feet or less what he should be able to see at forty feet. Similarly, 20/200 vision means seeing at twenty feet or less what a normal eye can see at 200 feet.

Abnormal vision—sight that is not 20/20—is usually due to *refractive* errors, such as nearsightedness and farsightedness. Such errors may result from inheritance of an eyeball that is deviant in size or shape.

Professionals who deal with eye problems and corrective lenses include ophthalmologists, oculists, optometrists, and opticians. The role each of these persons plays in eye care is outlined in Table 19.1.

NEARSIGHTEDNESS The eyeball of a nearsighted, or *myopic*, person is elongated from front to back, so that distant sources of light tend to form their

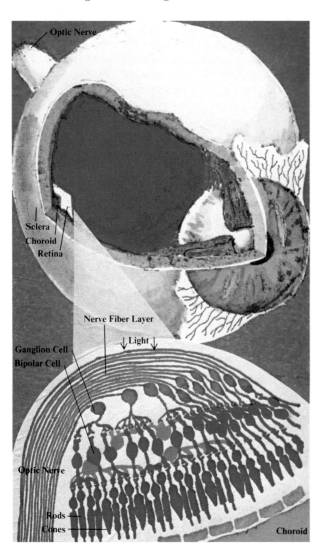

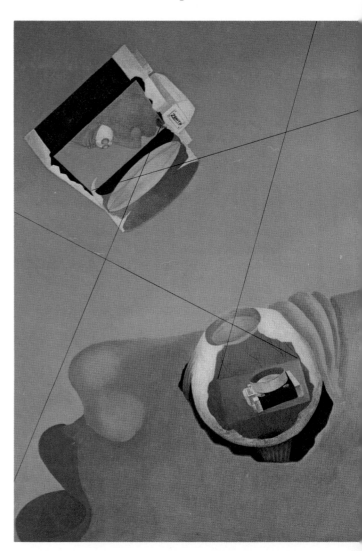

focal images in front of the retina rather than on it (see Figure 19.4). As a result, distant objects are blurred. The eye sees objects closer than twenty feet more clearly because their images are focused further back from the lens and therefore closer to or on the retina. A biconcave lens corrects myopia by spreading the parallel rays of light from distant objects further apart before they enter the lens, thereby permitting it to converge the rays to a focal point on the retina.

FARSIGHTEDNESS   The shape of the farsighted, or *hyperopic*, eye is opposite to that of nearsightedness. The farsighted eye is shorter than normal from front to back, so that parallel rays of light entering the eye tend to focus at a point beyond the retina (see Figure 19.4), because the eye lens cannot bend them inward enough. The more divergent the incoming rays (the closer the object), the greater the convergence necessary to focus them on the retina. A convex lens helps correct the condition by bringing the rays closer together before entering the eye, reducing the converging effort required of the eye lens. The hyperopic eye does not necessarily see distant objects clearly—it just sees them *more* clearly than near objects, and with less effort.

A hyperopic person under the age of forty-five can try to change the shape of his lens by performing eye exercises that will make the lens more convex. Such eye exercises take advantage of the process known as *accommodation*. Accommodation is the ability to control contraction of the ciliary muscles. Contraction of the muscles pulls the choroid forward, releases the tension of the lens ligament, and makes the lens bulge in the center, thus helping the eye to focus on near objects. Relaxation of the muscles aids the eye in distant focusing. When the ciliary muscles become fatigued, the person experiences "eye strain." In the hyperopic person, the ciliary muscles are constantly contracted in an effort to accommodate, hence eye strain occurs.

PRESBYOPIA   As a person ages, the eye lens loses some of its elasticity and no longer responds with adequate bulging to the contractions of the ciliary muscles. The resulting reduction in the ability of the eye to accommodate is called presbyopia. Many people who have no refractive errors in their vision become subject to presbyopia around age forty-five or older and frequently need biconvex eyeglasses for close vision, although their vision is normal for distant objects.

Table 19.1   Eye Doctors and Technicians

TITLE	*Requirements*	*Role*
Ophthalmologist or oculist	M.D. plus internship and 3 years additional study in eye diseases; must pass American Board examination	Diagnosis and treatment of diseases of the eye, including prescribing eyeglasses
Optometrist	Not an M.D.; usually has 2 years of college plus 3–4 years of training leading to Doctor of Optometry (O.D.); state board examination	Not licensed to care for diseases; measures refractive errors and eye-muscle disturbances, which he can treat with eyeglasses and eye exercises
Optician	Must have license in most states; must have training in grinding and preparation of lenses, usually on-the-job	Makes eyeglasses or contact lenses on prescription by ophthalmologist, oculist, or optometrist; fits and adjusts finished glasses; helps in selection of frames

Figure 19.2   (*left*) A schematic representation of the retina in cross section. The light does not immediately affect the receptor cells—it must first pass through the nerve fibers and blood vessels. At almost the last layer of the retina lie the rods and cones, the highly specialized cells containing pigments that, upon the absorption of light, undergo chemical changes that result in electrical neural impulses. The cones, which are thicker than the rods, generally connect with a single *bipolar* cell located in the next neural layer. Several rods share a single bipolar cell, which may send branches to cones as well. A second synapse in the retina occurs between the bipolar cells and the *ganglion* cells, whose axons are the fibers of the optic nerve. These fibers all collect at the *blind spot*, where they exit in a bundle.

Figure 19.3   (*right*) The functioning of the eye in many ways can be compared to that of a camera.

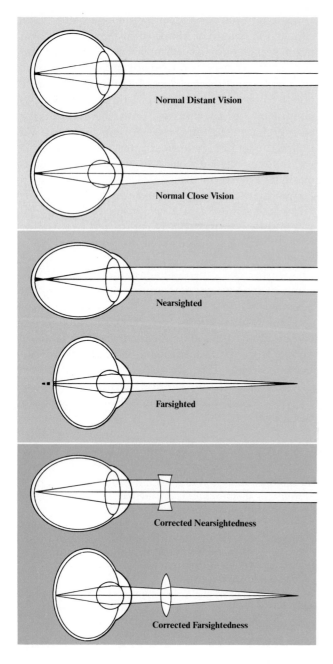

ASTIGMATISM Astigmatism is the result of a cornea that is curved unevenly. With this situation, rays of light entering the eye come to different focal points, resulting in blurred vision. A severe degree of astigmatism may be very disturbing and cause fatigue and chronic headaches. Astigmatism cannot be corrected simply with concave or convex lenses but must be compensated for with specially ground lenses. A person who is myopic or hyperopic and also astigmatic must wear lenses with a double correction.

CATARACTS Although the eye lens is normally transparent, aging sometimes causes a gradual development of opacity or cloudiness in one or both lenses. Senile cataract, as this disease is called, is thought to be inherited.

Once the cloudiness develops, there is no known way to reverse the process. The disease is usually allowed to progress until vision is seriously impeded. A cataract operation in which the lens is totally removed can then be carried out. An eyeglass lens is subsequently used to substitute for the natural lens. However, because accommodation cannot take place, adaptability is severely impaired.

GLAUCOMA Build-up of pressure in the anterior chamber of the eye is known as *glaucoma*. If untreated, glaucoma can eventually lead to blindness. Unfortunately, in some forms of the disease pressure increases so slowly that irreversible damage can be done before symptoms are severe enough to cause the victim to seek treatment.

Glaucoma also appears in an acute form that is characterized by abrupt onset of pain, perception of halos around light sources, and vomiting. If not treated immediately, acute glaucoma can cause blindness within days.

Tests for glaucoma are easily made in a doctor's office by measuring the degree of intraocular pres-

Figure 19.4   How light is focused on the retina and how the lens accommodates under normal vision, myopia, hyperopia, and corrective lenses.

sure with a small instrument (tonometer) placed over the cornea. Physicians recommend that this routine examination be carried out annually.

RETINAL ABNORMALITIES   A number of retinal abnormalities can affect vision. For instance, if the retina becomes partially detached, vision is impaired; if it is totally detached, blindness results. Surgery is required to correct this condition. Another retinal disorder is night blindness, usually caused by a deficiency of vitamin A. Vitamin A is necessary for the manufacture of rhodopsin, or visual purple, which is the material in the rod cells that allows one to see in dim light. Ingestion of vitamin A easily corrects the condition.

COLOR BLINDNESS   Color blindness in most cases is a sex-linked hereditary defect of the cone cells (see Chapter 14). About 8 percent of the male population has the defect, compared to .5 percent of the female population. The most common type of color blindness is an inability to distinguish red from green. Less common is confusion of other color pairs. Total color blindness, in which the individual perceives only black, white, and shades of gray, is extremely rare.

Contact Lenses

Contact lenses are usually circular bits of plastic, ground both to correct refractive errors and to fit the individual eye, that are held on the cornea primarily by the force of surface tension. Although most such lenses worn today cover only the cornea, scleral lenses are available that seem to be more advantageous in certain cases.

While regular eyeglasses act to change light refraction before it reaches the eye's surface in order to compensate for errors in the eye, contact lenses are designed to change the refractive power of the eye at its corneal surface. Contact lenses usually give the wearer a more natural picture of the world than do glasses, which tend to give the myopic person a smaller than normal image and the hyperopic person a larger than normal image.

Because the contact lens is a foreign body being introduced directly onto the eye, the healthy eye

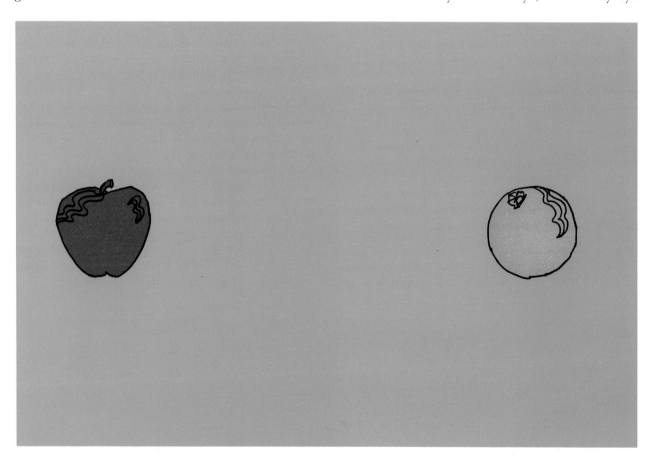

Figure 19.5   The blind spot. Closing your left eye, hold the book out at arm's length, focusing your right eye on the apple. As you pull the book toward you, the orange should disappear. The disappearance is due the the light rays falling on the head of the optic nerve, where there are no light-sensitive cells.

naturally tries to eliminate it. Thus contact-lens wearers must go through an adaptation process that may take as long as twelve weeks.

The primary motivation for wearing contact lenses is a cosmetic one—many people feel that eyeglasses detract from their appearance. In addition, contact lenses are extremely helpful to persons suffering from certain conditions, including extreme myopia and irregularities in the cornea.

The contact-lens wearer must be highly motivated, however, because of the disadvantages of the lenses. Among these problems are the high cost (150 to 300 dollars); the fact that they are easily lost or broken; the need for meticulous care; sensitivity to eye irritation such as from wind, dust, or air pollution; the danger to the eyes when improperly worn; and the need for a regular wearing schedule—sleeping with lenses on or wearing them too long may result in serious corneal abrasions.

Some people who desire to wear contact lenses are unable to because of conditions such as allergy, diabetes, anemia, use of certain medications, or working situations that would make wearing of lenses more harmful than helpful to the eye.

"Soft" lenses are now available that are less abrasive to the cornea and that allow eye tissue to "breathe" more freely because the lenses are permeable to oxygen and tears. However, soft lenses are more difficult to insert and remove than the conventional type and are more easily damaged.

THE EARS

The sensitivity of the human ear is truly amazing. It can distinguish about 1,600 different frequencies (from a low of 20 cycles per second to a high of 20,000) and about 350 different intensities, from soft to loud. But hearing is not the only function of the ear—it also controls equilibrium, or balance.

Structure and Function

The ear is divided into three main parts, as shown in Figure 19.7. The external and middle sections function solely for hearing; the inner ear has a dual role, functioning in part as a hearing organ and in part as the organ of balance.

THE EXTERNAL EAR   The *conchus*, or visible portion of the ear, functions to collect sound waves and funnel them internally through the large external auditory canal to the eardrum (the *tympanic membrane*), which separates external and middle ears. Sound waves strike the drum and cause it to vibrate.

The auditory canal is coated with wax secreted by the cells lining the canal. This wax protects the underlying skin from drying and scaling. Normally, just enough wax is produced to adequately coat the canal. Occasionally an excessive amount of wax accumulates and obstructs the canal, thereby preventing sound waves from impinging on the taut membrane of the drum.

THE MIDDLE EAR   The middle ear is a small cavity containing three little bones (or ossicles)—the *malleus*, the *incus*, and the *stapes*—intricately articulated with one another. The vibrating eardrum, in response to sound waves, sets up movements in the three bones, arranged in a chain behind it. The extent to which the ossicle articulation is sensitive to the vibratory eardrum depends on the state of contraction of two muscles, which are under reflex control. This "attenuation reflex" allows the ear to tolerate sounds of different intensities. The stapes, which is the smallest bone in the body, is the last to receive the auditory signal. It then taps its message through the *oval window* that separates the middle ear from the inner ear.

A delicate balance of pressure must be maintained between the air outside and inside the eardrum. The healthy ear maintains this pressure by means of the *eustachian tube*, which links the middle ear to the throat, opening and closing by means of the muscles of the palate when one swallows or yawns. The eustachian tube also serves to drain secretions that accumulate in the middle ear.

Figure 19.6   The contact lens fits over the iris. Between the lens and the eye is a tear layer that allows the eye to receive necessary oxygen and cleansing.

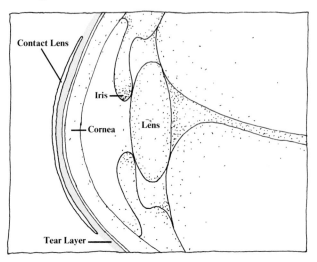

Contact Lens

Iris

Cornea

Lens

Tear Layer

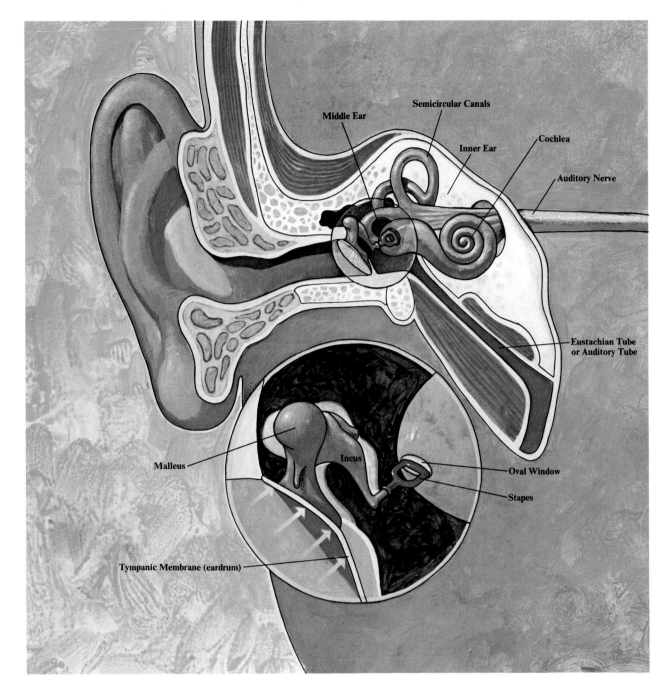

Figure 19.7   Ear structure and function.

If pressure in the middle ear is lower than the outside pressure, the drum is sucked inward, causing considerable pain. Similarly, if the pressure in the middle ear is greater than outside pressure, the drum is stretched in the opposite direction, also causing pain. Any condition that occludes the opening of the eustachian canal, such as colds, allergies, or infected adenoids, will result in pressure differences between the middle and outer ear.

Vigorous nose blowing or holding one's nose when sneezing can force bacteria into the eustachian tube and can result in infection of the middle ear. Infection also can occur if the air space of the middle ear becomes moist due to eustachian canal blockage, so that surfaces of the middle ear serve as a breeding ground for bacteria. Middle-ear infection, known as *otitis media*, can be acute or chronic. Acute otitis media is usually accompanied by build-up of pus. If pressures in the middle ear become great enough, the eardrum may perforate, allowing the pus to drain out. If not adequately treated, the infection may persist, becoming chronic and causing hearing loss.

THE INNER EAR The inner ear (or *labyrinth*) is essentially a fluid-filled, compartmentalized chamber containing two structures side by side. Sound-wave reception is carried out in a spiral-shaped structure known as the *cochlea*, while the function of equilibrium is carried out in a structure called the *vestibular apparatus.*

The vestibular apparatus, shown in Figure 19.8, consists of three semicircular canals (oriented at right angles to one another) and the vestibular *utricle* (through which their fluids communicate). These structures contain delicate nerve fibers that are stimulated by the movement of the fluid (*endolymph*) inside the canals each time the head moves. These nerve fibers are connected to the brain and thus relay to it information regarding

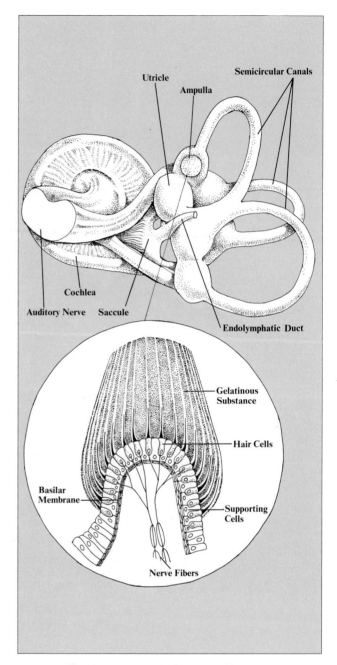

Figure 19.8 The vestibular apparatus of the inner ear. Movement affects the endolymph, which in turn bends the hair cells. These cells synapse with the bipolar cells of the vestibular nerve.

such movements as turning and bending. Any impairment of the functioning of this apparatus leads to dizziness, and if severe enough, to nausea and vomiting.

The second part of the inner ear, or cochlea, is concerned with hearing. The space inside the cochlea is divided into three portions by two membranes, the *Reissner* (or vestibular) and the *basilar* membranes. All three portions run the whole spiral length of the cochlea, hence their name of *scala* (ramp) *vestibuli* (between bone and vestibular membrane), *scala media* (between the vestibular and basilar membranes), and *scala tympani* (between basilar membrane and bone). The two outer ramps communicate with each other at the tip of the cochlea and are filled with a fluid called *perilymph*. The scala media is filled with endolymph, continuous with that of the vestibular apparatus.

When the sound vibration moves the stapes against the oval window, waves of movement are generated in the perilymph of the scala vestibuli (whose base lies at the oval window), propagate to the perilymph of the scala tympani, and dissipate on a mucous membrane at its base, or round window. During their travel along the scala tympani, the waves set into vibration the *basilar membrane*, located between the scala tympani and the scala media. Anchored to the basilar membrane, on the scala media side, is the *organ of Corti*, the specialized receptor organ for hearing. This tiny structure contains thousands of sensory receptor cells each with many delicate hairs (or *hair cells*). It is the movement of the basilar membrane that activates these hair cells and causes them to fire *bipolar neurons* connected to them. The neural impulses in these neurons are then relayed through their axons—the *auditory nerve*—to the auditory parts of the brain. Thus the initial sound waves in the air are converted into fluid waves that in turn are converted into electrical impulses perceivable to the brain.

Hearing Losses

It is estimated that about 3 million persons in the United States have major hearing losses. Because little routine testing of hearing is done, many children have undiscovered hearing defects. At times, such children may even be regarded as mentally retarded. The earlier that hearing defects are discovered, the greater the likelihood of their being corrected.

Professional attention to hearing disability can frequently lead to a marked improvement in the hearing abilities of persons of all age groups. If the defect itself cannot be repaired through treatment, it often can be compensated for by means of a wide variety of sophisticated electronic devices now being manufactured.

CONDUCTION LOSSES Anything that interferes with the transmission of sound waves through the external and middle ears is regarded as producing a conduction loss. Conduction losses can be due to either mechanical impediments or disease processes. If a large plug of wax occludes the auditory canal, sound waves cannot be propagated beyond the block, and a conduction loss occurs. It is easily

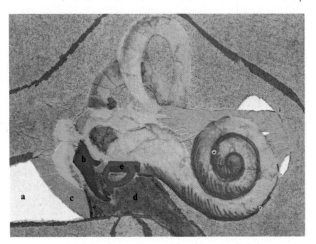

Figure 19.9 Sites of conduction hearing losses: (a) wax may occlude the ear canal; (b) there may be a congenital malformation of one of the bones of the middle ear; (c) the eardrum may rupture; (d) changes in pressure may occur as the result of a blocked eustachian tube; (e) otosclerosis may deposit calcium on bones, preventing them from vibrating.

treatable through removal of the impediment. Not so simple to treat, however, is a congenital malformation, for example, of one of the bones in the middle ear chain.

Disease processes also can lead to conduction losses. A *ruptured eardrum*, for example, may cause major or minor hearing loss, depending on the size of the lesion. A small rupture of the eardrum usually will heal. But if the rupture is extensive and does not heal, surgery can repair the defect. Changes in pressure due to blockage of the eustachian canal, discussed earlier, also produces a conduction defect, although it usually is a temporary one.

Otosclerosis is a common disease causing loss of hearing through conduction. It is characterized by deposition of new bone or calcium-containing materials on the bony elements responsible for sound transmission. If the addition is slight, there may be no noticeable effect on hearing. If the deposit is considerable, the stapes becomes immobilized and is unable to move in response to sound waves, thereby preventing them from being conveyed to the inner ear. The cause of otosclerosis is unknown, but it appears more frequently in women and it seems to have some hereditary basis. New surgical techniques are able to correct this problem in a large percentage of cases.

SENSORINEURAL LOSSES Conduction defects result ultimately from mechanical interference with the progression of sound waves as they are transmitted into the inner ear. Once in the cochlea, where wave patterns are converted into nerve impulses, which are relayed to the brain, interference with auditory transmission is known as sensorineural hearing loss. Although surgery can be successful in treating mechanical defects, it is unsuccessful at treating the nerve-type hearing loss of sensorineural defects.

There are many causes of this type of hearing loss, ranging from physical damage to the cochlea or the auditory nerve as a result of injury to the head, through tumors that interfere with the functioning of the auditory nerve, to overuse by sensitive individuals of certain medications such as aspirin, quinine, or streptomycin, which may induce toxic degeneration of the auditory nerve. Less common causes of deafness are mumps, measles, Ménière's disease (primarily affecting equilibrium, secondarily hearing), and atherosclerosis, which limits the blood supply and leads to tissue death.

Presbycusis, deafness in the elderly, is estimated to account for 16 percent of all deafness. It is a particularly frustrating disorder because the person claims he can hear and indeed he can. He complains, however, that he cannot *understand* the words that are spoken. People with presbycusis lose the ability to hear high-pitched sounds. As a result they can hear *speech*, which consists of both low-pitched and high-pitched sounds, but the *words* they hear are distorted because they cannot hear the upper-range sounds. Unfortunately, there is no medical or surgical treatment for this problem, although hearing aids are sometimes helpful.

Noise pollution also can lead to deafness. Increasing numbers of bus drivers, taxi drivers, road builders, traffic policemen, musicians, and workers in noisy factories are subject to progressive hearing losses. Post-mortem examinations of the ears of such people indicate that the cochlea is frequently broken as the result of excessive vibrations generated by loud noise. This kind of defect also leads to the loss of ability to hear high-pitched tones. In theory, the quieter one's environment, the less hearing loss he will suffer in time.

CENTRAL HEARING LOSS Because the transmission of sound must be relayed to the auditory centers of

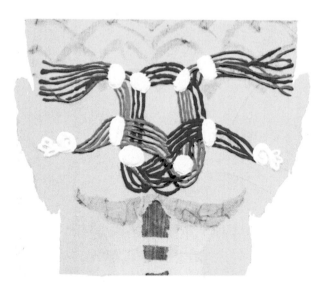

Figure 19.10 Sensorineural losses are caused by injury to or degeneration of the auditory nerve. Central hearing loss is due to interference with the functioning of brain centers involved in hearing.

the brain for hearing to occur, any interference with the functioning of the brain regions involved in hearing also will lead to deafness. Thus, such problems as brain injury, tumors, and strokes can result in hearing impairment.

Hearing Tests and Aids

Hearing losses frequently occur gradually and often go unnoticed until a considerable disability is manifested. Thus many processes that could have been treated and reversed in their early stages are allowed to become permanent and irreversible. If a hearing loss is discovered, the defect can usually be at least partly corrected either through medical treatment, surgery, or a hearing aid.

Tuning forks and audiometers are the principal "machines" for measuring hearing losses. The tuning fork can distinguish between a conduction defect and a sensorineural defect. The audiometer, a more complicated instrument that actually measures the intensity of sound, detects the degree as well as the type of hearing loss.

When medical and surgical treatment cannot bring improvement, hearing aids frequently can. Hearing aids are electronic devices consisting of a microphone to pick up the sound wave, an amplifier to increase the intensity of the sound, and a speaker. The microphone converts the sound wave to electrical current just as the organ of Corti converts waves to neural impulses; the amplifier increases the intensity of this electrical current, and the speaker converts the electrical current back to sound again. The aid is powered by small, electronic batteries. A plastic plug fits into the canal of the external ear and directs sound inward. The hearing aid has a volume control and some have a tone control. It can amplify sounds between 300 cycles per second and 3300 cycles per second—a range approximately between middle C on the piano and four octaves above.

Like corrective lenses, hearing aids can make up for sensory deficiencies but they can never totally replace the organs they are aiding. Sight and hearing will always be man's most precious senses and deserve all the care he can give them.

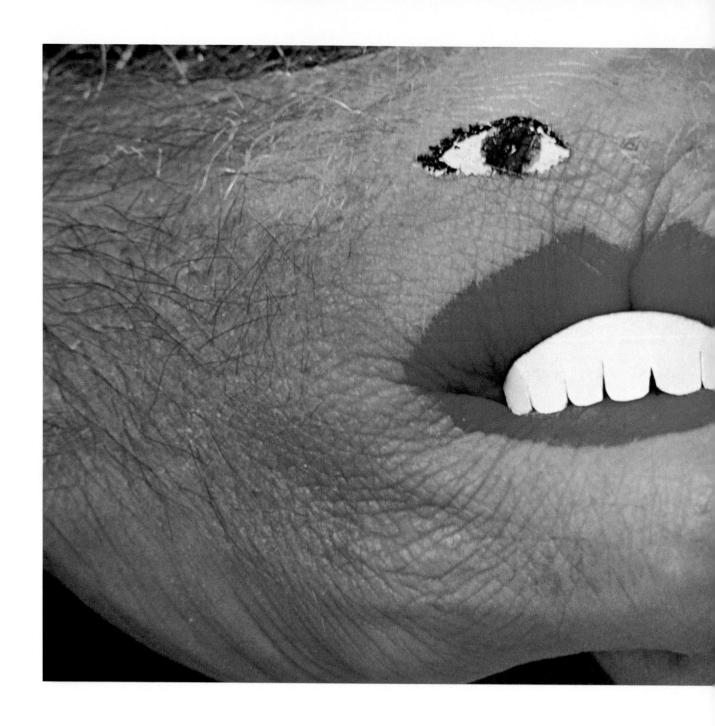

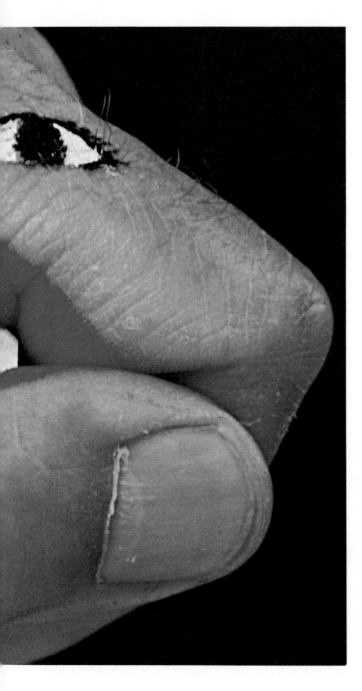

20

Among the traditional outward signs of health are bright, sparkling teeth, rosy complexion, and shining hair. These aspects of appearance have perhaps been overemphasized by advertisements for cosmetics, deodorants, suntan lotions, mouthwashes, toothpastes, hair dyes, shampoos, and numerous other products designed to create an appearance of health.

If one begins to investigate advertising promises in light of what is known about the body, he will find that most such products are unnecessary for his well-being and in some cases may even be harmful. Germ-killing mouthwashes may destroy beneficial bacteria in the mouth, upsetting its ecological balance; toothpastes that contain abrasives may hurt teeth more than they help; some hair preparations may cause hair to become brittle and break. Furthermore, many such products are used to cover up or hide problems that need professional attention—mouthwashes cannot cure pyorrhea, a disease that causes mouth odor and that if untreated, can do untold damage in the mouth. It is therefore important to understand how such structures as the teeth, skin, and hair function, how they can malfunction, and how they can best be cared for.

THE TEETH AND SUPPORTING STRUCTURES

The mouth and its various structures form a remarkably complex and essential organ system, responsible for evaluating, manipulating, masticating,

The Teeth, Skin, and Hair

and swallowing food. The mouth is amazingly resilient—it is exposed to temperature extremes ranging from iced drinks to scalding coffee; it is continually being dried by air and remoistened by saliva; and it frequently harbors dental restorations of varying plastic and metallic materials, some of which, when bathed in the electrolytic saliva, often produce electric current. In addition, the mouth ecosystem normally comprises more than eighty varieties of microorganisms.

The teeth are the largest single factor in the health and appearance of the mouth and face. Well-cared-for teeth contribute to the maintenance of a youthful and vital appearance. Unchecked dental disease leads to facial deformities, mouth odors, skin wrinkles, and premature signs of aging. People often view the loss of teeth as the loss of youth—to many people the construction of dentures represents the advent of old age. Yet with proper methods of oral hygiene and with quality dental care, teeth should virtually never be lost. Considering the advantages of being able to eat every kind of food (which the denture wearer can-

not do), enjoying good appearance, and being free of dental-related disorders, it is the wise individual who, early in life, makes a commitment to the health of his teeth.

Structure and Function

Man gets two sets of natural teeth during his lifetime: the primary or *deciduous* teeth and the permanent or *succedaneous* teeth. The deciduous teeth, popularly known as "baby" teeth, are much smaller and lighter in color than their successors. Many parents are startled by the first appearance of their child's permanent front teeth, which are three times as large and considerably darker and yellower than the tiny, blue-white primary incisors they are replacing.

The formation of the primary teeth in the embryo begins as early as the seventh week of pregnancy. For this reason fluoride pills or fluoridated water is often administered to women early in pregnancy so that the teeth being formed can have the cavity-inhibiting benefit that fluoride affords.

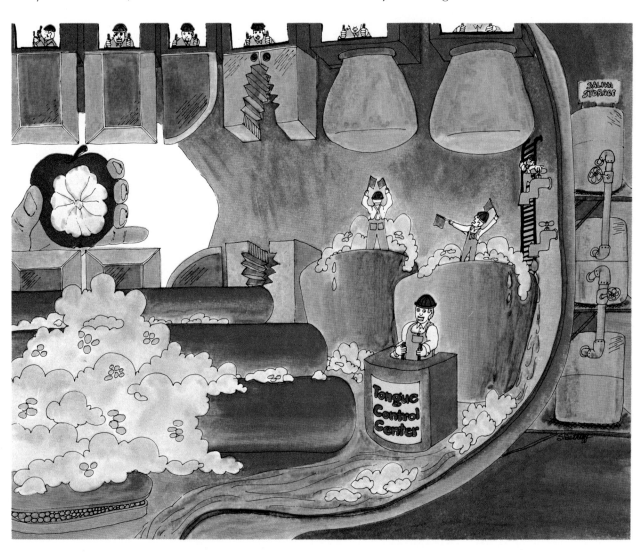

The first teeth to come through the gums usually appear at about six months of age. The chronological development of a tooth can be summed up as follows: tooth-bud formation, beginning of crown formation, completion of crown, beginning of root formation, eruption of tooth, completion of root. It is important to notice that it is an incomplete tooth that erupts—the root is not completed for some time afterward.

In addition to chewing food, the baby teeth also guide the development of the jaws and help to maintain sufficient space for the eruption of the permanent teeth. A baby tooth that is prematurely lost can no longer serve this function because adjacent teeth may crowd into the gap. The consequences can be serious: the tooth may be prevented from erupting at all, it may erupt in the wrong location, or it may be forced out of line, causing crowding and possibly a general deformation, which is a major problem requiring orthodontic repair (braces).

Because the developing teeth serve to guide the development of the jaws and profile, irregularities can lead to profile distortions. The personality development of an individual is profoundly affected by personal appearance. This fact alone should resolve any doubts about the need to care for a child's teeth from their first appearance.

In the mouth, *saliva* lubricates food, begins the digestive breakdown of starches, neutralizes strong acids and bases, and is a natural disinfectant. Even the gaping hole in bone and tissue left by an extraction rarely gets infected, which is remarkable considering the huge population of microorganisms normally present in the mouth.

The *periodontium*, the area immediately around the teeth, is comprised of the *gingivae*, or *gums*, the *periodontal ligament*, and the *alveolar jawbone*, which are the supporting structures of the teeth. The al-veolar bone is unique among body bone tissue; it can change its shape by the processes of resorption and rebuilding. These properties of the alveolar bone allow for a child's teeth to erupt through the bone and gums and develop normally; they are also responsible for the lateral movement of adjacent teeth when a tooth has been extracted and not replaced; for the damage inflicted by an irregularity in the way the teeth come together when biting (malocclusion); and for the tissue destruction of periodontal disease.

The tooth itself is divided into two major parts (see Figure 20.3): the *root*, set inside the bone beneath the gum, and the *crown*, visible above the gum. Inside the tooth is a soft, blood-filled, highly sensitive tissue called the *pulp*, which performs several defensive functions for the living tooth. The pulp is sometimes called the "nerve"; however, it is not a nerve but a very sensitive living tissue. The pulp is entirely enclosed by the hard inner walls of the tooth in the pulp canal, or root canal. When the pulp becomes inflamed due to caries (cavities), periodontal disease, or physical trauma, an excruciating toothache can result because the pulp cannot expand within the inflexible walls of the tooth, causing tremendous pressure. Often in such cases the dentist must drill into the pulp canal to release the pressure caused by the inflamed tissue.

Surrounding the pulp is the inner layer of the tooth, called *dentin*. Covering the dentin in the root area of the tooth is a substance somewhat related to bone called *cementum*. Covering the visible part of the tooth (the crown), is *enamel*. Tooth enamel is extremely dense and strong and is the second-hardest naturally occurring substance in nature—only diamond is harder. This hardness is necessary considering the chewing, grinding, and gnashing actions of the teeth. It is paradoxical that such a hard substance should be such easy prey to decay.

Figure 20.1 (*left*) A mechanistic overview of the functions of the mouth, as seen from the inside of the mouth of a person eating an apple. The front teeth act as chisels, chopping up food, while the side teeth work like mortars to grind the food. The cylinderlike tongue kneads and pushes the food against the roof of the mouth. On the right are the salivary glands, which secrete the saliva that helps to break down the starches and liquify the food.

Figure 20.2 (*right*) The right side of the skull of a seven-and-one-half-year-old showing the developing dentition. (a) Permanent centrals and laterals and (b) permanent first molars are erupted and in place. (c) Deciduous canines and (d) molars still in place will in a few years be replaced by (e) the permanent canines and (f) premolars seen developing within the jawbones. As these tooth buds develop and move mouthward they cause progressive resorption of the roots of the baby teeth, which they will eventually replace.

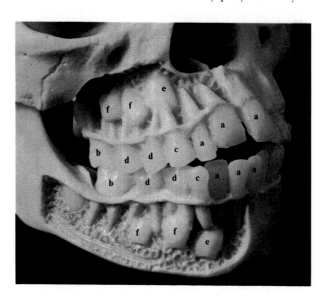

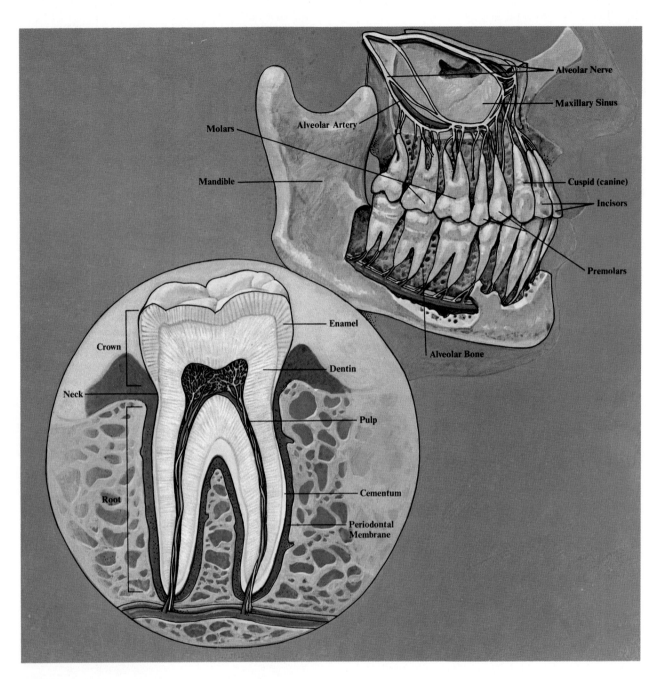

Figure 20.3 The supporting structure of the teeth, with a close-up of a tooth.

Major Dental Diseases

DENTAL CARIES   Although little is known about the exact causes of decay, much is known concerning its progress and prevention. Decay progresses at different rates—in some mouths a small cavity will show no change for years, yet in others an identical cavity may reach serious proportions in a matter of months. No doubt mouth chemistry and composition of the saliva (both factors affected by oral hygiene) play an important role in these differences. To give an oversimplified example, if one's saliva tends to be acidic, decay will probably occur more rapidly. People whose saliva tends to be less acidic are more resistant to decay but are more prone to formation of the white, crusty material called calculus and resultant periodontal disease.

A viscous, sticky saliva retains food in the mouth and aids in forming whitish food residues called *materia alba*. This residue adheres to the necks of teeth and to the gum margins and is a factor in the formation of *plaque*, a composite of debris on the surface of the tooth (see Figure 20.4). On the other hand, a serous, watery saliva tends to wash away food debris and thus to lower the incidence of dental caries.

Diet is another important factor in decay, but surprisingly, once the teeth are formed, nutrition is not. The typical American diet, high in refined carbohydrates, is highly conducive to caries. Sugars, sweets, and pastries form the tacky food residues that are hard to remove from the teeth and gums, and they contribute to the formation of materia alba and plaque, which accelerate the cariogenic process. It is the food remaining *in the mouth* and not the food in the stomach that is dangerous—prompt and thorough oral hygiene procedures after eating can theoretically reduce if not eliminate the caries-producing activity of the diet. Lack of oral hygiene and improper dental treatment, not poor nutrition, are to blame for decayed teeth. Nutrition can play a part in other mouth disorders such as periodontal disease, however.

Habits of good oral hygiene (proper brushing or rinsing after each meal) are difficult enough for adults to establish; for the child they are doubly difficult. Not only does the child lack the dexterity to properly brush his teeth, but such skill would be virtually useless to the typical young "continuous eater." Parents should not only instruct their small children in the brushing technique, but should strive to break the pattern of continuous eating. In particular, children should not be given candies such as lollipops that produce a sugary acid component that remains in the saliva for a long time.

The role of heredity in dental disease is not understood. Despite seemingly inherited bad gums or proneness to decay, neglect and poor quality dentistry are the leading causes of bad teeth. Experience does indicate that some mouths are more prone to decay than others, but not because of "soft teeth." People who believe they have "soft teeth" (there is no such thing) often despair of their chances to keep their teeth. This despair usually reflects poor oral hygiene, dental neglect, or experience with poor quality dentistry. With good home care and the conscientious application of the principles of modern dentistry, no one should lose teeth, "soft teeth" notwithstanding.

Another old-wives' tale that has been perpetuated is that during pregnancy a woman's teeth are weakened. If the mother's diet is deficient in calcium, the calcium requirements of the embryo will indeed be met first. The mother may lose some calcium from her bones, but not from her teeth. It is possible, however, that some pregnant women (particularly in their first pregnancy) are so concerned with the changes taking place in their bodies that they tend to neglect their oral hygiene and therefore cavities result. In other cases it may be coincidence: the age at which a woman is likely

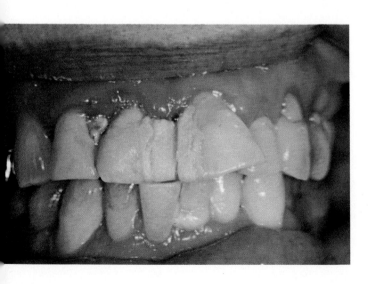

Figure 20.4   The unaesthetic, malodorous, and unhealthy effects of poor oral hygiene. These teeth bear a conglomerate of oral debris, plaque, and calculus, which are the major causes of dental disease. Gums are discolored, puffy, and oozing blood and pus.

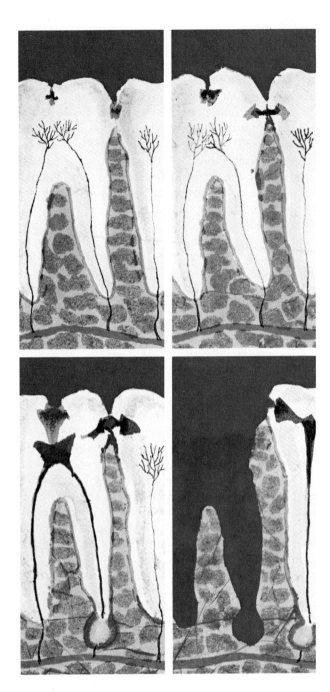

to be pregnant coincides with the time that neglected teeth begin to be extracted. In any case, this complaint is never heard from mothers who had practiced good oral hygiene and received competent dental care before, during, and after pregnancy.

PERIODONTAL DISEASE   The other major disease involving the teeth is periodontal disease, which affects the supporting structures of the teeth: the gums, periodontal ligament, and the alveolar bone. Periodontal disease, also called "pyorrhea," is the single most important cause of lost teeth. Like any chronic infectious condition, periodontal disease is uncomfortable, unaesthetic, and damaging to the individual's general health and sense of well-being. In advanced stages the gums may be festering, red, spongy, tender, and oozing pus that is swallowed with every meal. The mouth feels generally uncomfortable—the gums feel tight, weak, and tender, and a highly offensive breath is common. Many people go through life with such discomfort, ending in the loss of their teeth, never knowing the relief that can be obtained by proper and timely periodontal treatment.

Calculus, plaque, oral debris, and their associated irritants are the major factors involved in periodontal disease, but they are not the only factors. Irregularities in occlusion (the way the teeth come together when biting) can set up stresses to particular teeth that can weaken their support and cause periodontal damage. The deformations of the dental arch resulting from extractions and the subsequent shifting in position of the remaining teeth can result in periodontal damage, which is a prime reason why teeth should not be extracted or, if the extraction has already been done, why the tooth should be promptly replaced.

Facial-muscular habits, such as a tongue thrust, can produce periodontal damage, as can the tension-induced habit of grinding the teeth. Systemic conditions, metabolic disorders such as diabetes,

Figure 20.5   An extreme example of the tooth-decay mechanism. A small cavity becomes larger, eventually attacking the dentin and the pulp. An abscess forms, and the tooth finally becomes so ravaged by decay that it must be removed.

and defective circulation can complicate the periodontal situation. The caries-producing diet can be equally implicated in the cause of periodontal disease. Perhaps poor oral hygiene is the most important cause, leading to accumulations of oral debris and the consequent formation of calculus and plaque. The progress of periodontal disease often follows the course illustrated in Figure 20.6.

The presence and progress of periodontal disease also can be contributed to by a dentist who fails to perform thorough preventive calculus removal, neglects to instruct his patients in the correct methods of oral hygiene, and who, when decay does appear, fails to properly restore the teeth. If he is not the cause, the poor dentist can certainly be an accomplice in the disease process.

Treatment of periodontal disease includes thorough removal of calculus by scaling, the reshaping of teeth in the case of malocclusion, splinting of weak teeth to strong teeth if necessary, analysis and attempted correction of damaging habits, surgical correction of tissue defects if necessary, and, most important, the institution of meticulous oral hygiene techniques by the patient.

Restorative Dental Procedures

Restoring the teeth to proper form and function is a difficult and delicate job. The problems of restoring a tooth can be exceedingly complex, but even if nothing more than a root stump remains, most of the time a tooth can be restored. There are rare occasions, however, when so little of the root is left that the tooth must be extracted. In such cases the restorative problem involves replacing the missing tooth. If the decay has infected the pulp, root-canal procedures will be necessary. If the tooth has been much ravaged by decay, a major restoration such as a full crown may be necessary, although for most carious lesions the most common dental restoration, the filling, is the treatment of choice.

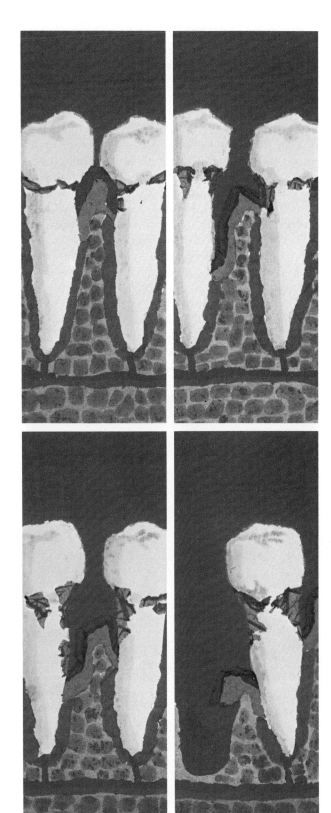

Figure 20.6 Periodontal disease. First tartar forms about the necks of the teeth and at the gum line. The tartar works its way deeper into the gum crevices, carrying with it debris and dental plaque, which act as chemical and mechanical irritants to the tissues. The periodontal tissue breaks down due to this irritation. The gingival tissues become inflamed and prone to hemorrhage; the fibers of the periodontal ligament are progressively destroyed to the point where it no longer is able to support the tooth. The tooth becomes loose and eventually must be removed.

The "simple" filling is actually quite a complex procedure that requires careful attention to a number of detailed steps, which are necessary to remove decay, minimize its chance of occurrence, and engineer a restoration that will be strong enough to withstand the powerful chewing forces without breaking or falling out. Aside from patient neglect, the most common cause of failure of fillings is the dentist who does not spend enough time on the many details of proper filling procedure. Because of its strength and durability, silver amalgam, an alloy formed by dissolving powdered silver and other elements in mercury, is the most common material used in filling teeth.

An *inlay* is a filling made outside of the mouth from measurements of the tooth and then cemented into place. Gold inlays, properly done, are excellent restorations and can be used for certain extensive restorative problems in which the properties of silver amalgam are inadequate.

For restoring front teeth, aesthetic considerations become important and compromises have to be made with respect to materials used—gold or silver is unsuitable for use in front teeth where the results will be visible. Synthetic materials such as cements, plastics, and composites are used for frontal fillings. These materials often are referred to collectively as "porcelain" fillings, but they are not porcelain—a material that must be fired and glazed at temperatures upward of 1,000 degrees and therefore cannot be made in the mouth. Recently, composite materials of plastics with glass and polycarbonate fillers have been developed. These materials offer some improvements but still fall far short of the desirable properties of metal fillings and are not satisfactory restorations for the back teeth.

The *crown* is a major dental restoration used when the tooth has been so badly ravaged by decay that there is not enough tooth structure left to support a filling or an inlay. The crown (known to the layman by the incorrect term "cap") replaces and completely covers the natural crown of the tooth and requires bulk removal of tooth structure in its preparation. Depending on its location, a crown can be covered with a gold, plastic, or porcelain veneer. Crowns can be reinforced when there is nothing left of the tooth but the root; in such cases the root canal is used for anchorage of the crown.

When the pulp within the tooth becomes infected or degenerates, severe pain, along with abscess or cyst formation, usually results. Although many dental practitioners rely on the extraction, the proper treatment is root-canal therapy (illustrated in Figure 20.8), which can save nearly any tooth.

Dental Prosthetics

The field of *dental prosthetics* concerns itself with the replacement of missing teeth. The best way to replace a missing tooth is with a fixed bridge, thus called because it "bridges" the gap between two teeth. The fixed bridge is cemented in place and is not removed, unlike the removable bridge, which is

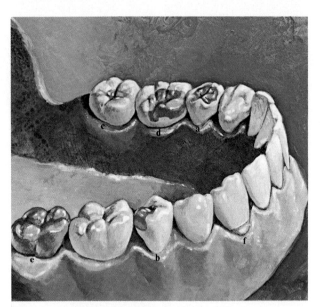

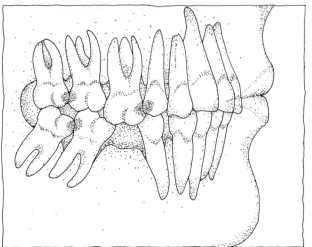

Figure 20.7 (*top*) Dental restorations. Various materials are used in restoring the teeth; the choice depends upon both functional and aesthetic considerations. Silver amalgam is suitable for most back-tooth restorations. (a) One-surface and (b) two-surface silver amalgam fillings. If decay has ravaged an extensive amount of the tooth, gold inlays (c, d) are used. Occasionally, so much of the tooth is destroyed that a full crown (e) must be used. With anterior teeth, aesthetic considerations demand restorations that can be blended to match tooth color. For this purpose, restorations of silicate cement or newly developed composite plastic materials (f) should be used. (*bottom*) What happens when a missing tooth is not replaced. The remaining teeth tend to drift into the empty space, and the opposing tooth, having nothing to bite against, starts to move out of its socket.

The Dr. Poorwork Affair

by Paul Revere

The typical dental patient would be shocked to learn that he might be getting less than a high level of care from his dentist. Yet the quality of dental service in America varies from excellent to disgraceful. Moreover, it is difficult to impossible for an uninformed layman to tell the difference—and the difference is important. A patient who receives good care has an excellent chance of keeping his teeth and maintaining good oral health indefinitely, while the patient who receives poor dentistry has little chance of doing either.

Organized dentistry has only recently begun to give attention to this question of quality, and no reliable statistics have yet been developed to tell how much of American dentistry is good and how much is substandard. My own estimate, based on observations as a practicing dentist and communication with dentists from all over the country, is that too many Americans have had dental work that falls so far short of minimum standards as to be disgraceful. A great many dentists routinely treat diseased teeth in such a manner that it is highly probable their patients will later suffer infection and loss of teeth. Yet all of these licensed dentists have proved their ability to practice good dentistry by passing rigorous dental school and state board licensing examinations. How, then, does one account for so much substandard dentistry?

The basic reason is economic. The dentist who tries to maintain high quality in a neighborhood accustomed to poor dentistry often finds himself at a powerful economic disadvantage. Suppose you live in a working-class neighborhood of apartments and private homes and are trying to decide between two local dentists. By inquiring you find out that although both men are licensed, experienced dentists, one man charges more, takes longer to do most procedures, and, especially with new patients, tends to prescribe a great deal of work. The other dentist charges less, works quickly, and seems to be more popular, because his waiting room is usually full. Which dentist would you choose?

But there are other, more important facts about these two dentists that would surely affect your choice if you knew them but that you are unlikely ever to learn. Patients of the less-expensive dentist, let's call him Dr. Poorwork, usually have increasing troubles with their teeth and finally lose them, while the patients of Dr. Goodwork have relatively trouble-free mouths and keep their teeth. Moreover, the patients of Dr. Goodwork are usually faced with less dental expense in the long run than the patients of Dr. Poorwork, who pay more and more as they gradually lose their teeth. These facts are unavailable to patients in general because Dr. Poorwork will not tell you, and Dr. Goodwork, restrained by the archaic code of ethics of dentistry, is not permitted to. Under this

Adapted from Revere, P. *Dentistry and Its Victims.* New York: St. Martin's Press, 1970.

code Dr. Goodwork may claim that his own work is good, but he must not even hint that Dr. Poorwork's care has been substandard.

It is a fact that good dentistry takes time and care, and the results are worth it. A "simple" silver filling, upon analysis, is revealed to be an intricate procedure involving many steps, inattention to any of which results in a tooth likely to give trouble. But, because dentists have been traditionally compensated on a fee-for-unit-service basis, Dr. Poorwork soon discovers that the less time he spends on any particular service, the more fees he can collect, and the temptation to cut corners to accelerate production can become irresistible. In a neighborhood where the Poorwork tradition is entrenched, where patients want dentistry that is fast, cheap, and painless, and where people are accustomed to accept the gradual loss of teeth as inevitable, it is most difficult for a dentist to strive for high ideals of practice. And the code of "ethics" completely protects Dr. Poorwork.

Although there is no foolproof method of finding good dental care, there are a number of steps you can take that will considerably increase your chances of finding a good dentist. One way is to contact a local dental school for a referral to a faculty member (Dr. Poorwork is rarely associated with a dental school). Whichever dentist you consider, try to talk with some of his patients. Make sure that the dentist schedules patients for a specific time and then allots sufficient time for proper treatment. Be wary of a crowded waiting room, which too often means the dentist's time is being spread too thinly. Beware of the factory-style office, where a patient goes from the x-ray technician to the hygienist to the cashier in rapid succession, with just a brief stopover with the dentist.

Beware of a dentist who enjoys a reputation for "painless" extractions. The extraction of a tooth is probably the easiest job in dentistry, involving the least skill and intelligence. With proper anesthesia, all extractions are painless. The good dentist does not enjoy a reputation as a fine extractor, because he rarely is called upon to pull a tooth. He may be equally or more skilled in extractions than Dr. Poorwork, but most of his patients will never get the opportunity to evaluate this skill, while extractions are always prominent in any discussion concerning Dr. Poorwork.

The type of initial examination can provide considerable insight into the expected quality of care. The examination should include full mouth x-rays and a careful clinical check with eyes, instruments, and fingers, and, for the more complex cases, study impressions. The dentist should then take time to explain your condition and his planned treatment. If you have any questions not explained by the dentist, it would be wise to seek another opinion or even be examined by a dental-school diagnostic clinic. An honest dentist will not object to this and will probably welcome the opportunity to have your doubts relieved. As work progresses, if you find that the dentist is rushed, spends little time with you, neglects gum conditions, or is eager to extract teeth, ask for an explanation and, if it is not convincing, consider changing dentists.

The mouth should generally feel comfortable after dental care; the gums should not bleed, and the bite should be comfortable. But some discomfort after routine dental treatment is common. A newly filled tooth may be sensitive to cold and hot for a few days, and gums are often sore after periodontal treatment. But these discomforts should not last long and can usually be controlled with aspirin. If the pain cannot be controlled in this way, something may be wrong and the dentist should be notified, even at night, if pain is severe. The responsible dentist does not want his patients to suffer and will arrange for the patient to receive help.

If, in the months and years after treatment, fillings fall out, the gums bleed frequently, pain is common, and extractions suggested, it is more than time to find another dentist.

The unit-fee-for-service tradition in dentistry (so much per filling, so much per "cleaning," and so on) is the cause of most of dentistry's ills. If a standard neighborhood fee for a "filling" is five dollars, for example, it stands to reason that a dentist who makes ten fillings in an hour earns twice as much in gross income as the dentist making five fillings in the hour, so the temptation is to reduce the time needed for a filling, sacrificing quality if necessary. It is depressing to find that nearly all of the many public, social, and insurance programs recently instituted to provide broader dental care for the public have adopted the quality-killing unit-fee system. Establishing a fixed fee for a "filling" makes as little sense as a fixed fee for mowing a lawn. Some lawns can be mowed in ten minutes, others in a day; similarly, some fillings can be accomplished in a few minutes while others can take ten times as long. And it is certainly irrational to pay to a good dentist who spends an hour on a tedious and difficult restoration the same fee that one pays to Dr. Poorwork for his five-minute mishandling of the same job.

Originally, the unit fees actually were worked out on a time basis: dentists approximated the time a typical procedure would take and charged accordingly. Instead of charging for fillings, dentists came to charge for "surfaces." For example, instead of five dollars a filling, fifteen dollars would be charged for a filling that extends over three sides (surfaces) of the tooth. Over a period of time the discrepancies of time required to treat various fillings or surfaces would average out. In practice, however, the unit-fee system provides a continuing incentive to the dentist to speed up his work, at the expense of quality.

These considerations suggest a novel approach that might be effective in securing quality dental service. This idea is to deal with the dentist on a time basis: a fee-for-time rather than a fee-for-unit-service basis. This approach would eliminate most of the incentives for poor dentistry. When he is scheduled and paid for a specific time period, the dentist is freed from the pressure of other patients piling up in the waiting room, he will not begrudge the extra time needed to properly complete a difficult filling, and, if he has easier work to do, he will complete as much as he can within the time period and at a saving to the patient.

If you are fortunate enough to find a dentist willing to treat you on a time basis, the per-time fee asked by the dentist might seem high. In fact, this is the reason most dentists haven't considered this approach, because the patient may feel that the fee is enormous. But consider this: the dentist's overhead is high, and his productive working hours are limited to the actual time he spends with his patients. He is not paid for time doing laboratory work, diagnostic procedures, business records, and so on, but only for what he calls "chair time." If a dentist averages 1,200 "chair-hours" a year, his office overhead comes to fifteen dollars an hour, and his fee is fifteen dollars per half-hour visit, his income will come to $18,000 a year. A patient earning seven dollars per hour, which, with fringe benefits, bonuses, and so on amounts to an income equivalent to the hypothetical dentist's $18,000, may think that thirty dollars per hour is a huge fee compared to his own seven dollars an hour, and many dentists are afraid to present a time-based fee because of this misunderstanding. But if one compares the work done under this method with the number of poor fillings done and number of patients seen by Dr. Poorwork in an hour, it will be evident that dealing with a good dentist on a time basis is best and actually least expensive in the long run.

a less efficient and desirable restoration. The adjacent teeth are prepared, by grinding down, to receive crowns, and the false tooth is attached to the abutment crowns, the whole assembly then being cemented into place. This procedure involves a great deal of time, effort, and expense, which is another reason to avoid the loss of the tooth in the first place.

Removable bridgework and dentures are the least desirable, poorest functioning, least comfortable, and least attractive dental restorations. They should only be made as a last resort. The full denture represents the ultimate failure of dentistry—the loss of all the teeth in an arch. Full dentures are far less efficient than the natural dentition for chewing; they are unsanitary, uncomfortable, annoying, and require constant care and cleaning. Again, reasonable oral hygiene and quality dental care are effective insurance against ever needing dentures.

Prevention

Dental research recently has focused on prevention as an attempt to reduce dental need. Among the areas being explored are fluoridation of community water supplies and the study of dental plaque, which is thought to play a significant role in the formation of caries and periodontal disease.

Fluoridation is by far the most extensively studied and documented scientific program in history. Fluoridation has been shown to reduce caries by 50 to 70 percent. The research effort focusing on the activity and effects of dental plaque may provide insight into new preventive measures.

The most important form of prevention of dental disease yet discovered is meticulous oral hygiene. Even if the researchers succeed in pinpointing plaque as the major cause of dental disease, the only way to remove plaque would be to use the methods of oral hygiene. The purpose of oral hygiene is to remove all food residues from the mouth; if the individual succeeds in this task, dental disease definitely will be reduced. The critical oral hygiene tool is the toothbrush, which requires a considerable amount of training and skill to use properly. There are several different methods of toothbrushing all of which are effective. One popular method is shown in Figure 20.9. All good dentists are willing to spend time instructing their patients in proper oral hygiene—there is no more important service they can perform. Many persons lacking the dexterity to brush really effectively have found the electric toothbrush a great help in improving their oral hygiene performance. Water jet appliances, used under a dentist's supervision, also can be helpful for some persons.

Timing is important. Because the only source of trouble-producing oral debris is ingested food, it stands to reason that the mouth should be brushed immediately after eating. Many people brush before they retire and again in the morning. After the morning brushing, which is performed on an essentially clean mouth, the individual eats breakfast, making the mouth filthy again, and then goes off to school or work. Obviously it is sensible to brush *after* breakfast, and not before, but too many people do the reverse and damage their mouths as a result. If one rinses his mouth with plain water upon arising he will eliminate that horrible taste that compels him to brushing his teeth before breakfast. Unlike plain water, chemical mouthwashes can be useless and even dangerous: they can upset the ecological balance of the mouth and saliva and lead to dangerous fungal infections.

It is most important to brush the gum crevices as well as the surfaces of the teeth because most oral debris accumulates at the gum line. Any standard, mild toothpaste is of some assistance in oral hygiene, but it is the action of the brush that does the important work. One should beware of the so-called "tooth-whitening" toothpastes—they are

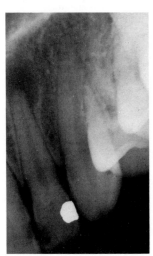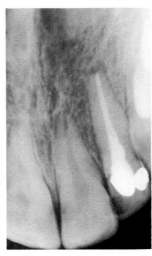

Figure 20.8 These x-ray pictures demonstrate the treatment of an abscessed tooth by endodontia (root-canal therapy). The picture on the left shows a lateral incisor (front tooth) with a large abscess around the root end (apex). The abscessed area is full of exudate (pus), which is damaging the jawbone at the root apex. The photograph on the right shows the tooth after root-canal treatment. The abscessed area has been drained, and the root canal has been cleaned, widened, filled, and sealed.

usually too abrasive for routine use. There are no magic ingredients in toothpastes to protect against caries or dispel mouth odors, despite what advertisements may say. And no toothpaste will make teeth white, because the natural color of teeth is not white, but yellowish, ranging from a gray-yellow to a light reddish-yellow. Although the ads proclaim the merits of using whatever product is being touted, all toothpastes, mouthwashes, and drugs are useless in fighting periodontal disease once it has started. The only effective therapy is through treatment by a capable dentist. In young people especially, halitosis (mouth odor) is invariably a sign of periodontal troubles and can be treated.

THE SKIN AND HAIR

The skin is the body's buffer against the adversities of the outside world. It protects one from mechanical injury, blocks penetration of microorganisms, is responsible for maintaining body temperature within a wide range of environmental temperatures, and helps maintain water balance despite air dryness or humidity.

Skin is a dynamic structure, renewing itself and changing constantly. The structure and function of the skin over the body varies, often considerably. Skin over joints such as knuckles, knees, and elbows, for example, has the ability to stretch when the joint is flexed. The skin on the palms of the hands and on the scalp, however, is designed to withstand considerable trauma. Even within the relatively small area of the face, the skin ranges from being thick, coarse, and hairy (at the eyebrows) to thin and smooth (forehead and cheeks).

In addition, skin can regenerate itself and heal the wounds inflicted upon it. The mechanism of wound healing is at once a marvel of biological skill and a marvel of engineering. The power of the skin to heal has enormous survival value. A. E.

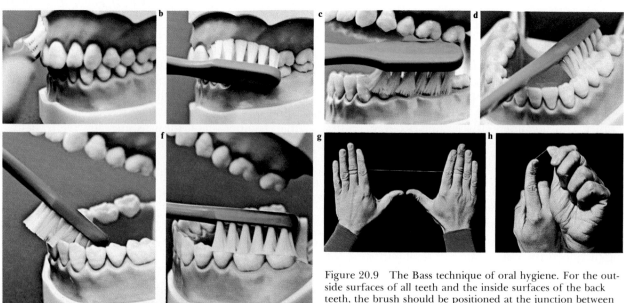
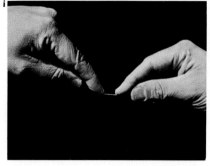
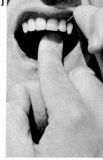

Figure 20.9   The Bass technique of oral hygiene. For the outside surfaces of all teeth and the inside surfaces of the back teeth, the brush should be positioned at the junction between the teeth and gums (a). Short back-and-forth strokes should be used. One should first do the outer surfaces (b, c) and then the inner surfaces (d, e) in the same manner. For the inner surface of the upper front teeth, the brush should be held vertically, using several gentle back-and-forth strokes over gums and teeth. One should brush back and forth on biting surfaces (f). After brushing, one should rinse the mouth vigorously to remove the loosened plaque from the teeth and mouth. The use of dental floss is encouraged for getting into the crevices between teeth. Wrapping the floss around the middle fingers (g), one should pass the floss over his right thumb and the forefinger of his left hand (h) for cleaning the upper right back teeth and reverse the hold for the upper left back teeth (j). The floss should be held between the forefingers of both hands (i) for cleaning the bottom teeth.

Needham of the University of Oxford estimates that a man suffers an average of one minor wound per week, or 4,000 or more in a lifetime of seventy years. All skin, whether of man or other animals, is composed of two distinct layers: the superficial *epidermis* and the underlying *dermis*.

The Epidermis

The epidermis covers the entire external surface of the body and consists of four successive cellular strata (see Figure 20.10). The top layer of flattened, dead cells is the stratum corneum, or *horny layer*. Under it are the stratum granulosum, the stratum spinosum, and the stratum germinativum, or *basal layer*. The epidermis is a self-contained system that continually replaces itself by the cellular proliferation of the basal layer. New basal cells move up-

ward toward the surface as they gradually differentiate into thin, flexible flakes of horny material. Human epidermis has intricate understructures of branching ridges and valleys, columns and pits, as is shown in Figure 20.12. The epidermis is the principal defense against invasions and infections and is a barrier against injury from the environment.

The Dermis

Much thicker than the epidermis, the dermis consists of coarse, branching *collagenous fibers* and a varying number of *elastic fibers*. Both collagenous and elastic fibers make the dermis tough and resilient. Connective-tissue cells, such as fibroblasts, macrophages, and mast cells, also are present. Dermis and epidermis are bound together by the interlocking of the descending epidermal ridges

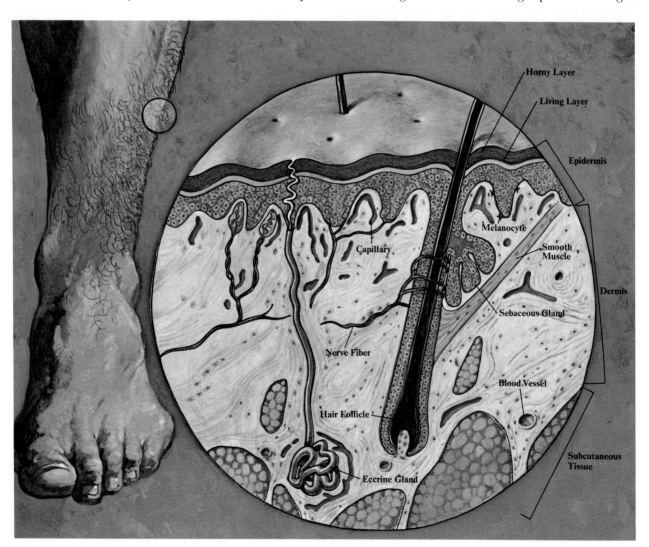

Figure 20.10   Structure of the skin.

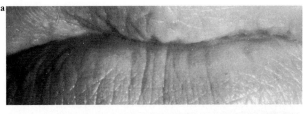

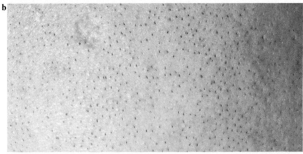

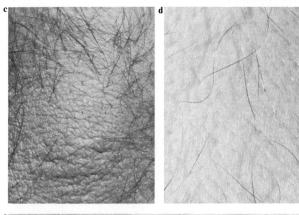

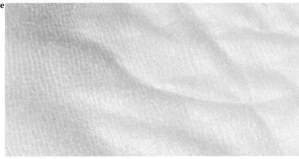

Figure 20.11 Variations in the skin on different parts of the body: (a) lips, (b) cheek, (c) knee, (d) stomach area, (e) bottom of foot. Note the differences in texture and hair distribution.

and the ascending protrusion of the dermis (see Figure 20.12).

Throughout the body, a luxuriant network of blood vessels courses through the dermis. This massive blood supply far exceeds the skin's metabolic needs and acts as a temperature regulator by transferring the internal heat of the body to the surface of the skin. The dermis also houses the cutaneous appendages: hair, sebaceous glands, and sweat glands.

THE HAIR Hairs are nonliving structures composed of hardened cells tightly cemented together. Found exclusively in mammals, they are the products of the skin and grow out of hair follicles embedded in the dermis.

In contrast to nails, which grow continuously throughout life, hairs have definite growth cycles ranging from a few weeks to several years. Hair growth is a matter of alternate growing and resting periods, with new hairs arising periodically. During these periods or phases, both the hair shafts and the hair follicles undergo characteristic changes commonly referred to as the *hair cycle*. A hair cycle begins with the formation and growth of a new hair, followed by a resting stage, and ending with the growth of another hair from the same follicle.

THE SEBACEOUS GLANDS These glands are present over the entire surface of the body except in the palms and the soles. They lie in the dermis and their excretory ducts open into the necks of hair follicles. The glands secrete fatty substances called *sebum*, which emulsifies and retains water in the skin, thereby making it soft and pliable. Sebaceous glands are largest and most numerous in the face, scalp, and midline of the chest and back.

THE SWEAT GLANDS One of the outstanding features of man's skin is its ability to sweat profusely. Man has approximately 3 million sweat glands in

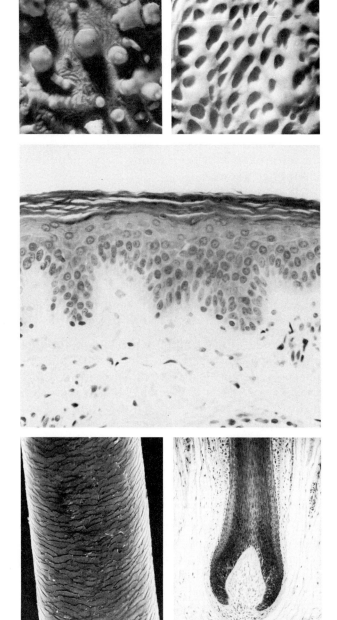

his skin. They are simple, tubular structures that originate in the epidermis and extend into the dermis. Sweat glands are composed of an upper duct lined by two cell layers and a twisted and coiled secretory part in the deep dermis (see Figure 20.13). There are two kinds of sweat glands: *apocrine*, which are usually associated with hair follicles, and *eccrine*, which are not.

Apocrine glands are found in the armpit, breast, genital, and pubic areas. They are primarily scent glands and secrete their products largely in response to stress or sexual stimulation. Although the glands are relatively large, they secrete only small amounts of substance.

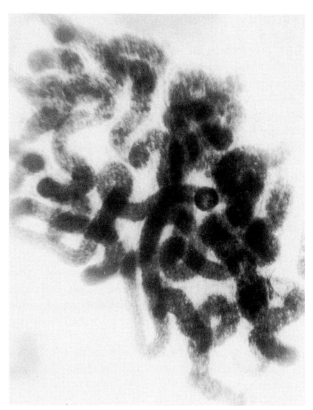

Figure 20.12 (*top*) The epidermis varies from one area of the skin to another as shown in these two photographs, one of the undersurface of the lip (*left*) and the other of the undersurface of the cheek (*right*). (*center*) How the epidermis and dermis interlock. (*bottom*) Close-ups of a hair and a hair follicle. Note how the scales on the hair shaft are oriented toward the tip of the hair.

Figure 20.13   The coiled segment of an eccrine sweat gland.

Smaller but more numerous than the apocrine glands are the eccrine sweat glands, found over the entire body surface. They are the source of most of man's sweat, which has two essential functions: (1) to reduce body temperature by evaporation, and (2) to moisten the skin and thereby to prevent scaling of the horny layer. Heat is the major stimulus for eccrine sweating, but emotions also cause it. The palms, soles, underarms, and forehead are the primary sites for this type of sweating.

The Pigment System

Pigment cells, or *melanocytes*, which produce dark-colored pigment, or *melanin*, are scattered throughout the epidermal-dermal junction. Branched and spider-shaped, these cells inject granules of melanin into the neighboring epidermal cells. A prime function of melanin pigment is to protect the cells by absorbing the ultraviolet rays of the sun. The phenomenon of tanning on exposure to sunlight results from an immediate darkening of the existing melanin and later an increased activity in the melanocytes themselves, leading to the formation of new melanin.

By giving the skin a tan, brown, or black color, melanocytes provide some of the most striking differences in the outward appearance of the human race. In spite of these differences, all human beings, regardless of race, have about the same number of melanocytes; those in the skins of darker races simply produce more pigment.

In albinos, however, there is no pigment. Albinos have melanocytes, but as pointed out in Chapter 14, they lack the enzyme tyrosinase responsible for the conversion of tyrosine into the necessary precursors of melanin. Because melanin serves as protection from the harmful effects of ultraviolet radiation, albinos must be cautious about their exposure to the sun.

Nerve Endings

A dense network of nerves traverses the dermis throughout the body. Much of this nervous system is concerned with the control of glands, blood vessels, and other skin organs. *Mechanoreceptors*, a vast complex of sensory nerve endings, are specialized sense organs that respond to such mechanical stimuli as touch, pressure, and tension. For example, hair follicles are surrounded by a complex of nerve fibers; when the hair is bent, it stimulates the nerves around it. The resulting nerve impulse is interpreted as touch.

Common Skin Disorders

The range of skin disorders in man is as large and complex as the skin itself. Skin diseases account for almost 12 percent of all human pathological conditions. The following brief descriptions include the most common skin disorders. Skin cancer is discussed in Chapter 23; less common disorders are described in Appendix A.

DERMATITIS Although this general term includes any inflammatory skin disorder, for therapeutic purposes dermatologists (skin specialists) distinguish several categories, among them contact dermatitis, atopic eczema, seborrheic dermatitis, and so on, depending on the area of the skin affected and the possible causes. Dermatitis in many cases may be an allergic response (see Chapter 25) in which chemicals in perfumes, cosmetics, soaps, or other materials that come in contact with the skin cause a reaction in sensitive persons.

ACNE Acne is a chronic inflammatory disease that results from overactivity of the sebaceous glands. Greater activity of these glands occurs along with other physiological changes associated with adolescence. The sebum secreted from the glands begins to clog the ducts, causing a bump under the skin. If the bump becomes infected, it forms a pimple. The infection may become so serious that it destroys the gland cells, leaving a disfiguring scar.

Squeezing of pimples is destructive to the skin and contributes further to scarring. In milder cases, it is helpful to keep the face clean and free of excess oil. In more severe cases, one should see his physician or dermatologist, who can remove the cores of pimples without damaging the skin and who can give advice on cleaning and eating habits tailored to the individual.

WARTS These domelike projections are induced by a virus and occur most commonly on the hands and on the soles of the feet, although they can appear anywhere on the skin surface. Treatment consists of surgical removal and destruction through chemicals or cauterization.

HERPES SIMPLEX The *herpes simplex* virus, which is constantly present on the skin, sometimes gets out of hand and forms "cold sores," usually around the mouth and nose. The process is poorly understood, but current experiments with vaccines offer promise for ultimate control in highly susceptible individuals. Without treatment, these sores generally vanish within ten days after they appear.

Plastic Surgery

Used for more than a century, plastic surgery is successfully employed in the treatment of large wounds, severe injuries, and burns. Basically, plastic surgery consists of autografting and homografting. An *autograft* is a transplant of tissue from one site to another in the same individual. In cases of skin loss from injuries, burns, and ulceration, plastic surgeons remove a flap of skin, usually from the abdomen or thigh, and transplant it to the injured sites. Skin grafts are applied in large sheets, strips, or small rectangles known as "postage stamp" grafts. A *homograft* is a transplant made from one person to another. Skin grafts between identical twins behave like autografts and may survive permanently. Except for such cases, homografts between related or unrelated persons grow initially but usually are rejected within two to four weeks.

Plastic surgery becomes necessary only in major injuries, for most of the time the skin exhibits a remarkable ability to heal scrapes, minor burns, cuts, and other such wounds. But in order to carry out these and its other important functions, the skin needs the nourishment derived from a balanced diet and daily cleansing to remove harmful bacteria and cells shed from the horny layer.

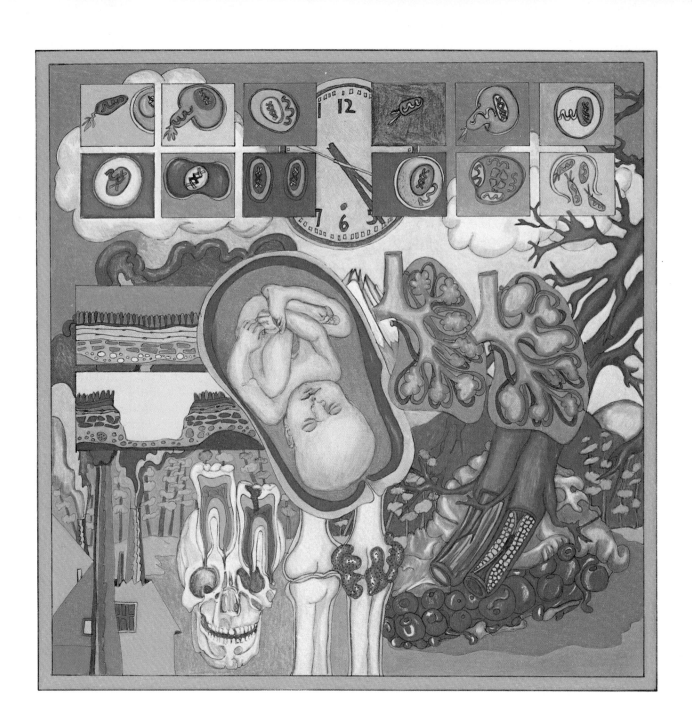

VI HEALTH AND DISEASE

For most of man's million or more years on earth, he has been relatively helpless in the face of the natural forces that threaten his individual, group, and species survival. Although the intelligent use of tools and evolving technology and social structures have afforded greater and greater protection from starvation and exposure, until recently man remained hopelessly victimized by disease. In the past century most of the historically dreaded afflictions of mankind have yielded in varying degrees to the applications of health science. ¶ So successful has man been in controlling disease and early death that the most pressing disasters facing man today now result from population growth and the scientific technology responsible for that growth. Biologically the primary goal of human life is clear—survival. That survival is basic seems almost too self-evident to mention, yet modern man behaves frequently, if not dominantly, as if his survival is independent of his behavior. Witness, for example, people who smoke. ¶ Modern health science seeks not only to understand the causes and cures of illness and suffering but to influence the adoption of behavior consistent with those understandings. Choices among alternative behaviors are central to the process and include levels of decision making from international programs affecting all of mankind to individual choices facilitating individual health. ¶ The concept of disease encompasses a variety of disorders with a variety of causes. Disease includes not only such infections as colds and influenza but chronic and degenerative diseases such as cancer and atherosclerosis. And disease causes include not only bacteria and other parasites but heredity, stress, pollution, accidents, and poor diet. Many of these disease factors can be brought under control and minimized by each individual. Other factors, such as air pollution, require an informed and committed social effort to control or eliminate.

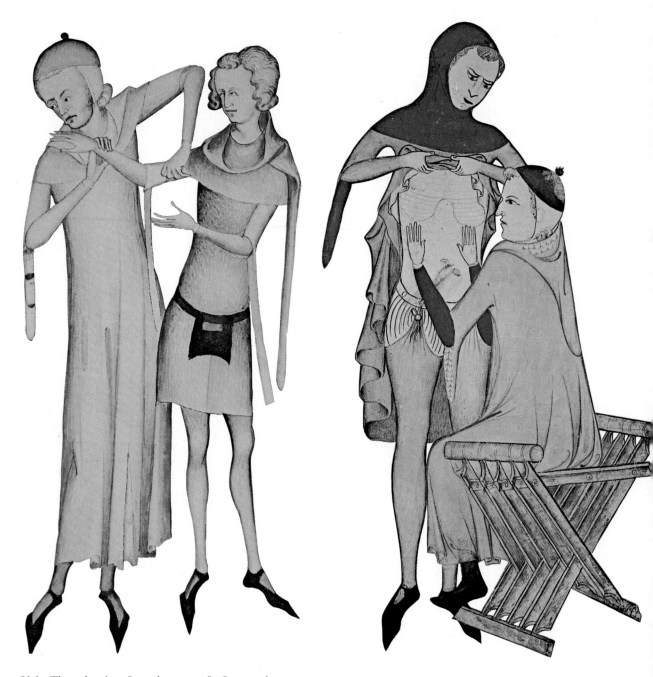

Figure 21.1   These drawings from the pages of a fourteenth-century manuscript on anatomy show two types of physical examination and an operation to open the skull.

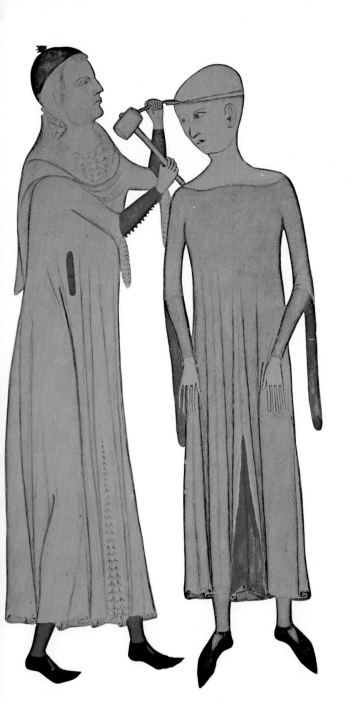

21

"Houses were filled with dead bodies and the streets with funerals." This description of the bubonic plague that ravaged early Rome came from Publius Cornelius Tacitus, a first-hand observer of the daily events occurring in the then capital of a great empire. It was the golden age of Roman civilization, from A.D. 96 to 180, hailed by British historian Edward Gibbon sixteen centuries later as "the period in the history of the world during which the conditions of the human race were most happy and prosperous . . ." Yet this golden era began with an outbreak of plague so devastating that during its peak it claimed 10,000 lives a day in Rome alone, a city with a population of about 700,000. During the last sixteen years of Gibbon's favored period, the Roman army was nearly wiped out by plague.

Dramatic though the Roman pestilence had been, it was but a pale episode when compared with the outbreak of the Black Death, as the bubonic plague was called, that spread throughout Europe in the fourteenth century. In 1346, the Tartar army was besieging an important Black Sea port when it was hit by the plague. As perhaps the first example of "bacteriological warfare," the besieging army catapulted its dead bodies into the besieged city, thus spreading the pestilence among the city's defenders. Supply ships carried the plague to other Mediterranean ports. Year after year, the waves of Black Death spread wider and wider: in 1347, the plague ravaged Constantinople and invaded the Mediterranean islands (Sicily, Sardinia, Corsica); in 1348,

The Conquest of Disease

Italy, France, and Spain succumbed to it; by 1350, all of Europe to the northmost regions of Scandinavia was devastated. In England, the population fell from 3.8 million in 1348 to 2.1 million in 1374. One-third or more of all the people in Europe died, and it took more than 200 years for the population to return to its preplague level. The impact on the economic, moral, religious, and social structures and the changes that the plague's devastation caused to the course of history were enormous.

It was only at the end of the nineteenth century, after the work of Pasteur and many others, that it was discovered that the plague is due to a small bacterium called *Pasturella pestis* (the infective agent), conveyed to humans by fleas (the vector), that picked it up from other infected organisms, mainly rats (the carriers). Today bubonic plague is rarely found in the Western countries, and if it should appear, physicians know how to stop its spread and how to treat infected individuals.

The scourges of infection that once decimated cities more thoroughly than did conquering armies are rarely found in modern, industrialized nations, but the scourges nevertheless still exist in the world. An epidemic of the dreaded killer cholera struck the southern resort area of Russia in 1970, causing officials to restrict travel in and out of the popular Black Sea vacationland. Millions of Russians were cautioned to take special care with their food and drinking supplies. This outbreak of cholera was traced back to an original focus of infection in the Celebes Islands of Indonesia. First identified there in 1935, it eventually began spreading through Asia in 1961. Public health officials estimate that since 1935 this strain of bacteria has killed millions in the seventh world-wide pandemic of cholera since 1817. Cholera is fatal in about two-thirds of all cases if untreated. Ninety-nine out of one hundred cases, however can now be helped to recover with the proper treatment. The spread of cholera can be prevented by good sanitation, particularly the protection of public water supplies.

EPIDEMIOLOGY

Tracing the causes and spread of such diseases as plague and cholera is part of the branch of medicine known as *epidemiology*. Epidemiology is the study of the distribution and dynamics of disease. It examines the frequency of occurrence of a disease and its correlation with geographical, ethnic, economic, social, and other parameters; it also considers disease causes and the modes by which disease can be prevented before it takes hold or brought under control once it is started. The epidemiology of yellow fever, for example, would include the recognition that it is spread by a certain species of mosquito and that it can be prevented by draining swamps and removing other bodies of

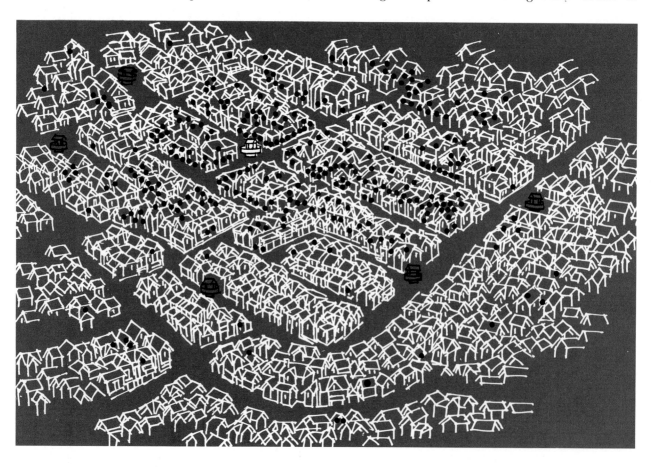

water that serve as breeding grounds for the insects. Thus the epidemiologist must consider environmental and ecological influences as well as specifically medical ones.

Today, epidemiology is being utilized increasingly to study and control such noninfectious disorders as coronary artery disease, cancer, drug addiction, and suicide. With such health problems, as with infectious disease, the classic epidemiological model based on the host-agent-environment relationship is relevant. For example, it is necessary for the victim of an infectious disease such as smallpox (1) to be living within an *environment* that provides a source of the infectious agent and favors its development and transmission, (2) to have come in *contact* with the infectious agent, and (3) to be *susceptible* as a host to the disease. Likewise, coronary artery disease results from (1) psychosocial and economic *environments* that cause or reinforce behaviors leading to development of the ailment, (2) *contact* with specific disease-inducing factors (fats in diet, lack of exercise, high blood pressure, smoking, obesity, for example), and (3) individual *susceptibility* (genetic predisposition, undermining influence of other diseases, and so on).

One of the difficulties that epidemiologists encounter in attempting to obtain useful statistics is the relative reliability of the statistics themselves. A study of the historical or the geographical distribution of a disease depends critically on the recognition and faithful reporting that went into the making of available records on the diseases in question, and these records may vary with the medical awareness present in different societies. Similarly, the sampling on which the statistics are based must be truly representative of the population, and this information, too, may depend on the extent to which data are available on the characteristics of both the disease and the populations involved. Finally, death rates, or *mortality* rates, while most readily assessed, do not tell the whole story. A disease may be prevalent but not cause many deaths. The common cold is such an ailment. And yet, colds keep many people from work every day, and they significantly affect the nation's health and well-being. Accordingly, epidemiologists also attempt to determine the occurrence of a disease—its *morbidity*. Morbidity statistics are more difficult to obtain than those for mortality because some illnesses may go unreported, while others may be incorrectly diagnosed.

Nevertheless, examining epidemiological data can lead to certain generalizations. In regions where people have high standards of living, nutritional and infectious diseases seem to have both low morbidity and low mortality, while heart disease, cancer, stroke, and accidents show high morbidity and mortality. Underdeveloped nations, on the other hand, must cope primarily with nutritional deficiencies and infectious diseases. Undernutrition, protein deficiencies, malaria, tuberculosis, and parasites are the greatest killers there. Other nations in various stages of development experience a variety of disease patterns, with the major killers varying somewhat from culture to culture.

Epidemiology is particularly useful in relation to outbreaks of disease. Such outbreaks usually involve a communicable disease, but they also may be caused by a poisonous agent, either natural or introduced into the environment by man. An *epidemic* occurs when a disease affects a larger number of people in one area than it normally would. This concept usually is thought of in terms of hundreds or thousands of victims, but often it is used relatively. One case of yellow fever or a few cases of plague in the United States might be considered an outbreak today simply because those diseases are so rare here; on the other hand, thousands of colds on a winter day in New York City would not be considered abnormal.

An epidemic that becomes geographically widespread is described as *pandemic*. It may affect a country, a continent, or much of the world. Dis-

Figure 21.2 Epidemiology was advanced in 1854 by Dr. John Snow, who theorized that cholera was a water-borne disease. On a map of his district in London he plotted each house where one of his patients had died recently of cholera. The map showed a concentration of deaths around a particular water pump. When the pump handle was removed at Snow's insistence, new cases of cholera dropped abruptly and soon ceased. It was later learned that the pump water had been contaminated by an overflowing cesspool. Snow was correct in his theory, but his ideas were not accepted by scientists until many years later.

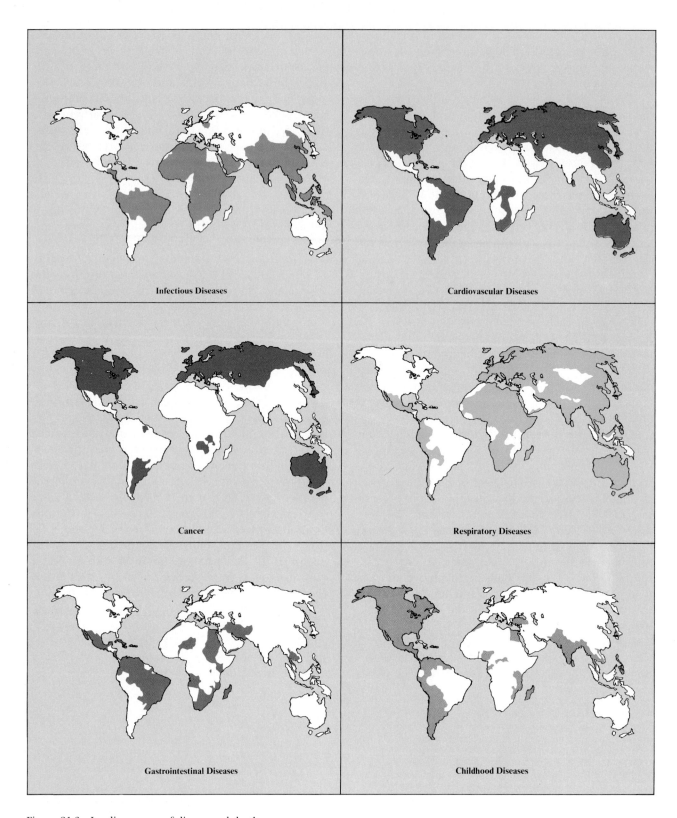

Figure 21.3 Leading causes of disease and death
for various areas of the world. This representation is
limited by the fact that statistics for undeveloped areas
are scarce or nonexistent.

Rx DRUGS

by Donald Robinson

The next time you go to the druggist to have a prescription filled, think about this word: "equivalency."

It is the newest temper-triggering expression about a subject in which heated words are as plentiful as pink pills. It is causing more frayed nerves among people who have to do with prescription drugs than almost any word since "thalidomide." It may soon have a major effect on the drugs your physician may prescribe for you, how useful these drugs will be, and how much they will cost you.

The meaning of "equivalency" takes some explaining, but the following dramatic case report gives some idea of the problem.

A man suffering from agonizing arthritis had kept the pain in check for many years through the use of a steroid hormone called prednisone, a drug taken regularly by millions of Americans. But one day, the man suddenly found that the drug wasn't working for him any more.

Almost frantic with pain, he doubled the dosage without asking his doctor. This didn't help. In desperation, he took four times as much as usual. Still no relief. Finally, he telephoned the doctor, who began to investigate.

The findings were startling. The man's druggist had simply switched drugs—not to a different kind of drug, but to the same drug from a different manufacturer. The substitute prednisone had exactly the same chemical ingredients, but it acted differently in the patient's body. The regular prednisone tablets had dissolved in 4.3 minutes; the substitute prednisone took two hours and 53 minutes!

One drug was the product of the company that had originally developed the drug. The other was from another company that had entered the market later with a competitive brand. The drugs were chemically the same, but they were not therapeutically "equivalent."

Until lately, it was generally assumed that any two drugs with precisely the same active chemical ingredients would perform in precisely the same way inside the human body. Now evidence is building up to indicate that some makes of the same drug don't do the therapeutic job they're supposed to.

This realization could affect one of the biggest controversies in the field of pharmacy—the battle over so-called generic versus brand-name drugs. For the most part, the controversy rages over perhaps twenty-five to thirty of the most commonly prescribed drugs. Most other drugs are one-of-a-kind, available only from a single com-

pany. But these twenty-five to thirty drugs are among the most widely used prescription pharmaceuticals. They include life-savers like penicillin and tetracycline, the digitalis family of drugs, the cortisone steroids, and nitroglycerin, used by hundreds of thousands of people to control the pain of angina pectoris.

All these drugs—brand and generic alike— are federally approved. But the original versions were approved only after lengthy and thorough testing by the manufacturer, which had been scrutinized by the Food and Drug Administration in Washington. If a prescription product has already been on the market and the developing company's exclusive patent expires, another company can get government clearance to market it under its official, generic name. Generally, the extent of the data required for clearance is vastly smaller. In effect, this second company has basically only to demonstrate that its drug is the same chemically. It does not have to conduct costly tests to show that its product is therapeutically as effective as the original.

Some leaders in the medical field as well as in Congress steadfastly hold that chemical equivalency is proof enough and that chemical equivalence and therapeutic equivalence are the same. But more and more experts are beginning to bring forth evidence to show that it just isn't always so. For example, the respected Food and Drug Directorate of Canada examined ten different manufacturers' tablets of hydrochlorothiazide, the most widely prescribed drug for lowering blood pressure. All ten tablets had identical chemical ingredients, but they dissolved at varying speeds, from a rapid two minutes to a slow five hours. This meant that one pill could commence to help a sick person immediately. Another wouldn't do any good for many long hours, if ever.

As Dr. Peter J. Lemy of the University of Maryland School of Pharmacy explains the process:

"The effect of a drug depends not only upon how much of the drug reaches the blood, but also on how fast it is absorbed. It is entirely possible that a drug, if absorbed too slowly, will never establish a therapeutic blood level—and although all of the drug may be absorbed, a therapeutic effect never occurs."

There are many reasons why a compound can differ so widely. The noted University of Illinois researcher, Dr. Max S. Sadove, has described twenty-four different production factors that can alter the physiological action of a drug. They include such things as

Adapted from Robinson, D. "The Big Question About Rx Drugs," *Family Health* (April 1971), pp. 16–19.

the coating of a tablet, its viscosity, the dissolving point, flavoring and coloring agents, even the amount of pressure exerted by the machinery used to shape the tablet.

But why should government-licensed-and-regulated companies produce such different results? Not surprisingly, economics is a major reason. The nation's well-established manufacturers of pharmaceuticals have greater resources for ensuring the quality of the medicines they make. The Pharmaceutical Manufacturers Association reports that its sixty member firms expend more than $100 million a year on controlling the quality of their products. Yet more than one-third of all drugs taken off the market in 1970 were ineffective simply because of unsatisfactory manufacturing processes. The manufacturers involved did not spend the money needed to improve their plants, did not make adequate laboratory checks on every batch of drugs, did not keep watch over long-standing drugs to make sure they hadn't deteriorated, and "skimped" on scientific personnel. With minimal expenses for research, development, and federal clearance, any company can produce cheaper drugs. And there's a big market for them.

The biggest purchaser is the government itself. The Veterans Administration, the Department of Defense, and public health agencies that use drugs in clinics, hospitals, and armed forces installations are the nation's—perhaps the world's—largest buyers of pharmaceuticals. The Defense Department alone spends more than $100 million a year on drugs. By law, these agencies are supposed to buy their drugs from the lowest bidder among qualified companies. Traditionally, the government tries to buy the most acceptable drug at the lowest price by applying the so-called cost/effectiveness ratio. When a generic drug is available, it is most often chosen on the assumption that it is just as effective.

But unsettling reports began surfacing as a result of VA and Defense Department purchasing policies. The commanding officer of the Fitzsimons General Hospital in Denver made one such revelation. Several epilepsy patients in his hospital had been taking Dilantin, the Parke, Davis-developed antiepileptic drug. They had gone for six years without a single epileptic seizure. Then, the Department of Defense allowed the hospital to stock and dispense only generic makes of

the drug diphenyl-hydantoin. Every one of the patients soon began having seizures again, and only when the hospital resumed the use of Dilantin did the symptoms stop. "No seizures have occurred since then," the hospital's chief reported.

The situation was even more critical with nitrofurantoin, a drug that is widely employed against infections of the urinary tract. Patients with chronic urinary infections require this drug over long periods of time. After using a brand-name drug called Furadantin in its hospitals for several years, the Department of Defense decided to try a foreign generic make because it cost less.

Military hospitals began reporting that the generic nitrofurantoin was dangerously unsatisfactory. The Army's famous Walter Reed General Hospital in Washington, D.C. submitted evidence that it "almost invariably" caused nausea and vomiting. The Sheppard Air Force Base in Texas described cases of severe rashes from its use.

Lately, the debate over equivalency has intensified, and now seems to be heading toward a climax on four fronts.

On one front, FDA Commissioner Charles Edwards is trying to hammer out a long-range program to make sure all important medicines with the same active chemical ingredients are therapeutically equivalent. This program calls for more market surveillance, more FDA testing, reassessment of many drugs by the prestigious National Academy of Sciences/National Research Council, a closer check on manufacturing methods, and most significantly, a requirement that all manufacturers submit demonstrable proof to the FDA of the biological availability of their products.

The second front involves some politically potent forces who are pushing for greater discretion for the retail pharmacist in dispensing medicines. At its recent convention, the American Pharmaceutical Association voted to demand immediate repeal of the so-called "antisubstitution laws." At the moment, if your doctor writes out a prescription for a specific brand of a drug, in forty-eight states the druggist is legally required to give you that particular brand product, and nothing else. But if the doctor simply orders the drug by its generic name, the druggist may give you any legally available form of the drug, from any licensed manufacturer. The

pharmacists want the law changed so that the druggist may decide which manufacturer's version of a drug he will use to fill a prescription, regardless of what brand the doctor orders.

The American Medical Association is alarmed at the prospect of repeal. An editorial in the journal of the AMA stated: "Such ill-conceived action by a segment of the pharmacy profession denigrates the profession itself and indicates a disrespect for the patients the profession serves. The antisubstitution laws protect patient, pharmacist, and physician. Their repeal would effectively remove such protection. It would permit a pharmacist who chooses to do so to dispense substitutes in defiance of the physician's best therapeutic judgment without the physician knowing when a substitute or what substitute is dispensed."

Repeal of these laws in some states is likely, in view of the heavy influence of pharmacists in most legislatures.

The third area of action is Congress. Senator Russell Long of Louisiana, chairman of the powerful Senate Finance Committee and a strong critic of brand-name drugs, has been pushing a bill to establish a National Formulary Committee. Such a committee would evaluate all drugs, branded and unbranded, and decide which ones among them could be purchased with federal funds. At the same time, other congressmen are proposing legislation that would require the generic name of the drug to be on the labels of containers dispensed by the retail pharmacist to the patient.

The fourth and final arena of action is the marketplace. Drugs distributed without a brand name have usually cost less than those with brand names. At the same time, the druggist can make a bigger profit selling unbranded drugs—since he can buy them for a lot less than branded drugs and charge you a little less. But in recent years, the price of unbranded generics has been slowly climbing, while the price of brand-name pharmaceuticals has been falling. If the margin becomes quite narrow, one point of contention would be reduced.

Many participants in the controversy feel, however, that cost is the least important point. Price is always of some consideration, of course. But in matters of health, the ultimate and most significant question will be: which drug will do you the most good?

eases become pandemic when they spread beyond their usual geographic confines. Diseases that occur normally in a given area and at a relatively consistent level are considered to be *endemic* to that area. Cholera was endemic in the Celebes Islands of Indonesia but has become pandemic since 1961.

When one considers the frequency with which pandemic infectious diseases occurred until the last century, one can appreciate the tremendous contribution made by the scientific researchers who investigated their causes and liberated many millions from the constant fear of death. Some of these pioneers, as well as other historic figures of medicine, are shown in Figure 21.4.

CHANGING PATTERNS OF DISEASE

Man will always fear disease. In the past he particularly dreaded the mass killers—plague, diphtheria, tuberculosis, malaria, typhoid fever, yellow fever, and others. Although in many parts of the world today these traditional killers still threaten life, in the United States and many other countries these infections have been controlled. Nevertheless, infectious diseases such as pneumonia and influenza

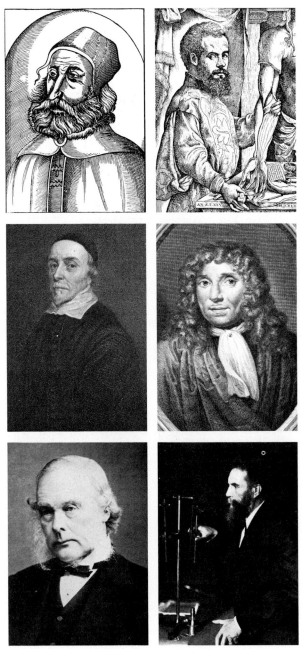

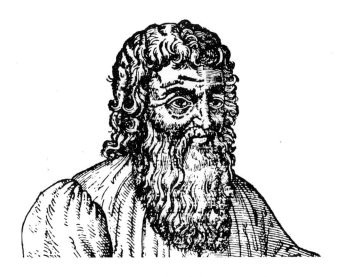

Figure 21.4 (*above*) The art of medicine in the ancient world developed to its highest point in Greece between 500 B.C. and A.D. 500. This creative period is symbolized by Hippocrates, whose works include the Hippocratic oath and descriptions of various aspects of medicine including lengthy passages devoted to the etiology of epilepsy. (*top left*) Galen (A.D. 130–200), Greek physician and founder of experimental physiology, is considered, after Hippocrates, the most distinguished physician of antiquity. His writings—which consist of some 300 treatises—were the bases for medical diagnosis and treatment for 1400 years. (*top right*) Andreas Vesalius, a sixteenth-century Flemish physician, pioneered the study of the structure (anatomy) and function (physiology) of the human body. Because of strict law forbidding the dissection of human corpses, Vesalius routinely collected his cadavers from the public gallows. (*center left*) In the early seventeenth century William Harvey uncovered the mysteries of the circulatory system. Al-

though his explanation of how the circulatory system works was a major landmark in medical history, of equal importance were his studies of human anatomy and physiology, which determined that structure and function are totally interrelated. (*center right*) Antony van Leeuwenhoek, the Dutch microscopist who lived from 1632 to 1723, was the first to describe red blood cells. Because of Leeuwenhoek's construction of the first microscope the human organism could now be examined on the cellular level. (*bottom left*) Joseph Lister (1845–1923) was the first to conclude that bacteria cause infection. Surgical instruments were washed with an acid solution; the same solution was sprayed into operating rooms. After Lister's presentation and application of the "germ theory," 50 percent fewer surgical patients died from postoperative infection. (*bottom right*) With the discovery of the x-ray by Wilhelm Roentgen in 1895, physicians were presented with a remarkable aid to what is still the physician's most difficult task—proper diagnosis.

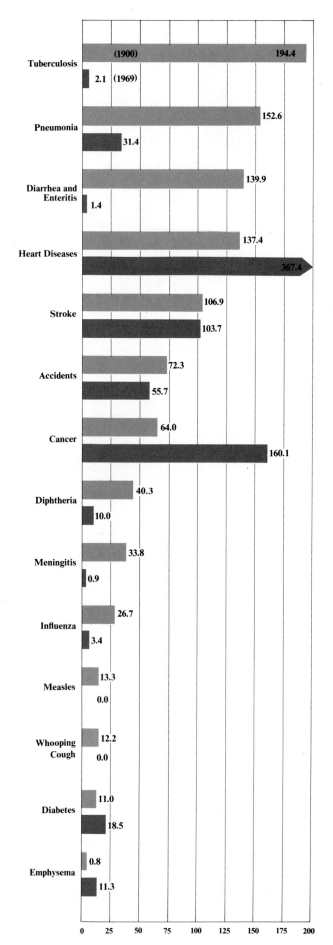

Tuberculosis	(1900) 194.4
	2.1 (1969)
Pneumonia	152.6
	31.4
Diarrhea and Enteritis	139.9
	1.4
Heart Diseases	137.4
	367.4
Stroke	106.9
	103.7
Accidents	72.3
	55.7
Cancer	64.0
	160.1
Diphtheria	40.3
	10.0
Meningitis	33.8
	0.9
Influenza	26.7
	3.4
Measles	13.3
	0.0
Whooping Cough	12.2
	0.0
Diabetes	11.0
	18.5
Emphysema	0.8
	11.3

0 25 50 75 100 125 150 175 200

may still kill. Tuberculosis remains a debilitating chronic disease and a not infrequent cause of death, especially among the poor. And, in recent years, venereal diseases, while rarely fatal, have been on such a dramatic rise in the United States that they have officially acquired epidemic or even pandemic ratings.

Influenza, pneumonia, tuberculosis, and diphtheria, leading causes of death in the United States a century ago, no longer take many lives, as Figure 21.5 shows. However, as one group of problems comes under some degree of control, something new becomes a significant threat. Today, a new group of diseases predominates among the leading causes of death in the United States: heart disease, cancer, and stroke, in particular.

These diseases are new in the sense that they were not as important decades or centuries ago, partly because people rarely lived long enough to develop them, but also because they did not live in ways that predisposed them to these newly significant diseases.

Climate, social custom, technology, and living standards as well as longevity affect the patterns of disease, as Figure 21.6 illustrates. Although people in the United States had a relatively long life expectancy in 1968, it was not as long as for those persons living in many European countries. In contrast with the populations of these advanced nations, the citizens of most South American, African, and Asian countries have shorter life expectancies. Infectious diseases and nutritional deficiencies take more lives in the less advanced nations, while heart disease and cancer seem to be the major killers of people in highly technological nations.

Each culture has its own characteristic pattern of disease, and although there is a correlation between the kinds of disease that will strike a population and the life expectancy of its members, many other factors are involved, as the comparisons of nations with similar life expectancy in Figure 21.6

Figure 21.5 Leading causes of death in the United States, 1900 and 1969.

Figure 21.6 Death rates for selected countries.

show. These other factors are attributable to differences in life styles among various cultures, although the mechanisms by which these factors work are poorly understood.

The national figures used so far do have important limitations. They do not suggest, for example, the variations that may exist in different parts of the same country. Some of these differences are illustrated in Figure 21.7. When one looks at life expectancy, death rates, and the frequency of given diseases, it becomes clear that nonwhite Americans, who primarily make up the lowest socioeconomic levels in the United States, suffer illnesses commonly found in underdeveloped nations. On the average, a nonwhite American can expect to live between six and seven years less than a white American, which in part helps to explain the relatively shorter overall life expectancy in the United States relative to other countries (see Figure 21.8). The comparatively high infant mortality rate among the poor also affects this figure.

CAUSES OF DISEASE

So far this discussion has focused on the existence of disease, its spread, and what is known about the patterns of appearance of different kinds of diseases in different cultures and under different living conditions. But what exactly is disease? Everyone has at least some idea of what is meant when the term is used, but before going any further perhaps a more precise definition should be offered. *Disease*, then, is incorrect functioning of an organ, part, structure, or system of the body. Disease results from (1) heredity, (2) diet, (3) infection, (4) stress, (5) environment, (6) degenerative processes as yet poorly understood, or some combination of these factors.

Following is a more detailed explanation of the various causes of disease. One must remember, however, that they also may play supportive, rather than causal roles toward one another. Often an illness results not from just one disease-causing agent but from a combination of several of the factors. One individual might develop heart disease through a combination of hereditary factors, poor eating habits, stress, smoking, and lack of exercise. Similarly, some cancers may involve viruses interacting with environmental irritants and stress. Thus, besides the specific treatment required for a given disease, it is often crucial also to provide adequate protection of the sick person against other agents that might take advantage of his debilitated condition to impose their own damaging, even lethal, effects.

Heredity

A child receives exact copies of half the DNA from each parent (as described in Chapter 14). Therefore, a defect in the parental genetic material will

	Mexico Life Expectancy 58-64	Colombia Life Expectancy 60	Mauritius (Africa) Life Expectancy 58-65	Ceylon Life Expectancy 62	United States Life Expectancy 71	Netherlands Life Expectancy 74
TB	20.7	22.3	11.7	14.1	3.5	.3
Pneumonia	107.9	59.8	34.4	37.6	24.0	10.1
Gastroenteritis and Colitis	89.0	108.2	126.2	34.9	3.6	3.5
Heart Diseases	42.6	81.3	93.6	58.6	373.3	243.6
Cancers	38.5	54.6	40.7	27.2	156.6	186.4
Cirrhosis of the Liver	20.2	4.4	3.5	4.7	14.1	3.5

be passed on from generation to generation. The defect in the DNA causes a defective production of a particular protein and hence an impairment of all the body functions in which this protein is involved. Some such function may be critical for life, and the inherited defect leads to death before or shortly after birth. In other cases, the inherited defect is not lethal and only causes an impairment of the health of the affected individual.

Certain diseases can be quite obvious at birth; others are so subtle that they do not overtly affect a person's health until late in life. Thus, a person with a genetic disease may well reach reproductive age and pass the genetic defect on to his or her progeny. Some genetically caused diseases were described in Chapter 14.

Heredity also can serve as a *predisposing* factor in a variety of diseases and ailments; that is, persons who have relatives with these diseases are more likely to get them than are persons with no afflicted relatives. Such diseases include heart disease and stomach and breast cancers.

Diet

The United States has one of the highest standards of living in the world. As a result, Americans are, on the average, well fed. This generalization can be viewed as an example of how deceiving general statistical statements may be, because in actuality, and paradoxically, some Americans are too well fed, while a large number of others are underfed or poorly fed.

Overeating, or eating too much of certain foods, may contribute to heart disease. In addition, obesity can contribute to a variety of health problems, as was discussed in Chapter 17. Abundance has allowed many prosperous persons to dig their graves with their forks. At the same time, the poor in America often are undernourished. Some simply receive too few calories to function well, while others lack certain essential food substances, such as vitamins or proteins.

A 1965 U.S. Department of Agriculture survey of American eating habits showed that a surprising number of people at all economic levels had diets low in two or more nutrients. In this category were 39 percent of low-income families, 21 percent of families with incomes of 7,000 to 10,000 dollars, and 18 percent with yearly incomes of 10,000 dollars. Thus, although there seems to be a general rule that the higher the income, the better the nutritional quality of the diet, high income itself does not insure a good diet.

The National Nutrition Survey, begun in 1968 under the auspices of the U.S. Department of Health, Education and Welfare, has documented

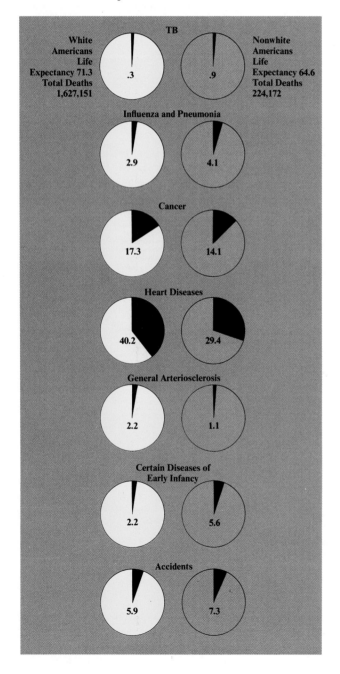

Figure 21.7 Comparison of life expectancy and death rates for different diseases among white and nonwhite Americans.

widespread malnutrition among American poor. It reports that in the population studied, of which the majority were families with incomes of less than 3,000 dollars, almost 4 percent of children under six were deficient in vitamin D. Such deficiency can result in the bone-deforming disease known as rickets. One-third of children under six were found to have low levels of vitamin A, lack of which may lead to night-blindness (see Chapter 19).

The national study also found that from 12 to 16 percent of the population in all age groups were deficient in vitamin C, and 4 percent showed symptoms of the nutritional disease scurvy, caused by insufficient vitamin C. Kwashiorkor, a protein-deficiency disease frequently affecting children of underdeveloped nations, discussed in Chapter 17, also is found in the urban slums and among the rural poor of America.

Even less severe diet deficiencies during the infant years, when the brain is undergoing critical development, may cause important mental impairment, ranging from the lethargic behavior typical of kwashiorkor children up to 20 percent IQ defi-

cits from other severe dietary deficiencies. Malnutrition (the wrong diet ingredients) or undernutrition (insufficient amounts of food) at all ages often sets the base for the high incidence of other diseases among the poor.

Infection

An infectious disease (see Chapter 22) is one that is caused by an agent capable of reproducing within the host: it could be a living cell, like a bacterium, or a nucleic-acid-containing particle, like a virus. Bacteria and viruses cause most of these ailments, but there are other organisms involved, too—plantlike fungi that cause athlete's foot as well as more serious infections; rickettsiae, which cause typhus fever and Rocky Mountain spotted fever, among others; single-celled animals known as protozoa, responsible for such tropical diseases as malaria and sleeping sickness; and metazoa, or many-celled animals, such as flukes and tapeworms, which can reside as parasites within human organs.

Although it is generally thought that infectious diseases are largely conquered in the United States,

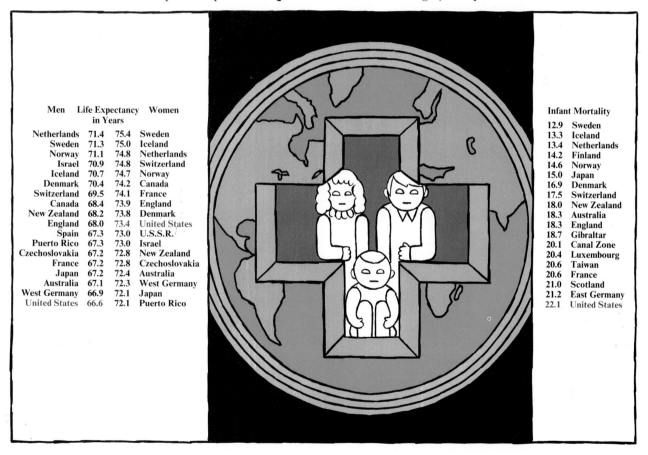

Men	Life Expectancy in Years	Women
Netherlands	71.4 75.4	Sweden
Sweden	71.3 75.0	Iceland
Norway	71.1 74.8	Netherlands
Israel	70.9 74.8	Switzerland
Iceland	70.7 74.7	Norway
Denmark	70.4 74.2	Canada
Switzerland	69.5 74.1	France
Canada	68.4 73.9	England
New Zealand	68.2 73.8	Denmark
England	68.0 73.4	United States
Spain	67.3 73.0	U.S.S.R.
Puerto Rico	67.3 73.0	Israel
Czechoslovakia	67.2 72.8	New Zealand
France	67.2 72.8	Czechoslovakia
Japan	67.2 72.4	Australia
Australia	67.1 72.3	West Germany
West Germany	66.9 72.1	Japan
United States	66.6 72.1	Puerto Rico

Infant Mortality	
12.9	Sweden
13.3	Iceland
13.4	Netherlands
14.2	Finland
14.6	Norway
15.0	Japan
16.9	Denmark
17.5	Switzerland
18.0	New Zealand
18.3	Australia
18.3	England
18.7	Gibraltar
20.1	Canal Zone
20.4	Luxembourg
20.6	Taiwan
20.6	France
21.0	Scotland
21.2	East Germany
22.1	United States

Figure 21.8 Life expectancies and infant mortality rates for selected countries. Note the low comparative position of the United States.

there are some such diseases that are still major killers, particularly among certain segments of the population. The venereal disease gonorrhea, almost eradicated after World War II, has spread dramatically over the past few years and is now the most commonly recorded infection among American adolescents, with true epidemic character. Tuberculosis as a cause of death is three times higher among nonwhite than white Americans.

Despite advances in medicine, man still is unable to control many viral diseases, the most common type of illness. In 1968 more than 100 million work days were lost from virus-caused colds and influenza alone. Every five to seven years in America's recent past there has been an epidemic of German measles, a virus-caused disease. Also known as rubella, German measles is usually very mild in children, less so in adults. Most importantly, it may cripple an unborn baby if its mother contracts the disease during the first three months of pregnancy. During the epidemic of 1963 to 1965, an estimated 20,000 infants born in the United States had birth defects, and another 30,000 stillbirths and miscarriages occurred as a result of maternal German measles. The federal government is supporting an effort to vaccinate children in order to reduce the carriers from which this disease could be transmitted to expectant mothers and to create an immune population.

As medicine improves, fewer persons die of infections. Ironically, however, some of the treatments that must be used for certain other diseases, such as cancer or kidney disease, actually inhibit or knock out one's natural defenses against microorganisms. Patients who have received x-ray treatments for cancer, for example, may become susceptible to infections that would normally not make them sick, because the x-rays weaken their natural defense mechanisms. Individuals who have received heart transplants must take drugs that leave them open to infections that doctors have never seen before. One patient whose transplanted heart was functioning well died sometime later as a result of six simultaneous infections. Although each was extremely rare as a cause of death, all six infections in combination had a fatal effect. Experts in the field say that doctors will see more and more patients with unusual if not bizarre infections as medicine continues its attempts to manipulate the body's protective mechanisms.

Environment

Just as infection was a universal hazard in the past, so are environmental nuisances that interfere with life and health in the world of today. The chemicals found in polluted air are one kind of environmental irritant. Air pollution has been implicated as triggering or accelerating serious respiratory ailments, heart disease, and cancer.

America's waters also are being fouled by chemical poisons. Lake Erie is now a receptacle for human, agricultural, and industrial wastes. In 1970 officials of the World Health Organization declared that most of the peoples of the world do not have safe drinking water. Contaminated water was an important factor contributing to the cholera pandemic. Even the oceans are not safe, as the government confiscation of mercury-contaminated tuna and swordfish in 1970 and 1971 demonstrated.

Just as the air and water are polluted, so is much of America's food. It is now virtually impossible to buy vegetables or meats that are uncontaminated by pesticides. Even if the foods themselves are not treated with these compounds, the chemicals are so plentiful in the environment that plants and animals destined for America's dinner tables absorb them. It should be all too apparent that chemical agents are not just part of the environment today—they are part of man. This pervasiveness of chemicals is due to the fact that as one

Figure 21.9 Environmental elements, such as population density, air pollution, and sanitation, are all factors that can lead to disease.

moves up the food chain (from plant to animal to man), chemicals like pesticides may be accumulated as much as ten times at each step (see Chapter 26). But food pollution is not limited to the chemicals picked up by organisms from the environment. Industrial and marketing treatments introduce additional chemical contaminants (such as preservatives, flavors and colors, packaging materials), the health consequences of which are only beginning to be assessed.

A variety of other external factors can either cause or provoke disease. Certain chemicals, for example, are known to be carcinogenic (cancer causing), and others are clearly poisonous to the body in certain dosages. In addition, the environment in which fetal development takes place is of-

ten affected by the maternal use of certain chemicals or drugs, which may lead to serious birth defects. Another form of environmental assault on the body can be considered the physical damage from heat and cold, or the fracturing, cutting, or crushing of tissues. Accidents are still the fourth highest cause of death in this country (see Chapter 27), half of them from cars, and war injuries are affecting millions of human beings, world-wide.

Stress

Life is largely a continuing series of adaptations to stresses from the environment. When one adapts well, life is enjoyable. But when one is unable to adapt to stress, physical and emotional complications may develop. The resistance to infectious and

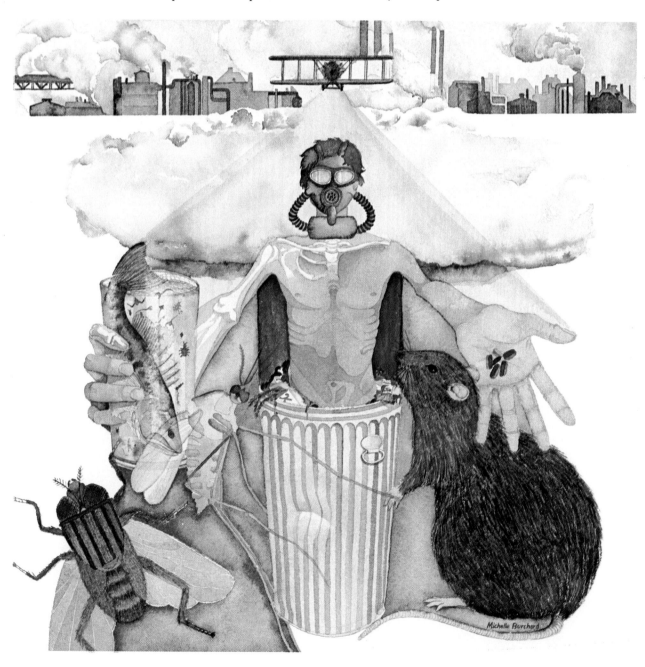

other diseases is reduced. Furthermore, many common ailments are suspected to result from poor adjustment to stress—certain ulcers, arthritis, asthma, cardiovascular conditions, and kidney disorders, for example. It has been estimated that from one-half to two-thirds of the patients seen by family doctors have ailments that are at least partially brought on this way. There also are distinct emotional adaptations to stress, some of which are described in Chapter 5.

The ways in which stress can affect the body are poorly understood, but they are thought to be associated with the secretion of epinephrine from the adrenal glands. As described in Chapter 3, this hormone is called into play in stressful situations and in part acts to increase heart rate, raise blood pressure by selective arteriole constriction, and mobilize glucose and lipids from storage sites.

Long-term exposure to stressful stimuli, particularly when there is no corresponding physical "working off" of the tensions involved, can contrib-

ute to permanent changes in body tissues and function, particularly in the heart and vessels. This is probably the cause of long-term psychological and psychosocial stress, and the source of many psychosomatic disorders, an area of disease that appears to be gaining increasing importance in today's American society.

Degenerative Processes

Degenerative diseases are poorly understood but are really separate from any of the other categories, although an interaction of other factors can certainly affect these diseases. Some of the ailments included in this category are degenerative arthritis (osteoarthritis), certain forms of emphysema, menopausal disorders, cataracts, and certain kinds of cancers. To some extent these diseases are considered inevitable because they accompany the gradual deterioration of the bodily machinery with age. Nevertheless, many Americans die much earlier than they should, or suffer chronic disease need-

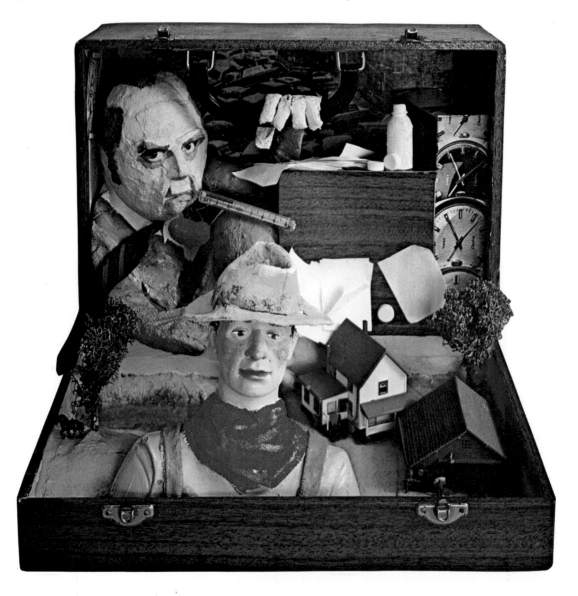

lessly, because of the American way of life. More and more atherosclerosis, hypertension, and cancer, among other "old age" diseases, are viewed as resulting not from age but from accumulated stress or "insults" with age.

It is now believed that a large portion of heart conditions could be prevented or delayed significantly if people would acquire good health habits. The wrong diet (including eating too much), cigarette smoking, overdependence on the automobile, sedentary work, and the psychological stresses of industrialized society among other factors are thought by some to accelerate the appearance of degenerative disease.

CHEMOTHERAPY

The dramatic decrease in infectious diseases, and the consequent shift in the disease pattern of America, would not have been possible without the discovery and use of selectively active chemicals, or drugs. *Chemotherapy*, the treatment of a disease by chemical means, has become the predominant approach of medical care, extending beyond the attack against infective agents to the treatment of degenerative disease and mental disorders.

Like many other sciences, chemotherapy has long roots in the past: in every civilization, potions and powders, plant extracts and animal materials have been attributed generic or specific curative properties, and some of them are eventually confirmed by modern science as well. Among the most threatening and ubiquitous diseases, for example, has been malaria—a blood infection caused by a protozoan parasite and transmitted by a mosquito. One of the Vedas of ancient Indian culture refers to malaria as the "King of Diseases," and the Babylonian god of pestilence, Nergal, was depicted in the form of an insect. Yet it appears that a cure for malaria was discovered by only one among all the threatened cultures. Early Peruvians successfully used the bark of the chincona tree against malaria.

Figure 21.10 One's life style must be examined in order to understand his particular health problems. The businessman whose frantic pace includes tremendous pressures, lunchtime cocktails, and improperly balanced meals will have a list of health problems that differ markedly from those of the farmer whose pace is relatively relaxed.

It is recorded that in 1619 the wife of the Spanish governor of Peru was cured from malaria by treatment with an extract from this bark—possibly the first documented practice of chemotherapy.

However, it was only after the basic discoveries of Louis Pasteur, Robert Koch, and many others in the nineteenth century that a systematic search for chemotherapeutic substances could be launched with a greater insight for the pathology of infectious disease. The first successes came early in the twentieth century, primarily through the work of German chemists and medical researchers. Paul Ehrlich showed the way with his studies on the chemotherapeutic effects of vital stains (organic compounds capable of staining living cells)—that led to the chemical treatment of trypanosomiasis (a group of protozoan infectious diseases)—and the use of metal-containing chemicals against the agent of syphilis.

Up to 1930 the successes of chemotherapy were mainly against diseases caused by protozoans. There was widespread belief that bacteria, which were the agents of the major diseases of Europe and America, were not susceptible to any drug that was not also toxic to man. This belief was proved false in 1932 by the introduction of the antibacterial drug Prontosil, the forerunner of *sulfonilamide* or sulfa drugs. During the following years several derivatives of sulfonilamide proved successful against many bacterial diseases, including pneumococcal pneumonia, gonorrhea, and puerperal fever.

The mechanism of the antibacterial action of the sulfonilamides is based on the principle of competitive inhibition, by which structurally analogous compounds inhibit or block the utilization of molecules necessary for the life processes of bacteria. This is a theory upon which much subsequent chemotherapeutic research has been directed.

Certainly the greatest success of chemotherapy has been the development of *antibiotic* drugs. Antibiotics differ from synthetic chemotherapeutic agents (such as the sulfonilamides) in that they are produced by living organisms. Antibiotics are substances produced by microorganisms that, in dilute solution, can kill or inhibit other microorganisms.

In 1877 Louis Pasteur found that two different microbes cultured together often inhibited each others' growth, even when excess food was available. He summarized his observations with the statement: "Life hinders life." By 1885 it had been suggested that one microorganism could stop the growth of another by the secretion of toxic substances. In 1897 Ernest Duchesne performed an amazing experiment in which one group of mice were inoculated with a pathogenic bacterium while others were inoculated with the bacterium and also a broth in which the mold *Penicillium glaucum* had grown. All of the mice that had been inoculated with only the bacteria died, whereas those animals that had received injections of the broth lived.

Unfortunately, this experiment was ignored,

and it was only by accident that Alexander Fleming rediscovered the antibiotic properties of secretions of *Penicillium* in 1928. Even at this time there was reluctance in the scientific community to accept the idea that substances toxic to bacteria would not also be harmful to host organisms. Fleming himself was afraid that the extract, which he named penicillin, would be too toxic to be of clinical use, and he gave up in his attempts at purification. Finally, in 1940, Sir Howard Florey showed, by experimentation remarkably similar in principle to Duchesne's, that a purified form of penicillin could be used as an antibacterial agent without producing harmful effects in laboratory animals. Further studies by other researchers elucidated the chemical nature of the agent and its mechanism of action as an antibiotic. It was through such efforts that the world came to accept this "wonder" drug.

Following this initial success, many new antibiotics were introduced. Antibiotic drugs developed

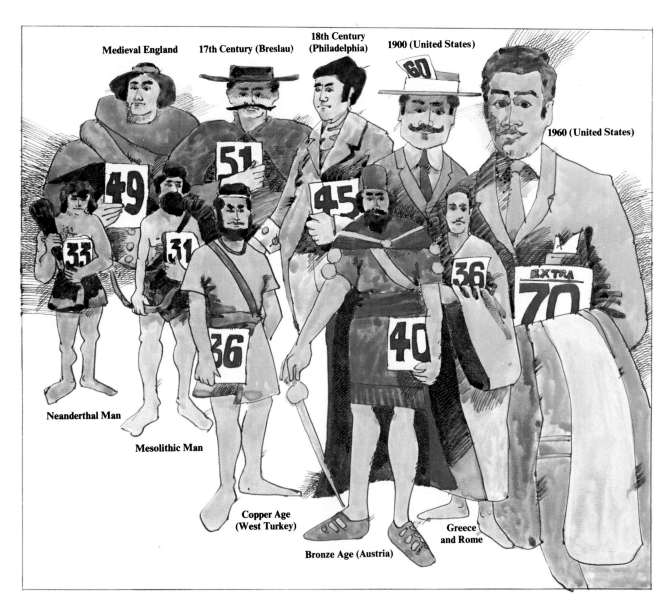

since penicillin include streptomycin, the tetracyclines, and erythromycin. The successful applications of antibiotics have served to reduce such threats to world health as pneumonia, bubonic and pneumonic plagues, tuberculosis, scarlet fever, rheumatic fever, and many other diseases.

Although antibiotics have greatly reduced the threat of infectious disease, they have by no means been totally successful. In some ways antibiotics have introduced new problems to medical care. The incidence of directly toxic or allergic reactions to certain antibiotics has shown the need for extreme caution in their use. For example, serious skin reactions and anaphylactic shock have resulted from the use of penicillin in certain patients. Another problem that has arisen is the appearance of strains of bacteria that are resistant to a given antibiotic. That is, within a species of bacteria, there are certain individual bacterium on whom a specific antibiotic fails to act. As these individuals grow and reproduce, they give rise to whole populations that are not affected by the antibiotic. To combat this problem, a doctor must have a series of antibiotics at his disposal, so that if one fails others may be tried. Therefore, there is a continuing need for research toward the development of new and effective antibiotics.

Although the search for new antibiotics continues, the frontiers of chemotherapeutic research have shifted to research directed toward the development of antiviral and anticancer drugs. Some successes have been made in both fields, most notably against viral diseases. Cancer research, at present, is in much the same state of development as bacterial research was late in the nineteenth century. That is, the basic causes of cancer are still being defined. Although some cancer-inducing agents have been identified (as will be described in Chapter 23), much basic research into the causes of many types of cancer remains to be done.

CONQUEST – OR PARTIAL TRUCE?

Has man conquered disease? Of course not, and perhaps he never will. But he certainly has achieved a partial truce that enables many individuals to live far healthier lives than their grandparents did and vastly healthier ones than their great-great-grandparents did.

As has been true throughout the course of human history, disease patterns are altered by social, cultural, and economic factors, and the diseases of each era relate specifically to how people live in those times. Eighteenth-century Philadelphians, for example, could expect to die six years younger, on the average, than their counterparts among the burghers of Breslau, Germany, a century before them (see Figure 21.11), probably because of the poor conditions in the New World and the attacks of epidemics such as yellow fever. Today in the United States, an even larger difference continues to separate the life expectancy of white and non-white citizens living at the same time in history.

Each person would do well to remember that he has some say, at least in statistical terms, about the sorts of diseases that will afflict him. With proper concern for social conditions, the environment, and his own personal health, the average American could help to alter the patterns of illness in this country for the last quarter of the twentieth century, and thus to reduce his own risk of encountering the most common health problems of today.

Figure 21.11 As is pointed out in the chapter, there are several factors that affect how long one will live: the geographical area in which one lives, the immediate environmental conditions, the dissemination and application of medical knowledge, and, as illustrated here, the culture into which one is born. Note that the life expectancy during the Bronze Age was forty years but dropped to thirty-six in the cities of Greece and Rome, where epidemics were common. Note also that an eighteenth-century Philadelphian had a shorter life span than his seventeenth-century forefather, whose shorter life probably reflects the squalid conditions that prevailed in many cities of the New World.

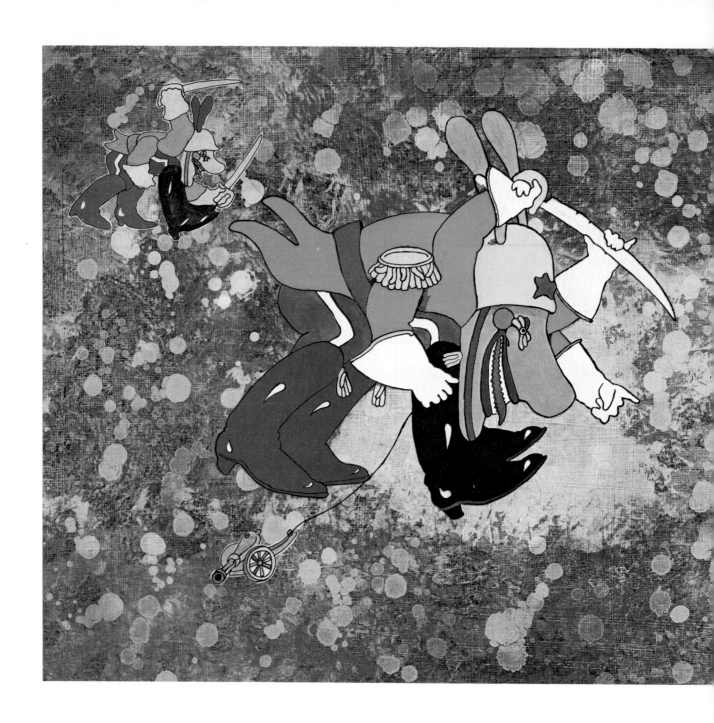

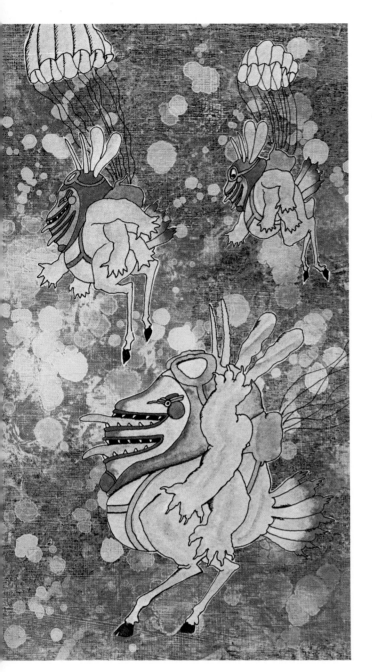

22

The concept of environment is generally thought to refer to that which is outside the human body. But the body is itself an environment, teeming with a variety of living microorganisms. A typical human body houses a number of organisms—probably on the order of 15 million million. There are billions in the mouth alone, perhaps 100 billion on the skin, and most of the rest are in the intestines. That they are so remarkably plentiful was actually recognized 300 years ago by the first man ever to see bacteria, Antony van Leeuwenhoek. Leeuwenhoek wrote in 1683 that there "are more animals living in the scum on the teeth in a man's mouth, than there are men in a whole kingdom . . ."

Many people fear microorganisms, or microbes, whether from the external or the internal environments, and refer to them as "germs." But despite the exaggerations of television commercials, not all microbes are harmful. Specialists have estimated that actually only a limited number of the known microbial species are *pathogens*, that is, organisms that regularly cause disease.

Those organisms with which men live most intimately and harmoniously are called resident, or *endogenous*, microbes, meaning that they reside within the human host. These microbes are so small that the billions of them in one body combined probably would not take up much more than one and a quarter measuring cups. Most of them are quite compatible with the health of the human body and in fact may contribute to its welfare—for

Infectious Diseases

example, by manufacturing essential vitamins and amino acids in the intestines. However, endogenous microbes cannot be regarded as completely or permanently harmless simply because they are inoffensive under normal circumstances. When these circumstances change, serious diseases may result.

Other organisms are *exogenous*; that is, they normally live outside the body. They include microbes that cause plague, cholera, influenza, tetanus, and venereal disease, among others. Such organisms will cause disease if they gain a foothold of any kind. But even when they invade, a variety of circumstances may determine whether the invasion will lead to disease. The number of organisms present, the health of the individual exposed (including fatigue, resistance, and so on), and even the individual's environment are often involved.

Infection is the attack that these exogenous agents wage against the body. Disease occurs only when the infectious agent originally *presents itself* in such great numbers or *multiplies* to such an extent within the infected body that it can cause harm to it. The microbes may produce damage simply because of their numbers, as is the case with pneumonia, or because they release poisons, or *toxins*, like those given off by the bacteria responsible for tetanus or diphtheria. In other cases, both mechanisms are involved. Disease usually becomes apparent when the body fights the invader. The site of infection may become sore, hot, and swollen, or other parts of the body may be reached by the infection and become involved.

AGENTS OF INFECTION

As described in Chapter 21, infectious agents are of six main types: bacteria, viruses, rickettsiae, fungi, protozoa, and metazoa. These agents are depicted in Figure 22.1. Many common diseases caused by the six main types of pathogens are described in Appendix A.

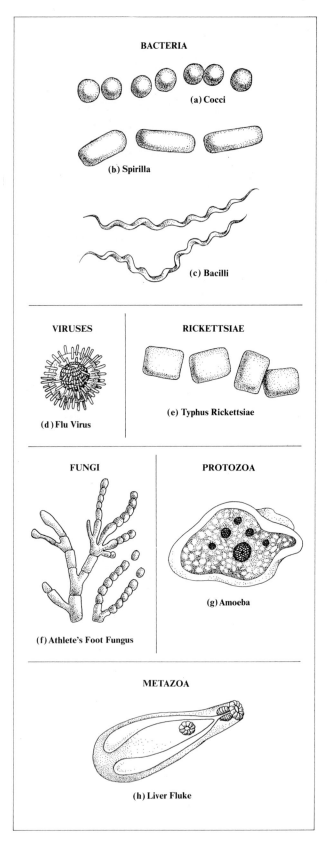

Figure 22.1 The six main pathogens. Examples include (a) the bacterium that causes strep throat and other streptococcal infections; (b) the tuberculosis bacillus; (c) the spirochete of syphilis; (d) the influenza virus; (e) the rickettsia that causes typhus; (f) athlete's foot fungus; (g) the amoeba causing amoebic dysentery; (h) the liver fluke that causes schistosomiasis.

Life on Man

by Theodore Rosebury

The color and odor of the fluid suggest cleanliness, and the bottle is pretty but austere, like a starched nurse. The voice on TV says it kills germs, kills them by the million.

This is today's mythology. Cleanliness has moved up from being merely next to godliness into a religion in itself. We are becoming a nation of tubbed, scrubbed, deodorized neurotics. Once it was only pleasure that was dirty and sinful. Now there is dirt everywhere, and there are germs to prove it. How irrational can we get?

If you are healthy and your teeth are clean, unless you have been eating onions, your mouth doesn't smell. If it does, you should see a dentist. Perfectly healthy young adult mouths contain germs by the billion—which means, of course, by the thousand million. No mouth is without them. Even if something really did kill them by the million it would be doing only one-thousandth of the job. But as it kills a few germs it also damages the cells of your mouth and interferes with other things provided by nature that

Adapted from Rosebury, T. "Preview," in *Life on Man*. New York: Viking, 1969, pp. xiii–xv.

need no help in keeping your mouth healthy—including some of the microbes, which destroy other microbes. Not only are you wasting your money on this beautiful rubbish, but it would not be worth using if you got it for nothing. It does harm without doing good. At best the harm is not noticed, and you may settle for a clean sensation. You may mask an odor, but if it didn't come from something you ate, the odor should be treated, not masked.

The same goes for other body odors. Blood and sweat do not smell until they are decomposed. Up to a point there is nothing unhealthy about the decomposition, even though microbes bring it about. But the use of a deodorant within bounds is a cosmetic act, like the use of lipstick and perfume. Only when it is done excessively, obsessively, does it become neurotic. The use of antiseptics, however, can hardly ever be justified. The attempt to kill the microbes that normally live on us is a mistake.

We have become too fastidious. Our noses have become so absurdly sensitive that we wrinkle them at the slightest hint of a healthy smell, which is not too strong a term for the smell of sweat from hard work or active play. We don't object to these smells in ourselves or in people we love unless they are forced on our attention. In learning to find them intolerable we are aping the dandified, exquisite aristocrat of the seventeenth century in his powdered wig, his laces and satins. There wasn't much plumbing then either for him or for the sweaty peasant. He shared the peasant's lice and fleas as well as his smells. But he masked his superior status by wearing ornate dress and strong perfume. We do things differently now, pretending to have the support of science. But our excesses are no more scientific than his were, and they are even further from common sense, since we ought to know better.

Most body odors are produced by microbes; and although we objected to some of them long before microbes were discovered, we have come to associate the two things. Germs produce disease, and so we think of them as nasty little things in their own right. Traces remain of the puritan notion that our bodies, or parts of them, their functions and products, are ugly, dirty. Sex has been entangled in this notion. Feces, filth, dirt, soil, earth—these are all related. Now that we know that germs are active in all of them, it looks as though there may be sense in the whole idea. But microbiologically speaking—and for other good reasons as well—it just isn't so.

Some of the other good reasons have been contributed by Freud rather than by Pasteur. Some of them have come from anthropologists and archaeologists. And, in fact, some of the most telling reasons have been given to us by artists, poets.

Freud has made us see, for instance, that our reaction to excrement tends to go far beyond the bounds of rationality. We all share in some degree the delusion of the "anal" person who keeps washing his hands and picking threads off his clothing, trying desperately to hide from the world an unconscious notion of inescapable filthiness. We are all in some degree compelled toward a spotlessness we can never achieve in fancy or in fact, nor would there by any sense in it if we could.

The anthropologists tell us that primitive man tended—just as infants do today—to venerate his body and to cherish what it produced. It is characteristic of Western civilized man that he has become extraordinarily anal in Freud's sense. Young people today, including many college students, often prefer to emulate the more alienated hippies rather than their elders, rejecting many of our values, including the whole business of neatness. They see cleanliness as part of the sham of a hypocritical world. They are also forcing a sexual revolution upon us; and we are inclined to sympathize with part of it, since the irrationality of regarding sex as something dirty is becoming inescapable. Yet the dimensions of our irrationality extend

well beyond sex—which is certainly part of what poets and artists have been trying to tell us since long before Rabelais, before Chaucer, since the times of Aristophanes and Praxiteles and Sappho, of Solomon's Song of Songs.

We are starting to teach the biology of reproduction to children and hope for rationality and sanity in generations to come. Perhaps we ought to do the same with the microbiology of man, for the same purpose of encouraging rational behavior. We ought to reconcile the science of epidemic disease with that of soil fertility, and show that the microbes living normally on man are a kind of bridge between these two, an aspect of the overall scheme of living things in the world. These microbes fall neatly between the "evil" of disease and the "good" of the earth's fertility. They are closer to the second, since in the normal course they do us no harm. In fact we know now, from experiments with animals we can make and keep free from germs—they turn out to be miserable, deprived things—that we could not get along without microbes.

"Dirt," considered as "earth," is not evil. The myth that germs and dirt are always our enemies is harmful and costly. We ought to get rid of it. The evil of disease remains, of course. We need to put it in perspective. Disease lends itself to measurement and analysis by the methods of science. It has shown itself to be amenable to understanding, treatment, control, even the possibility of eradication. For our purposes we can point out the connection between disease and cleanliness and set limits to it. It can be made clear that too much cleanliness is as sick as too little.

Bacteria, a type of single-celled plant life, are the most plentiful of such microorganisms and comprise the major portion of organisms endogenous to man. Most bacteria are either nonharmful or are vital to man's existence. The bacterium *E. coli*, for example, plays an important role in digestion; other bacteria perform such functions as vitamin production and destruction of potential pathogens.

Some diseases are caused by endogenous bacteria that for various reasons get out of hand. For instance, bacteria normally found on the skin may have a role in acne, bacteria endogenous to the mouth are involved in the serious gum disease pyorrhea, and intestinal bacteria, particularly in women, may be transferred from feces to the urethra and cause urinary tract infections. An upset in normal balances between tissues and the flora that inhabit them is thought to play a role in such problems. Harmful bacteria, on the other hand, are responsible for such diseases as gonorrhea, meningitis, tuberculosis, tetanus, and syphilis. Fortunately, bacteria are susceptible to antibiotics, so that bacterial diseases can largely be brought under control.

Viruses are the most minute and primitive form of life. They consist essentially of a bit of nucleic acid within a protein coat. Once a single virus enters a cell, it takes over the cell's machinery and directs it to produce many hundreds of new viral particles. A single cell thus engorged with viruses breaks aparts, spewing its hundreds of viruses in all directions, each virus having the ability to again enter a cell, capture its machinery, and start the cycle again. Among the many virus-caused diseases are smallpox, rubella, measles, mumps, influenza, the common cold, and some forms of hepatitis. Because viruses are in many ways similar to human cells, science has been hard put to come up with a method of destroying a virus without also harming the human cells. The answer may lie in the interferon story, described later in this chapter.

Rickettsiae are considered intermediate between bacteria and viruses. Most of these organisms grow in the intestinal tracts of insects that carry them to their human host. Such blood-sucking insects as lice, rat fleas, mites, and ticks spread these infectious agents to man. Typhus fever is transmitted by lice; Rocky Mountain spotted fever is transmitted by mites.

Fungi are plants that lack chlorophyll and must obtain their food from organic material—in some cases from man. Ringworm and athlete's foot are infections caused by fungi.

Animal parasites, including certain types of *protozoa* and *metazoa*, are organisms that have developed the capacity to live in or on the body of another animal, known as the *host*. Most parasites have acquired the remarkable ability of spending part of their life in one host (man) and the rest of their life in another host (which can range from a mosquito to a cow). Protozoa are responsible for such diseases as amoebic dysentery and malaria. Metazoa that make their home on man include pinworms, tapeworms, and flukes.

HOW INFECTION SPREADS

Acne, pyorrhea, and urinary tract infections are examples of situations where endogenous, normally harmless microbes cause their own host to become diseased. Or, possibly, the host person has become diseased and that causes its own endogenous microbes to proliferate and cause further ailments. In any case, the resulting disease remains restricted to that one person. But other infectious ailments from exogenous microbes, such as colds, tuberculosis, venereal disease, malaria, and so on, can be passed from individual to individual, either directly or through such intermediaries as insects, air, or drinking water: they are *communicable*.

Pathogenic agents may enter the body either through breaks in the skin or through any of the

Figure 22.2   How a virus invades a cell, taking over the cell's machinery to reproduce more copies of the virus, which in turn invade more cells.

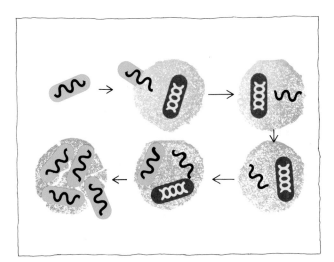

natural openings of the body, such as those of the respiratory tract, the alimentary tract, or the urogenital tract. Pathogens also are often *released* from these same parts of the body, to be picked up by other persons.

Certain infections are spread by direct physical contact—venereal disease, for example. Others may be spread by objects such as clothing or eating utensils that have been touched or used by an infected individual. Some organisms travel through the air attached to dust particles or water droplets. One sneeze can account for approximately 20,000 droplets, which may cover a range of fifteen feet and which contain large numbers of microorganisms, many of them capable of causing disease. Food and water also can transmit infectious agents, as occurs in cholera, typhoid, and dysentery. In addition, insects act as *vectors* (intermediaries) for such diseases as plague, yellow fever, and malaria.

THE COURSE OF AN INFECTION

Because all these infections depend upon basically the same mechanism—invasion by foreign organisms and the reaction of the invaded body to them—a common pattern can be recognized when disease develops. The course of an infectious disease has five broad phases:

1. The *incubation period* begins with the invasion. During this phase the organisms multiply in the host. The length of the incubation period varies from disease to disease and from one person to another for the same disease.
2. The *prodrome* period is a short interval characterized by general symptoms such as headache, fever, nasal discharge, malaise, irritability, and discomfort. Diagnosis is difficult because the symptoms are so similar for most diseases. The disease is highly communicable during prodrome.
3. *Clinical disease* occurs when illness is at its height. The characteristic symptoms appear during this

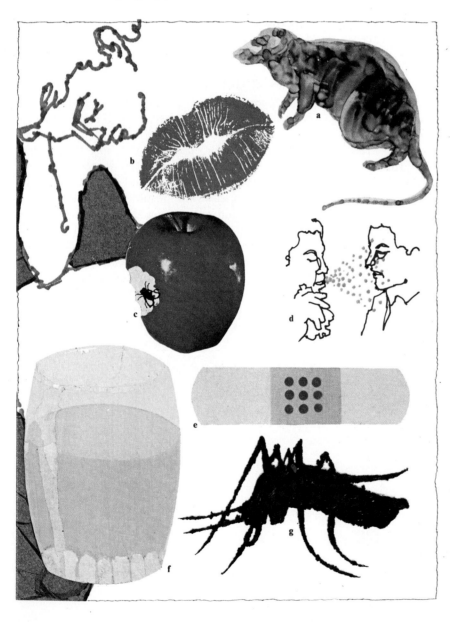

Figure 22.3 How infectious invaders gain access to the human body. (a) Animals may be a source of infectious disease. Rodents serve as a reservoir for plague; dogs and squirrels are common sources for rabies; brucellosis, or undulant fever, is acquired from drinking the raw milk of infected cows or by handling the diseased animals. (b) Direct contact is the most frequent method by which one individual infects another. Some of the diseases transmitted by this means are colds, influenza, pneumonia, tuberculosis, syphilis, and gonorrhea. (c) Flies and other insects transfer disease-producing microorganisms on their feet or other appendages or by using their bodies as mechanical means of transfer. (d) Microorganisms can be spread by the droplets that are constantly projected into the air by sneezing, coughing, breathing, and talking. (e) Transmission of microorganisms to the new host is in itself not sufficient to produce infection. The microorganisms must gain entrance to the body before they can multiply and cause infection. A cut, an abrasion, or an open wound will provide a means of breaking through the protective mechanism of the skin. (f) Microorganisms are transmitted indirectly by vehicles of infection such as water, milk, other food, and inanimate objects such as clothing and eating utensils. Typhoid fever, dysentery, and cholera are spread through water. (g) The transfer of disease by certain insects requires that the microorganisms undergo changes within the insect vectors. Such a process occurs in one species of mosquito that carries malaria-causing protozoa.

phase, and specific diagnosis becomes possible. A disease that is *subclinical* presents few symptoms and therefore may be undiagnosed.

4. The *decline stage* is marked by subsiding symptoms. The patient may feel well enough to become active before he is recovered, which may increase the danger of relapse.

5. *Convalescence* is the recovery period. The disease may still be communicable. If the patient recovers but still gives off disease-causing organisms, he then becomes one form of *carrier* of that disease.

BODY DEFENSES

The body is exposed to an almost infinite number and variety of organisms, many of which are capable of causing disease. To combat these agents, the body mobilizes a system of natural defenses. One must remember, however, that the strength with which these defenses will operate will be greatly influenced by the health conditions of the whole body or of the body systems that are involved in individual defense mechanisms.

The skin is the first line of defense. An invading microbe must find its way inside the skin or the mucosae, the mucus-coated membranes that make an "inner skin" for the body by lining the respiratory, digestive, and urogenital tracts. Secretions such as tears, sweat, and urine can flush bacteria away. In addition, respiratory passages have fine, short, moving hairs—cilia—that trap disease organisms or other foreign particles and beat them back toward the outside. Enzymes and the acidity of the stomach destroy still more.

Microorganisms sometimes get beyond these first defenses—through a cut in the skin, for example. They then face a second line of defense in the blood and the tissues. The blood, like some external secretions, contains bacteria- and virus-killing chemicals. It also contains cells (a variety of white blood cells) that engulf bacteria and foreign particles and digest them. Cells that do so are called *phagocytes*. Although these cells normally circulate in the blood, they also can squeeze through the

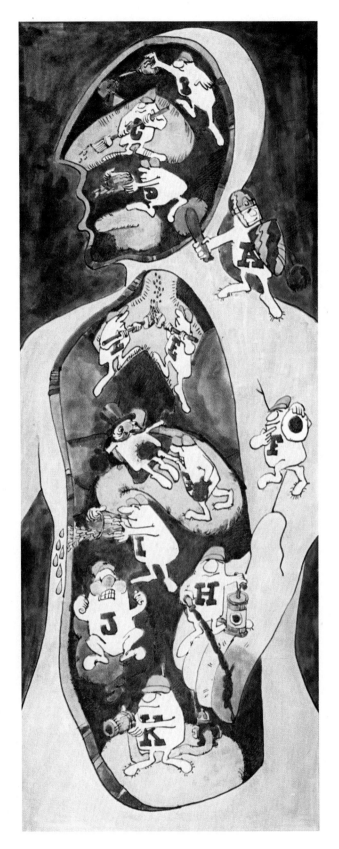

Figure 22.4 Body defenses: (a) The skin defends the body from disease and injury by acting as a physical barrier. (b) Tears help to wash away foreign material and contain bactericidal substances. (c) The cilia of the nasal passages keep foreign particles from irritating sensitive nasal membranes. (d) The saliva is highly bactericidal. (e) Cilia of the trachea and lungs prevent foreign particles from irritating the tissue. (f) White blood cells surround and ingest foreign bodies and disease organisms. (g) Stomach acids and enzymes destroy most disease organisms that are found in food and water. (h) When the skin is cut or punctured, bleeding acts as a mechanical "wash" and begins clotting at the injured area, thus inhibiting the passage of foreign material into the body. (i) The sweat glands help maintain normal body temperature and secrete bactericidal substances. (j) Pain helps defend against problems becoming critical by alerting the person that there is infection of injury. (k) The urine acts as a mechanical wash and has some bactericidal capacity.

walls of a blood vessel, migrate to the site in the tissue where microorganisms have entered, and there wage their fight against the invaders. Tissues, too, contain phagocytic cells of a larger size—*macrophages*—that contribute to the local fight. Thus, many bacteria never gain a foothold in the body.

Suppose, however, that microbes do become established and begin to multiply. The body must then resort to a third line of defense, which is part of a complex phenomenon called *inflammation*. The inflammatory response is not specifically directed against infectious agents. It is a response to any irritant, whether physical, chemical, or microbial. A splinter would be just as effective in eliciting the response. The blood supply to the endangered area increases and, at the same time, the blood flow through it slows down, resulting in a leakage into intercellular spaces of tissue fluids (exudate), which accumulate at the site together with antibacterial and antitoxic proteins. The rush into the tissue of blood phagocytes also is greatly increased, while mechanisms come into play to continually replace them in the circulating blood.

The outward signs of inflammation are usually redness and local warmth, swelling, and pain. Though discomfort is produced, the action is beneficial. Generalized *fever*, on the other hand, is a sign that a battle is being waged all over the body. Fever is, at least in part, caused by toxic materials produced by the invaders or released from them during their destruction that interfere with the regulatory mechanisms that normally control the temperature of the body. The results of an inflammatory response vary considerably, depending on the balance between the numbers and virulence of the

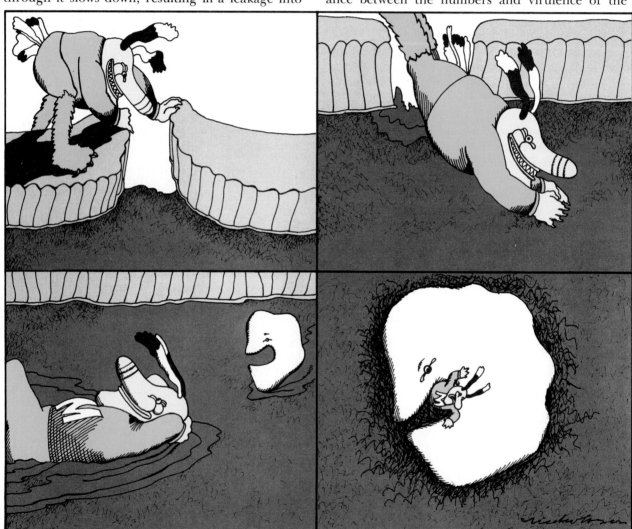

Figure 22.5 When the skin is punctured, the alert goes out to the immune system, which reacts by sending large clumps of white blood cells to the injured area. The cells ingest the foreign material. Due to the large concentration of these cells, the injured area usually is swollen and painful from added pressure on surrounding nerves.

invaders and the strength of the body defense mechanism. In the most severe cases, this third line of defense may fold, the invaders spread through the tissues and even into the bloodstream, and the infection becomes a generalized and highly dangerous one. In other cases, the local battle may go on and on, at a standstill. More and more of the local tissue gets destroyed, and a cavity, or *abscess*, is formed that fills with fluid, battling cells, and white blood cells that have died in the attack (*pus*). The abscess may eventually be walled in, drained, and replaced with scar tissue, or pockets of it may persist, converting the acute (short-term) inflammatory process into a chronic (long-term) inflammation. Full victory, that is, resolution to normal, occurs when all the invaders are killed.

The body also has a defense mechanism directed entirely against viruses. This mechanism, still only partially understood, results in the formation of a small protein known as *interferon*, which is manufactured mainly by various types of lymphoid cells, the same kind of cells that are involved in the immune mechanism (described in the next section). These cells occur in great numbers in the bone marrow, spleen, lymph nodes, lung, and liver tissue. Other similar cells, or lymphocytes (another variety of white blood cell), constantly circulate through the bloodstream, from the blood vessels into the tissues, from the tissues into the lymphatic vessels and lymph node, and eventually back to the bloodstream. The trigger for the production of interferon by these cells is provided by the virus itself or, more precisely, by its nucleic acid; even an inactivated virus—one incapable of multiplying inside an infected cell—can act as such a trigger. Viruses differ in their effectiveness as interferon triggers, but the interferon manufactured under the influence of one virus can be used by the body to protect itself against other viruses as well. It is believed that interferon, by reaching potential target cells ahead of an invading virus, makes them manufacture a substance that will prevent the infecting virus from multiplying within them.

IMMUNITY

While the inflammation battle rages at the site of invasion, the body is marshalling yet another defensive system, the *immune mechanism*. The immune response provides protection against a specific invader by manufacturing an *antibody* that fights only against that foreign organism or one of its chemical products. Antibodies are produced in increasing amounts over a period ranging from several days to several weeks.

Antibodies, like so many of the important products of the body, are proteins. They are manufactured by certain types of lymphoid cells, called *plasma cells*, and many of them circulate freely in the blood. Antibodies help in dealing with bacteria in several ways. They cause bacteria to clump together, making it easier to remove them from the bloodstream before the reach into the tissues.

Figure 22.6 Where blood components are made. The red blood cells (erythrocytes) are manufactured in the bone marrow. The blood platelets are small cellular bodies (not actually cells) that are derived from the largest cells of the bone marrow. The leukocytes, which also are manufactured in the bone marrow, are an important factor in the cellular defense mechanism of the body. When infection is introduced into the body, the lymphocytes, produced in the lymph nodes, increase in size and transform into large phagocytic cells (macrophages) that engulf foreign material and inhibit the growth of pathogens.

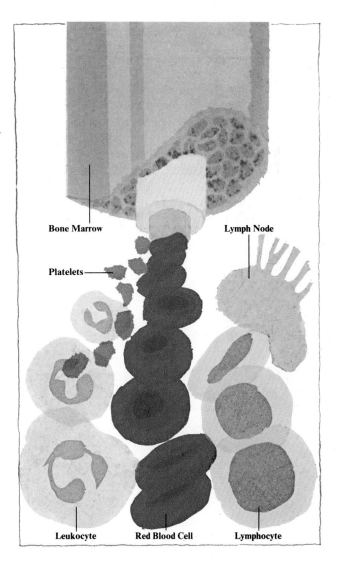

Bone Marrow

Lymph Node

Platelets

Leukocyte

Red Blood Cell

Lymphocyte

When bacteria are coated with antibody they are more readily ingested by the phagocytic cells. Antibodies attached to the bacterium activate certain bactericidal substances of the blood and bring about their distinctive action on the invading organisms. In addition, antibodies may combine with viruses and prevent them from entering their target cells.

The most remarkable thing about these antibody proteins is their *specificity*, a property lacking in the interferon proteins. The body has the capacity to make innumerable antibodies—at least one kind for each different infectious agent, regardless of what it is. Antibodies destroy only the agent that evoked the antibody or one closely related to that agent. Antibody-inducing agents are called *antigens*. The specificity of the immune response can be illustrated with almost any virus. Suppose one is exposed to measles and the body produces antibodies against measles virus. If now a mumps virus infection becomes established in the body, the antibodies synthesized against the measles virus cannot attack it. In order to cope with the mumps virus, the body must synthesize a new set of antibodies that will inactivate only the mumps virus.

Immunity is acquired naturally when one develops a disease. In the course of an illness, antibodies appear, and one begins to recover. Not many years ago, having the disease was the only way people could develop immunity. Today immunity may be induced artificially by means of vaccines injected into the body. In several days or weeks, specific antibodies in large amounts circulate in the bloodstream, ready to attack the initiating microbe (antigen).

Some vaccines contain living infectious agents; included in this group are those used against smallpox, yellow fever, and measles, as well as the Sabin oral polio vaccine. These living agents have been weakened (attenuated) in the laboratory but still provoke the formation of specific antibodies. Other vaccines contain killed infectious agents; included in this group are the whooping cough and Salk polio vaccines. The killed microbes will not produce the disease but will stimulate production of specific antibodies against the same organism, thereby protecting the body from future infection.

Based on similar principles, acquired immunity can be induced against certain microbial *toxins* that produce disease. Diphtheria and tetanus produce disease through their toxins. Modified toxins, called *toxoids*, that are no longer poisonous, are used to induce antibodies that will inactivate the poisons if the invading organism strikes.

Having the disease or receiving a vaccine produces *active* immunity. Occasionally someone is exposed to a disease and cannot wait for his own antibodies to form. In this instance, antibodies formed by another person or an animal can be given, using the process called *passive immunization*. These antibodies come from a protein fraction of blood serum called gamma globulin. It is used for passive immunization against such diseases as infectious hepatitis, for which an effective vaccine for humans has not yet been devised.

Effective and safe vaccines for most common viral diseases are available today. In general, active immunity is long term and in some cases lifelong, while passive immunity lasts only a few weeks or months. Table 22.1 gives a schedule for recommended immunizations and boosters. A physician should be consulted for any variations.

PREVENTION AND TREATMENT

One can prevent many infectious diseases just by taking a few simple precautions. Some are based on what is known about the transmission of disease—avoiding food and water suspected of being contaminated, for example, will spare one many a

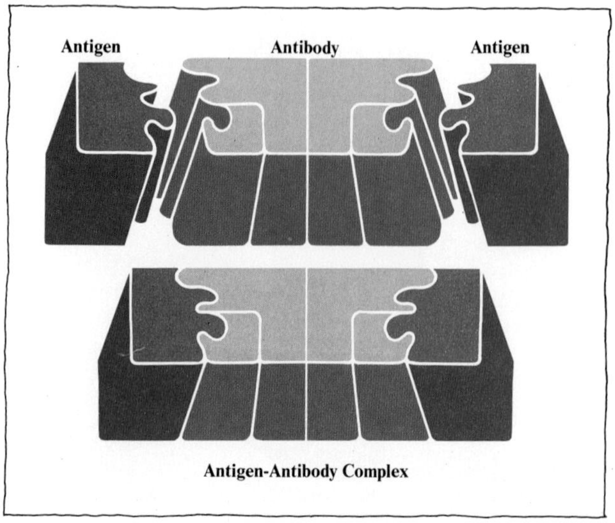

Antigen   Antibody   Antigen

Antigen-Antibody Complex

Figure 22.7 Antigen-antibody reaction. Contemporary research evidence indicates that an antibody molecule has two identical halves, each with one large and one small component. Each antibody has only one antigen that fits with it. The two surfaces of the antibody molecule fit against the surface of two antigen molecules, thus inactivating them.

stomach or intestinal upset and may prevent serious diseases as well. Other precautions are based on what is known about the relationships between the human body and invading organisms.

Because there frequently seems to be a relationship between the initial number of infecting microbes and the severity of disease, such simple precautions as cleanliness and protection from contact with infected persons may limit the number of infecting agents in contact with the body. It is also important to be sure that one has been protected from certain communicable diseases by the proper immunizations.

Vaccination is a way of preventing some infectious diseases and passive immunization can be used to provide temporary immunity. But what sorts of treatment are available when one has already come down with the symptoms of infectious disease? Although every disease demands specific treatment, there are several general steps that are followed for all such diseases.

The major goal in the treatment of an infectious disease is accurate diagnosis, based on examination of the stricken person's urine, sputum, blood, or similar material. When the results of such tests have been returned, the most specific and effective

Table 22.1   Recommended Immunization Schedule

DISEASE	*Age of First Dose*	*Boosters*
Diphtheria Whooping cough Tetanus	6 weeks to 2 months; series: 3 injections one month apart	At 1 year and before entering school; tetanus every 4 years
Polio Sabin (oral)	6 weeks to 3 months; three doses 6 to 8 weeks apart	At 12 to 15 months and on entering school
Measles	1 vaccination at 12 months	As yet, no recommendation
Mumps	1 vaccination in preadolescence	As yet, no recommendation
Influenza	Any age past 3 months; series: 2 shots one month apart for person exposed to flu in their work	Annually for person exposed or endangered
German measles	1 vaccination at 12 months	As yet, no recommendation
Typhoid and paratyphoid A and B	After 3 months; series: 3 shots one to four weeks apart for persons taking trips where water supply is questionable	One shot every three years if visiting frequently or living in typhoid area
Tuberculosis	After 3 months; series: 1 shot BCG vaccine for selected persons unavoidably exposed to continuous contact with TB	BCG only on recommendation of the U.S.P.H.S.
Rabies	Any age; series: up to 14 injections after being bitten by a rabid animal or one suspected of being rabid	None
Yellow fever	After age 6 months; series: 1 shot if going to yellow fever area	One, if remaining in a yellow fever area for prolonged period
Cholera	After age 6 months; series: 2 shots 7 to 10 days apart if traveling to cholera area	Boosters 4 to 6 months apart if living in cholera area; after 4 years repeat immunization

Source: Adapted from U.S. Public Health Service, Communicable Disease Center, Atlanta, Ga. and from Metropolitan Life Insurance Company.

drug can be chosen and administered. Other general measures include (1) drainage—the opening of an abscess or the encouragement of coughing to get rid of infected material; (2) rest—of the total body with generalized infections, or of the affected part with localized problems; (3) administration of fluids—especially important with urinary tract infections; (4) local heat—to promote circulation in the infected area; (5) elevation—to accelerate drainage of tissue fluids collecting in an inflamed (swollen) area. Proprietary medicines such as cold remedies and aspirin do little to control the infection process, although they often make the sufferer more comfortable.

COMMON INFECTIOUS DISEASES

This discussion has focused on the spread, effects, prevention, and treatment of infectious diseases in general. A description of the major human infectious diseases is provided in Appendix A. Nevertheless, there are some diseases that are so prevalent that they warrant special attention in this chapter. These common infections include colds, flu, pneumonia, tuberculosis, and mononucleosis. Special attention will be given to syphilis and gonorrhea, the most common venereal diseases. In addition, these discussions should help illuminate some of the general points about disease just discussed.

The Common Cold

The common cold is practically a universal nuisance and contributes heavily to the amount of time lost each year because of viral diseases. One theory suggests that healthy people carry cold viruses in their noses and throats all the time but only exhibit cold symptoms when something like fatigue or lowered resistance produces favorable circumstances for the viruses to proliferate and get out of hand. Cold viruses seem to survive in the air, beginning their journey to another person either in the spray of droplets resulting from a sneeze or in the air exhaled when a cold victim talks or breathes. The period of time between first exposure to the virus and the appearance of symptoms—the incubation period—is short, on the order of eighteen to forty-eight hours.

One would think that with so many people having colds and so many man-hours of productivity being lost, scientists would know more about the common cold than they do. But the disease is more complicated than it appears at first. Only in the last few years have researchers gained any certain knowledge about the agents responsible for it. For one thing, there are many viruses that cause colds. So far more than thirty have been implicated, and more may still be discovered. Each of these viruses can be grown in the laboratory and will produce certain recognizable results in experimental human subjects. Cold viruses appear to differ from other viruses in that they do not confer long-lasting immunity. It also is possible that cold viruses mutate rapidly. If that is the case, then each successive cold could be caused by a different virus, resulting in an endless series of apparently similar diseases.

The fact that colds are caused by viruses suggests some means of prevention and treatment. Because so many different viruses are involved and because the environmental and physiological circumstances for the development of colds are still so poorly understood, there is little one can do to prevent them beyond avoiding persons with "new colds" (the first twenty-four hours is the most communicable stage) or staying away from others when one has a new cold. It is also useful to maintain one's resistance to infection through adequate nutrition, rest, and exercise, although expert opinion on the values of such measures varies widely.

Once a cold has developed, one's main concern is to keep it from leading to more serious illness. No chemicals or antibiotics are effective against the common cold, although aspirin may be useful in easing discomfort. Nasal sprays, nose drops, decongestants, cough medicines, or other proprietary remedies should not be used without medical supervision because most of them are useless, and some may create conditions favoring more serious infection. Some decongestants, for example, may dry and crack the mucous membrane of the bronchi and make it more vulnerable to bacterial infection. Over-the-counter cough medicine is rarely strong enough to offer much relief but on occasion may interact harmfully with other drugs one is taking. Cough drops are relatively expensive and offer no advantages over ordinary hard candy in stimulating saliva flow to relieve a mild tickling cough. When one blows his nose, he should do so gently with his mouth open, to avoid forcing congestion and infection up the eustachian tubes to the middle ear. Steam breathing is useful in loosening nasal congestion.

Occasionally the attack by a cold virus is followed by a secondary invader, usually bacterial, taking advantage of the lowered defense barriers. Once the new organism establishes itself, a long-lasting chronic condition may develop unless proper treatment is instituted. The most common secondary invaders are cocci—pneumococci, staphylococci, and streptococci. Judicious treatment with antibiotics under medical supervision should serve to eliminate such infections. Nevertheless, indiscriminate self-administration of antibiotics for every passing infection, whether viral or bacterial, is not recommended; constant medication with antibiotics may produce drug allergy in some people so that when a serious infection does occur, the drug cannot be used.

Influenza

Influenza, or flu, is not usually a serious disease when uncomplicated by secondary infection. But when bacteria become involved, or when the flu virus spreads to the lung, the condition may be lethal. Several viruses are responsible for influenza. There are two major types, A and B, as well as numerous strains within each type. When epidemics occur, the viruses seem to cause more serious forms of the disease than they do during the lulls between major outbreaks.

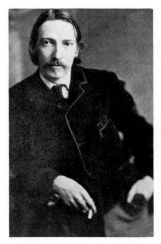 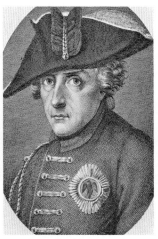 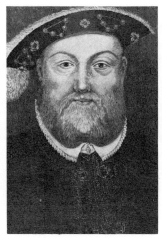 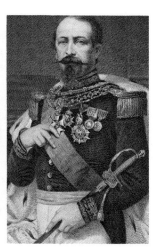

Figure 22.8 *(from left to right)* Before modern medicine conquered the "white plague" of tuberculosis, this disease claimed the lives of countless people, including such famous artists as Keats, Schubert, Chopin, Modigliani, Kafka, and Robert Louis Stevenson (pictured here), Scottish man of letters, who died of tuberculosis in 1894 at the age of forty-four. Frederick "the Great," enlightened and cultured eighteenth-century despot of Prussia, suffered from gonorrhea. Henry VIII, much married and high-living king of England, died in 1547 of syphilis and cirrhosis of the liver. Napoleon III, French president and emperor, suffered from gonorrhea and kidney disorders. He died of uremia in 1873.

The early symptoms of influenza resemble those of the common cold, but in addition there is often sudden fever, weakness, coughing, and aching pain in the back and extremities. Incubation is brief, requiring only one to three days. The infected individual is able to communicate the infection to others from just before symptoms appear until approximately a week later. Frequently, a great physical and mental depression accompanies influenza, often persisting long after the infection itself is over.

There are vaccines against specific strains of influenza virus, but they are not effective against other strains. Accordingly, vaccination will not protect susceptible individuals if an outbreak involves a different viral strain. Nevertheless, the Surgeon General's Advisory Committee on Influenza suggests that persons over sixty-five, those with chronic cardiovascular disease and certain other diseases, and pregnant women be vaccinated. The components of the vaccine are changed periodically, so individuals must be revaccinated each year.

Tuberculosis

Half a century ago about 80 percent of all Americans became infected with the tubercle bacillus before they were twenty years old. By 1940 the total infected by that age had dropped to 40 percent. Today the figure is 5 percent or less in most parts of the United States.

This changing pattern of infection does not mean that tuberculosis (TB) is under control. It is still a major problem in urban ghettos and among the rural poor, both in the United States and in underdeveloped nations of the world, and it is a significant medical problem for the elderly.

The tubercle bacillus causes chronic inflammation in many organs of the body. The lungs are the primary sites for tubercle infection, but other tissues, as shown in Figure 22.9, also come under attack. The victim of tuberculosis can cough and

breathe out 2 to 4 billion tubercle bacilli over a twenty-four-hour period, so it is essential that he observe such elementary rules of hygiene as covering his mouth when he coughs.

Fortunately, a high percentage of TB cases yield to careful treatment of the disease. Because of the highly contagious nature of TB, all family members and close contacts of the infected individual should undergo routine checks for the disease.

Pneumonia

Pneumonia, too, used to be a scourge of the world's population. With the advent of antibiotics, pneumonia became a far less serious disease. Nevertheless, it remains a leading cause of death in the United States, particularly among the very old and the very young. Unlike influenza or even the common cold, it is not a disease caused by one specific type of agent. It is a disease characterized by inflammation of the lungs, and this inflammation may result from infection or may be caused by exposure to all sorts of irritants, including dust and chemicals.

Bacterial pneumonia responds to antibiotic therapy. The most common pneumonia-causing bacteria are pneumococci. They produce sudden illness with chills, fever, shortness of breath, and coughing. The illness is diagnosed by laboratory tests or with x-rays. Viral pneumonia, of course,

Figure 22.9 Common sites of tuberculosis infection. The lungs are the sites of approximately 93 percent of all TB cases. It can also attack the kidneys, spine, and parts of the skeletal system.

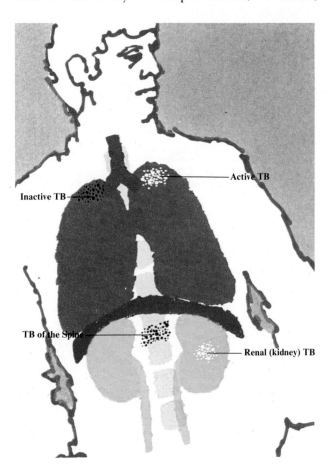

cannot be treated with antibiotics. Influenzal pneumonia frequently occurs in epidemic form and can be produced by many of the influenza viruses. It is best diagnosed by x-ray. Other viruses, such as those that cause measles and chickenpox, also can initiate pneumonia. Bacteria and viruses are not the only infectious agents that can cause pneumonia—fungi and other parasites also may cause it.

Mononucleosis

Probably every college student has heard of "mono"—infectious mononucleosis. Sometimes it is called "the college disease" or "the kissing disease" because it occurs so frequently during the college years and for a long time was thought to be transmitted principally by kissing.

The greatest incidence of mononucleosis in the United States is among those fifteen to nineteen, followed by the twenty to twenty-four age group. It can produce severe, if relatively short-lived symptoms, such as fever, sore throat, nausea, chills, and general weakness. Fortunately, permanent disability following mononucleosis is rare. But a lingering weakness is common and may last a few weeks or several months. The symptoms closely resemble those of several more serious diseases, among them polio, meningitis, tuberculosis, diphtheria, and even leukemia. A clear-cut diagnosis can be made with a simple blood test, however.

Until recently the cause of the disease could not be identified. An infectious agent was suspected because of characteristic changes produced in the blood—raised levels of disease-fighting white cells and antibodies. Research in the late 1960s, however, began to implicate a specific organism, the Epstein-Barr virus, as the cause of the most common form of infectious mononucleosis. One or two other forms may exist, caused by other viruses, but they appear to be quite rare.

The poor, both in America and abroad, are apparently exposed to Epstein-Barr virus early in

Figure 22.10 The incidence of reported cases of gonorrhea (*top*) and of primary and secondary syphilis (*bottom*) in the United States, 1950–1970.

life and often contract a mild form of the disease that usually goes unnoticed. But people who have more protected lives, medically speaking—middle-class families, for instance—are not generally exposed to the virus until later in their lives and seem to get much sicker when they do contract it. They tend to be exposed as adolescents and young adults, in high school, college, and military service. The exact methods by which the virus spreads are not known, but kissing is probably only one of several ways. The disease does not spread easily by ordinary contact; in fact, it is rare to have more than one case in a household.

VENEREAL DISEASE

Most of the common infectious diseases that now plague the average American are viral in origin—colds, flu, and so on. Bacterial diseases have been largely conquered through the use of antibiotics. It is therefore surprising to find that one of the most common types of infectious disease continuing to ravage the American population is bacterial in origin—venereal disease.

Veneral diseases are infectious diseases that are almost always transmitted during sexual intercourse, homosexual relations, or other sexual activity. *Syphilis* and *gonorrhea* are by far the two most fearsome diseases of this category, and, while other

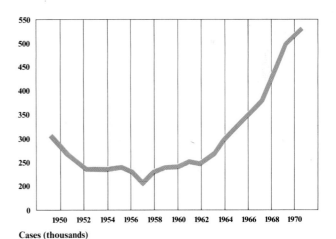

Cases (thousands)

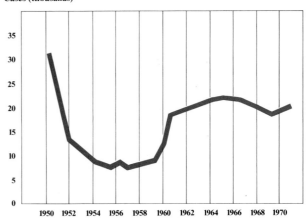

types of genital infections are known, it is for these two that the common use of the term "venereal disease," or VD, is reserved.

In the late 1950s, after a decade of reasonable control of venereal disease through antibiotics, VD, primarily gonorrhea, began showing dramatic increases that have continued, resulting today in a problem of epidemic proportions. In most communities today gonorrhea cases alone outnumber all other reportable infectious diseases combined. There will be more than 1 million new cases of venereal disease in the United States this year, and cases among persons fifteen to nineteen years of age will outnumber all other age groups combined more than two to one. Currently, one of every fifty teen-agers contracts gonorrhea.

Figure 22.11 illustrates how a venereal disease spreads. This illustration depicts a local epidemic of syphilis. Notice that the disease is not limited to those with many sexual partners—many of those found to be infected in this epidemic apparently had sexual contact only once, but it was unfortunately with an infected partner. There seem to be two main reasons why VD has been on the upswing even though the two most common types of VD can easily be cured with antibiotics: (1) many are infected but do not know it, and (2) many persons aware of being infected do not seek treatment even though they know that venereal disease can cause severe, permanent damage if not treated.

Syphilis

The spiral-shaped bacterium (spirochete) that causes syphilis—*Treponema pallidum*—does not long survive the drying effects of air, but it will grow profusely in the warm, moist tissues of the body. The

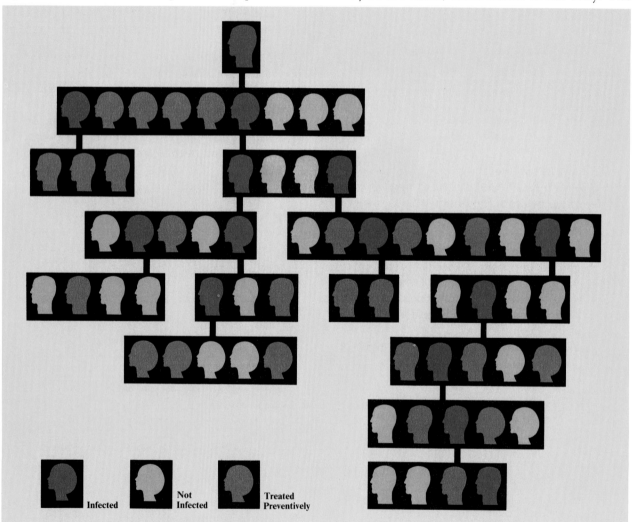

Figure 22.11   How an outbreak of syphilis was spread at a high school. The contacts of each infected person were traced in order to treat them and prevent further spread of the disease.

mucous membranes of the genital tract, the rectum, and the mouth are perfect breeding grounds. It is thus easy to see why sexual intercourse provides the best mode of transfer.

PRIMARY SYPHILIS   The disease begins when a spirochete enters a tiny break in the skin. The infected person may show no sign of the disease for from ten to twenty-eight days. When he does, the sign is in the form of a lesion known as a *chancre* (pronounced shank-er). The chancre of syphilis is often an open lump or swelling about the size of a dime or smaller, teeming with microscopic spirochetes. The sore is moist, although there is no discharge, and is generally painless. It often appears at the site of infection, usually in the genital region—on the shaft of the penis or on the vulva. Unfortunately, it also can develop out of sight and never be noticed: deep in the recesses of the vagina, the rectum, or the male urethra. Thus many infected persons, women in particular, never know they have the disease during the initial phase. But visible or hidden, the chancre is dangerously infectious and readily transmits the organism from person to person.

At this stage a diagnosis can easily be made by a doctor, and the disease can then be treated. Even without treatment, the chancre disappears within several weeks. Many persons therefore gain a false sense of security, thinking the chancre was nothing more than a minor nuisance that disappeared leaving only a small scar and an unpleasant memory. But, in fact, the infection has entered the blood and the spirochetes are being carried to all parts of the body. The primary stage of syphilis has ended, and the secondary stage has begun.

SECONDARY SYPHILIS   Secondary-stage symptoms appear anywhere from a few weeks to six months and occasionally even a year after the appearance of the chancre. The symptoms vary greatly in intensity—many people show no symptoms at all while others become disabled. The symptoms may last only a few days or may persist for several months. If lesions develop, they may heal and leave no scars even without treatment, again lulling the afflicted person into a false sense of security.

Symptoms and signs of secondary syphilis may include a skin rash; the development of small, flat lesions in regions where the skin is moist; whitish patches on the mucous membranes in the mouth and throat; spotty, temporary baldness; and such constitutional symptoms as general discomfort and uneasiness, low-grade fevers, headaches, and swollen glands. These symptoms are easily mistaken for those of other diseases. It is therefore important to

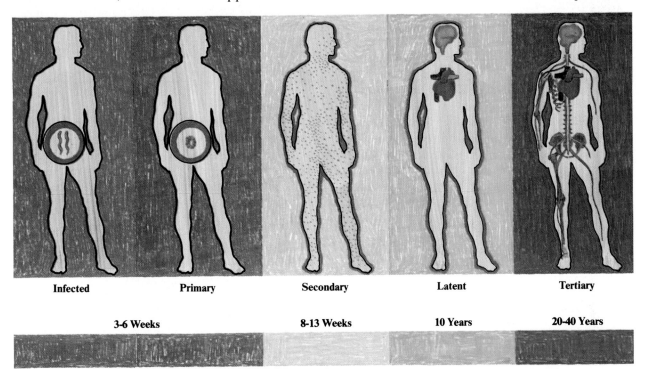

Infected	Primary	Secondary	Latent	Tertiary
3-6 Weeks		8-13 Weeks	10 Years	20-40 Years

Figure 22.12   The stages of syphilis. In the early stages, syphilis is easily diagnosed and treated. Unfortunately, in the later stages signs and symptoms are far less obvious and treatment is difficult because the infection has invaded and damaged vital body systems.

consult one's physician if any of these signs appear, particularly if one has been exposed to syphilis at any time during the preceding six months or so. Secondary syphilis, which lasts from three to six months, can always be diagnosed by blood tests.

During the secondary stage the disease is more contagious than at any other phase of its development. All the lesions are filled with spirochetes, hence any contact with open lesions—even without sexual intercourse—can transmit the disease.

LATENT SYPHILIS The third stage of syphilis is called the latent period because all signs and symptoms of the disease disappear. Essentially the disease is hidden, but it is not gone. Spirochetes are actively invading various organs, including the heart and the brain. This phase of the disease sometimes lasts only a few months, but it also can last for twenty years or until the end of life. In this stage the infected individual appears disease free and is usually not infectious, with an important exception: a pregnant woman can pass the infection to her unborn child. Although there are no symptoms, a blood test during this stage will reveal syphilis. The infected person is still *potentially* contagious, however, for within the first two years a relapse may occur, with the redevelopment of the highly contagious secondary stage.

LATE SYPHILIS The late stage of syphilis generally begins ten to twenty years after the beginning of the latent phase, but can occasionally occur much earlier. For the infected person, it is the most dangerous stage of the disease. The disabling effects of late syphilis depend on which organ or organs the spirochetes settle in during the latent period. In late syphilis, twenty-three out of every one hundred untreated patients become incapacitated. Thirteen of the twenty-three develop serious cardiovascular disease; many die of severe heart damage or rupture of the aorta. The other ten have slowly pro-gressive brain or spinal cord damage, eventually leading to blindness, insanity, or crippling.

CONGENITAL SYPHILIS Congenital syphilis results from the transmission of the disease from pregnant mother to unborn child. If the fetus is exposed to the disease in its fourth month of development, the infection may kill it, may produce various disfigurations, or may cause an obviously diseased baby. If the fetus is infected late in pregnancy, the infection may not be apparent for several months or years after birth, when the child may become disabled as in late syphilis. Treatment of the infected pregnant woman within the first four months of pregnancy halts the spread of the disease in the unborn child.

TREATMENT Syphilis is easily cured with antibiotics when the treatment is begun in the first two stages or even in the latent phase. Penicillin is the drug used most often, but other antibiotics may be used when the patient is sensitive to penicillin. The infection will not recur unless one contracts the disease again from an infected person. An individual can be reinfected over and over again—syphilis confers no immunity to succeeding infections, and there are no preventive vaccines. Thus continual caution must be taken to ensure prompt and effective diagnosis and treatment after each possible exposure to syphilis. To reduce the spread of the disease, prenatal as well as premarital tests are required by law in forty-five states.

Gonorrhea

Gonococci, the bacteria that cause gonorrhea, initially multiply in the lower urogenital tract of both sexes—the urethra of the male and the urethra, vaginal glands, and cervix of the female. If untreated, the infection spreads upward along the passageways of the genital tract and may produce sterility in both males and females, as well as other serious effects on all the reproductive organs. In addition, the bacteria may enter the bloodstream and cause a severe arthritis (inflammation of the joints) and a type of heart inflammation known as endocarditis. Gonorrhea is thus potentially a serious illness and one that affects many parts of the body. It has a short incubation period (three to fourteen days) and becomes contagious after incubation. Gonorrhea is easily treated, particularly if caught in its early stages.

GONORRHEA IN WOMEN Gonorrhea affects men and women in different ways because of their anatomical differences. Because early symptoms frequently are not pronounced, women may not be aware of infection. Often a woman does not suspect she has gonorrhea until a man reports he contracted the infection from her. A few days after exposure, a mild burning sensation in the genital· region, with or without discharge, may be noticed. If the infected woman were examined at the time, the physician might find a mild inflammation of the vagina and cervix. The disease subsequently spreads from the vagina through the uterus and into the Fallopian tubes and ovaries. Inflammation of the Fallopian tubes frequently is quite painful. Pain and fever can either be severe or be mild enough to be passed off as·a stomach upset. If the infection continues untreated, the symptoms may diminish, though the disease continues unabated. The whole pelvis can become inflamed, pus oozing from the Fallopian tubes or ovaries into the peritoneum (the lining of the abdominal cavity), sometimes causing a serious inflammation there.

The acute infection can subside after a few weeks. It is followed by a chronic infection that can last for many years, causing extensive damage to the reproductive tract. Sterility frequently follows inflammation of the Fallopian tubes.

Although gonococci may be detected in a discharge or grown in cultures, the disease is not as easily diagnosed as syphilis, particularly in women.

When a woman suspects exposure to gonorrhea or if she has a vaginal discharge, she should be examined promptly by a physician. He will be able to examine the discharge microscopically and confirm the diagnosis. If no organisms are found, he may wish to repeat the tests once again or to have other tests run. There are many other causes of vaginal discharge besides gonorrhea, and many different organisms other than gonococci can be responsible. Each organism may require a different treatment. Nevertheless, the consequences of gonorrhea are so serious that until laboratory confirmation is available a physician may treat the discharge as if it were due to gonorrhea. Some authorities suggest treating suspected contacts for gonorrhea even before symptoms appear.

GONORRHEA IN MEN The early symptoms of gonorrhea are more evident in men. About three to eight days after exposure men experience a sharp, burning pain during urination. At about the same time pus begins oozing from the penis, which causes many men to seek treatment. If prompt treatment is not received, the infection spreads to the prostate gland and testicles, where it can cause sufficient damage to produce sterility. In time, the urethra can become narrowed, making it difficult for a man to urinate. If the infection is severe, men can also suffer arthritis as well as heart damage.

TRANSMISSION Gonorrhea is most often contracted or transmitted through sexual intercourse. But the pus often is so laden with gonococci that the infection can be transmitted by hand to susceptible tissues. Personal hygiene is accordingly an important factor in combatting the disease.

Gonorrhea from infected mothers used to be a frequent cause of blindness in children. The bacteria were transferred to the baby's eyes as it passed through the birth canal. Today newborn babies are routinely treated with penicillin and silver compounds to prevent subsequent blindness.

TREATMENT Penicillin is the first choice for treatment of gonorrhea, despite the recent appearance of strains of gonococci that are partially resistant. Other antibiotics also can be used with success, particularly for those persons who are sensitive or allergic to penicillin. The response to treatment is rapid. Prompt treatment of the early stages almost immediately clears up the discharge from the vagina or penis and kills the infecting bacteria. It is more difficult to treat more severe cases in which complications have appeared, and, of course, there is no repair of scarred tissue.

A patient may be infected with syphilis and gonorrhea at the same time. Although penicillin can kill both gonococci and spirochetes, the amounts required for the effective treatment are usually different, and treatment for one disease may leave the other uncured. Therefore, anyone suspected to suffer from one of these diseases should have routine examinations for both diseases before treatment as well as sometime after the prescribed course of therapy has been completed.

Prevention and Control of Venereal Disease

Gonorrhea and syphilis produce no immunity, so that reinfection is always possible. Their control, therefore, can only be achieved ultimately by preventive measures that will progressively reduce the number of infected persons, hence of carriers and sources of the infectious agents.

It is probably unrealistic to expect total prevention of venereal disease. But it could be curbed

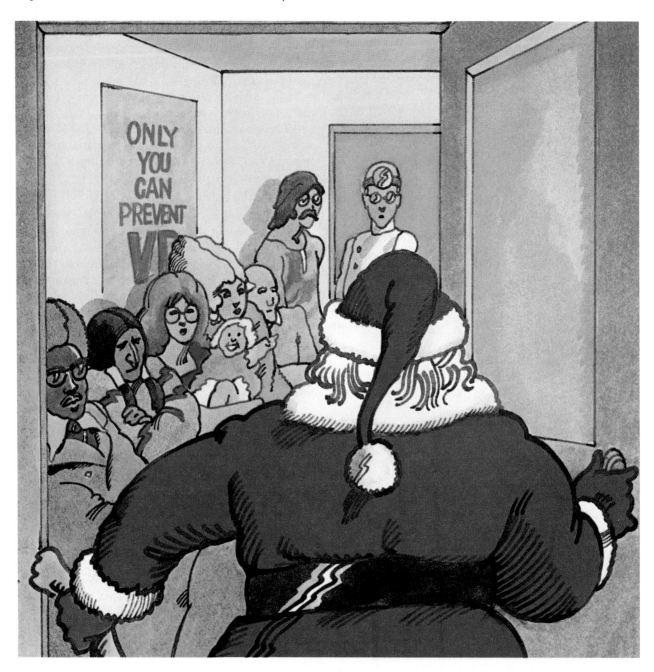

dramatically if people become sufficiently aware and concerned about its spread. Clearly, the only way to minimize the chances of getting VD is to confine one's sexual activity to uninfected partners, or have none at all. Those with many sexual partners are likely to become infected sooner or later. If one is going to have sex relations, however, certain precautions may help. Male use of condoms during any and all contact with persons who might be infected reduces the risk of infection, especially if combined with washing. Nevertheless, disease can still be transmitted through kissing or through contact with broken skin or sores. Despite these limitations, the use of prophylactics and washing is recommended when the VD status of one's partner is uncertain.

Public health workers also try to reduce the spread of VD by asking those seeking treatment to name all of their sexual contacts. Even when patients are cooperative, contact-tracing is time-consuming and expensive work, further hampered by a shortage of trained personnel. Obviously all who are infected cannot be discovered. Even though every state requires physicians to report all cases of syphilis and gonorrhea to the health department, case finding is further handicapped by massive failure to report.

Venereal infections represent a major social problem as well as a medical one. Unlike most other infectious diseases, venereal infections still carry a social stigma, which along with widespread ignorance reduces the likelihood that all with infections will seek treatment promptly, refer their contacts to physicians for treatment, and avoid sexual contact themselves until they are cured. Yet, an awareness of the symptoms, combined with prompt action when they appear, can save everyone involved much needless anxiety and future agony.

THE ROLE OF INFECTIOUS DISEASE

Although, as was pointed out in Chapter 21, infectious diseases are not the killers they once were in the United States, they still have a significant impact on the everyday life of the average American. Everyone suffers at least one cold a year, and most people are hit by the flu at periodic intervals. Nevertheless, today's children, through the use of vaccines, are avoiding many of the diseases their parents experienced as a "normal" part of childhood: measles (rubeola) and whopping cough, for example. The cases of such formerly feared diseases as smallpox, polio, diphtheria, and tetanus have dropped to almost nothing.

Within the next few decades science hopes to dramatically decrease the incidence of many more infectious diseases, through the use of vaccines, drugs, and epidemiological methods. As these diseases one by one come under control, medicine can then focus more and more on the noninfectious diseases that have been the new killers of mankind. Such diseases are discussed in the next three chapters.

Figure 22.13 Anyone can get VD.

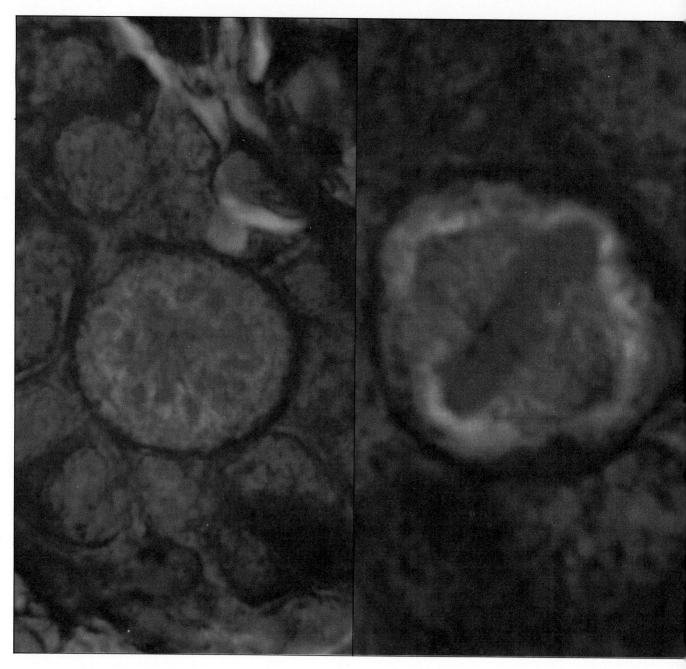

Figure 23.1   Cancer cells exhibiting abnormal cell division.

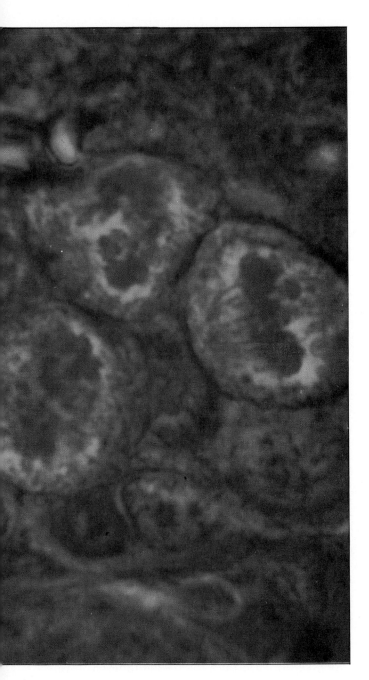

23 Although cancer is considered to be a disease of modern times, it apparently was not unknown in ancient times, for it was named by the Greeks (from a word meaning "crab") and is thought to be the condition referred to in several parts of the Old Testament. There is no question, however, that cancer has been on a dramatic rise in recent decades. As a cause of death in the United States, cancer has climbed from causing less than 6 percent of deaths in 1900 to causing nearly 20 percent in 1969. Today cancer is second only to heart disease as a killer of American men and women, accounting for more than 300,000 deaths per year.

Man's knowledge about cancer is still far from adequate. Nevertheless, there has been steady progress in recent years both in understanding of the disease and in finding ways to cope with it. Today about 35 percent of all cancer patients in this country live at least five years after the illness is diagnosed and treated, a survival span that is generally taken as an indication of successful treatment. In the 1940s, only 25 percent of cancer patients survived this long. A decade before that, the number was 20 percent. At the turn of the century, there was little hope of cure for any patient with cancer of internal organs. These overall figures, however, like those in the overall rise of cancer incidence, do not apply uniformly to all forms of cancer. Lung cancer now kills fourteen times as many men as it did in 1935; however, breast cancer, the leading cause of cancer death among women, has had about the same mortality rate for nearly forty years.

Cancer

Nevertheless, the cancer picture could be even better today than it is. Medical authorities estimate that 65 percent or more of patients with cancer could be saved with existing methods of treatment—instead of the present 35 percent. Why do so many with curable cancer have to die? The problem seems to be partly one of communication. More patients would be treated earlier, and more cured, if people (1) were aware of the danger signs of cancer, (2) would have an annual health examination, and (3) did not allow fear to keep them from seeking medical diagnosis. This is one situation in which it is profoundly dangerous to believe, "What you don't know can't hurt you."

Early recognition of the signs of cancer, prompt diagnosis, and aggressive treatment by the appropriate means have made the word "cancer" much less terrifying than it used to be. Even those persons with forms of cancer that are still difficult to treat today can live with the hope that current techniques may enable them to outwit the disease until better techniques become available through new research. Thus, for many cancer victims there is hope where there used to be only despair.

UNCONTROLLED GROWTH

Cancer is characterized by the abnormal growth and spread of cells. If the growth is not stopped, the patient dies. Accordingly, to understand the nature of cancer, it is necessary to understand how the physician (pathologist) distinguishes cancerous tissue from other kinds of tissue.

A *tumor* is a swelling or mass that is formed when cells that normally cooperate with each other in performing a useful function no longer cooperate but instead begin to multiply independently, often rapidly, taking nourishment from normal cells and no longer contributing to the functional activity of the tissue or organ. Such a group of cells, growing in an uncontrolled fashion, is called a tumor, or *neoplasm.*

A cancer is a tumor, but not all tumors are cancers. Tumors that are not cancers are termed *benign,* and they generally grow slowly, are surrounded by a capsule so they remain localized in the tissue that generated them, and do not recur once they are removed. The fact that they are benign does not mean that they do no damage. They can cause pressure and subsequent harm to surrounding structures, and they can rob normal tissues of their blood supply. It is obvious that a benign tumor can have serious consequences if it occurs in a vital organ such as the brain. Benign tumors are usually curable by surgical removal, however.

Malignant tumors, on the other hand, *are* cancers. Multiplying rapidly, free from the restraints of any capsule, they compress, invade, and ultimately kill surrounding tissues. Cancer cells also invade neighboring blood vessels and lymphatic channels, from which they can be swept into the bloodstream or the lymph fluid and be carried to distant parts of the body. There they settle, again multiplying rapidly and unrestrictedly, forming another tumor that invades and destroys neighboring tissues (see Figure 23.2).

Such secondary tumors, which may be of considerable distance from the original site, are called *metastases.* The process by which secondary growth is produced is called *metastatic growth.* Each metastasis and the original cancer itself are capable of seeding more sites. In this way, the entire body can become literally riddled with cancer.

The cure for cancer involves the complete removal or destruction of *every* malignant cell. Once the metastatic state is reached, it becomes difficult to remove all of the cancer from the body. Because there generally is a time lag before the metastatic state is reached, early diagnosis and treatment can eradicate the tumor before it has had a chance to spread.

The value of early detection is demonstrated by the different cure rates for certain different forms

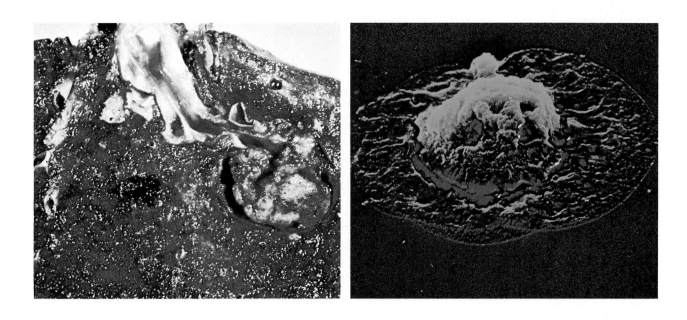

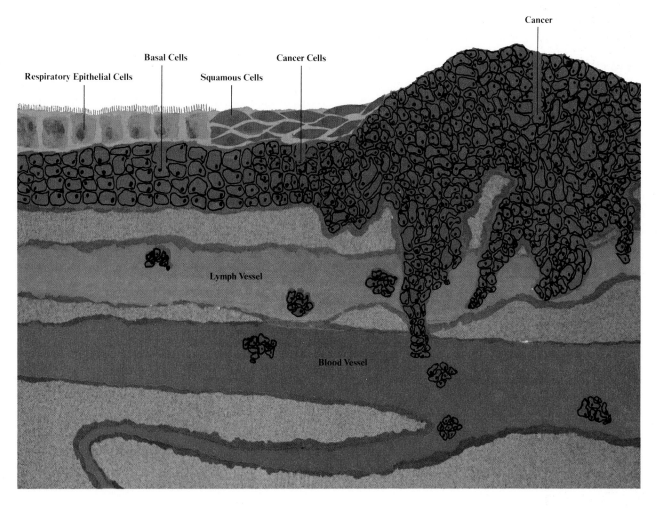

Figure 23.2 (*above left*) A benign tumor. (*above right*) A malignant tumor being attacked by the body's immune mechanism. (*bottom*) How cancer cells multiply and metastasize.

of cancer. Skin cancers are easily seen and frequently get early attention; in addition, they are readily accessible to treatment. With the exception of one rare form that is particularly resistant to treatment, the cure rate is more than 90 percent. For lung cancer, on the other hand, the overall cure rate is less than 10 percent. This disease is not immediately apparent and produces symptoms that a patient may not take seriously for some time. Lung cancers are treated surgically; often one lobe of a lung or an entire lung must be removed. If the tumor at surgery appears to be confined to the lung, almost 30 percent of patients will survive five years and be considered "cured."

The poor cure rates for lung cancer are due in part to the fact that the usual diagnostic procedures—x-ray and microscopic examination of a specimen of lung tissue—detect the disease too late. Sputum cytology is designed to pick up early signs of cancer and earlier precancerous cell changes. It calls for regular microscopic examinations of sputum coughed up from the lungs by high-risk patients (such as cigarette smokers).

TYPES OF CANCER

Malignant tumors are classified according to the cells from which they arise and to their appearance under the microscope. Those that arise from epithelium—the cells forming the skin, glands, and the membranes lining the respiratory, urinary, and gastrointestinal tracts—are called *carcinomas*. Those that arise from supporting or connective tissues—such as bones, cartilage, and the membranes covering muscles and fat—are called *sarcomas*. In cancer of the breast, for example, cancers derived from cells lining the milk ducts are called *adenocarcinomas*, meaning that they are composed of glandular (*adeno-*) epithelial cells. Other breast cancers might arise from the connective tissue of the breast, in which case they are called sarcomas.

Further subdivisions identify cancers from lymphatic cells as *lymphoma* (Hodgkin's disease is a dramatic example) or as *lymphosarcoma*; cancers from blood-forming cells as *leukemia*; cancers from pigment-carrying cells of the skin as *melanoma;* and so on. By these criteria, more than one hundred cancer entities can be identified. There also are cancers whose cellular structure is so altered that they no longer resemble the cells from which they originated, so that no identification is possible. Such cancers are termed *anaplastic.*

DISTRIBUTION OF CANCER

Figure 23.3 indicates by sex and by site the most common forms of cancer among the 200 million people of the United States. The gastrointestinal tract as a whole is the most common cancer site. The incidence of all cancers in women exceeds that of men until the age of fifty-five. This difference primarily is due to the fact that the most common forms of cancer in women attack the breast and the genital organs (especially the uterine cervix). Except for these sex-specific sites and the thyroid and gall bladder, men have more cancer than women when compared by the sites they share. This difference may be due to the greater exposure of men to environmental cancer-producing agents, or it may be due to greater genetic susceptibility. After fifty-five, men have a higher overall incidence of cancer than women.

Most cancers occur more frequently among older people. However, there are some types of cancer that occur frequently among children; these childhood problems include acute leukemia and certain cancers of bone, nerve, and kidney tissue. Fortunately, these cancers are relatively rare.

HEREDITY AND ENVIRONMENT

As in any disease, cancer depends on both the environment and the genetic consitution of the host. A clear example of genetic and environmental interplay is found in carcinoma of the skin. A large proportion of skin cancers are due to exposure to sunlight, expecially ultraviolet light. Persons with light skin, particularly the freckled type, are about ten times more likely to develop skin cancer after prolonged exposure to sunlight than are persons with heavy pigment, such as Negroes. Nevertheless, American Negroes are as susceptible as Caucasians to most other forms of cancer. The relationship between skin lightness (a genetic trait) and sunlight (an environmental agent) in the production of can-

cer has been reproduced successfully with mice and rats under laboratory conditions.

Human beings of all races, colors, and environmental habits have been known to develop cancer of one type or another. There are, however, intriguing differences in the occurrence of some cancers among different human populations. As compared with the United States, stomach cancer is more frequent in Scandinavia and Japan, cancer of the cervix and of the penis are much more frequent in India, and cancer of the breast and prostate are one-fourth as frequent in Japan as in the

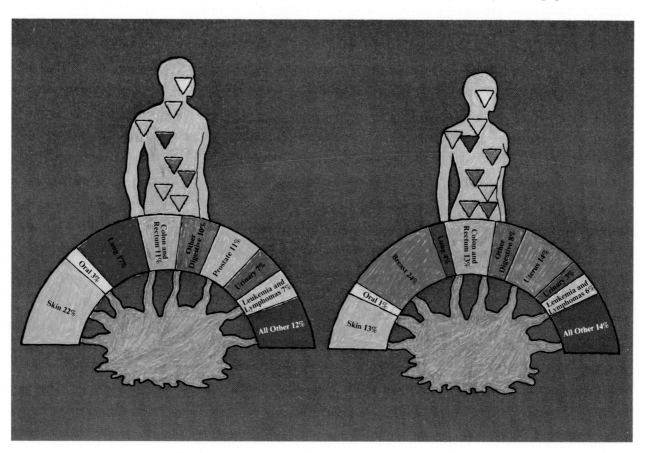

Figure 23.3   Incidence of cancer by sex and by site.

United States. The relative involvement of genetic and environmental factors in these differences has not been established and is an important area for continuing research.

CAUSES OF CANCER

There are many known factors promoting cancer in man and experimental animals. For a long time these diverse conditions seemed unrelated. Today scientists are trying to find a unifying hypothesis—one explanation that will account for the fact that such different agents as cigarette smoke and x-rays can produce uncontrolled cellular growth. Recent research encourages the idea that the unifying theme may be found in the virus story. The various other agents may simply open the door for a latent or hidden cancer-inducing virus that can, under certain circumstances, transform normal, regulated body cells into wildly growing parasites that destroy surrounding tissues, metastasize, and finally kill their host. Another promising and related theory holds that cancer may result from a defect in the body's immune system.

Chemical Agents

Several hundred chemicals are now known to possess carcinogenic (cancer-producing) properties. Workers in a number of occupations have an increased incidence of cancer. Those exposed to petroleum and its products may develop skin cancer, but it may be prevented by good hygiene, if workers are careful to bathe regularly after their job. Similarly, those who may inhale substances at work need to be particularly careful—uranium and other radioactive ores, asbestos, and chromium compounds, for instance, markedly increase the risk of lung cancer.

As was discussed in Chapter 9, tobacco smoke is one of the most common carcinogens. Tobacco tar contains cancer-producing chemicals. The polluted air of cities also contains related chemicals, resulting in a higher rate of lung cancer among city dwellers than among rural inhabitants. Of course, urban cigarette smokers run the greatest risk of all.

The evidence indicates that carcinogenic irritants inhaled over a period of time trigger the cancerous potential in susceptible lung-tissue cells. In the case of cigarette smoke, the smoke inhaled paralyzes the bronchial cilia, interfering with the natural cleansing mechanism. The carcinogenic dusts, gases, and tars linger to irritate and to cause precancerous alterations in lung-cell structure and thus eventually trigger the cancer mechanism. Cancer of the lung has reached near epidemic proportions, particularly in the male population over forty years of age and most particularly among men who have smoked cigarettes for twenty or more years. Currently, more Americans (60,000 plus) die of lung cancer than die in automobile accidents.

Estrogen, one of the female sex hormones, readily triggers cancers of the breast, uterus, and testes in mice and other rodents, but its role in human cancer is still unclear. Evidence to date points to low risks when estrogen is taken in contraceptive pills or as hormone-replacement therapy for postmenopausal women.

Chemicals that induce cancer trigger complex interactions within cells. The nature of the interaction is not known, but the final outcome is presumably a permanent change in the genetic elements of the cell; such changes are then transmitted to the daughter cells during cell division, and a new population of cells, the cancer cells, becomes established in the body.

Radiation

Two forms of physical energy also are cancer producing. Radiation from x-ray tubes, radium, or atomic-bomb explosions increases the occurrence of leukemia (cancer of the blood) and cancers of the thyroid, skin, and bone. Ultraviolet irradiation also has been shown to cause skin cancer, as was discussed earlier. The chain of events between exposure to radiation and onset of cancer has not been established. Radiation increases the percentage of genetic errors (mutations) in cells and thus could directly induce the first cancer cell; on the other hand, it might make cells more sensitive to a cancer-inducing agent or might activate a cancer-inducing virus.

Viruses

The most exciting and promising area of research trying to track down the causes of cancer is in the study of viruses. Viruses have been found to cause at least a dozen types of cancers in animals as diverse as frogs, mice, and cats. Up to the present, however, no human cancer has been demonstrated to be caused by a virus, although such an event seems only a matter of time. Acute leukemia, sarcoma, and melanoma are the cancers most likely to be initially linked with viruses.

The question now is not whether viruses cause some cancers—it is known that they do. Rather, the problem is *how* viruses transform normal cells into cancer cells, with all their properties of malignant growth and metastasis. Scientists know that all viruses, themselves made up of nucleic acids, establish an intimate relationship with the nucleic acids of the cell, that is, its hereditary machinery. Cancer viruses function no differently. It also is known that certain noncancer viruses can infect cells but remain hidden or latent for a period of time until they are unmasked by ultraviolet radiation or chemical agents. It is likely that a parallel situation could exist for animal tumor viruses—the inducer, such as radiation, might unmask the hidden virus and allow it to alter the host cell. Knowledge of the mechanisms by which viruses and chemicals transform normal cells into cancer cells would allow

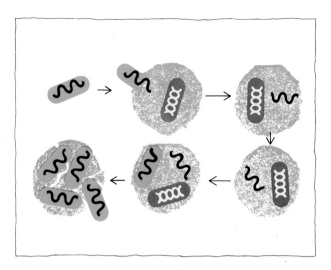

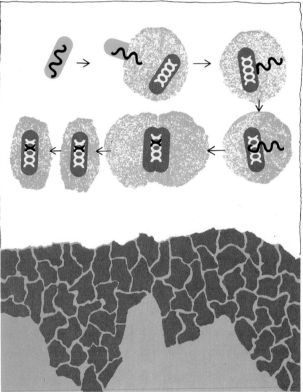

Figure 23.4   Normal viral infection compared to cancer-virus theory. (*top*) In a normal viral infection (flu, viral pneumonia, etc.) the virus injects its nucleic acid into the body cell. This material moves within the cell, but *does not* penetrate the nucleus. The virus material multiplies within the host cell and destroys it by initially crowding and eventually bursting out of the cell. (*bottom*) With the virus theory of cancer, the genetic material of the virus moves into the cell, but unlike the "normal" virus, the cancer virus moves into the cell nucleus and disrupts healthy genetic coding so that the body cell produces new cells that no longer resemble the parent cell—it has a new set of genetic instructions—and reproduces at an accelerated rate, causing the malignant tumor.

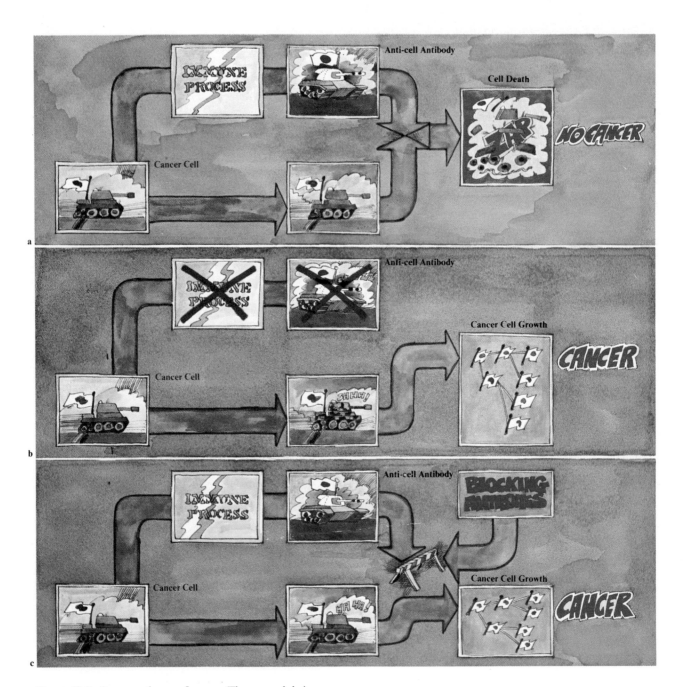

Figure 23.5   Immune theory of cancer. The research being done in the area of the immune response is highly complex — the explanation presented here is an attempt to summarize several possible explanations. (a) When cells extracted from a cancerous (malignant) tumor are exposed to lymphocytes isolated from other blood components, the cancer cells should be destroyed if they are like the cells of most infectious agents. (b) One theory that explains why cancer cells are not destroyed by the immunological process is that something in the nature of the cancer cell "tricks" the body's defense system so that it doesn't recognize a cancer cell as a foreign "enemy." (c) A second theory postulates that while the immunological process recognizes cancer cells as enemy invaders, something in the serum of the blood, called "blocking antibodies," inactivates normal production and the cancer continues to grow unimpeded.

meaningful approaches toward interfering with and even reversing the cancer-formation process.

Defective Immune Mechanism

Another theory proposes a relationship between cancer and the *immune* mechanisms of the body. According to this theory, most persons may be harboring throughout life individual tumor cells that are destroyed or repressed by normal immunological defenses. Occasionally, such defenses may become defective, possibly under the influence of one or another of the cancer-inducing conditions, and cancer flares up. There is a basic difference between the viral and the immune hypotheses, as they have been proposed: in one, the instructions for becoming an active cancer element come to the cell from a foreign agent, the virus, while in the other they result from an occasional mistake, or mutation, during cell reproduction. However, the viral and immune involvements in cancer need not be mutually exclusive; it is readily conceivable that either one may play a supportive role to the other, rather than being itself the primary cause.

PREVENTION OF CANCER

Prevention as well as treatment or cure in any disease depends upon three factors: the state of the practical knowledge available at the time, the state of public education and motivation to use the knowledge, and the availability of an adequate medical system to apply the knowledge. In the case of cancer, science does not yet understand the mechanism responsible for the disease. Nevertheless, true prevention, in the sense of preventing the occurrence of the disease, can be carried out by avoiding known carcinogens.

The single most important carcinogen in the environment of the United States is the smoke of tobacco, especially from deeply inhaled cigarettes.

It is estimated that at least 75 percent of lung cancer, now the number-one malignant killer of man, could be prevented if this habit were terminated. There would also be a reduction in cancers of the mouth, throat, larynx, esophagus, and bladder.

Chronic, excessive alcohol consumption, a major social and health problem in itself (see Chapter 8), also is related to the higher risk of cancer in the mouth, throat, larynx, and esophagus, when combined with the effects of tobacco smoking and defective nutrition.

Good hygiene of the genitalia, mouth, throat, and skin will help reduce the likelihood of cancer in those locations. Early circumcision helps prevent cancer of the penis, but meticulous cleanliness also is effective. Repair of jagged teeth helps prevent cancer of the tongue. In general, being observant about one's body and seeking prompt care when anything unusual develops is sound preventive medicine.

X-rays and other sources of ionizing radiation are to be avoided as much as possible because of the additional risk of developing leukemia and cancer of the thyroid and perhaps of the breast and lung. Such exposure is especially dangerous in children and in the developing fetus. This warning does not mean that x-rays should never be used diagnostically but it does mean that they should be used with discretion and that exposure rates should be kept as low as is practicable. Poorly shielded equipment, in the home and at work, may be another source of radiation, and effective production controls should be rigorously enforced.

It is not possible nor desirable to avoid ultraviolet radiation completely. Nevertheless, individuals with particularly susceptible skin, such as albinos or light-complexioned persons, should protect themselves from overexposure to the sun by appropriate cover and salves.

DETECTION AND DIAGNOSIS

The greatest hope for the cancer victim remains in early diagnosis and prompt treatment. Individuals who are alert to the signals that may mean cancer and to the need for regular medical checkups are most likely to have cancers detected early enough to be successfully treated.

The American Cancer Society emphasizes seven warning signals of cancer, shown in Figure 23.6. They should be known and remembered by every-

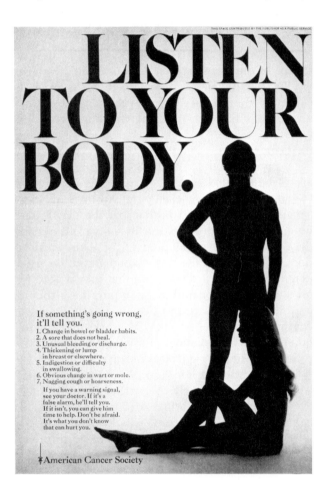

If something's going wrong, it'll tell you.
1. Change in bowel or bladder habits.
2. A sore that does not heal.
3. Unusual bleeding or discharge.
4. Thickening or lump in breast or elsewhere.
5. Indigestion or difficulty in swallowing.
6. Obvious change in wart or mole.
7. Nagging cough or hoarseness.
If you have a warning signal, see your doctor. If it's a false alarm, he'll tell you. If it isn't, you can give him time to help. Don't be afraid. It's what you don't know that can hurt you.

American Cancer Society

Figure 23.6   Cancer's seven warning signals.

one. *None of these symptoms means cancer—most often they do not.* But they *are* warning signals, and if they progress or last for longer than *two weeks*, they demand medical attention.

The most curable cancers usually are those that are detected earliest, that is, before actual symptoms appear. There is a good chance that an individual can detect some of the early warning signs by examining himself periodically. With the aid of a mirror, he should observe his skin, mouth, and scalp. Men should examine the penis and testes, women their breasts and vulva. Women should make a habit of examining their breasts every month, preferably between menstrual periods. The suggested method is shown in Figure 23.7.

Personal examinations should be supplemented with an annual physical checkup by a physician. If one of the warning signs develops between visits to the doctor—even shortly after one has just seen him—it should be reported to him immediately.

During the physical checkup the doctor should examine a woman's breasts and cervix. Specimens should be obtained from the vagina and cervix for a Papanicolaou test, or *Pap smear*, which is used to detect early signs of cancer of the cervix. Deaths from cervical cancer could be reduced 90 percent if all women had this test annually and were promptly and adequately treated when abnormalities were noted. Both men and women periodically should have a rectal examination.

Cancer patients should have periodic x-rays of the chest, and all women over forty years old should have a soft-tissue x-ray of the breast, or *mammography*, which is useful in revealing possible cancer deep within the breast. As a result of early detection through mammograms, 25 percent more cures are obtained.

The diagnosis of cancer is based upon a *biopsy* of the tumor—the examination under a microscope of a bit of tissue suspected to be diseased. The tissue is

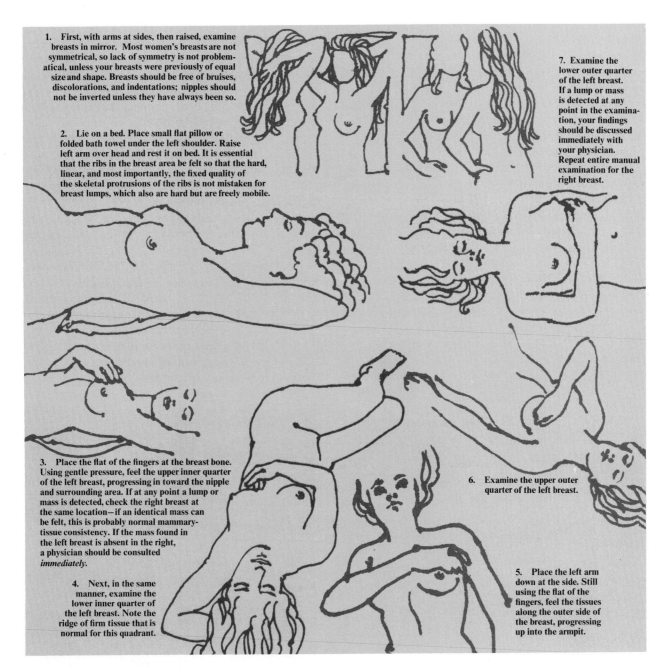

1. First, with arms at sides, then raised, examine breasts in mirror. Most women's breasts are not symmetrical, so lack of symmetry is not problematical, unless your breasts were previously of equal size and shape. Breasts should be free of bruises, discolorations, and indentations; nipples should not be inverted unless they have always been so.

2. Lie on a bed. Place small flat pillow or folded bath towel under the left shoulder. Raise left arm over head and rest it on bed. It is essential that the ribs in the breast area be felt so that the hard, linear, and most importantly, the fixed quality of the skeletal protrusions of the ribs is not mistaken for breast lumps, which also are hard but are freely mobile.

3. Place the flat of the fingers at the breast bone. Using gentle pressure, feel the upper inner quarter of the left breast, progressing in toward the nipple and surrounding area. If at any point a lump or mass is detected, check the right breast at the same location—if an identical mass can be felt, this is probably normal mammary-tissue consistency. If the mass found in the left breast is absent in the right, a physician should be consulted *immediately*.

4. Next, in the same manner, examine the lower inner quarter of the left breast. Note the ridge of firm tissue that is normal for this quadrant.

5. Place the left arm down at the side. Still using the flat of the fingers, feel the tissues along the outer side of the breast, progressing up into the armpit.

6. Examine the upper outer quarter of the left breast.

7. Examine the lower outer quarter of the left breast. If a lump or mass is detected at any point in the examination, your findings should be discussed immediately with your physician. Repeat entire manual examination for the right breast.

Figure 23.7 Breast self-examination. The breasts should be examined at the same time each month—one week after the end of the menstrual period.

preserved or "fixed," cut into tiny slices, placed on a glass slide, and stained with dyes. Interpretation of the biopsy is made by a pathologist. Microscopic examinations of cells taken from the patient by means of the Pap smear or sputum sample also can be used to determine the existence of cancer, but these methods must be subsequently confirmed by acutal biopsy. Surgery, one of the two main approaches to cancer cure, can also be used to prevent cancer. Prophylactic (preventive) surgery consists in removing tissue known, from past medical experience, to have a potential for developing into cancer. Such tissues include warts or moles in areas that are subjected to constant irritation and abnormalities in the mouth, vagina, and rectum.

CANCER TREATMENT

The key to successful treatment of cancer is to diagnose it at a stage when it can be completely removed from the body or destroyed, leaving no malignant cell behind. Unfortunately, with only rare exceptions, the only techniques available today to accomplish this task are surgery and x-ray thera-

py. The sad fact is that in order to be absolutely sure that all the cancer cells are eradicated, surgery and radiation usually must remove or destroy a considerable area of normal tissue surrounding the tumor along with the malignant tissue. It is the hope of physicians and scientists that eventually a therapeutic agent can be developed that will selectively kill the malignant cells without interfering with normal cells. To date, this task has not been accomplished and physicians must struggle with the existing methods of surgery and x-irradiation, drastic as they may have to be.

Most patients with cancer require careful management by their physician. Often the knowledge and skills of several specialists are needed, and the patient may benefit from a team approach that marshals the talents of a surgeon, radiologist (a specialist dealing with all forms of irradiation therapy: x-rays, radium, or radioactive isotopes), internist (an expert on the internal organs of the body), and pathologist. Most cancer patients are best handled in cancer centers or by medical groups whose main focus is in neoplastic disease. The American

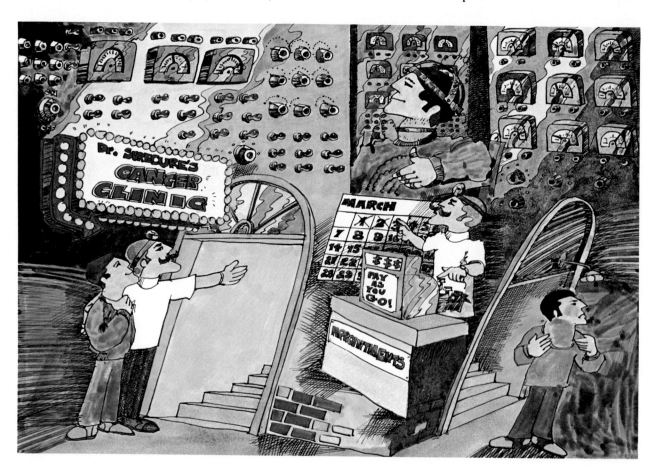

Figure 23.8 Cancer quacks not only do not heal cancer, they often delay the patient from seeking proper treatment until it is too late.

College of Surgeons lists more than 900 cancer clinics in the United States and Canada where proper treatment can be obtained.

Some cancers do not respond adequately to x-ray treatments and must be primarily treated by surgery, although x-rays may be used in combination with it as a supportive treatment. Such cancers include those of the stomach, rectum, and breast. In some cancers, such as Hodgkin's disease (a generalized cancer condition affecting the lymphoid tissue), lymphosarcoma, and leukemia, x-rays are considered as the preferable method. Modern x-ray treatment depends upon powerful sources of radiation, such as cobalt machines utilizing radioactive cobalt or electronic equipment such as linear accelerators. Because this equipment is large and expensive, it is usually limited to larger institutions staffed with radiotherapists specially trained to use such tools.

There are, up to now, no curative chemotherapeutic agents for cancer, except for the treatment of a rare tumor in women and for a small proportion of the cases of leukemia in children. However, several dozen chemical agents have proved to be useful in producing temporary recoveries from a variety of cancers. The present trend is to ulitize several chemical agents either in sequence or in combination.

The results of cancer therapy are judged by the proportion of patients who survive for at least five years without recurrence of cancer. Unfortunately, some cancers recur even after five years, so that most physicians avoid the word "cure." All cancer patients should receive regular, periodic examinations to assure that the cancer has been eradicated and to permit further treatments if there is evidence of recurrence.

CANCER QUACKERY

Although surgery and x-irradiation are the only present methods used to cure cancer, some Americans do not go to physicians and hospitals where they can be treated. They go instead to quacks, on whose advice they spend an estimated 100 million dollars annually on medicine, diets, and all forms of bizarre treatment. Cancer quacks prosper not only because people are ignorant but because they are afraid or desperate. Victims who fear they have incurable cancer or who have had those fears confirmed by medical means often will grasp at any straw. The greatest tragedy of cancer quackery is that the patient who might be cured often delays a trip to his physician and instead relies on useless drugs and treatments. When he does finally seek appropriate treatment, it may be too late to stop the disease.

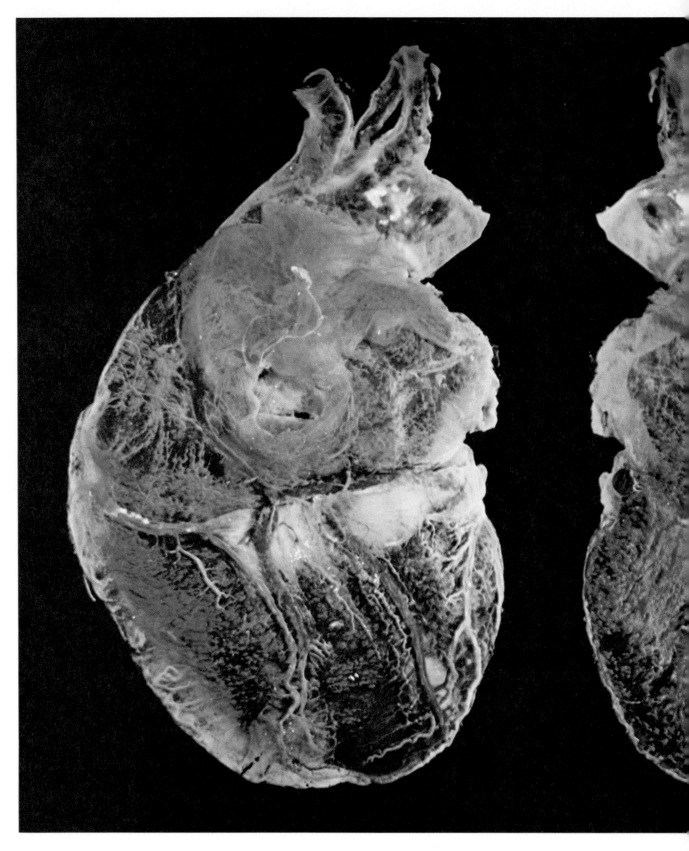

Figure 24.1   Ventral and dorsal views of the human heart.

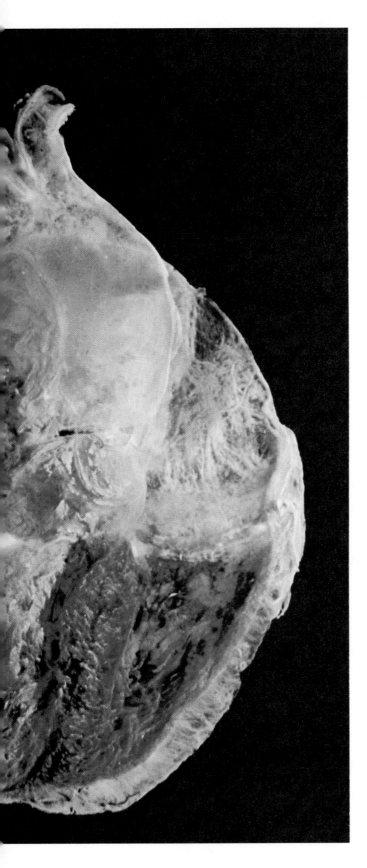

24

Modern industrial culture has brought many changes to both Western and non-Western societies. Western man has prospered in terms of physical wealth and a longer life span. But economic and technological development also has brought with it problems poorly recognized by man in earlier centuries. Among these problems are the so-called chronic and degenerative diseases that can affect entire systems of the body but that are most frequently associated with the cardiovascular system.

Most people consider afflictions such as cardiovascular diseases and cancer to be inevitable with middle or old age but irrelevant to children, adolescents, or young adults. As will soon be shown, however, even a small child may be on the way to a heart attack if various factors—such as heredity and diet—are working against him. Because such action as dietary changes or modified habits may help such a child to reduce his lifetime risks, it is obvious that behavior can play a large role in whether or how severely one will suffer from coronary atherosclerotic heart disease and similar degenerative disorders.

Considering the central role that the circulatory system plays in the body, it is no wonder that impairment of its function will also profoundly affect the activity of other body systems or that the malfunction of these other systems will in turn markedly influence cardiovascular performance and health. In Western countries, cardiovascular disease is the most drastic killer of modern times. In the United States, it alone is responsible for 60 per-

Cardiovascular Diseases

cent of all deaths. Cardiovascular disease and cancer together take the lives of four out of five Americans who die each year.

ATHEROSCLEROSIS

Atherosclerosis is the narrowing or thickening of arterial blood vessels due to build-up of fatty deposits. In the United States and other similarly industrialized nations, atherosclerosis probably begins before most people are twenty years old. Heart attacks, which alone claim more than 600,000 lives in the United States each year, are a complication of *coronary* atherosclerosis—fatty thickening of the inner lining of the coronary arteries, which carry the blood supply for the heart tissue. Without sufficient blood the heart muscle may stop working entirely, may falter in its regular rhythm, or may beat so weakly that it is useless. The flow of blood to the heart muscle can easily be halted by a small clot caught in an already-narrowed atherosclerotic coronary artery, often resulting in a heart attack. A similar clot in the brain can cause a stroke.

Coronary artery disease is the leading cause of death among American men over the age of thirty-five. Caucasian women in the United States are far less prone than men to develop atherosclerosis and heart attacks unless they have underlying diseases such as high blood pressure, diabetes, or a kidney ailment. Before menopause coronary artery disease is unusual. After menopause women still have only half the number of heart attacks as men, but the rates become equal at the age of sixty-five. Among American Negroes, however, men and women have coronary artery disease and heart attacks at almost the same rates.

The incidence of heart attacks and strokes may be increased by a number of *risk factors* to which the potential victims have been exposed. Specialists cannot yet agree which of the many factors involved in the disease is the most important single

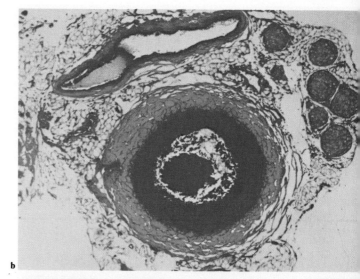

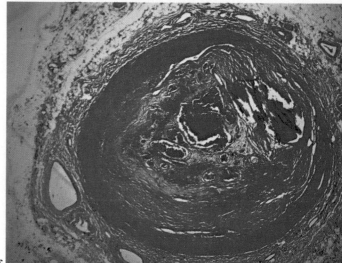

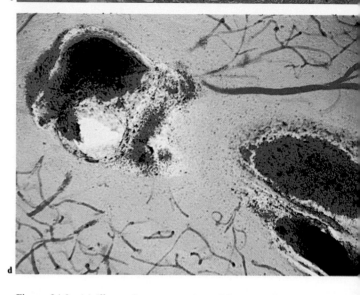

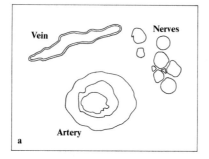

Figure 24.2 (a) Illustrative cross-section of the normal artery. Note location of vein and nerves. (b) Photographic cross-section of normal artery. (c) Atherosclerotic artery. (d) Blood clot in artery.

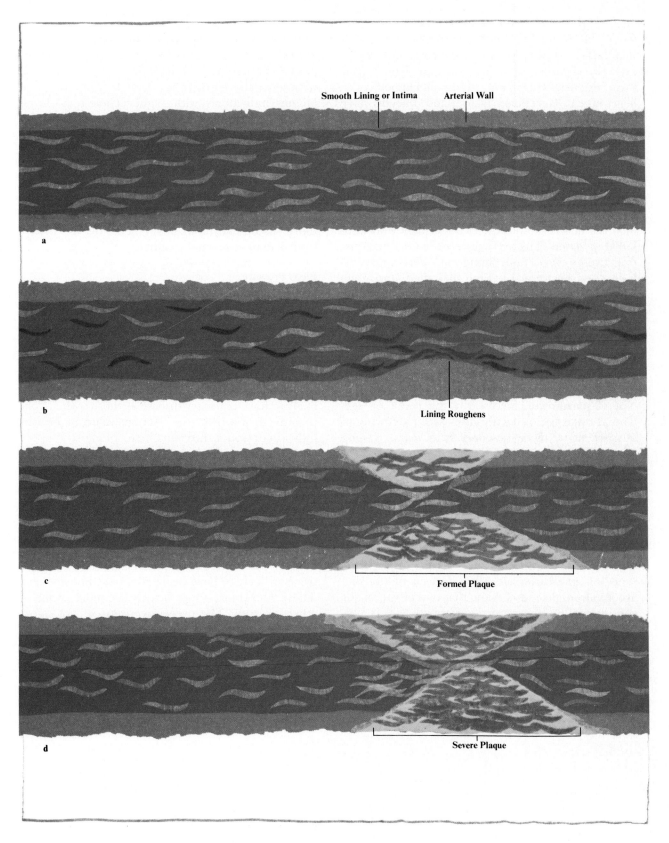

Figure 24.3   The mechanism of atherosclerosis. Atherosclerosis may develop when (a) normally smooth intima (the innermost lining of the artery) (b) becomes irregular and attracts fibrin. (c) This fibrin matrix then collects fat particles and other debris, thus producing plaque. (d) Later in this degenerative condition, calcium is deposited and the plaque hardens.

one, but they have identified several of them. Content of fat in the diet is under suspicion, along with such factors as obesity, excessive eating, and lack of exercise. Cigarette smoking and high blood pressure seriously contribute to the likelihood of a heart attack. Hereditary factors and diabetes have been implicated. Psychological stress also may play a role. The reduction of risk factors, in the opinion of many physicians, could considerably decrease the number of heart attacks.

Diet

During the Korean War, Army pathologists examined the hearts of 300 American soldiers who were killed in action. The average recorded age was just over twenty-two. These young men were apparently in good health at the time they died, and none had previous signs of coronary disease. And yet the coronary arteries of more than three-fourths of them (77.3 percent) already were thickened or narrowed, clearly manifesting early signs of atherosclerosis. More than 15 percent had an artery that was narrowed by one-half or more; in 3 percent of the cases one blood vessel was completely obstructed. Nor was narrowing necessarily the result of age. The average age of twenty cases with narrowing of 50 percent or more was only 22.6 years. Among young Japanese men studied by the same researchers, no arterial narrowing exceeding 50 percent was observed. Some investigators believe that the differences found in the American and Japanese arteries are related to the high-fat diet of the Americans.

A number of specialists regard diet as one of the single most important influences in the occurrence of atherosclerosis. Many aspects of the diet are involved. Scientists know that one of the major constituents of atherosclerotic fatty deposits is cholesterol, as was discussed in Chapter 17. Although the experts cannot agree about convicting cholesterol for its role in narrowing and hardening of the arteries, it at least may be an accomplice in the crime: Numerous investigations have shown that disease of the coronary arteries is more frequent among individuals with higher cholesterol levels than among those with lower cholesterol levels.

A problem associated with diet that contributes heavily to the risk of coronary artery disease is obesity. By itself obesity can make one more susceptible to high blood pressure, high blood cholesterol, strokes, diabetes, and kidney disease. The middle-aged, overweight man is two to three times more susceptible to coronary heart disease than a similar man of normal weight.

Blood Pressure

High blood pressure (which will be discussed in more detail later in this chapter), also increases the likelihood of atherosclerosis. In both men and women, the higher the pressure, the greater the risk of coronary artery disease. One study showed that those with systolic pressure (maximum pressure in the artery) above 180 were seven times as likely to have coronary disease as those with systolic pressure below 120 (the average value in healthy individuals under thirty-five years of age).

High blood pressure often can be prevented. Regular physical examinations should be obtained in order to reveal any inordinate changes in blood pressure. If it is elevated, most forms of the condition can be controlled with medication.

Cigarette Smoking

Persons who smoke one pack of cigarettes a day are twice as likely to have heart attacks as nonsmokers. Those who smoke more heavily are more prone to atherosclerosis. The preventive value of not smoking has been clearly demonstrated. Three years

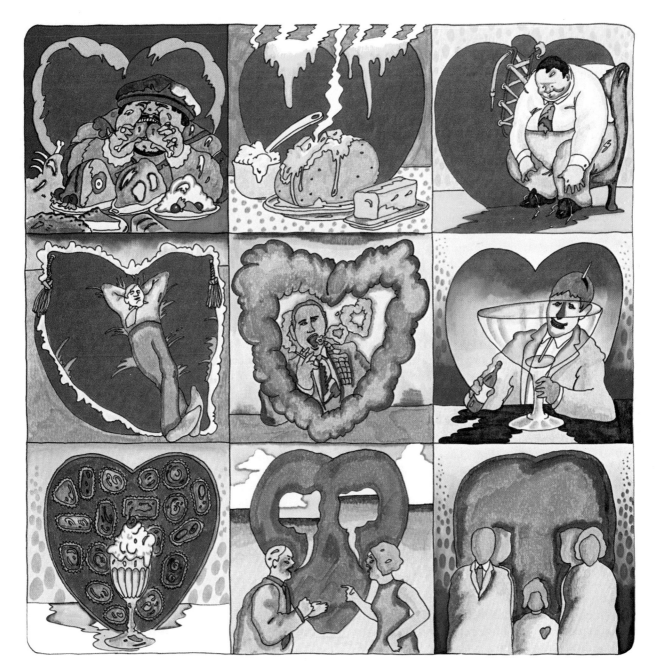

Figure 24.4   The nine contributing factors to heart disease include overeating, saturated fats and cholesterol, obesity, sedentary living, smoking, alcohol, diabetes, stress, and a family history that exhibits tendencies toward heart disease.

after a smoker has given up cigarettes entirely, his risk of getting a heart attack can drop back to that of a nonsmoker. The role of smoking in heart disease also was discussed in Chapter 9.

Exercise

People who are physically active seem to be less prone to heart attacks than those who lead sedentary lives, as has been suggested many times in studies comparing active and less active workers, often in the same occupational field. The sort of physical activity involved also is important; endurance training of the sort described in Chapter 18 provides the best protection. Besides any effects on fat consumption or accumulation, appropriate physical activity may improve blood circulation in the heart tissue, as well as in arteries throughout the body.

Multiplying the Risks

Any one of the risk factors so far discussed adds significantly to the chances of getting a heart attack. But when several are combined, the danger is greatly multiplied—up to seven times with high cholesterol, multiplied by up to seven times more for high blood pressure, multiplied by two for smoking a pack of cigarettes a day. When the risks are multiplied this way one can see even more clearly the consequences of the high-calorie, high-fat, inactive style of life of affluent societies.

There is no scientific proof that these are the only or even the most important factors involved in the development of atherosclerotic heart disease. Without controlled experiments with large numbers of human subjects over a period of many years, science probably will not know all the answers about the causes of this disease. Until more knowledge becomes available, however, the principles of living outlined above represent the best current medical knowledge. Following these recommendations will not guarantee protection against atherosclerotic heart disease, but it will certainly do no harm and will reduce the risks substantially.

HEART ATTACKS

In medicine, prevention is never perfect. Even the safest vaccines may make a few people ill, and individuals who eat properly, have low blood pressure, do not smoke, and exercise regularly may still have a heart attack (though the chances are much less). Everyone should therefore be aware of what happens during a heart attack and of how it is treated.

The symptoms of a heart attack are sometimes mistaken by the patient for something else. By and large, they consist of a constricting, squeezing, or crushing pain in the middle of the chest. The pain may radiate down the left arm or be felt in the back, shoulders, or jaw. The victim becomes pale, sweats profusely, grows short of breath, and may vomit. The symptoms, however, may vary greatly from patient to patient. Some patients feel no pain but experience sudden fatigue, anxiety, or general discomfort. A heart attack also may be so mild one never feels it at all, or one may confuse it with something like indigestion. These "silent" heart attacks may only be recognized later by studying the electrical activity of the heart with the electrocardiograph, or at autopsy.

The symptoms a patient feels are the expression of damage to the heart muscle when the coronary blood flow becomes reduced by a narrowing of coronary vessels. The narrowing may be accentuated by a temporary contraction of the blood vessel (spasm) and is sometimes associated with the establishment of a blood clot, or *thrombus*, which may precede or follow the attack. Heart attacks are therefore sometimes called *coronary thromboses*. If the damage is serious enough, a part of the heart muscle that has been denied its blood supply may die. The dead area is called an *infarct*; this sort of heart attack is thus termed a *myocardial* (muscle of the heart) *infarction*. When part of the muscle dies, scar tissue forms. Scar tissue does not contract, but if the scar is not too large the heart may continue to function, and the patient may recover. One of the reasons patients are required to rest for some time after a heart attack is to reduce the work load on the heart so it can heal the wound.

A Faltering Heartbeat

A heart attack not only damages the muscle physically, it also may drastically alter the rhythm of the heartbeat. The heart is a mechanical pump with its own electrical system. The muscle cells are highly specialized and, unlike those in the muscles that move an arm or leg, can contract even without an initiating nerve stimulus. The rate at which the heart beats (normally, about seventy times a minute) is regulated by a tiny area of specialized tissue known as the *pacemaker*. It sends a current of electricity over the heart. First the upper two chambers (the right and left atria) contract. After a very slight pause, the lower chambers (the right and left ventricles) follow suit (as described in Chapter 2).

Sometimes a heart attack may produce little or no damage to the heart muscle but still cause the ventricles to go out of control. They beat hundreds of times a minute, so rapidly the heart is incapable of pumping blood. Unless such *fibrillation* can be stopped and normal circulation restored, the patient will die. One of the major reasons for the need to get a heart-attack victim to a hospital as soon as possible is that ventricular fibrillation can be immediately recognized and treated with special equipment there. Carefully controlled electric shock is usually required to stop the fibrillation, and the heart may have to be stimulated electrically before it beats normally. Many heart-attack victims succumb to ventricular fibrillation even though their heart muscle is not permanently damaged.

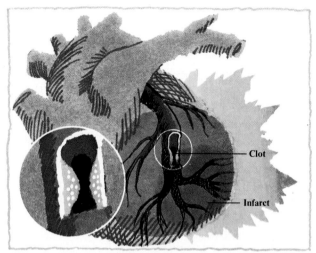

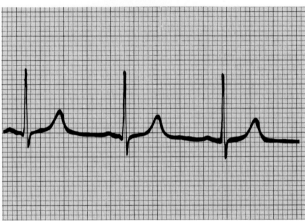

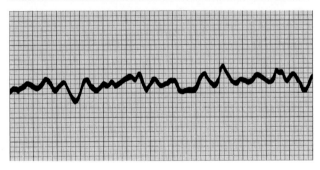

Figure 24.5 (*top*) Coronary thrombosis. When a clot suddenly forms or migrates to a part of the heart muscle, the central area deprived of blood may die. The dead tissue is called myocardial infarction or infarct.

Figure 24.6 (*bottom*) An ECG, that exhibits the regular waves of a normal heartbeat is compared to the wild, irregular rhythm of a heart muscle during fibrillation.

Heart Block

Sometimes a heart-attack victim who seems to be recovering will experience a sudden slowing of his heartbeat. It may drop to thirty beats a minute, or stop altogether. This condition is known as *heart block*. It also may occur for reasons other than a heart attack and most typically affects patients in their sixties or older.

Heart block results when the electrical connection between the main atrial pacemaker and the ventricles fails. Impulses do not reach the main pumping chambers often enough. The normal rate can be restored with an electronic pacemaker. Usually the heart can repair itself within a few days, and the natural rhythm returns. When it fails to do so, an artificial pacemaker can be implanted and take over the job for many years.

OTHER HEART PROBLEMS

Angina Pectoris

Pain, pressure, or tightness in the front part of the chest may be a sign that the heart is not getting enough oxygen. When a person regularly has such pain following exertion, excitement, or overeating, he may have *angina pectoris*. Angina is not really a disease but is a symptom of oxygen deprivation. Angina pains may occur in persons who have recovered from a heart attack or in those who have never had such an attack and may never have one. They are usually due to cornonary atherosclerosis. The reduced blood flow through the narrowed arteries carries sufficient oxygen for normal, but not for overloaded, heart activity. An increased demand on the heart will reveal this deficiency and trigger the angina attack.

The outlook for persons with angina pectoris varies greatly with the individual. They may have to restrict their activity to avoid pain, or they may hardly be aware of the problem. In any case, most people are able to carry on normal lives for many years. Use of nitroglycerine tablets, which dilate the arteries, is the best and fastest remedy for angina being used today.

Heart Failure

Angina pectoris is but one example of a condition that might lead to heart failure. The term "heart failure" does not refer to a heart that has stopped but to a heart that cannot pump enough blood to meet all the demands put on it. Practically every known type of heart disease may produce heart failure. Sometimes it can be triggered by high blood pressure, which forces the heart to work extra hard to overcome it and still deliver blood to the body's organs and tissues. At other times it can be due to defective heart valves, damaged heart muscle, or weakening of the entire heart by disease or poison.

Some of these defects may be alleviated by surgical procedures or medical treatment. When the underlying disease cannot be remedied, the physician can still improve the action of the heart by administering digitalis or a similar drug that strengthens the heart's contractions. Certain drugs can be administered to remove the excess water; restricted salt intake is also beneficial.

Cardiac Arrest and Emergency Treatment

Anytime the heart stops beating the condition is called *cardiac arrest*. The heart may stop because of a heart attack or for many other reasons—drowning, electrocution, or strangulation, among others. Immediate action is necessary or the patient may die, for the brain can survive without damage only for about four minutes after the circulation is stopped.

In the absence of immediate medical attention, resuscitation that includes ventilating the lungs and cardiac massage can save the patient. Mouth-to-

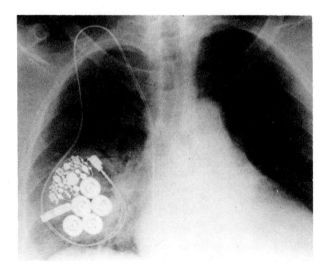

Figure 24.7 This x-ray shows an artificial pacemaker positioned in the chest. This prosthetic device has proven to be highly successful in patients whose cardiac electrical system no longer delivers electrical impulses strong enough or regular enough to maintain the rhythmic contractions of the heart. The active life of Justice William O. Douglas, a recipient of the artificial pacemaker, is illustrative of the success of modern medical advances. See Chapter 2 for further discussion of the regulatory influences on the heart.

mouth breathing forces the victim's lungs to continue supplying the needed oxygen to his body. Cardiac massage squeezes blood out of the heart and forces it into the arteries and thus to the tissues. These techniques should be known by all adults.

Congenital Heart Disease

Congenital defects (see Chapter 14) can affect all structures of the heart or its emerging vessels. They may come in combination as well as singly. *Septal* defects result from small holes in the walls separating the left and right chambers of the heart. One of the most common congenital defects is a hole in the atrial septum, the wall between left and right atria. A ventricular septal defect also is common. By themselves, these defects appear to have little effect on the circulation at least for a period of time. Some of the blood flows back from left to right chambers, reducing the overall efficiency of the heart cycle. Some of the blood may also flow directly from right to left chamber, diluting the oxygen-rich blood coming from the lungs with deoxygenated blood from the veins.

Much more serious are the defects involving an obstruction or narrowing of the valve between the right ventricle and the pulmonary artery, or *pulmonary stenosis*, coupled with septal defects. The most common combination is the *tetralogy of Fallot*, involving four defects: a ventricular septal defect, pulmonary stenosis, a consequent thickening of the right ventricle, and a shifted position of the aorta (the main artery leading away from the heart). The seriousness of these defects derives from the fact that a considerable portion of the blood, prevented from entering the pulmonary artery, is diverted directly into the left ventricle and pumped out to the body without having had a chance to become oxygenated. The poorly oxygenated blood mixture reaching the tissues confers to the baby

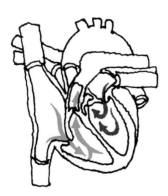

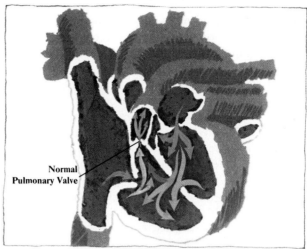

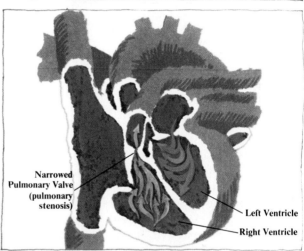

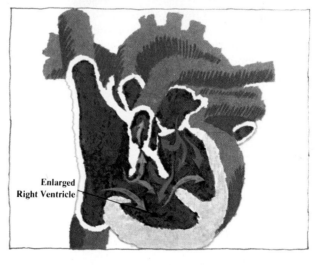

Figure 24.8 (*top*) Ventricular septal defect. (*center*) Pulmonary stenosis. (*bottom*) Tetralogy of Fallot. The diagram (*left*) indicates the normal cardiac circulation pathway.

(particularly at the lips and fingertips) a dusky, bluish color instead of its normal pinkishness. Such a child is commonly called a "blue baby." The degree of cyanosis, or bluish color, depends on the severity of the defects.

New techniques of diagnosis and therapy are saving many individuals with congenital heart defects from early death or a lifetime spent as an invalid. Sophisticated x-ray methods and techniques for sampling pressures within the heart now enable physicians to identify defects precisely and to determine whether they can be corrected. Open-heart surgery, made possible by the development of the heart-lung machine, which can take over the functions of these two organs, can be used to correct many defects so the affected children can lead normal lives.

Rheumatic Heart Disease

Rheumatic fever is an inflammatory disease of connective tissues that may occasionally follow a streptococcal infection, usually of the throat. Today there is no reason why the serious heart complications of this infection cannot be prevented with appropriate early treatment. Nevertheless, rheumatic heart disease still accounts for much of the heart disease found in young children and adults.

Rheumatic fever is usually regarded as a disease of childhood, mostly affecting children between the ages of five and fifteen years, although it does occur in older people as well. It is a disease that has a great tendency to recur, however, and thus becomes a chronic ailment affecting all ages. Rheumatic fever affects many parts of the body—joints and muscles in particular—but damage to the heart from scarring of the heart muscle and the heart valves is its greatest danger. Depending on the extent of the scarring, rheumatic heart disease will interfere with the normal functioning of the heart, which will then be forced to do more work in supplying the body's needs. An attack of rheumatic fever does not necessarily mean that one is left with a damaged heart. Nevertheless, with each recurrence of the disease there is an increased chance that damage to the heart will ensue.

Rheumatic heart disease is virtually 100 percent preventable because penicillin can cure streptococcal infections; early treatment of the infection with antibiotics prevents heart damage. It is therefore extremely important to consult one's physician if one develops a sudden, severe sore throat or if one has been exposed to a strep infection. Patients who have had rheumatic fever once are given penicillin (or another appropriate antibiotic) for several years in order to prevent recurrence of the disease. Surgical operations are used to correct or remove already damaged valves.

HIGH BLOOD PRESSURE

When the powerful left ventricle pumps blood into the body, it produces a pulse and blood pressure. When the heart relaxes in preparation for the next contraction, the pressure drops somewhat. These two pressures are what a physician measures when he puts a blood pressure cuff around an arm. They are the *systolic pressure*, produced as a result of the heart's contraction, and the *diastolic* pressure that remains after the heart dilates and its muscle relaxes. Young adults have a normal systolic pressure of between 100 and 120, older adults from 120 to 140. Diastolic pressure is usually below 90 in a healthy individual. Thus a good average blood pressure for a college student might be 120/80.

The systolic pressure represents a marked increase within the arteries with each heartbeat, but healthy arteries are elastic and expand to accommodate the load. Blood-pressure readings normally vary from time to time. They may increase during excitement, decrease during rest. High blood pressure, known medically as *hypertension*, refers to a condition in which the blood pressure is always higher than it should be. Generally speaking, a continued blood pressure above 150/100 is considered abnormal.

About 22 million people in the United States have hypertension in one form or another. Many are free of symptoms and learn of their problem only during a routine physical checkup. There is a tendency for an increase in systolic blood pressure with age. Hypertension is rarely found in persons under twenty years of age but is common above that age. After fifty years of age approximately one-half of the population has this disease to some degree. There is no disease of abnormally *low* blood pressure (hypotension)—generally, only in certain drastic situations such as hemorrhage or shock is low blood pressure a problem.

By far the most common form of hypertension is known as *essential hypertension*. About 90 percent of persons with hypertension fall into this category. This condition is present in about 10 percent of the population (about 20 million Americans). Today it is known that essential hypertension is due to the sustained constriction of the smallest arteries all over the body, decreasing the amount of blood carried by the vessels. The reason why they become constricted is still not known, however.

Hypertension is often associated with atherosclerosis and is believed to augment it. High blood pressure can cause serious harm to the arteries of the kidneys or other organs. Dull headaches on awakening are a common symptom associated with hypertension, although many people have no symptoms at all.

The treatment of hypertension depends on the severity of the disease. Much of therapy is directed toward dilating and relaxing the constricted blood vessels. In addition, obese patients are directed to reduce, and those under excessive stress are asked to change their routine to provide substantial time for adequate rest and relaxation. Smoking, which constricts the arterioles, should be eliminated. Sometimes a low-salt diet is prescribed. Diuretics, drugs that help reduce the amount of body water, are frequently beneficial.

STROKES

Strokes occur because of clots or hemorrhage (uncontrolled bleeding) or other blood-vessel obstruction in the brain, causing the destruction of a significant amount of brain tissue. They constitute the third leading cause of death in the United States. In addition, about two-fifths of persons over age fifty have severe atherosclerosis (one or more arteries narrowed at least 50 percent) of vessels in or serving the brain.

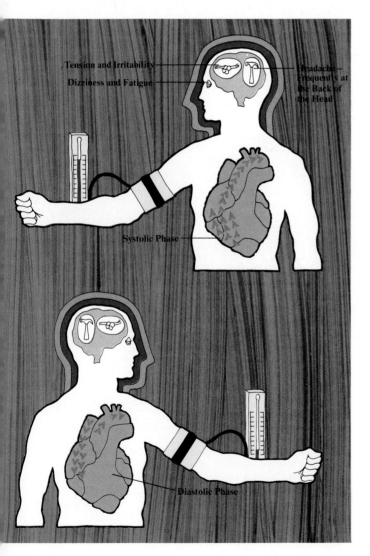

Tension and Irritability
Dizziness and Fatigue
Headache Frequently at the Back of the Head
Systolic Phase
Diastolic Phase

Figure 24.9 High blood pressure. The heart exerts its greatest pressure when pumping in a fresh supply of blood (systolic phase, *top*) and the least pressure when pausing between beats to fill with blood (diastolic phase, *bottom*). The blood pressure is the measurement of pressure on the arterial wall at the extreme points of the systolic and diastolic phases. Persistent high blood pressure (hypertension) often causes such symptoms as dizziness, persistent fatigue, irritability, and headaches, and, if allowed to continue untreated, may lead to hypertensive heart disease.

Medical terms used for various kinds of strokes are cerebral hemorrhage, cerebral thrombosis, and cerebral embolism. An *embolus* is a mass of abnormal material that comes through the bloodstream to clog a blood vessel. Often, the material is a fragment of a clot (thrombus) or an atherosclerotic thickening (plaque) broken off the original location. A diseased heart may be a cause of cerebral embolism in a brain whose arteries are still quite normal. But in many strokes, as in many heart attacks, the critical, crippling event occurs long after the underlying disease begins developing. A stroke may have been "incubating" for thirty or forty years before symptoms appear. Preventing atherosclerosis, or treating diseases such as diabetes or hypertension that may lead to strokes, can reduce the mortality rate from strokes.

When some of the nerve cells in the brain are deprived of their blood supply by a stroke, the parts of the body controlled by these nerve centers can no longer function normally. As a result, a stroke patient may be partly paralyzed, may have difficulty in speaking, or may suffer some loss of memory. The amount and location of damage to the brain will determine the extent of the difficulty experienced by the patient.

Some patients recover quickly and can resume normal activity. Others may never recover completely. Partial recovery takes a long time if serious damage has occurred. If the stroke is induced by a blood clot or a narrowed blood vessel, anticoagulants are sometimes prescribed. Occasionally, surgery is useful. On the whole, however, rest, good nursing care, and encouragement of earliest possible activity are the major forms of therapy in the beginning. Proper exercise and other forms of therapy can do much toward helping the patient reacquire speech and the use of muscles. Often an extensive period of retraining is required.

HEART TRANSPLANTATION AND ARTIFICIAL HEARTS

Surgery has made many contributions to the treatment of heart defects. Congenital conditions have been repaired and damaged heart valves replaced. Surgical repair of diseased coronary arteries has not developed to the same level of success but is being vigorously investigated at present. Many pa-

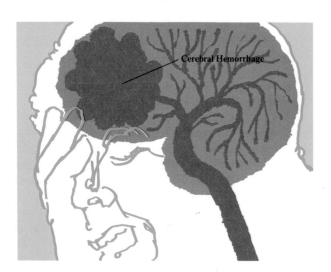

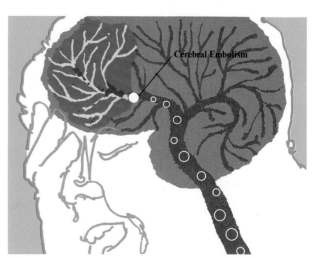

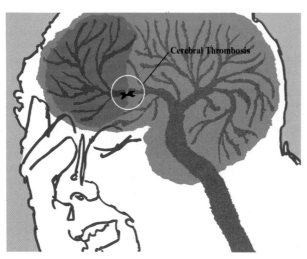

Figure 24.10   Three types of strokes. (*above left*) Cerebral hemorrhage, in which blood flow to the brain is impaired due to rupture of a diseased cerebral blood vessel. (*above right*) Cerebral embolism, in which a mass of abnormal material clogs a blood vessel. (*left*) Cerebral thrombosis, in which a blood clot forms in a cerebral blood vessel. In all cases, oxygen transport to parts of the brain is impaired, resulting in the death of some brain tissue.

tients die today whose hearts are simply so diseased they cannot continue to function.

Two particularly dramatic approaches to the problem have been tried — heart transplantation and the development of artificial hearts. Heart transplantation is beset with the same problems as many other forms of organ grafting, most of them resulting from the body's natural tendency to reject foreign tissue, even when it represents a beneficial replacement. Medicine is gradually improving its techniques for dealing with graft rejection, but it still represents a serious stumbling block for organ transplantation. Most physicians believe that many more years of research are needed before heart transplant can become a practical form of treatment. Even if this technique will prove workable for larger numbers of heart victims, it is estimated that only about 33,000 patients per year would benefit from the procedure in the United States.

Small mechanical pumps have been used as auxiliary circulatory devices to relieve diseased hearts temporarily while the heart muscle heals itself. The long-term potential of such equipment is uncertain, however. A true artificial heart, capable of functioning inside the body indefinitely, has not yet been developed. Although many investigators are studying the possibility, it seems unlikely that such a device will become a reality for many years.

Prevention is still the best weapon modern medicine has against heart disease. It is far easier to eliminate the causes than to have to depend upon surgery or medication after the fact. The risks of developing atherosclerosis may be considerably reduced by adopting healthier life habits. Many congenital heart defects can be avoided by preventing disease or intoxication of pregnant women. Rheumatic fever can be caught and treated before it attacks the heart. *Cor pulmonale* (or pulmonary heart), a condition induced by the high capillary resistance of diseased lungs, is aggravated if not actually caused by tobacco smoking. True prevention of heart disease, however, will depend in the final analysis on the commitment by potential victims to take full advantage of current medical knowledge and continue to support the research still necessary to further advance it.

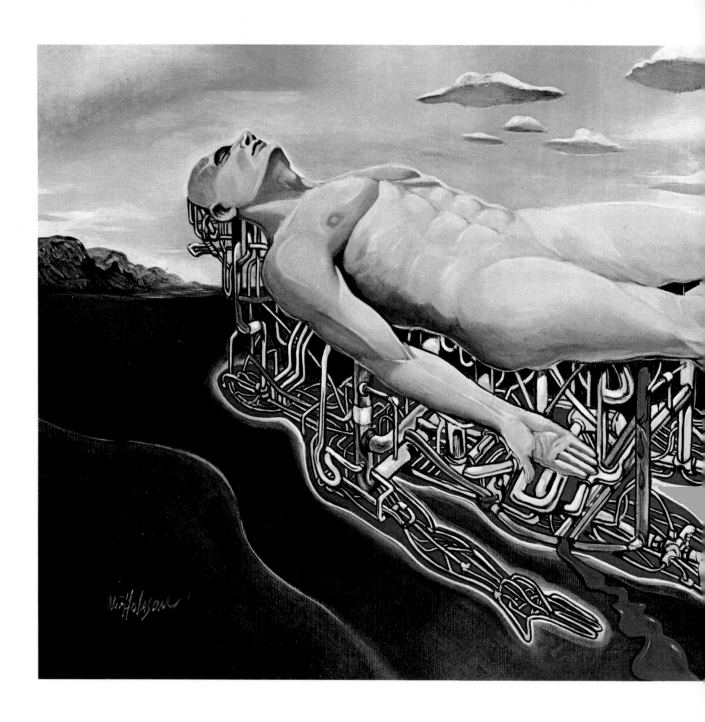

472

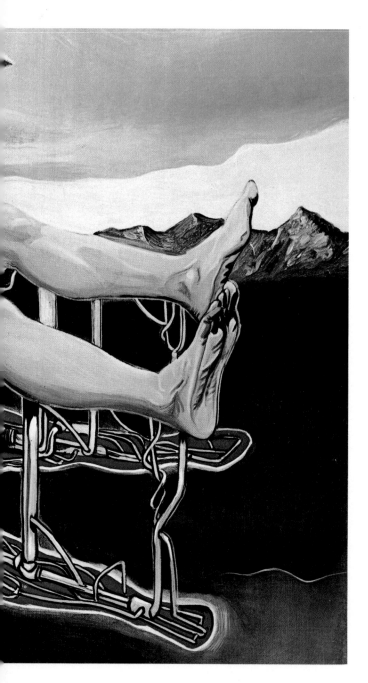

25

Like the cardiovascular system, other body systems are susceptible to chronic or degenerative disorders, besides specific infections. Sometimes the disorders affect primarily one segment of the system, although the disease of one segment may well lead to the secondary malfunction of the others, or even of many other systems or organs in the body. Sometimes, however, the disorder is truly *systemic*, in that it involves all the components of one system or a widespread tissue (such as lymph) regardless of its location in the body. An example of such systemic diseases has already been encountered in the case of atherosclerosis, of which coronary artery disease and certain cases of cerebral stroke are but local reflections. In the following sections, selected examples will be presented of both localized and generalized disorders more commonly affecting various body systems.

DISORDERS OF THE IMMUNE SYSTEM

Chapter 22 discussed the phenomenon of immunity, that is, the ability of a special type of lymphoid cells, or plasma cells, to counteract the appearance in the body of alien substances (antigens) with the production of specific antibodies to be released into the bloodstream. Besides these circulating or *humoral antibodies*, antibodies also are produced that will bind to tissue cells and remain fixed in these tissues (*cellular antibodies*). Modern theories of immunology—a science in which exciting advances

Systemic Diseases

are currently being made at a fast pace—conceive the involvement of at least two and probably three cell types in the immune mechanism.

Deficiency in antibody production may result from injury or disease of the tissues from which these cells originate—bone marrow, lymphoid tissue, and, possibly (only in early stages of development), the thymus. Body irradiation, for example, such as may be needed for the treatment of widespread cancer, will drastically reduce resistance to infection due to low or no production of humoral antibodies. By the same token, irradiation or treatment with certain drugs is used to reduce the immune defenses so as to permit a patient to avoid rejecting a newly transplanted organ.

Allergy

Rather than a specific disease, allergy—also known as *hypersensitivity*—is a body reaction that reflects an overcompensation, rather than a failure, on the part of the immune system. Exposed parts of the body may respond to contact with a foreign substance by releasing a chemical called *histamine*—the same chemical that most such cells would release upon other kinds of injury. Histamine is a powerful agent that affects the contraction of smooth muscle cells, for example, around blood vessels or in the walls of the respiratory canal. The massive release of histamine results, therefore, in local dilation of blood vessels, passage of fluid out of the capillary bed into the tissues, and production of the symptoms so commonly associated with allergy. The mucous lining of the nose and throat becomes swollen, and as the irritation moves into the lungs, wheezing and sneezing result. Similarly, the skin becomes red, itchy, and swollen and may develop hives. The eyes also may become red and vision blurred. This allergic response may be set off by pollen, the chemicals in fabrics and dyes, foods—especially shellfish—or drugs such as penicillin.

The mechanism, still poorly understood, depends on the formation of cellular antibodies to the alien substance, or *allergen*. When the body is again exposed to the allergen the antibody binds it, and this allergen-antibody reaction at the surface of the tissue cells causes the histamine release that sets off the allergic response in the region of entry, whether it be the skin, digestive tract, or respiratory system. Essentially, then, this mechanism is a protective one that by its violent response warns the body that it is being exposed to an unwelcome material. When this mechanism goes awry, a normal response becomes one of hypersensitivity.

Hay fever is typical of the hypersensitivity reaction. This common disorder, which occurs in 10 percent of the population, results when the individual becomes sensitized to normal pollens. Then, during the seasons in which pollens are prevalent, preformed antibodies bind the inhaled material, and the characteristic upper respiratory response results. To treat this disorder one can either avoid pollens by changing locations or take antihistamines to diminish the response. Alternatively, one can take a series of desensitization injections in an effort to familiarize the body to the specific allergen and thus reduce the response. This treatment, however, usually is reserved for severe allergies, because the time required for successful desensitization is quite long.

When bronchial passageways become exceedingly sensitive to foreign protein, *asthma* results. This complex and poorly understood disorder is characterized by attacks of severe airway obstruction. The bronchial passages become engorged, filled with mucus, and constricted. Soon the person develops respiratory distress because he cannot get enough air through his narrowed airways. The treatment is to administer epinephrine (adrenalin) either by injection or aerosol. This relaxes the bronchial muscles and opens the airways. Preven-

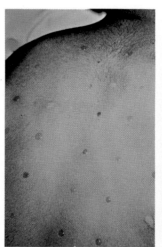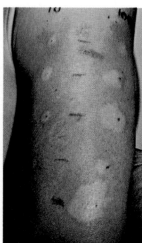

Figure 25.1 Allergy skin test. In both photos an array of allergens has been injected under the skin in different areas. The area is "mapped" so that if a response appears, the doctor will know what substance the patient is allergic to. The most common allergens are pollens, animal dander, and dust, but cases in which the allergen is milk, eggs, or common chemicals are far from rare.

tion of attacks involves avoidance of identified allergens as in hay fever, although an attack often may be precipitated by an emotional upset; in these instances psychological as well as pharmacological support is required.

Autoimmune Disease

The body normally recognizes its own antigenic determinants as "self" and does not make antibodies against its own cells or tissues. This immunological unresponsiveness, or *tolerance*, does, however, break down at times, and antibodies are made against a tissue or an organ and slowly damage or destroy it. The person is then said to be the victim of *autoimmune disease*. There is as yet no clear understanding of the circumstances and the process leading to it.

A widely held hypothesis is that the body's tissue becomes so altered that it will present alienlike antigens to the normally functioning immune mechanism of the body. This alteration of body tissue can occur after chemical injury such as in the drug-induced *hemolytic anemia*. In this disorder the body forms antibodies against its own red blood cells and then destroys them, producing a profound anemia. What is proposed here is that the drug becomes attached to the red cell, the altered cell is no longer recognized as self, and so it is destroyed. The treatment, of course, is to stop taking the offending agent and then temporarily depress the body's immune system with other drugs until all the affected cells have cleared. Bacteria also can institute the phenomenon of autoimmunity. In *rheumatic fever*, for example, the valves of the heart become slowly destroyed long after the acute illness has subsided. It is thought therefore that a bacterial toxin alters the valvular cells, makes them unrecognizable, and thus sets up an immune response.

When one considers *rheumatoid arthritis*, a possible autoimmune disease, the concept is more puzzling, because no triggering event has yet been clearly identified. Arthritis is a common, chronic, disabling, systemic inflammation of the joints that affects about 5 percent of the general population. The first symptoms include early fatigue, fever, morning stiffness, and swelling in the small joints of the hands and feet. Gradually the affected joints become more deformed and swollen and in the more extreme cases can render the limb useless. The theory of autoimmune disease in relation to rheumatoid arthritis is shown in Figure 25.2.

In most cases the disease is chronic, with alternating periods of remission and exacerbation. There is no cure and the best treatment includes rest, heat, aspirin, and certain antiinflammatory drugs that are reserved for severe attacks. One recent treatment for rheumatoid arthritis is surgical, and at present many hands have been returned to almost normal function after replacement with plastic joints.

DISORDERS OF THE RESPIRATORY SYSTEM

A number of infectious diseases involving the lung tissue, such as different types of pneumonia and tuberculosis, have already been mentioned. Cancer of the lung and its dramatic rise in recent years have been discussed in Chapter 23; its special relationship to tobacco smoking also was discussed in Chapter 9. Mention also has been made, in the section on immune system disorders, of the way in which the respiratory apparatus and functions are affected by asthma. Here, two other common respiratory diseases will be considered, chronic bronchitis and emphysema.

Chronic Bronchitis

The term *bronchitis*—like any other "itis" in the medical nomenclature—describes a state of tissue inflammation, irrespective of what has caused it. In the case of bronchitis, the affected tissue is the

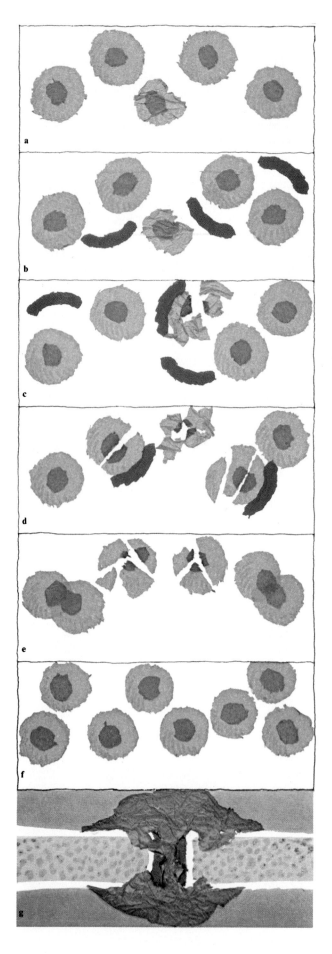

mucous membrane of the bronchi and their smaller subdivisions, the bronchioles, which constitute the lower portion of the airways to the lungs. Bronchitis is a common disease, both in the acute (viral or bacterial infections) and in the chronic forms. *Chronic bronchitis* rates among the top causes of working time losses by older workers. Toxic inhalation at work, tobacco smoking, and heavy atmospheric pollution are important contributing, if not causal, factors.

Irritation of the mucous lining produces excessive mucus discharge that fills and obstructs the smaller air passages, establishing a medium for infection. As the mucus becomes infected and pus is produced, it ultimately destroys the hairlike cilia of the lining cells, which normally work to clear the lungs by sweeping mucus and materials outward through the upper respiratory tract. Coughing then remains the only means of expelling these materials. As a result, more accumulation and obstruction is produced and the bronchioles become more irritated and swollen. The symptoms generally begin with a morning cough, trying to clear the secretions that have accumulated during the night. As the condition progresses, the cough worsens markedly through the day, and soon the sufferer is incapacitated by the inability to clear his secretions, the racking and frequent bouts of cough, and a shortness of breath. If untreated, chronic bronchitis becomes refractory (resistant to treatment), leading to progressive incapacitation and early death.

The best treatment is, of course, prevention by the avoidance of cigarette smoking and polluted environments. Such avoidance becomes an absolute necessity when the disease is already established, as is the avoidance of unnecessary exposure to adverse weather conditions. Various medications (expectorants, mucolytic agents, aerosols) are used to liquify and expel the sticky mucus. Further treatments include effective bronchial aerosol with ade-

Figure 25.2 Autoimmunity. The explanation of the process of rheumatoid arthritis, while still only theoretical, suggests that when (a) normal cells are injured or infected (b) antibodies are formed and (c) attack damaged or diseased cells; but due to some unknown cause (d) the antibody is unable to distinguish between normal and diseased cells and attacks both. Other adjacent cells begin rapidly reproducing (e) to replace damaged cells, and joint tissue proliferates (f) and eventually swells to the point where the joint is damaged and sometimes even immobilized.

quate hydration and use of antibiotics at the first sign of infection. In later stages, oxygen may have to be given continuously to keep the patient alive.

Emphysema

Emphysema is a common respiratory disease in America's elderly. It is best described as a loss of functioning lung volume, with an associated overinflation of remaining tissue. It often follows other chronic respiratory diseases such as asthma and

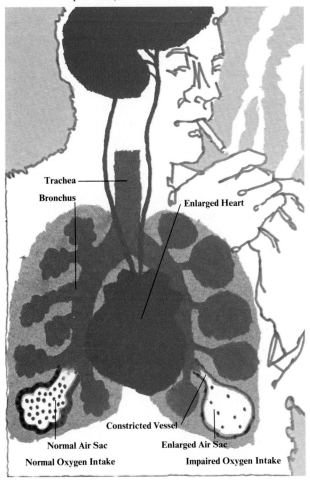

Trachea

Bronchus

Enlarged Heart

Constricted Vessel

Normal Air Sac

Enlarged Air Sac

Normal Oxygen Intake

Impaired Oxygen Intake

Figure 25.3 It is not known whether bronchial infection (bronchitis) first constricts passages leading to the air sacs, making the lungs highly susceptible to emphysema, or if emphysema causes alveolar malfunction leading to bronchial dysfunction. Note that in normal air sacs (alveoli) oxygen and carbon dioxide pass easily in and out of the thin membrane. In the diseased lung, however, little oxygen passes into the air sac and carbon dioxide accumulates.

bronchitis, and, of course, there is a high association with cigarette smoking and air pollution. Persons who have "dusty" occupations like mining, milling, or grinding, or who "breathe for a living," such as glass-blowers or wind-instrument musicians, also appear to be more frequently affected.

Persons with emphysema are short of breath and can tolerate only minimal activity. Both the mechanical events of respiration and the gas exchange between alveolar air and blood are impaired: the lungs cannot take in additional air and do not have enough functioning tissue to utilize the air they take in—patients may even be blue from lack of oxygen. The resulting strain on the right ventricle of the heart may further aggravate the patient's condition with impairment of heart function. Treatment is similar to that for chronic bronchitis, that is, adequate bronchial and pulmonary (aerosol) toilet so that whatever lung tissue remains may be used to its full extent.

KIDNEY DISORDERS

The kidney is an important organ because it functions to clear wastes from the body and to maintain fluid balance. It has a large reserve capacity and in fact a person can live a normal life with only one kidney. Thus, the normal, healthy kidney is well equipped to handle the extra load placed on it when other parts of the body become diseased and release excess amounts of toxins and degradation products to be eliminated.

Diseased kidneys, however, have a reduced capacity to fulfill even their normal role. Deficient functioning is reflected in more abundant and frequent urination and the pale color of the urine. Swelling of body tissues, reflecting an excessive retention of salt and therefore of fluid, is another important indication of some sort of kidney trouble. In more serious kidney diseases, the drastic reduction in the number of functioning units, or

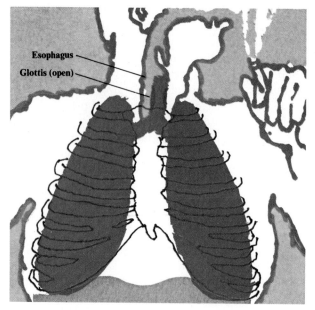

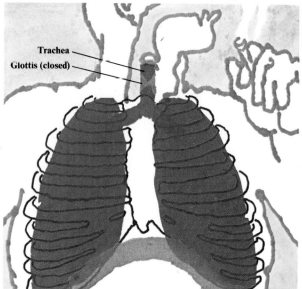

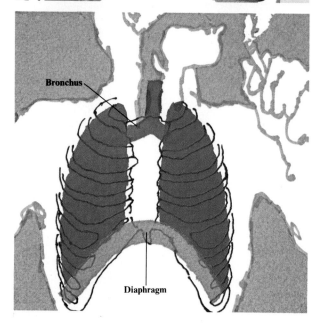

nephrons, is expressed by a progressive *decrease*, or even cessation, of urine output. Most dangerously, failure to excrete urea (the final product of protein breakdown within cells) and other products of metabolism leads to their accumulation in the blood and causes a general systemic poisoning, known as *uremia*, which can be fatal. The uremic stage is characterized by muscle twitching, vomiting, lethargy, mental confusion, and—in extreme cases—coma and death.

Kidney (*renal*) disease is of two types—glomerular and tubular; both may result in severe disorders. The first is best represented by *glomerulonephritis*, which can follow a streptococcal infection of the throat or skin. Usually it is an acute, self-limiting illness, but if repeated attacks are allowed to occur, *chronic nephritis* sets in. Progressively more of the filtering glomeruli are destroyed, and the kidney ultimately fails. There is no real treatment for this problem except early administration of antibiotics when a strep infection is diagnosed.

When the tubules are diseased, the ability to secrete and reabsorb and thus to alter the concentration of the urine is affected, so that even though the plasma is being filtered effectively through the glomeruli, proper urine is not made in that nephron. In *pyelonephritis*, the consequence of a severe urinary tract infection, the tubules are infected and filled with pus. With recurrent infections enough tubules can be destroyed to result in the loss of a functional kidney.

The term *nephrosis* is often used to indicate a noninflammatory, degenerative alteration of the tubules, resulting in losses of protein from the blood into the urine.

Persons with debilitating kidney disorders or with temporary renal failure are now benefiting from scientific advances in treatment. *Artificial kidneys* are machines that can filter wastes out of the bloodstream using a process called *hemodialysis*. If treated two or three times a week, persons with no

Figure 25.4 The cough mechanism occurs in three distinct phases: (*top*) A large breath is taken to fill the lungs with air. Note that the glottis is open so that air can pass from the outside in; the chest wall expands and the diaphragm moves down causing air to move into the lungs. (*center*) In the second phase the glottis closes so that no more air passes in or out; the chest wall and diaphragm move inward, thus increasing the pressure within the chest cavity. (*bottom*) In the third phase the glottis opens and, because the pressure within the chest cavity and lungs is so much greater than the atmospheric pressure, the air rushes out.

kidneys can lead almost normal lives. Unfortunately, the present treatment is essentially limited to medical centers and is quite expensive, therefore only a fraction of the thousands of uremic patients can benefit from it. Efforts are in progress to develop effective home-care units that could put hemodialysis in the hands of family physicians and thus extend indefinitely lives that are now doomed.

Renal transplantation has become a more frequently used method of treatment in kidney failure. Viable kidneys are much easier to obtain than other organs for transplant, because the donor can live with only one kidney. More importantly, though, the recipient can be kept alive on hemodialysis until there is a donor kidney—a luxury not yet available in heart and liver disease. Of course, as with all transplants, the body's rejection of foreign tissue is a problem, but this mechanism is slowly being overcome with better tissue matching and the use of immunosuppressive therapy.

DISEASES OF THE DIGESTIVE TRACT

Inflammations

Inflammatory diseases of the stomach (*gastritis*) and the intestines (*enteritis*, *colitis*) are the most common disorders of this system, particularly for the infant. Inflammation can be caused by a number of agents, including bacteria, viruses, or chemicals. Infectious diseases of the stomach are considerably rarer than those of the intestines.

Inflammation of the intestines is manifested by a rather constant set of symptoms: cramping abdominal pain (*colic*), fever, loss of appetite, and a severe diarrhea that can be bloody. The definitive treatment depends on the identification of the causative agent but must include supportive measures such as adequate rehydration to compensate for the extensive fluid losses along with medications that ease the pain and allow the bowels to rest.

One segment of the intestines that is frequently subject to infection is the *appendix*, a tubelike exten-

sion from the first segment of the large intestine. *Acute appendicitis* can be a serious problem because of its possible complications. When inflamed, the appendix is swollen, tense, and markedly congested, with sharp localized pain that the body attempts to relieve by contracting the abdominal musculature. The inflamed appendix can readily become infected, with heavy pus production, which may lead to the formation of an *abscess* in its wall, the rupture of the wall (*perforation*), and the generalized infection (*peritonitis*) of the peritoneum, the abdominal lining that envelops most of the abdominal viscera. These serious, and occasionally fatal, complications can be avoided by a timely surgical removal of the diseased appendix (appendectomy).

Gastric (Peptic) Ulcer

In the stomach, there is normally a balance between the acid (hydrochloric acid) and enzymes that digest the food and the mucus—also secreted by the gastric wall—that coats and protects the stomach lining. Hydrochloric acid functions to promote chemical breakdown of certain food molecules and, more importantly, to activate some of

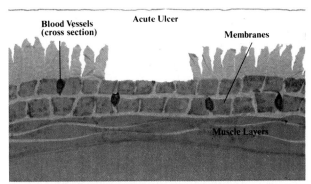

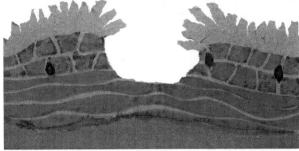

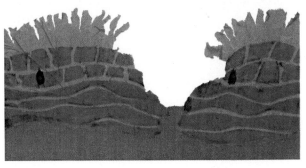

Figure 25.5 Formation of peptic ulcer. Although the precise cause of peptic ulcers is not known, emotional stress appears to contribute to their formation and often precipitates ulcer attacks. The action of the gastric acid destroys the membrane of the stomach or the duodenum. (*top*) The acid first destroys the surface membrane. (*center*) If the production of acid continues or is produced in excessive quantities, the ulcer soon invades the underlying muscle tissue. (*bottom*) Eventually, if allowed to go untreated, it will perforate the stomach wall, and gastric juices will escape into the abdominal cavity. At this point surgery is necessary to close the perforation or the ulcer may be fatal.

the digestive enzymes secreted by other cells of the gastric wall. In persons suffering from *gastritis*, the acid secretion can be reduced, leading to impaired digestion, or it can be exaggerated, producing the symptom improperly called "heartburn." Excess acid production is often related to the ingestion of acid-stimulating substances, such as coffee.

Excess acid production and a defective or insufficient mucus production may combine to upset the balance protecting the mucous membrane of the stomach wall, and localized lesions of the wall can develop that are known as *ulcers*. The person with ulcers has gnawing pains in his stomach that are quickly relieved by either antacid pills or milk. The pains can awaken him in the night, and he finds he is most comfortable if he eats continuously. Should an ulcer erode a blood vessel, hemorrhage can occur and the person vomits blood. An ulcer also can perforate the gastric wall, causing stomach contents to spill into the abdominal cavity.

The treatment against acid gastritis and mild ulcers is to avoid acid-stimulating foods and to take antacids to neutralize the stomach excess. If these methods fail, there are several surgical interventions that can repair the damage and avoid the more extreme complications.

The Liver

The liver, like the kidney, has a large reserve capacity, but due to its multiple involvements it is liable to injury from many causes—infection, circulatory disturbances, dietary deficiencies or imbalances, intoxication (alcohol, chloroform, mercury), and so on.

In *acute hepatitis* after viral infection, for example, the inflammation of the tissue reduces the functional ability of the liver cells to the point that they can no longer cope with hemoglobin breakdown. Bile pigments—the degradation products from hemoglobin—increase in the blood, escape through capillary walls, and accumulate in the tissues, conferring upon them a characteristic yellow tinge. This occurrence, known as *jaundice*, also may be brought about, in the absence of a primary liver cell lesion, by obstruction of the bile tract (for example, with gallstones) or an excessive destruction of red blood cells (as is the case with hemolytic anemia). The person affected by hepatitis, besides becoming jaundiced, fatigues readily, loses his appetite, and gets progressively weaker. Usually, the inflammation subsides and the jaundice clears on no treatment except good food and vitamins, but in severe cases antiinflammatory drugs such as cortisone must be used to slow down liver-cell destruction.

In *cirrhosis* of the liver the process is chronic and slow and may take thirty years to develop. This disease, which is caused by either excessive alcohol or the nutritional deficiencies associated with alcoholism, is characterized by a hardened, enlarged liver filled with scar tissue. (See photograph in Chapter 8, Figure 8.2.) As the amount of scar tissue increases, more functioning liver cells are lost and hepatic failure develops. Unlike what happens with hepatitis, jaundice is a late complication of cirrhosis and is usually preceded by evidence of muscle wasting and abdominal fluid collection, as the diseased liver cannot supply the body with eough protein to build new tissue and retain fluid within the vascular bed. Treatment is based on good nutrition and the avoidance of alcohol. Sometimes this treatment is successful in the motivated individual, but usually the disease is preterminal and little can be done to reverse it.

The Pancreas

The pancreas, which is located behind the stomach, serves two functions. The first is the supply of digestive enzymes to the small intestine and the second, to produce the hormone insulin in special islet cells. When the pancreas becomes inflamed, the person has severe abdominal pain that causes repeated vomiting. High fevers are common, and peritonitis and hemorrhage complicate severe cases. The usual cause is an overindulgence in alcohol, but pancreatitis also can accompany gall bladder disease when a stone from the gall bladder obstructs the duct that drains the pancreas. There is no specific treatment for pancreatitis, and most attacks subside after a few days of fluid support and pain relievers. The real danger is in repeated attacks, for if the pancreas becomes scarred, not enough enzymes can be made to digest the intestinal contents adequately. When islet-tissue destruction becomes advanced, a diabetic syndrome (to be discussed later in this chapter) can ensue.

DISEASES OF THE ENDOCRINE SYSTEM

The endocrine glands together form a group of intricately connected organs whose individual products, the hormones, are discharged into the bloodstream to affect many aspects of body metabolism. Diseases of these glands are important because of what the changes in hormone level do to the rest of the body. The basic defects can be either an under- or overproduction of hormone; the prefixes hypo- and hyper- are used to identify each of them respectively. Only the major examples of endocrine disorders will be mentioned here; a more comprehensive list is given in Table 25.1. Only hormones that have been linked to disease or disorders have been included.

The Pituitary

The pituitary gland (or hypophysis) is located at the base of the brain and is interrelated through feedback mechanisms with many other endocrine glands such as the thyroid and the gonads. Because of these connections, pituitary disease can cause dysfunction in any of the other glands, some of which will be discussed later. The pituitary, however, produces specific hormones other than the "tropins" directed to endocrine glands elsewhere. Among them are GSH (growth-stimulating hormone) and ADH (antidiuretic hormone).

Insufficient production of GHS at birth will result in a *pituitary dwarf*—an individual who never achieves normal adult size. Excessive production will lead to *gigantism*—though it is a rare phenomenon. There also may be an increase in GSH production in adulthood caused by certain pituitary tumors. Called *acromegaly*, the disease manifests itself with increases in the size of the hands and feet, the jaw becomes prominent, and there is a coarseness to all features. The treatment is to remove the tumor or destroy it with irradiation, which will halt progression of the disease in 70 percent of patients but will not reverse the changes that have already occurred.

Underproduction of ADH causes the disease *diabetes insipidus*, which is characterized by the excretion of large volumes of dilute urine to the point of dehydration. This condition can be acute or chronic and when it occurs must be treated with rehydration and supplements of ADH.

Adrenals

The adrenal glands, located above the kidneys, produce two sets of hormones. Within the center of the gland, or medulla, epinephrine and norepinephrine are made. There are no deficiency diseases of the medullary hormones, as the deficit can be made up from other production centers. However, overproduction can induce severe episodic high blood pressure.

The outer portion of the gland, or cortex, produces several hormones. Excess production of cortical hormones results in *Cushing's syndrome*, or hyperadrenocorticism. The person develops obesity of the trunk, with skinny arms and legs. The face becomes moon shaped, and a large fat pad de-

Table 25.1   Endocrine Disorders

GLAND OR TISSUE	Hormones	Physiological Role	Effects of Deficiency	Effects of Excess
Island of Langerhans (pancreas)	Insulin	Storage and mobilization of glucose; glucose transport into cells	Diabetes mellitus	Low blood sugar
Ovaries	Estrogens	Stimulates development of female organs and secondary sexual characteristics	Tendencies to masculinity	Precocious sexual development
Testes	Androgens	Stimulates development of male secondary sexual characteristics	Tendencies to feminity	Precocious sexual development
Pituitary	Growth hormone (GSH)	Affects growth, especially of the skeleton	Dwarfism	Gigantism, acromegaly
	Thyrotropic	Stimulates activity of the thyroid	Decreased activity of thyroid	Increased activity of thyroid
	Adenocorticotropic	Stimulates activity of adrenal cortex	Decreased output of corticosteroids	Increased output of corticosteroids
	Diabetogenic	Increases blood glucose	Reduction of blood glucose	Permanent diabetes mellitus
	Prolan A	Stimulates ripening of Graafian follicles in the ovaries	Atrophy of the ovaries	Precocious sexual development
	Prolan B	Production of yellow bodies after release of eggs	Indirectly causes miscarriage	None known
	Prolactin	Production of milk in the mammary glands	Very little milk secretion	Excessive milk secretion
	Male gonadotropic hormone	Stimulates development of sperm and the hormone tissue of the testes	Atrophy of testes	Precocious sexual development
	Antidiuretic hormone (ADH)	Controls resorption of water by the kidney tubules	Excessive dilute urine (diabetes insipidus)	
Thyroid	Thyroxin	Controls rate of metabolism and hence of growth	Cretinism, myxedema	Goiter, speeded metabolism
Parathyroids	Parathormone	Controls exchange of calcium and phosphate between bones and blood	Tetany, muscular spasms of varying severity	Muscular weakness; kidney stones in gut
Adrenals	Aldosterone, corticosterones	Control salt and water content of blood; cell metabolism	Addison's disease	Cushing's syndrome
	Epinephrine (adrenalin) Norepinephrine (noradrenalin)	Controls reactions to shock and stress		Hypertension

Source: Adapted from A. E. Vines and N. Rees. *Human Biology.* London: Pitman, 1966, pp. 295–296.

Figure 25.6   The mechanism of diabetes mellitus. In normal metabolism (*left*), fuel in the form of blood glucose enters the cell in sufficient amounts to operate the turbine (the Krebs cycle) and to maintain a reserve supply in the storage tanks. The entrance of the glucose is regulated by insulin secreted by the pancreas. In diabetic metabolism, little or no insulin is produced, so that little glucose enters the cell. The turbine can work only by depleting the reserves, particularly those from the fat reservoir.

velops behind the neck. The victim also has severe acne and purple stripes that cover his abdominal wall. High blood pressure is also common, and there is tendency toward holding salt and water in the tissues.

In *Addison's disease* the opposite happens; there is too little of the cortical hormones. The affected individual is dramatically thin, with darkly pigmented skin. He has a low blood pressure and loses salt into his urine. Most importantly, he has no capacity for stress and can become critically ill or die from mild infections. The treatment is to give cortisone replacement to cure the problem.

Thyroid

Hyperthyroidism occurs when too much of the hormone thyroxin is produced by the thyroid. Usually a mass (or *goiter*) appears in the neck, and the victim exhibits all the symptoms one would expect from overactive body metabolism. He has a fast pulse and is always hot and sweaty. Weight loss accompanies an increased appetite, and there is nervousness and a constant tremor. The treatment

is to slow the thyroid down with drugs or to remove most of the functioning tissue with surgery.

In hypothyroidism, or *myxedema*, the opposite effects are seen. The individual is lethargic, mentally dulled, and slow of speech. He always feels cold, complains of constant fatigue, and lacks drive. His skin is swollen, and he is usually obese. Administration of thyroid hormone reverses all these symptoms.

Islet Cells of the Pancreas

As already mentioned, certain specialized cells of the pancreas—or islet cells—have endocrine functions. Excess production of the islet-cell hormone, insulin, is sometimes caused by tumors of the islet cells. All symptoms are related to low blood sugar. The person has to eat continuously to keep from being dizzy or fainting.

Insulin deficiency is the basis of *diabetes mellitus* (sweet diabetes). Insulin deficiency interferes with sugar metabolism, is associated with the inability of the body to store carbohydrates as glycogen, and causes excessive accumulation of sugar in the blood

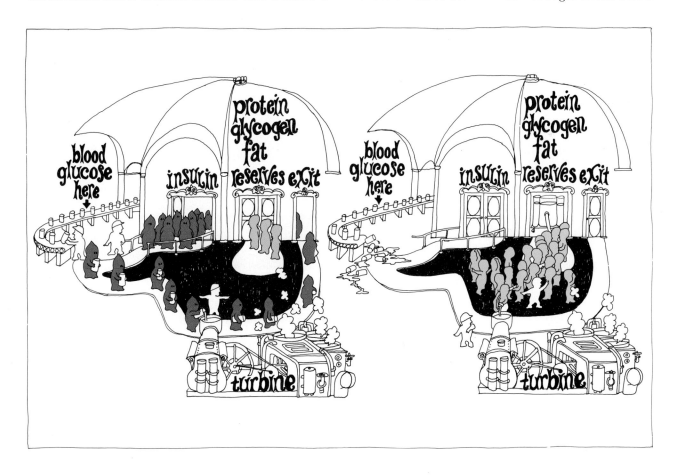

and the excretion of excessive sugar in the urine. The utilization of fat also is impaired. Of the 2 million Americans who have diabetes, only about one-half know it.

There are two basic types of diabetes—juvenile and adult. The juvenile type occurs during the childhood or early-adult years, with the average age of onset being ten to twelve years of age. About two-thirds of juvenile diabetics have a diabetic relative. The basic defect appears to be a severe deficit in the synthesis of insulin by the pancreas. The adult type of diabetes most commonly develops in obese individuals after age forty. Adult diabetes appears to be caused by insufficient insulin production rather than lack of insulin and is not as severe as the juvenile type. Some forms of diabetes may be due to the destruction of islet cells as a consequence of pancreatic diseases, rather than a genetic defect.

The onset of diabetes is often indefinite and insidious. Common symptoms include increased urinary output, increased thirst and appetite, and fatigue. The complications of diabetes involve all body systems, particularly the cardiovascular, endocrine, and nervous systems. Diseases of these systems are complicated or accelerated by diabetes. The objective of treatment is to correct the disturbed metabolism by the administration of insulin and the restriction of dietary carbohydrates, to maintain normal nutrition and reasonable weight by dietary alterations and exercise, and to prevent or slow down the progress of any complications.

DISEASES OF THE NERVOUS SYSTEM

The central nervous system is subject to the same disease processes as the other parts of the body. Vitamin deficiencies, especially of thiamin, produce a severe *neuritis*. The feet become tender and painful and there is a constant sensation of burning. With prolonged deficiencies, especially in association with alcohol abuse, cerebellar function is impaired, and the gait becomes unsteady. Cognitive and emotive functions also are affected.

Infections by viruses and bacteria can produce *meningitis* or *encephalitis*. In the former, the covering of the brain and spinal cord (the meninges) becomes inflamed. The afflicted person develops stiff neck, fever, and headache and can rapidly slip into coma and die if not treated quickly. Encephalitis, on the other hand, involves the substance of the brain tissue. It is usually a viral infection so there is no specific treatment. Again, fever, headache, and stupor are common, with coma being the final step leading to death. *Polio* also is a viral infection but is located more peripherally. It attacks the nerves as they leave the spinal cord and in this way produces paralysis. Prevention is the best treatment with the use of vaccine. Fortunately, vaccination has been effective, and the disease has become a rarity.

Another viral disease is *rabies*, which occurs after the bite of an infected animal. From the bitten site, the virus travels up the nerve fiber until it reaches the brain. Along the way it produces pain and spasms in associated muscles, and after reaching the brain develops into a frank encephalitis with the frightening symptom of hydrophobia (fear

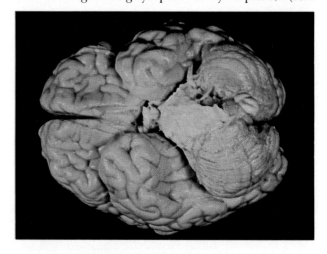

Figure 25.7 Meningitis, an inflammation of the meninges of the brain, is characterized by swelling and, in severe cases, destruction of delicate brain tissue. The importance of meningitis as a threat to health was reduced considerably with the advent of penicillin and other antibiotics.

of water) that causes the person to convulse at the sight or taste of fluid. Once the disease sets in it is fatal, so prevention is the only treatment. Proper wound care and vaccination must be quickly performed if an infection is suspected.

Tetanus and botulism are two diseases produced by neurotoxins. These substances, which are lethal even in very small doses, are released by two species of bacteria from the genus Clostridium. *Tetanus* comes from dirty wounds in which clostridia live. The toxin is released and travels along the nerves, stimulating muscle spasms. However, the brain is not involved, and the afflicted person experiences these horrible contractions with a clear mind. Fortunately, the disease is not fatal with the early administration of antitoxin. However, the victim must be paralyzed and sedated with drugs and supported by an artificial respirator until the toxin clears. The toxin of *botulism* is liberated in contaminated canned or preserved foods. When ingested even in minute amounts it produces a severe diarrhea, with abdominal pain and associated feeling of weakness and lassitude. If allowed to progress, respiratory paralysis and death result. This disease also is treated with an antitoxin and respiratory support if needed.

Multiple sclerosis is a disease of unknown cause, although autoimmunity has been implicated. It starts in the young with signs of eye weakness, which later disappears as the chronic disease becomes established. If it is severe, it can progress to complete paralysis and death within a year. Usually, however, there are long periods when the person is symptom free or at most has only minor complaints. The basic defect is a loss of the myelin substance that insulates the nerve processes. No one knows why or how this loss happens, and there is yet no treatment.

Epilepsy is not a disease but rather an expression of irritation within the brain. It can be caused by a scar, brain tumor, infection, or toxin and cannot be appropriately treated until the cause is determined. An abnormal electrical focus establishes itself at this area of irritation, and when it discharges the typical seizure is seen. The symptoms can now be fully controlled by appropriate drug treatment and, when properly handled, the epileptic can lead an essentially normal life. One approach to treatment of epilepsy was presented in Chapter 3.

The diseases outlined in this chapter are not, of course, the only diseases to attack the system involved (additional common diseases are presented in the Appendix). They do show, however, the variety of ways in which body mechanisms can go awry. The next two chapters will explore environmental circumstances that can contribute to or cause the kinds of noninfectious diseases that are now plaguing mankind.

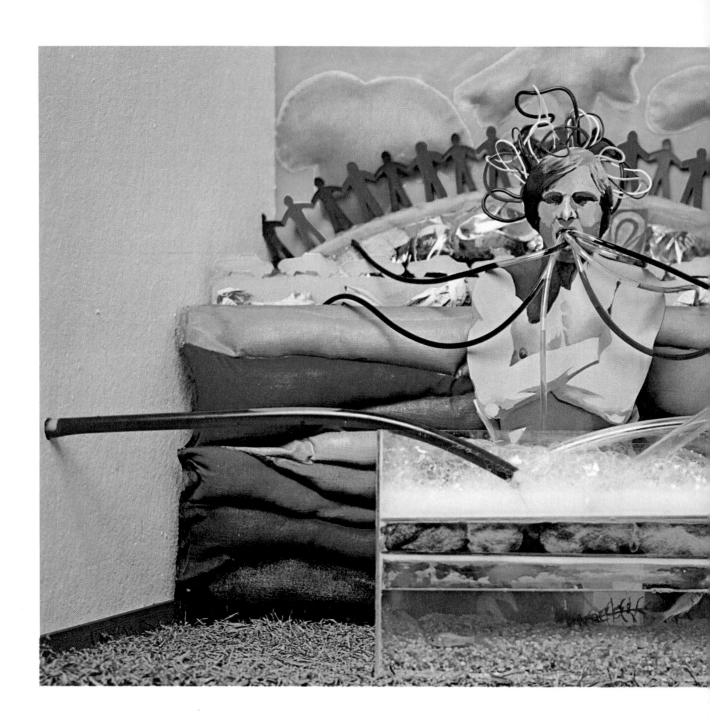

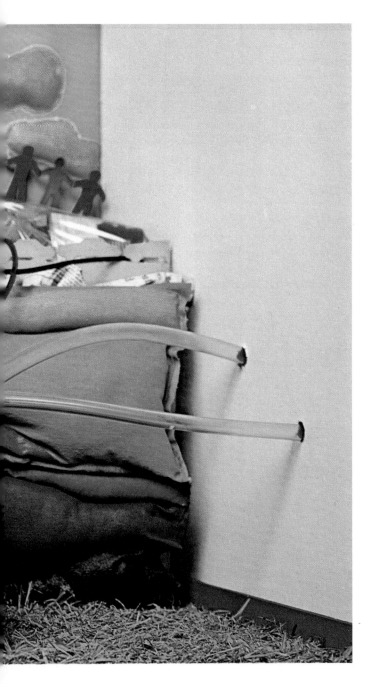

26

Hardly anyone would question the statement that health and pollution are tightly interrelated. Certainly not the thirty-five dock workers in Houston, Texas who suddenly began gasping for air and were rushed to hospitals for emergency treatment, when a yellowish smog probably fed by the acid fumes of a nearby chemical plant hung over the area where they were working. Certainly not the couple in San Jose, California who were forced to move from their comfortable home on a busy streetcorner, when the exhaust of passing cars began to give them constant, throbbing headaches. Nor would anyone who has spent time in Manhattan, Los Angeles, or Denver and felt the raw sore throats and the itching eyes that air pollution inflicts on so many citizens. Pollution of air, water, soil, and food supplies is a national health crisis today.

Environmental pollution is not only national; it is a world-wide problem. Air pollution in Tokyo is second only to that of New York but surpasses that of Los Angeles. Traces of DDT have been found in ice at the South Pole. The crisis is massive both because the world's *population* has grown so enormously and because the *technology* of the so-called "more developed" nations is dumping billions of tons of wastes into rivers, oceans, and skies.

It would be a grave mistake, however, to think of pollution as merely a *physical* problem, the replacement of clean air, clean waters, and clean space with the dirty or toxic products of man's activities.

Pollution and Health

Pollution has a *biological* dimension, the critical importance of which only begins to reach the awareness of the average person.

POLLUTION AND POPULATION

Population has historically been limited by the nature of agricultural technology. When men hunted animals or gathered wild plants for food, they needed much more land to support their small population. Scientists have inferred from the average population density of hunting and gathering tribes today that 20 million square miles of the earth's land surface would have supported only 5 million people. When more stable, agricultural societies evolved, a denser population could be supported. Archaeologists have estimated, by counting rooms in ruins of villages, that there may have been a quarter of a billion people on earth for the first century A.D.

The results of the first census in 1650 showed a population of half a billion people in the "civilized" world. By 1850, world population had grown to a billion, and had doubled by 1930. By the 1970s it doubled again, and will again by the year 2000, and again by the year 2015, when the world population is predicted to be 16 billion people. The question of whether or not the earth can support such a massive number of people has been the subject of wide debate. Most experts suggest that man reevaluate his relation to the environment and determine ways to change his present trend toward a human population too large to be supported by environment.

The pollution that resulted from the early societies was both minimal in amounts and highly localized. The advent of industrial societies has enormously expanded the amounts of pollution. In the nineteenth century, industrial cities had already-serious coal smoke problems, but the problem remained local. People often moved away from a polluted area. With today's population density, people cannot move to get away from their wastes, and neither can the large quantities of waste be contained in any one locality.

The population-environmental crisis has many different aspects. One is the energy aspect: the possibility that man is approaching the day when the oil, coal, and gas deposits beneath the earth's surface may be exhausted. Man has only just begun to turn his attention to new energy sources, such as atomic power and solar power, but even these are limited sources for future demands.

Overpopulation not only brings the threat of food shortages and the disappearance of natural resources but the threat to survival posed by the contamination of air, water, and food by the by-products of man's expanded industrial technology.

While man is affected by an adverse environment mainly through the media of air, water, and food, these media themselves suffer not only from direct pollution but from the consequences of the despoilment of the land. Destruction of forests (to feed paper and other industries) and strip mining for coal and minerals ravage the land's surface, erode the soil, change the subsurface water flow, and alter water contents, atmospheric humidity, and wind patterns. Vast tracts of the livable surface of industrialized countries are increasingly covered with asphalt and cement and thus subtracted from both food- and oxygen-producing capacities. In the United States alone, industry dumps 110 million tons yearly of solid waste that chokes the land, fills the waterways, and releases abnormal chemicals into air, water, and food. And every one of these actions modifies the environment for living organisms that are integral components of man's life.

All living beings "pollute" their environment, but the animal waste and plant destruction produced by nonhuman beings are easily absorbed into nature's cyclical pattern of growth and decay; that is, they are *biodegradable* in quantities that do not upset

Figure 26.1   Man's manipulation of his environment through such activities as land development has resulted in unbalance in many ecosystems.

natural equilibrium. Nature maintains a balance in her system. Man, however, in his increasing ability to manipulate nature, has upset this balance. If nature's balance is upset too drastically, *no* life will survive. People must find ways to rebalance natural phenomena if they are to remain compatible with their environment. Because *ecology* is the science that studies this relationship between living things and their environment, ecology is clearly a field with important implications for health.

ECOLOGY AS A SCIENCE

Biologists have long recognized that all living things are intricately interrelated. Flowers depend on bees and butterflies for pollination, while the insects in turn depend on the flowers for food. Green plants capture energy from the sun. Plants are eaten by animals, which are eaten by other animals. Some plant-eaters (*herbivores*) eat only certain types or parts of plants, while others eat only one species. Some animals eat only other animals (are *carnivores*), while others eat both plants and animals (are *omnivores*). Ecologists believe that such complex interrelated *food webs* are in part responsible for the stability of most ecological communities, or *ecosystems.* The more cross-connecting strands a web has, the more able it will be to compensate for changes imposed upon it. In some simplified webs, such as in certain types of agriculture, the system is less stable and an insect pest or disease attacking the

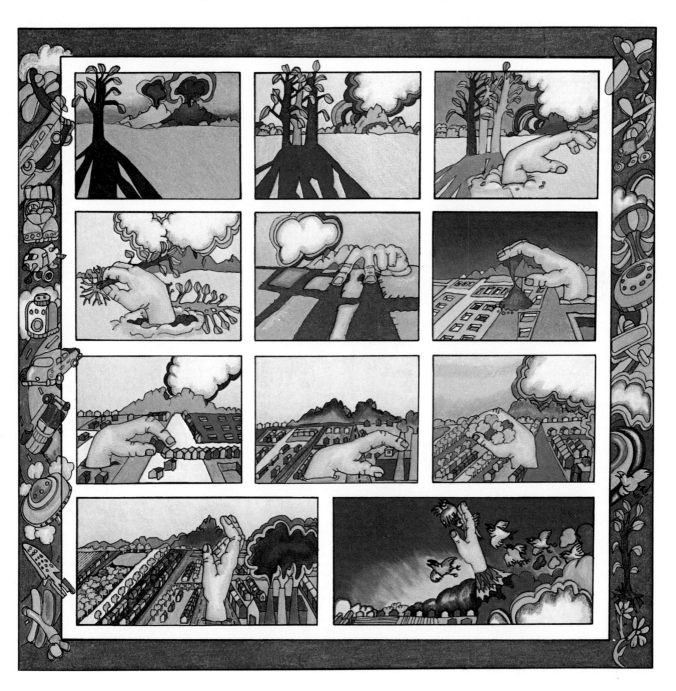

Figure 26.2   Various components of air, land, and water pollution.

AIR POLLUTION   Most atmospheric pollutants are gases or dusts emitted when coal, oil, or natural gas is burned. DDT and other organochlorine pesticides are distributed mainly by air, since they readily evaporate, but are extremely insoluble in water. Some pollutants, such as the particles of carbon known as smoke, fall to the ground within 100 miles of emission. Others, particularly minute radioactive particles, can circle the globe for months. Some pollutants undergo chemical change in the air; sulfur dioxide is oxidized and then hydrolized to fall in rain as dilute sulfuric acid.

LAND POLLUTION   The soil is a living organic layer, in dynamic equilibrium with, and continually being replenished by, the rocks beneath it and the air above it. Pollution affects it in many ways. The farmer who sprays plants with insecticides may leave residues in the soil for thirty years, impoverishing the microorganisms that contribute to the ecology on which the crops depend. The delicate chemical balance of the soil may be disrupted by rain loaded with nitrates and sulfates from polluted air. But the land also is a depollutant. Some substances can be buried with the knowledge that before they can reappear they will have been oxidized to harmless compounds.

WATER POLLUTION   Water is a great transporter. Agricultural runoff joins sewage and industrial wastes in their journey down the rivers. Although some organic pollutants decay or settle into mud, most end up in lakes, estuaries, and shallow seas. These are the very waters that have the highest productivity, and already the spawning grounds of fish and shellfish have been seriously damaged in some enclosed waters. Today man treats the deep seas as his final dust bin. Radioactive wastes are dumped in containers, and drums of sulfuric acid are tipped overboard. The sea is the main transport route for bulk materials, notably crude oil. As the size and speed of bulk carriers increase, so does accidental pollution of busy waterways become more frequent and more severe.

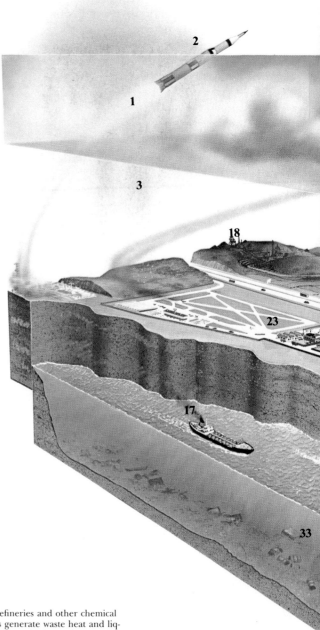

AIR POLLUTION

1. Rocket exhaust contains a variety of combustion products.
2. Space launchings leave jettisoned propellents and other debris orbiting above the atmosphere.
3. Nuclear weapon testing can leave fallout on a global scale.
4. Jet efflux contains kerosene combustion products, unburned fuel, and particles of soot.
5. Nuclear weapons can cause radioactive contamination.
6. Jet aircraft and supersonic aircraft are large contributors to noise pollution.
7. Large-scale aerial transport of pollutants distributes particles and gaseous matter.
8. Carbon dioxide build-up and the "greenhouse effect" trap solar heat within the atmosphere.
9. Pesticide spraying can cause widespread contamination, and organochlorine residues (such as DDT) can build up in animals and disrupt natural food chains.
10. Nuclear power stations are a potential source of escaping radioactive or liquid coolant.
11. Thermal power stations cause thermal and chemical pollution from exhaust stacks.
12. Power station cooling towers transfer waste heat to the air.
13. Sulfur dioxide from high chimneys falls into "canyon streets," causing irritation to eyes and lungs.
14. Refinery waste gases burned in the air cause heavy pollution unless the flame is extremely hot.
15. Motor-vehicle exhausts and crankcase gases contain lead, unburned hydrocarbons, carbon monoxide, and nitrogen oxides; action of sunlight on nitrogen oxides causes smog.

16. Most domestic fuels are inefficiently burned, causing smoke and chemical pollution.
17. Steam boilers or diesel smoke can cause persistent trails of gaseous and particulate matter.

LAND POLLUTION

18. Coal mining leaves unsightly and potentially dangerous wastes.
19. Utility poles are a classic example of visual pollution.
20. Powerful air conditioning cools buildings but heats the immediate surroundings.
21. Unreclaimed wastes are often dumped and not recycled.
22. Quarrying leaves unsightly scars.
23. An increasing number of large airports occupy otherwise valuable land.
24. Even modern industrial parks cause chemical and thermal pollution and pose waste-disposal problems.
25. Large freeways, especially interchanges, occupy large areas of land.
26. Modern litter includes a high proportion of nonbiodegradable materials.

WATER POLLUTION

27. Nuclear power stations discharge waste heat into rivers and can cause radioactive contamination.
28. Untreated industrial wastes are often poured into rivers.
29. Cooling water from thermal power stations can cause large-scale heating of rivers, changing or destroying natural organisms.

30. Refineries and other chemical plants generate waste heat and liquid refuse, which may be discharged directly into rivers.
31. When it reaches the sea, the river is heavily polluted by nitrates and phosphates from fertilizers and treated sewage, as well as by heavy toxic metals.
32. Tankers too close to shore cause beach pollution from accidental release of cargo.
33. Radioactive wastes often are dumped without detailed knowledge of local conditions and without maximum precautions.
34. The main influx of pollutants into the sea is via rivers.
35. Excess nutrients from untreated sewage can lead to "blooms" of toxic marine plankton or, through oxidation and decay, to severely reduced oxygen levels in the water.
36. Sewage sludge dumped into the sea contains persistent chemicals.

37. Large oil slicks are released by tanker accidents and by oil-rig blowouts.
38. Sediments stirred by mineral exploitation may form thick layers on the ocean floor, suffocating the organisms living there.
39. Clouds of particulate matter reduce the penetration of sunlight and sharply curtail marine productivity.
40. In some waters, wrecks pose hazards to fishing, which may lead to further pollution.
41. Traces of organic chemicals may confuse or disrupt the mating behavior of fish that normally make use of related chemicals.

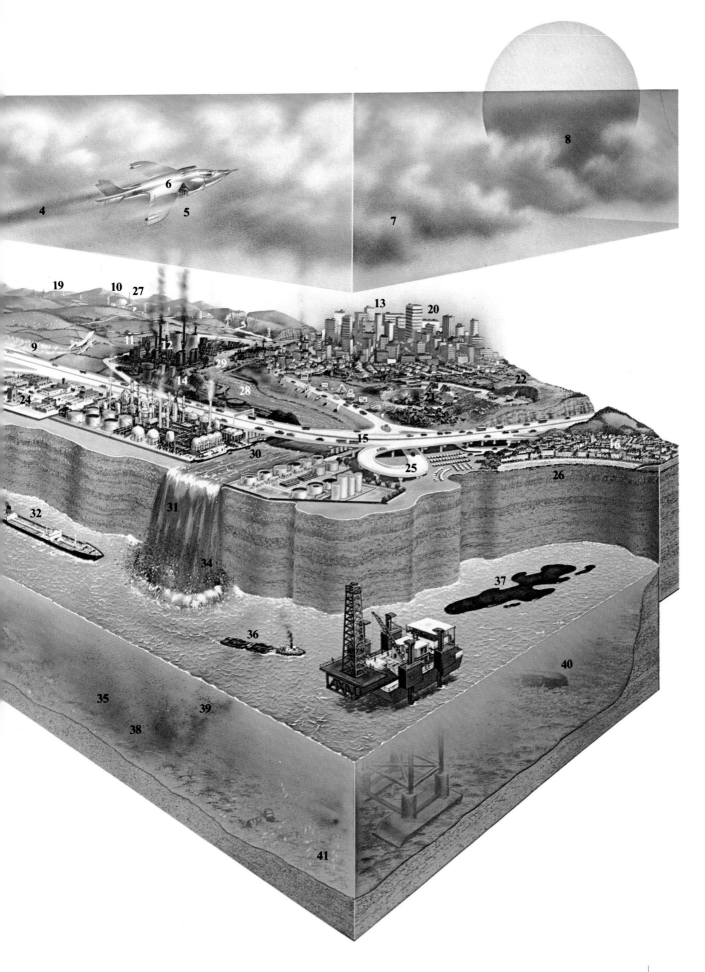

system can affect a large portion of the population.

Energy relationships within an ecosystem can be envisioned in terms of a series of levels. Organisms whose food is obtained from the same number of steps are said to belong to the same *trophic level*. Green plants are on the first trophic level, herbivores on the second level, carnivores on the third level, and secondary carnivores on the fourth level (see Figure 26.3). A given species may occupy one or more trophic levels.

In order for an organism on one trophic level to gain one pound, it must consume about ten pounds from a lower trophic level (see Figure 26.3). Thus, in order for a man to gain one pound it takes about ten pounds of tuna, which have eaten about one hundred pounds of smaller organisms (such as sardines), which in turn have eaten about 1,000 pounds of plankton. DDT and other persistent toxic chemicals can be deposited in small amounts in plankton and other plants and become concentrated considerably as they move up to higher trophic levels. This process is called *biomagnification*.

A current problem is the danger for bird species because of DDT biomagnification. DDT is an insecticide that when ingested by most organisms is absorbed into fatty tissues and is not easily excreted or modified. It was found that insects killed by DDT were eaten by birds. The DDT did not kill the birds or any higher forms of life. However, it accumulated in the birds and interfered with the calcium metabolism, resulting in delicate eggshells that broke so readily that many of the young birds did not survive the incubation period. In a relatively short time, there were so few adult birds of some species that predation, which had previously served to control excess population, now threatened to produce extinction.

But DDT has also been a savior rather than a killer for mankind. In 1966, 2.8 million people had malaria on the island of Ceylon. When DDT spray-

ing was instituted in 1967 and 1968, the malaria morbidity rate dropped to 128 in 1968. When DDT spraying was stopped in 1969, the malaria incidence again soared to a staggering 2.5 million cases in 1970.

Within every ecosystem, cyclical and evolutionary changes occur constantly. For example, although a pond looks the same from year to year, many of the individual organisms are different. Birds have eaten some of the fish, frogs have eaten the insects, last year's flowers have been replaced by this year's. Despite all these changes, some kind of process of balance preserves the pond environment. This balance does not prevent gradual changes from occurring, however. At different

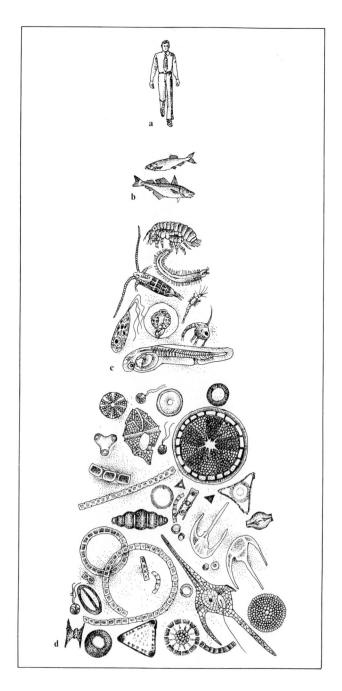

Figure 26.3 Trophic levels. The dependence of one trophic level on another is depicted in this schematic illustration. The sea must produce 1,000 pounds of phytoplankton (d), which is fed upon by tiny herbivores (c), 100 pounds of which is necessary to feed carnivorous fish (b), 10 pounds of which are needed for a man (a) to gain 1 pound. So, for a man to gain a pound the sea must produce a ton of living matter.

Survival is Not Enough

by René Dubos

I am tired of hearing that man is on his way to extinction, along with most other forms of life. Like many others, I am alarmed by the destructive effects of our power-intoxicated technology and of our ungoverned population growth; I know that scientists have even worked out a specific timetable for the extinction of mankind. But my own view of man as a biological animal suggests that something other than extinction is in store for us.

Man will survive as a species for one reason: He can adapt to almost anything. I am sure we can adapt to the dirt, pollution, and noise of a New York or Tokyo. But that is the real tragedy—we can adapt to it. It is not man the ecological crisis threatens to destroy but the quality of human life, the attributes that make human life different from animal life.

Wild animals can survive and even multiply in city zoos, but at the cost of losing the physical and behavioral splendor they possess in their natural habitat. Similarly, human beings can almost certainly survive and multiply in the polluted cage of technological civilization, but we may sacrifice much of our humanness in adapting to such conditions.

The dangers inherent in adaptability were dramatically shown by the illustrious French bacteriologist Louis Pasteur in a lecture to students of the Ecole des Beaux Arts in Paris, in 1864. Pasteur pointed out that most human beings crowded in a poorly ventilated room usually fail to notice that the quality of the air they breathe deteriorates progressively; they are unaware of this deterioration because the change takes place by imperceptible steps.

Then, to illustrate the danger of such adaptation to an objectionable environment, Pasteur placed a bird in a closed container

Adapted from Dubos, R. "Mere Survival is Not Enough for Man," Life (July 24, 1970), p. 2.

and allowed it to remain in the confined atmosphere for several hours. The bird became rather inactive but survived. In contrast, when a new bird of the same species was introduced into the same cage where the first bird remained alive, it immediately died.

The precise interpretation of this experiment is complex, but the lesson is clear. Like animals, men tend to make some form of adjustment to dangerous conditions, when these develop slowly without giving clear signs of the deleterious effects. Paradoxically, most of the threatening situations we face today have their origins in the immense adaptability of mankind.

The worst effects of environmental pollution are probably yet to come, since it is only during recent decades that certain chemical pollutants have reached high levels almost everywhere and that children have been exposed to these pollutants almost constantly from the time of birth.

But the quality of the environment cannot be measured only in terms of gross defects such as air, water, or food pollution. Environmental conditions experienced early in life (including the formative months before birth) cause the most profound and lasting changes in man. But human beings continue to be shaped by their environment throughout their lives. What we call humanness is the expression of the interplay between man's nature and the environment, an interplay that is as old as life itself and that is the mechanism for creation on earth. Rational and blasé as we may be, and scornful of any thought that there is a "ghost in the machine," we still believe deeply that life is governed by forces that have their roots in the sky, soil, and water around us. And there is, in fact, a profound biological basis for this belief. Many basic biological rhythms in man, such as body temperature, hormone secretion, blood pressure, vary with the seasons or other cosmic forces. Some of man's deepest biological traits are governed by the movement of the earth around the sun, others are connected with the movement of the moon around the earth, and still others result from the daily rotation of the earth on its axis. All of these fluctuations in biological characteristics probably derive from the fact that the human species evolved under the influence of cosmic forces that have not changed. These mechanisms became inscribed in the genetic code and persist today even when they are no longer needed under the conditions of modern life.

We have retained so many behavioral traits inherited from our Stone Age ancestors that, according to Dr. David Hamburg, professor of psychiatry at Stanford University, the best relic we have of early man is modern man.

The survival of the distant past in human nature manifests itself at almost every moment of our daily life. We build wood fires in steam-heated city apartments; we keep plants and animals around us as if to maintain direct contact with our own origins; we travel long and far on weekends to recapture some aspect of the wilderness from which our ancestors emerged centuries ago. When we can afford it, we go back to hunting, first using guns, then bows and arrows; very soon, I am sure, we shall use spears armed with points that we shall fashion from stones with our own hands—not out of necessity, but as a symbol of return to the Stone Age.

Our genetic make-up and therefore our most basic needs are still essentially the same as those of the Paleolithic hunters from whom we originated. Those early hunters moved freely among trees and grass, streams and rocks, tame and wild animals. They engaged in occupations that were at times dangerous and that always sharpened their wits. They had to make decisions on their own, rather than being entirely programmed for a limited social role. The maintenance of biological and mental health requires that technological societies provide in some form the biological freedom enjoyed by our Paleolithic ancestors.

The primordial habitat in which the human race evolved still shapes man's most basic responses in adapting to conditions of modern life. Our reaction to crowding and to strangers, our sense of social order, even our forms of conflict, are conditioned by deep imprints from the biological past. A human environment must allow ways for man to express his aboriginal nature, to satisfy those needs that are rooted in the Stone Age, however great the outward changes brought by urbanization and technology.

Ecologists and medical scientists have been chiefly concerned with the undesirable effects of the physical environment of man. But the creative aspects are more interesting and more important in the long run. The problem of the environment involves the salvation and enhancement of those positive values that man uses to develop his humanness. It involves, ultimately, a social organization in which each person has much freedom in selecting the stage on which to act his life: a peaceful village green, the banks of a river, the exciting plaza in a great city. Survival is not enough. Seeing the Milky Way, experiencing the fragrance of spring, and observing other forms of life continue to play an immense role in the development of humanness. Man can use many different aspects of reality to make his life, not by imposing himself as a conqueror on nature, but by participating in the continuous act of creation in which all living things are engaged. Otherwise, man may be doomed to survive as something less than human.

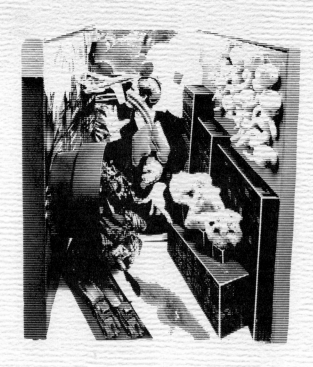

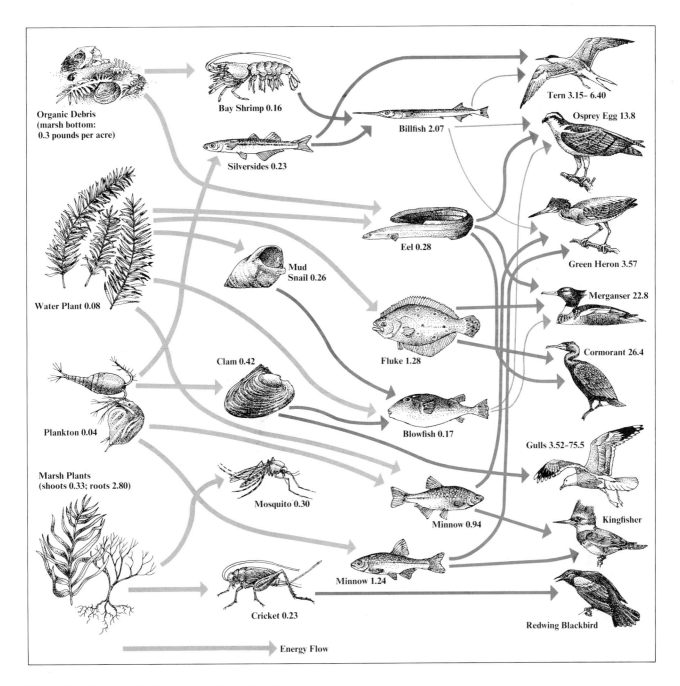

Organic Debris
(marsh bottom:
0.3 pounds per acre)

Bay Shrimp 0.16

Billfish 2.07

Tern 3.15– 6.40

Silversides 0.23

Osprey Egg 13.8

Water Plant 0.08

Eel 0.28

**Mud
Snail 0.26**

Green Heron 3.57

Merganser 22.8

Clam 0.42

Fluke 1.28

Cormorant 26.4

Plankton 0.04

Blowfish 0.17

Gulls 3.52–75.5

Marsh Plants
(shoots 0.33; roots 2.80)

Mosquito 0.30

Minnow 0.94

Kingfisher

Minnow 1.24

Cricket 0.23

Redwing Blackbird

Energy Flow

Figure 26.4   Portion of a food web in a Long Island estuary.
Arrows indicate flow of energy. The thickness of the arrows
indicates the amount of energy (food) passed on to the next
trophic level. Numbers are the parts per million of DDT found
in each kind of organism, to illustrate the concept of biomagnification. (After Woodwell, "Toxic Substances and Ecological
Cycles." Copyright © 1967 by Scientific American, Inc. All
Rights reserved.)

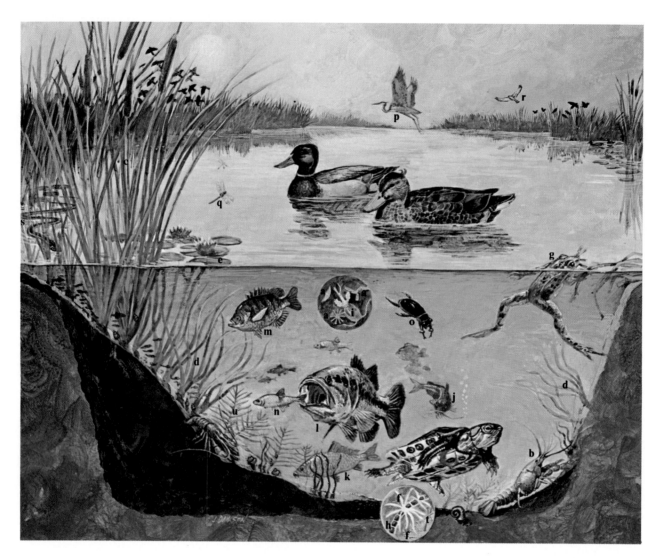

Figure 26.5 Comparative ecosystems—a typical pond ecosystem and a hypothetical urban ecosystem. Insight into the operation of ecosystems can be gained by considering the sources and transfers of energy and food material. The ultimate source of energy for all ecosystems (defined as a community of interacting organisms and the environment in which they live) is the sun. Plants use solar energy to drive the energy-requiring reaction called *photosynthesis*, which is the process by which simple carbohydrates are manufactured from carbon dioxide and water by chlorophyll-containing cells. Even electricity and gas—important as energy sources in urban ecosystems—can ultimately be traced to the sun. Electricity is often produced by generating plants that use fossil fuels (including coal and oil) to drive generators. Coal and oil are products of the decomposition of ancient plants, which originally obtained their energy from the sun by the process of photosynthesis. Only energy produced by nuclear reactions, such as in nuclear-powered electricity generating plants, *cannot* be traced to the sun. In the pond ecosystem plants include pond weeds such as water milfoil (u) and water celery (d) as well as microscopic, unicellular plants including diatoms (t) and other algae (h) that are collec-

tively termed phytoplankton (a). The urban ecosystem has far fewer species of plants within its confines. In fact, to supply food for their inhabitants, cities must bring in plant-produced material (including wheat and corn) from outside. One of the most significant cultural achievements of man has been the development of agricultural techniques that maximize the amount of food produced per unit of land area utilized. In a *food web*, plants are referred to as *primary producers*. The next level or link in the food web contains the *herbivores*, the plant-eating organisms. In the pond ecosystem herbivores include copepods (i) and other members of the zooplankton grouping (which feed on phytoplankton) and ducks (which feed primarily on pond weeds). In the urban ecosystem, the herbivores are cattle, which do not live in the city but certainly supply a good deal of its food. The next position in the food web consists of *carnivores*—animals that eat other animals. In the pond ecosystem, the carnivores are the larger fish such as catfish (j), bass (l), and sunfish (m); birds such as the heron (p) and osprey (r); water snakes (s); frogs (g); and dragonflies (q). In the urban ecosystem some species of birds and cats fill the role of carnivores. Animals that eat both plants and other animals are *omni-*

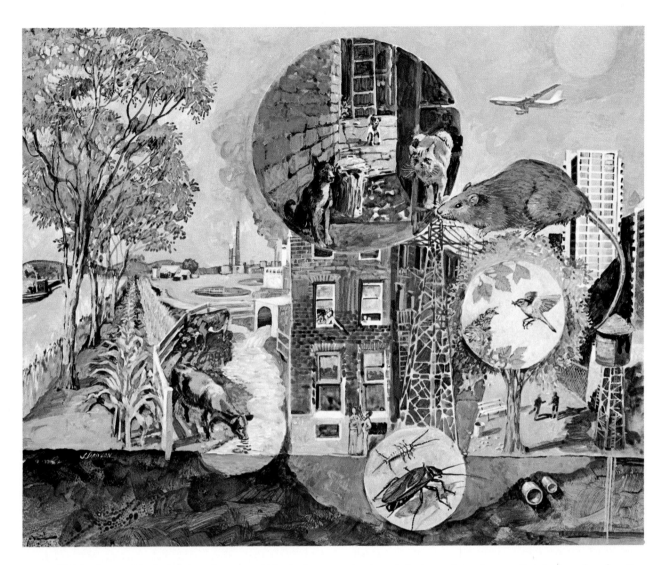

vores, which in the pond include fish such as carp (k) and minnows (n); water beetles (o); and some species of turtles. In the urban environment man is by far the most significant omnivore in terms of amount of consumption. Dogs, which are almost always supported by man, can also be considered omnivores. Another grouping of organisms that is extremely important in the cycling of organic matter and energy within ecosystems is the *scavengers*, which feed primarily on dead plant and animal matter. In ponds this grouping includes crayfish (b) and snails. In cities cockroaches, silverfish, and rats are scavengers. Again, it is important to realize that these animals depend almost entirely on the waste products of man for their source of food. All of these classifications are somewhat arbitrary. Often animals perform more than one function in any given ecosystem—carp (in ponds) and dogs (in cities) can be both omnivores and scavengers. A final grouping of organisms that perform an extremely important function in any ecosystem are the *decomposers*. Decomposition is the process by which organic material is broken down into smaller compounds, including carbon dioxide and water. Thus, keeping in mind that photosynthesis requires carbon dioxide and water to manufacture

simple carbohydrates, it can be seen that the transfer of matter and energy within ecosystems is cyclical. Bacteria (f) are, by far, the most important decomposers in any ecosystem. In ponds they are located either in the water or in bottom mud. In urban ecosystems the process of decomposition occurs to a large extent in sewage disposal plants where bacterial cultures are maintained by man. By keeping decomposition confined to small, isolated areas man also strives to minimize the spread of disease bacteria that may be carried with waste products. Every animal must have a place to live that provides shelter from climatic forces and refuge from predators. In ponds this important function is often performed by larger plants such as water lilies (e). cattails (c), and pond weeds (d) that provide shelter for birds, fish, and other animals. In cities, man has provided homes not only for himself but also for a large proportion of the other animals. Such structures as buildings and sewers provide homes for cats, dogs, birds, silverfish, and cockroaches. In the modification of the environment to suit his needs man has drastically changed the kinds and numbers of *ecological niches*, that is, the positions that specific organisms occupy in an ecosystem.

times of the year, different species of flowers predominate, which attract different species of birds and butterflies. Such orderly and progressive change is called *succession.* Over the years, the changes begin to alter the shape and the content of this one ecosystem. The pond becomes shallower, marshes develop around the edges, debris accumulates and fills it in. Gradually the pond turns to swamp, then to field, and ultimately to forest. Life forms change accordingly. Often it takes hundreds of years for the final maturation stages to be reached. Succession is one of the most important principles in ecology, for it explains nature in terms not of a static balance but a *dynamic* one. If man changes this balance or even the rate of succession, he can seriously affect the quality of his food, drinking water, and air.

The balance of nature appears to be a progression of coordinated changes. Long-term progression involves not only changes in the relative numbers of different life forms but also adaptations in the life forms themselves. Modification of environmental conditions has been a major cause of the evolution of new forms of life. The controlling mechanism of evolution has been *natural selection*: the relative reproductive success of those organisms that are best able to survive and compete against other organisms in particular environments. Evolution is the product of stress and threat to life; it has prevented environmental change from eliminating life. By diversifying its forms, life has increased the probability that it will survive environmental change. Nature's strategy has worked, but if man is to survive as part of nature, he must become aware of the consequences of his present course and change it.

The notion that "man is a threat to nature" is misleading, because man and everything he does are part of nature. Man, in expressing himself through his intellect, his skilled hands, his awesome technology, may seem at times to conquer or to destroy nature. When man alters the environment to the extent that he hastens the demise of his own species, he will have merely followed the course of countless other species that once inhabited the earth but specialized themselves into extinction.

AIR POLLUTION

The potential threat posed by urban air pollution was horribly dramatized in 1952 by the atmospheric inversion that forced foul air to remain for days over London, precipitating more than 4,500 deaths in a ten-day period. Noxious gases, such as sulfur dioxide, and irritating smoke hovered close to the ground, claiming as victims those people who were

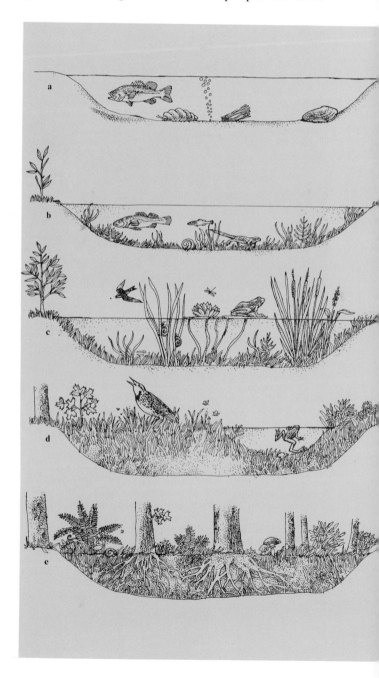

Figure 26.6 Biological succession. The gradual changes by which a pond becomes a forest: (a) bare bottom (pioneer) stage; (b) submerged vegetation; (c) emerging vegetation; (d) temporary pond and prairie; (e) beech and maple forest (climax) stage.

already weakened by cardiopulmonary diseases, red blood cell deficiencies, malnutrition, allergies, or other respiratory ailments.

Fossil fuels, such as soft coal and fuel oil, have been polluting the atmosphere longer than any others, rising from cottage chimneys through the centuries and pouring out of factory stacks during the industrial revolution. The combustion of these fuels, whether in fireplaces or power plants, produces *sulfur dioxide* and a cloud of particles. Although the sulfur dioxide level provides an index of how heavy the pollution is, the most harmful substances are not the sulfur dioxide but the combinations of sulfur oxides with small particles. The combination makes it hard for children to breathe, causes many people to cough up sputum, aggravates chronic bronchitis, and generally increases the mortality rate in the areas on which the particles fall. It may be that the particles act as the "carriers" for sulfur dioxide, which, once the particles are inhaled, is released to irritate lung tissue.

Carbon monoxide is a deadly pollutant emitted from fossil-fuel burning engines, especially those of automobiles. By disabling hemoglobin and thus hampering the oxygen-carrying function of red blood cells, carbon monoxide can seriously reduce the supply of oxygen to the brain and heart. The concentration of carbon monoxide in the nation's cities has increased dramatically in recent years. Amounts currently being recorded can recognizably

Pollutants	Where They Come From	What They Do
Aldehydes	Thermal decomposition of fats, oil, or glycerol	Irritate nasal and respiratory tracts
Ammonias	Chemical processes: dye-making, explosives, lacquer, fertilizer	Inflame upper respiratory passage
Arsines	Processes involving metals or acids containing arsenic; soldering	Break down red cells in blood; damage kidneys; cause jaundice
Carbon monoxides	Gasoline motor exhausts	Reduce the oxygen-carrying capacity of blood
Chlorines	Bleaching cotton and flour; many other chemical processes	Attack entire respiratory tract and mucous membranes of eyes
Hydrogen cyanides	Fumigation, blast furnaces, chemical manufacturing, metal plating	Interfere with nerve cells; produce dry throat, indistinct vision, headache
Hydrogen fluorides	Petroleum refining, glass etching, aluminum and fertilizer production	Irritate and corrode all body passages
Hydrogen sulfides	Refineries and chemical industries, bituminous fuels	Smell like rotten eggs; cause nausea; irritate eyes and throat
Nitrogen oxides	Motor-vehicle exhausts, soft coal	Inhibit cilia action so that soot and dust penetrate far into the lungs
Phosgenes	Chemical and dye manufacturing	Induce coughing and lung irritation
Sulfur dioxides	Coal and oil combustion	Cause chest constriction, headache, vomiting, and death from respiratory ailments
Suspended particles (ash, soot, smoke)	Incinerators, almost any manufacturing	Cause emphysema, eye irritations, and possibly cancer

Figure 26.7   Health hazards of filthy air.

impair central-nervous-system functioning in a healthy person. Because cigarettes also contain carbon monoxide, the smoker in an urban area is subjected to even greater quantities of this gas.

Although no serious health problems have been traced to the breathing of *lead compounds* (from the tetraethyl lead used in auto fuels), health professionals are worried about the possible relation between the level of lead in the body and high blood pressure. People living near smelters in Nevada have suffered *arsenic*-induced skin disorders. Workers in *asbestos* factories have suffered more from lung cancer than other individuals, and *beryllium* and *cadmium* are known to be poisonous to humans. As the percentage of these pollutants in the air increases and as they are studied more carefully, it will most likely be found that they are seriously damaging the people, animals, and plants that lie within their fallout area.

When combined with smoking or respiratory diseases, air pollution can cause severe chronic bronchitis and asthma. Even nonsmokers are 10 percent more likely to develop lung cancer if they live in a polluted environment than if they live where the air is relatively clean. Air pollution affects those people already suffering from chronic respiratory diseases most seriously; it is mainly these people who die from heavy pollution. Although most people are only irritated and inconvenienced by peak smog days, they may be more seriously affected by long-term exposure.

High-risk of pollution-associated diseases also falls to individuals who inhabit those urban areas that have the highest air pollution because of their proximity to industrial plants, the high concentration of pollutant-emitting vehicles, and their exposure to the burning of garbage and low-grade fuels.

Industry contributes about one-third of all air pollution; other major sources are electric power plants, municipal waste-disposal plants, and motor-vehicle exhausts. Mechanical ways are available to reduce air pollution. Emission standards can be set for refineries and power plants, the sulfur content of fuels can be limited, open-burning dumps can be banned, commercial and domestic incinerators can be controlled, and criteria can be set for emission levels of automobile engines.

Many of these measures require costly equipment. Who should pay for the measures? Who should decide what levels of pollution are acceptable? Who should decide whether new plants, industrial or others, should be built and where? These are all complex political questions in which consumers must become involved to insure that a safe limit is set on the ever-increasing amounts of pollutants in the air.

WATER POLLUTION

Water pollution highlights the dilemma man faces when he begins to tamper with the organic balance of his environment. For years, cities have added purifiers to their water systems to protect their citizens from the dangers of water-borne diseases. Concern has been primarily with killing bacteria, however, and thus some viruses, such as the type that causes hepatitis, are not necessarily removed in the treatment process, resulting in epidemics (usually caused by contaminated shellfish, which filter in the virus along with their food). It now appears that some of the chemicals used to purify water may themselves be pollutants. Chlorine is the traditional foe of sewage contamination of water, but scientists are today wondering about the potential genetic harm of constant intake of large amounts of chlorine.

Sewage contamination is only one way by which water resources become organically polluted. Pollution of surface waters now menaces every use of the vital resource: daily necessities, recreational and commercial fishing, agricultural irrigation, and the functioning of the very industries responsible for dumping their wastes into the country's rivers, lakes, and oceans. The President's Council on Environmental Quality estimates that industries alone generate five times more water pollution than all the rest of the population. Another important source is represented by municipal sewage systems. According to the Environmental Protection Agency, nearly half of all United States municipal waters do not meet federal health standards.

Chemical water pollutants include toxic compounds like cyanides, arsenic, acids, chromates, zinc, mercury, copper, and synthetic hydrocarbon detergents. These pollutants kill fish and vegetation or merely make them inedible, and they make water unfit for drinking.

At the end of World War II, synthetic hydrocarbon detergents replaced fatty-acid soaps. Tons of these new detergents were emptied into streams and rivers, but unlike their predecessors, they did not disappear. Finally scientists realized that these synthetic detergents do not decompose, as soaps do, because they are not susceptible to bacterial action. Communities began to outlaw the sale of synthetic detergents. Responding to public pressures, the detergent industry developed biodegradable products that are susceptible to bacterial action and that do disappear from the waters they are emptied into. However, in introducing even biodegradable detergents man still generates problems. In great quantities these new products destroy the natural balance in water systems by causing large masses of "algae blooms," which die and decay, using up much of the oxygen needed for fish and other aquatic animals.

Nitrates are another source of chemical pollution of water. So far no one has developed a satisfactory way of eliminating this pollutant. Farmers have been using nitrate fertilizers for years. The water of Elgin, Minnesota was so polluted with nitrates that a new source of water had to be found. Nontoxic nitrates in the water can be made toxic by bacterial action, either within the human gastrointestinal tract or in open food containers. Toxic nitrate compounds interfere with the oxygen-carrying capacity of red blood cells. In babies and small children, the oxygen deficit can cause suffocation.

Pollution can also result from *physical* agents that are not normally regarded as pollutants. Heat, for example, is a dangerous pollutant when the temperature of ecosystems such as lakes or rivers is raised by industrial waters. Nuclear power plants use water to cool off the reactors and dump the hot water into the bodies of water beside which they are always built. Thus game and food fish are limited in their ability to survive and compete and have already disappeared from many rivers and are threatened in many more.

Radioactive wastes are presently being buried or dumped in the oceans, but only a finite amount of waste can be disposed of in this way. In addition, radioactive sand from uranium mines has been washed into the Colorado River system, a major source of drinking water in the South. These wastes are known carcinogens and also may cause genetic alterations.

FOOD POLLUTION

The taboos against certain foods prescribed by ancient tribes show that man has long been concerned with the possible harmful effects of specific foods. In preparing meals, women used to face serious

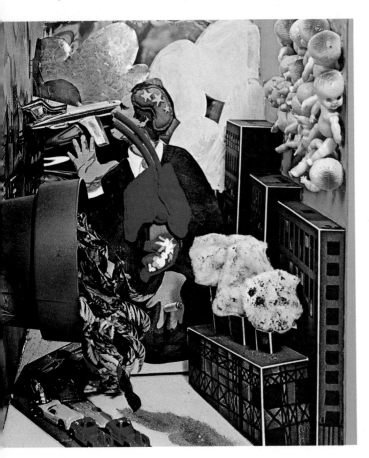

Figure 26.8 Water pollution, air pollution, noise pollution, overpopulation—all take their daily toll in deterioration of the individual's overall health.

danger of poisoning their families from spoiled or pathogen-laden food. Today refrigeration, public health measures, and food inspection have virtually eliminated these dangers, although occasionally the deadly botulism toxin gets by to the consumer.

Probably the most serious form of food pollution today is chemical poisoning that affects the whole chain of organisms from tiny microbes all the way up through fish and livestock to the human consumers. For years industrial plants have been dumping wastes into rivers that have flowed into oceans, assuming that the ocean contained enough water to dilute the wastes and render them harmless. Suddenly scientists are warning people not to eat tuna or swordfish because it contains a dangerous level of mercury. The mercury was absorbed by small organisms in the ocean, which were then eaten by crustaceans, then small fish, and then large fish, and the mercury built up its concentration through each organism's own life system (biomagnification).

Yet tuna fish probably always has contained from 10 to 100 parts of mercury per million—studies of tuna canned forty-five years ago found they contained the same level of mercury as the cans being rejected today. And the same level of mercury has been found in a seventy-year-old dehydrated tuna from a museum collection.

The crux of the food-web problem is that all forms of life interact with each other and with their physical environment. Man is totally dependent on other organisms for food. He can pick and choose, but he will never synthesize all his food from inorganic sources and thus become independent from the organic chain of foods. He must therefore adapt to the food available or adapt the food itself to his needs. He can adapt to the food by avoiding certain foods (such as tuna) and by seeking new food sources for the same nutrients (by eating vegetable protein instead of meat, for instance). He can adapt

the food itself by using genetic manipulation, fertilizers, preservatives, and so on to produce and maintain high-yield grains, produce, and meat animals.

NOISE POLLUTION

Like heat, noise has only recently been recognized as a pollutant. Deafness is an occupational hazard among taxi drivers, rock musicians, and construction workers. Industry makes a particularly large contribution to noise pollution. A major claim for workmen's compensation benefits comes from

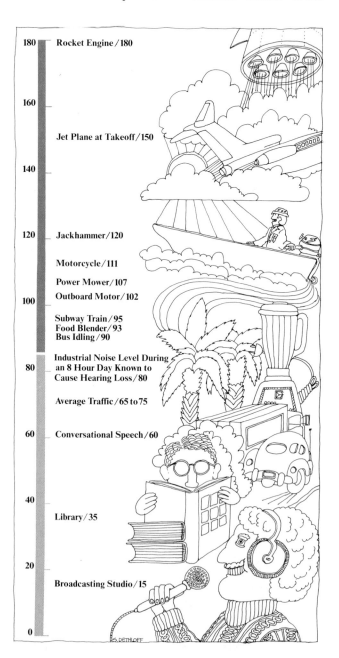

Figure 26.9   Noise pollution. The types of sounds that contribute to the noise level in urban communities, as measured in decibels. Sounds in the danger area in the top half can contribute to hearing losses.

ENERGY PRESERVATION

As with minerals, fossil-fuel consumption has grown at an astonishing exponential rate. Half the world's total consumption of petroleum occurred only during the last twelve years. Of fossil fuels in general, including coal, most of man's consumption took place during the last twenty-five years. The incredible acceleration of usage is expected to continue until the fossil fuels are completely gone.
THE ECOLOGICAL CITIZEN by Dirck Van Sickle

Extraction of fuel will continue to destroy land values. Thermal power plants, either fossil-fuel or nuclear, produce waste heat. By 1980 they are expected to use one-sixth of the average daily water-runoff for cooling, and by the year 2000 one-half of the available water.
THE USER'S GUIDE TO THE PROTECTION OF THE ENVIRONMENT by Paul Swatek

If you have it, do you need to use it?

Don't turn on the dishwasher or the washing machine until you have a full load.

Turn off unneeded lights.

Don't leave appliances and other equipment running when not in use.

If during the cold months you don't use a room, don't heat it.

Insulate your home so that less power is needed for heating and cooling.

Use higher wattage bulbs rather than several lower wattage combinations.

Conservation of petroleum products can be achieved by:

Driving less—walk, bike, jog, share a ride.

Establishment of bike lanes and mass transit.

Keeping car well tuned.

WATER CONSUMPTION

Unlike energy, water is not consumed; it is used. . . . [but] it depends on *how* it is used. Since pollution has destroyed much of our surface water supply, to meet residential water needs, many communities have turned to drilling wells to tap the groundwater supply. However, it takes a fair amount of land to provide enough groundwater for very many people. The dwindling supply of unpolluted surface water and the limited supply of groundwater conspire to make the supply of municipal water very short in most metropolitan areas.
THE USER'S GUIDE TO THE PROTECTION OF THE ENVIRONMENT by Paul Swatek

Minimize the amount of water you use and the waste burden you impose on the sewer system.

Fix leaky faucets and toilets. The steady flow uses up a considerable volume.

Food waste disposal units are about as ecologically unsound as an appliance can get. Garbage handled in this way contributes to the aging of streams and lakes. Instead, by starting a compost heap the organic matter and minerals can be returned to the soil to replenish and fertilize it.

Don't run water unnecessarily. For example, don't keep the water running the whole time you are brushing your teeth.

Take a shower and see how high the water level comes with the plug in the drain. If it is less than the water used when taking a bath—take showers.

The amount of soap, bubble bath, and water conditioners you use during a bath, shower, or doing a load of clothes or dishes is probably as important as how much water you use.*

Plant lawn covers and shrubs that will be able to get along with a minimal amount of sprinkling.

Don't move to an area where water is scarce.

Never use pesticides in such a way that would contaminate either ground or surface water.

Reducing your consumption of electricity will lessen the thermal pollution load on waters.

WASTE MANAGEMENT

We all take municipal refuse collection and disposal, like most public services, too much for granted . . . It costs us collectively in excess of $3 billion per year, more than anything else except schools and roads. It is the several hundred million tons produced each year in our homes and businesses and collected by municipal garbage collectors that contributes most heavily to the many environmental crises we face today.
THE USER'S GUIDE TO THE PROTECTION OF THE ENVIRONMENT by Paul Swatek

Use cloth napkins, handtowels, handkerchiefs, and diapers instead of throwaway paper ones.

Use a sponge rather than paper towels to sop up spills.

Use durable dishware rather than paper or plastic throwaways.

Avoid "overly" packaged products—such as individually wrapped slices of cheese, pieces of candy, etc.

Buy in bulk to reduce the proportion of packaging.

Share magazines and books.

Do something to stop junk mail. Ask that your name be taken off the mailing lists. Complain to the post office.

Buy quality. In the long run you will save money and reduce the amount of obsolete junk you have to toss out.

Don't discard anything that can be fixed or used by someone else.

Promote recycling of glass, paper, plastic, and metal products.

REDUCING AIR POLLUTION

Drive less or not at all.

Use low-lead gasoline.

Don't burn trash (and avoid plastics that, when burned, emit harmful chemicals into the air).

Stop smoking.

Avoid organochlorine pesticides (DDT).

Avoid burning fossil-fuels in fireplaces.

---

* Several years ago nonbiodegradable detergents were causing spectacular foams in rivers and lakes. The detergent industry complied by making all their products biodegradable. Now it is the phosphates which go right through our sewage systems and cause accelerated growth of water plants and algae. The decaying vegetation consumes the oxygen supply, killing the fish, and eventually takes over the body of water. Plants die and pile up, releasing more fertilizer into the deadly cycle. As the fish die and the dead plants accumulate, the lake becomes a swamp. Eventually as all growing things choke out each other and die, the swamp will dry up into a desert. This is *eutrophication*. ECOLOGY AT HOME

Figure 26.10 Suggested solutions to the pollution problem. The ecological approach to environmental problems requires that one work individually and through institutions—commerce, industry, and government. Some of the decisions one makes regarding his environment will have greater effects than others, but what must be kept in mind is that man is part of the environment and what he does or does not do will either bring about a better, cleaner environment, or he will bequeth to his children an environment fraught with foul air, unusable water, and depleted natural resources.

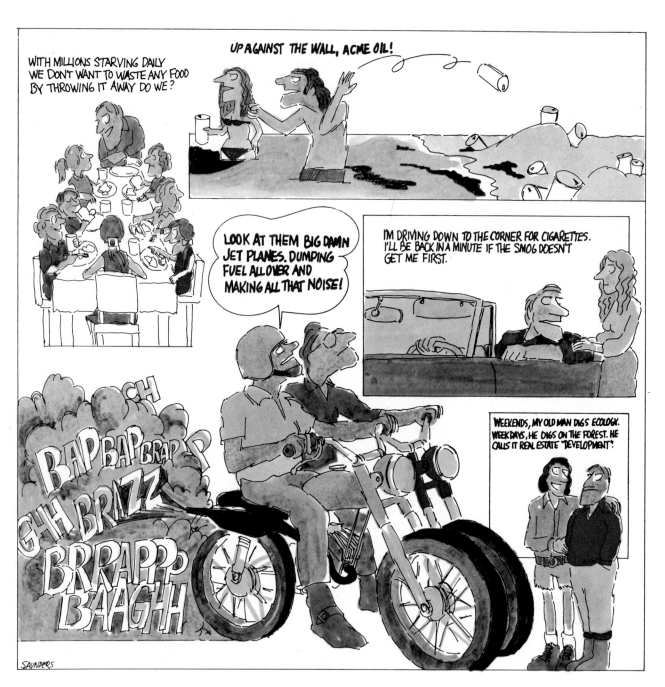

Figure 26.11   Pollution is a subject about which there often is more talk than action.

workers who have lost their hearing as a result of exposure to noise. Industries try to protect themselves by requiring workers to wear ear plugs.

People are increasingly besieged by noise at home as well as at work. Airplanes, cars, motorcycles, televisions, and power motors all contribute to a high level of background noise. At the least, they can interfere with sleep, and at the worst they aggravate such stress-related diseases as hypertension, colitis, and peptic ulcers. In addition, a high level of background noise is reflected in greater losses of hearing, greater irritability, and poorer efficiency and performance levels among city dwellers.

DIRECTIONS FOR THE FUTURE

If pollution is seen as a health problem, it clearly cannot be dealt with merely by seeking to cure the symptoms of those who are afflicted with lead or mercury poisoning or with asthma or bronchitis. These people must naturally be treated, but the underlying cause, the pollution itself, is the problem to be tackled.

Some people may try to dispose of the problem by claiming that, since evolution of life implies that man's fate is extinction, it is of no consequence whether he struggles or not. Fortunately, nobody knows what man's fate is. People who believe in the ability of man to survive—or even concern themselves about survival over the next few generations—must try and develop ways to meet the physical and biological threats of pollution.

Until now, organisms have always met stress from their environment by gradually adapting according to the rules of natural selection. Man is now facing a self-imposed stress—the consequences of contaminating his environment with his own effluvia. He is also facing an urgent, self-imposed necessity—to contain and eventually reverse this disastrous process.

The road to solving the problem is a long one, and involves many levels. At the level nearest to the concrete problems lies the human *technology* that will have to provide the physical solutions and the tools to implement them: human technology has been used to pollute, and it can be used to heal. The next level is the *economic* one, a formidable problem in itself according to a recent report by the President's Council on Environmental Quality: it estimates the cost of a clean-up over a six-year period at some 105 billion dollars—23 percent for air, 36 percent for water, and the rest for solid-waste pollution. Here too, one may claim that as industry has been a major culprit, so it ought to be a major sponsor, and indeed the Council's recommendation pegs industry's contribution at a hefty 42 percent of the total. Given the availability and the commitment of funds to research and execute the technological solutions, one still has to contend with the organizational task of merging different problems, different people, and different solutions into a balanced and coordinated program: this is a *political* level, involving the effectiveness of governmental structures at local, national, and supranational levels—and the sincere, selfless dedication of the individuals that operate them.

All that is necessary, but not sufficient unless the force is there that can make politicians truly operate for the welfare of the people, industry and other sources commit the necessary resources, and technologists embark on the quest for practical solutions. As has been recognized time and again with respect to so many other aspects of human health, it is ultimately up to individuals, each and every one of them, to recognize the life-and-death character of the problem and its increasing urgency, and to subordinate short-range advantages to the preservation of life and the establishment of a good life for future years and future generations.

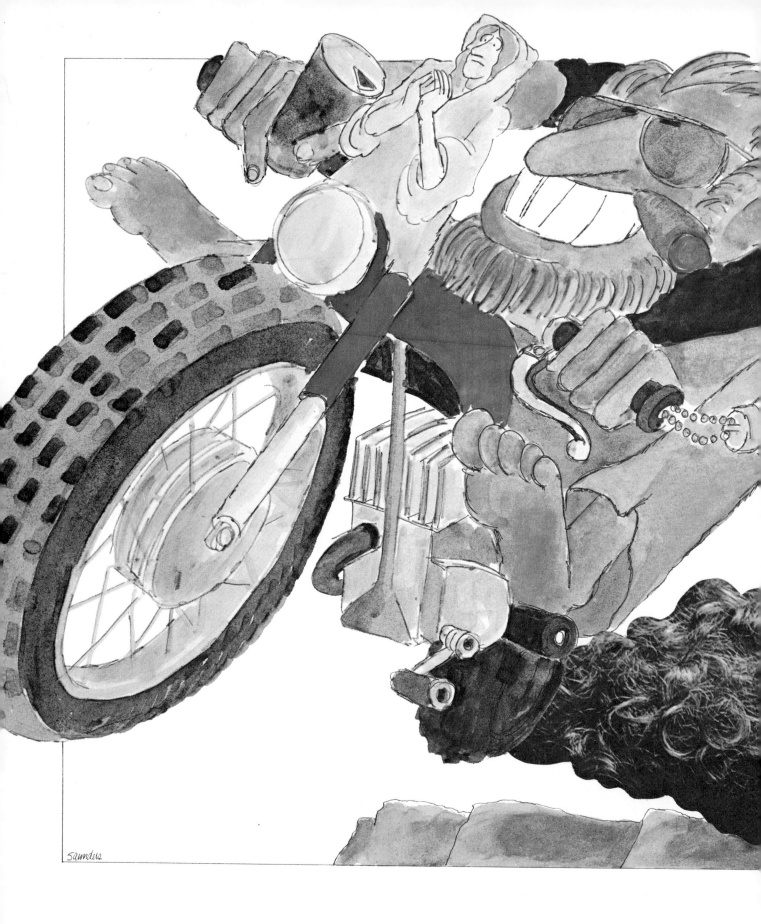

Saunders

506

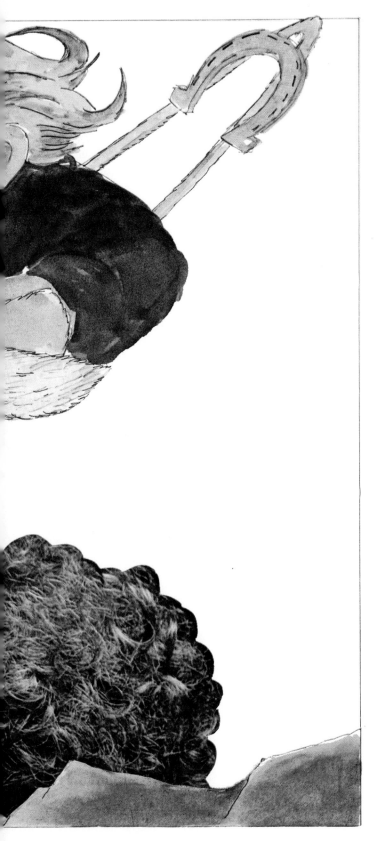

27

Man's conception of "safety" and of what constitutes an accident cover a wide field. On one hand there are those who would forbid a child to climb trees or participate in other kinds of "rough" but routine physical activities, or who would themselves refuse to fly on regularly scheduled airlines for fear of crashing. On the other hand, there are those who see accidents as "Acts of God" or "Fate" and therefore beyond human control; these are the people who drown because of their failure to wear life belts when riding in small boats, or who fatalistically refuse to use safety belts in autos because, "If my number is up, it's up."

The existence of either of these extreme positions appears incongruous in a world of alternatives in which people are constantly faced with critical decisions and choices, which almost always involve some risk and the consequences of which may often enough affect the lives not only of the individual who makes the decision but of various other persons. Incongruous as they are in the world of the average man, these extreme positions become terrifying when they are viewed in the context of decisions whose risks and consequences are nationwide or even world-wide. Nor is there any consolation in the fact that these are *extreme* positions, because to one degree or another—or in less crudely stated forms—they do reflect mental approaches shared by most people, whether engaged in private or in public activities. Although this chapter is involved with

Accidents and Safety

accidents and safety of the individual, some of the concepts to be discussed can be readily extended to a collective scale.

SCOPE OF THE ACCIDENT PROBLEM

Accidents probably touch the lives of more people than almost any other single malady. They are a psychological, social, economic, technological, and—given their overwhelming occurrence—epidemiological problem. In the United States, accidents rate as the fourth leading cause of death, after heart disease, cancer, and stroke, if the population is considered as a whole. In fact, accidents are the *leading* cause of death among both males and females through age thirty-seven. Among children aged one to fourteen, accidents claim more lives than all the five leading diseases combined. And within the fifteen-to-twenty-four age group, accidents not only claim more lives than *all* other causes combined (as shown in Table 27.1), but the death rate per 100,000 individuals has continued to worsen throughout this century, even though it has been improving in other age groups.

During 1968, the overall number of so-called accidental deaths exceeded 115,000—a slight decrease from 57 to 55.5 deaths per 100,000 population. In the same year, however, the recorded number of injurious mishaps approximated *50 million*. Of these mishaps, nearly 11 million caused injuries that incapacitated the victims for at least one day beyond the accident. And 400,000 people suffered some degree of permanent impairment.

The economic loss derived from accidents, including loss of wages, medical expenses, administrative and claim settlement costs, motor-vehicle property damage, fire, and so on, amounts to approximately 26 billion dollars annually. Other indirect costs, such as increased enforcement activities by police and courts arising out of automobile collisions, the drain on medical resources that could be used otherwise, social welfare expenditures, and

cost of family adjustments, are beyond calculation. Of the total direct economic loss, 97 percent is accounted for by *nonfatal* accidents, illustrating the dimension of the problem even if all fatalities could have been avoided.

THE CONCEPT OF ACCIDENT

To live is often to balance on the precarious edge of danger, to take those risks required in the activities that give or enhance life's meaning. *Risks,*

Table 27.1 Accidents Versus Other Causes of Death, 1968

AGE GROUP	Cause	Number of Deaths	Death Rates per 100,000 pop.
All Ages	All Causes	1,930,082	966
	Heart disease	744,658	373
	Cancer	318,547	159
	Stroke	211,390	106
	Accidents	114,864	57
	Motor-vehicle	*54,862*	*27*
	Pneumonia	66,430	33
	Diabetes mellitus	38,352	19
	Arteriosclerosis	33,568	17
Ages 1–14	All Causes	30,580	54.4
	Accidents	13,112	23.3
	Motor-vehicle	*5,773*	*10.3*
	Cancer	3,760	6.7
	Congenital malformations	2,442	4.3
	Pneumonia	2,062	3.7
	Heart disease	651	1.2
	Homicide	514	0.9
	Stroke	403	0.7
Ages 15–24	All Causes	41,140	124.4
	Accidents	23,012	69.6
	Motor-vehicle	*16,543*	*50.0*
	Homicide	3,357	10.1
	Cancer	2,731	8.3
	Suicide	2,357	7.1
	Heart disease	946	2.9
	Pneumonia	851	2.6

Source: National Safety Council. *Accident Facts,* 1971.

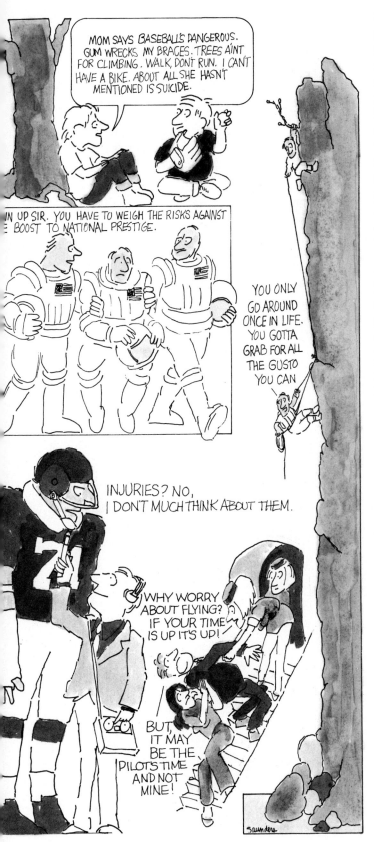

Figure 27.1 Each individual must determine his own safety goals. Some will prefer a low-risk existence, taking many precautions, while others may feel that to "live it up" they must take chances.

therefore, are unavoidable. But although risks cannot be avoided, they can be *chosen*. To do so, one must first of all understand them, that is, know as much as possible about the factors involved, recognize what the potentially injurious consequences of an action are—its hazards—and assess the probability that such consequences will occur. But one also must evaluate the rewards, or the prospects of reward, that would go with such an action, and pit their worth against the nature and size of the risks involved. A realistic appraisal of these two facets of a decision can make a *calculated* risk out of a careless one based on ignorance or foolhardiness.

One of the most hazardous challenges accepted in recent times, and known to be fraught with a high degree of risk at its inception, was the exploration of space, and particularly the first manned lunar landing. The potential rewards for the nation and for all mankind were measured against the immense effort, the delay that such effort might cause to the fight against other pressing national problems, and the perspective of the loss of human lives throughout the endeavors. These were calculated risks, and ones that deserved to be taken, at least in the judgment of the decision-makers.

But other risks also were taken on a more debatable level. By setting specific deadlines and allowing a time factor to take precedence over other considerations, further major risks were introduced that were considered justifiable in the light of less critical potential rewards—in this case, personal or national prestige. The tragic choice of a pure oxygen environment for the manned space capsule, for example, resulted in the fire destruction of Apollo 3 on the ground and the loss of its three astronauts.

It should be noted that the danger of a flash fire with a pure oxygen environment had in fact been shown on at least one occasion at the training facility. Thus, the technical choice was made with an awareness of the hazard involved, just as it involved a consideration of the time and dollar costs inherent to the development of alternative systems that would have removed it.

The Apollo 3 "accident" forcefully illustrates the need to challenge the overall concept of accidents. Is it the case, as it is usually assumed, that accidents are the results of unpredictable and uncontrollable, and thus unavoidable, circumstances? The truth of the matter is that accidents, while indeed *unplanned* events, are in most cases also *caused* occurrences. And their causes often *can* be predicted and controlled. Even natural catastrophes such as earthquakes, tidal waves, and tornados are, or will be with the advances of technology, increasingly anticipated and provided for. Because most accidents are from predictable and controllable causes, the fact that they are unplanned does not imply that they have to occur in an unexpected and unprovided-for manner. *Safety*, in fact, should consist in (1) expecting accidents, (2) reducing their probability, and (3) providing means to minimize their consequences.

A realistic philosophy of "accident prevention" and "safety" can be formulated. Both the successes and the failures of the space effort have contributed to the concept—and the acceptance by authorities and public alike—of "accident prevention" as a systematic process. Such a process holds that education can provide (1) the knowledge that will assist an individual to assume risks in full awareness of potential hazards, (2) the judgment of which risks are necessary for those activities that are worth having within the society one lives in, and (3) the experience to carry out such activities in the most competent manner.

ACCIDENTS AND THEIR VICTIMS

In American society, men are expected to take part in many activities, both occupational and recreational, that involve a higher degree of risk than those in which women are normally involved. This

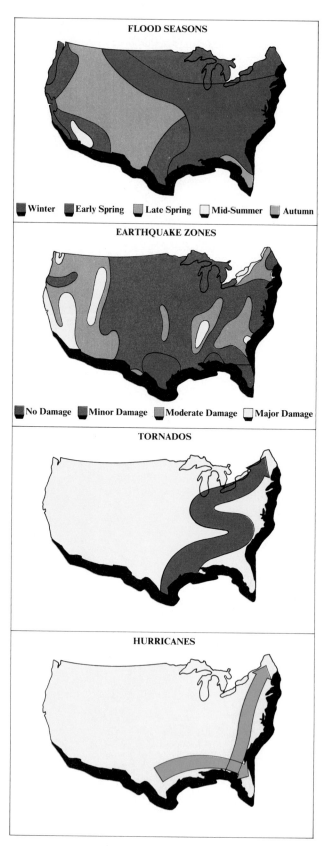

Figure 27.2   Areas of the United States with greatest danger of floods, earthquakes, tornados, and hurricanes.

difference is reflected in the accident rates for the two sexes. As shown in Table 27.2, the overall injury and fatality rates among males exceed those for females by more than two to one. The difference is even greater in certain age groups—among the fifteen- to thirty-four-year-olds, for instance, the ratio of male to female deaths is four to one—and for certain types of fatalities—97 percent of the deaths due to machinery and 85 percent of those due to firearms or drowning are male.

Rural residents have an accidental death rate of 69 per 100,000, about 20 percent higher than the national average. High-risk activities coupled with poor knowledge of their specific hazards, violation of safe practices, a lack of protective devices, and inadequate medical facilities within reasonable reach are the major factors responsible for this greater rate. Accident and death rates also are higher among the poor than in the middle classes, partly for similar reasons and partly because the poor have to cope with environmental hazards not usually confronted by the more affluent.

Accidents can be grouped in three major categories according to the environment in which they occur—home, work surroundings, and public places. The spectrum of people affected varies in the three categories, reflecting both the kind of hazards prevailing in each environment and the frequency or duration with which different types of people are exposed to them.

Deaths from *home accidents* represent some 24 percent of all accidental deaths. They are mainly due to falls and fire hazards (see Table 27.3). Less than a quarter of them occur in the age span between four and forty, and these include most of the deaths by poison. The very young die mainly of burns or suffocation, while the older people—particularly those above seventy-five—are principally victims of falls. Age rather than environmental hazards appears to determine the risk in this category.

Table 27.2   Accidental Deaths by Age, Sex, and Type, 1968

AGE AND SEX	All Types	Motor Vehicle	Falls	Fires, Burns	Drowning	Firearms	Ingest. of Food, Objects	Poison (solid, liquid)	Poison by Gas	% Male, All Types
All Ages	114,864	54,862	18,651	7,335	7,372	2,394	3,100	2,583	1,526	69%
Under 5	7,263	1,987	359	1,086	840	85	1,007	284	48	57%
5–14	8,369	4,105	193	686	1,670	421	115	37	71	69%
15–24	23,012	16,543	409	332	2,030	764	185	481	339	80%
25–34	12,444	7,727	399	438	750	318	131	440	212	81%
35–44	11,240	5,875	726	644	630	272	223	434	219	76%
45–54	12,193	5,875	1,180	900	580	230	317	396	208	75%
55–64	11,703	5,156	1,812	1,046	440	183	360	254	215	72%
65–74	10,961	4,261	2,990	993	270	87	343	158	130	63%
75 and over	17,603	3,309	10,577	1,198	150	32	419	80	83	45%
Age unknown	76	24	6	12	12	2	0	19	1	87%
Male	79,424	39,788	9,314	4,296	6,265	2,049	1,821	1,616	1,128	
Female	35,440	15,074	9,337	3,039	1,107	345	1,279	967	398	
Percent male	69%	73%	50%	59%	85%	86%	59%	63%	74%	

Source: National Safety Council. *Accident Facts,* 1971.

Occupational fatalities have decreased considerably over the last three decades, from about 75 per 100,000 (in 1936–1937) to 31 per 100,000 in 1969. They now account for about 12 percent of all accidental deaths. One-third of them occur in the manufacturing industries, the other two-thirds in the nonmanufacturing ones.

The category of *public accidents* is responsible for some 77,000 deaths every year, or 67 percent of all accidental fatalities. More than half of all accidental deaths are caused by *motor-vehicle* accidents. The death toll taken by car accidents in 1970 was great-er than the number of Americans who died in battle during either World War I or the Korean War.

Of the 107.5 million licensed drivers in the United States in 1969, one-quarter were involved in auto mishaps. Three-fourths of the auto casualties are male, presumably reflecting the greater number of male drivers. A comparison of types and degree of involvement by age (Table 27.4) shows the fifteen-to-twenty-four group to have the highest fatalities in all but two types of auto accidents—those involving pedestrians and bicyclists. Their fatalities are particularly high for overturning,

Table 27.3   Deaths from Home Accidents by Type and Age, 1970

AGE	Falls	Fires, Burns, and Deaths Associated with Fire	Suffocation — Ingested Object	Suffocation — Mechanical	Poisoning by Solids, Liquids	Firearms	Poisoning by Gases, Vapors	Other	Total
All Ages	9,600	5,600	2,300	1,100	2,500	1,200	1,200	3,000	26,500
0–4	300	800	900	600	200	90	60	1,050	4,000
5–14	120	600	110	250	50	300	60	110	1,600
15–24	80	300	140	80	750	300	300	250	2,200
25–44	300	750	300	60	800	250	250	190	2,900
45–64	1,100	1,500	350	40	450	190	300	470	4,400
65–74	1,600	750	150	40	150	40	110	260	3,100
75 and over	6,100	900	350	30	100	30	120	670	8,300

Source: Estimates by National Safety Council based on data from National Center for Health Statistics and state health departments.

Table 27.4   Motor-Vehicle Fatalities, 1969

AGE	All Motor Vehicle	Mot. Veh. Collisions	Overturn or Off Road	Pedestrian	Collision Fixed Object	Collision Train	Collision Bike
All Ages	56,400	24,000	16,000	9,800	4,200	1,500	820
0–4	2,100	700	300	1,000	50	30	20
5–14	4,100	900	650	1,800	100	100	530
15–24	17,700	7,100	7,000	1,050	1,900	480	150
25–44	13,900	6,500	4,300	1,450	1,200	400	40
45–64	11,300	5,500	2,600	2,100	700	310	40
65–74	4,100	1,850	750	1,200	150	100	20
75 and over	3,200	1,400	400	1,200	100	80	20

Source: National Safety Council. *Accident Facts*, 1970.

running off the road, and collision against fixed obstacles, namely those accidents that do not directly involve the actions of another vehicle. Lack of ability or experience, improper assessment or gross underassessment of potentially hazardous situations, and unreasonable acceptance of risks beyond the ability to cope are probably the main elements that lead young people to place themselves and others in a position of jeopardy. Night traffic fatalities also are in disproportionate numbers, suggesting the involvement of yet another set of influencing factors—such as limited visibility, distraction by passengers, effects of alcohol on drivers and pedestrians, and so on.

CAUSATION OF ACCIDENTS

The dimensions of the accident problem are such that only an epidemiological approach offers a possible solution. As with infectious and other diseases, epidemiology of accidents must first attempt to *identify* the causative elements of the problems, the ways they maintain themselves or even expand, and the circumstances under which they combine to produce their damage. Reality demonstrates, contrary to many public beliefs, that only rarely can an accident be attributed to a single cause. In fact, one may distinguish three main components in accident causation: the individual, the agent, and the environment.

The Individual

The individual contributes to accident causation both through *unsafe thinking*—improper assessment of hazards, underestimation of risks or overestimation of ability to cope—and through *unsafe acting*—use of improper tools; disregard or misuse of safety devices; ignorance, inexperience, or incompetence for a given activity. It is clear from the available statistics that certain groups within the society are more susceptible to accidents, or to a particular category of accidents, than is the society as a whole—approximately 15 percent of the population is responsible for approximately 85 percent of the accidents. Many investigators in the past believed in the concept of accident proneness as a persistent phenomenon. It is more accurate and productive to state that all individuals may be or become accident prone at one time or another, but that certain groups are more susceptible to involvement in an injury-producing situation because of physiological, psychological, or cultural predisposing factors, or a combination of them.

PHYSIOLOGICAL FACTORS Although physiological elements often are thought of as major contributors to accident involvement, research tends to show little relationship to such factors as auditory sensitivity, motor skills, or other bodily abilities above a certain minimal physical competence. In fact, there is reason to believe that physical abilities have an inverse effect at the psychological level: young drivers may overrely on their reaction time and physical ability, while individuals with a known physical handicap tend to exhibit superior performance in tasks fitted to their capabilities. However, overexertion and fatigue reduce the attention, sensory acuity, and reaction time of any individual and should always be taken into account in deciding what activity can be reasonably undertaken.

A review of injuries and fatalities by age reveals an overrepresentation at either end of the age scale. It also shows that, as the human organism ages, the probability of recovery from an injury is substantially reduced because of attendant complications—a consideration that may not affect the incidence of involvement in an accident but certainly does aggravate its consequences. General health also is an important consideration. Persons suffering from such diseases as epilepsy, heart disease, diabetes, and so on should consult their physicians before undertaking high-risk activities.

Prescription drugs can have a marked effect on human performance abilities. Few persons realize that antihistamines and other sedatives taken to alleviate the symptoms of even a common cold can be extremely hazardous. Drugs such as narcotics, barbiturates, tranquilizers, amphetamines, and hallucinogens are, of course, commonly known to affect performance of most activities. By far the most hazardous person to himself and others, however, is the person under the influence of alcohol. All indicators point to the fact that alcohol is a major contributor to at least half of all automobile fatalities and an extremely high percentage of on-the-job injuries (see Chapter 8).

PSYCHOLOGICAL FACTORS Investigators have found that chronic violators and accident repeaters share a number of psychological traits; it may be largely due to the prevalence of such traits among the under-twenty-four-year-olds that this group shows up so prominently in most accident fatality lists. One psychological factor is the exercise of bad judgment—insufficient seeking of adequate information, faulty expectations, impulsive decision. Another is an exaggerated opinion of self-importance, leading to lack of anticipation or actual disregard of other people's actions or reactions and to a deficient sense of responsibility for one's own activity. A third factor is overconfidence in one's ability, causing inadequate attentiveness and neglect of safety precautions.

Failure to practice safety procedures is largely responsible for drowning accidents—one should swim only where there is a lifeguard or employ the buddy system, one should use life jackets when riding in small boats or water skiing, and so on. Neglect of safety precautions also is an all-too-frequent cause of unnecessary harm in the case of automobile accidents. The most optimistic estimate places general use of lap safety belts at no better than 33 percent and shoulder belts at 2 to 3 percent; if all vehicle occupants used their safety belts 100 percent of the time, it is believed at least 9,000 lives could be saved annually—almost a 20 percent decrease in car casualties.

B. S. Birnbach, in a study on junior-high-school students, has compiled a profile of the accident-repeater that supports the three main psychological traits already discussed. Compared to the accident-free student, the accident-repeater shows poor attendance, lack of industriousness, and carelessness at school; decision-making based on superstition and ritualism rather than educated appraisal; recklessness and bravado acting; aggressiveness and physical bullying; and rebelliousness with little fear of punishment. Somewhat comparable traits were observed in the typical high-accident worker, including conflict with authority in both childhood and adulthood and an irregular work history.

CULTURAL FACTORS Cultural factors are, of course, interwoven with psychological and physiological elements of accident causation. Socioeconomic and family backgrounds contribute importantly to the intellectual and emotional make-up of the individual and often determine quantitatively and qualitatively his educational level. Many of the personality traits attributed to the high-accident worker and the accident-repeater student were found to be accompanied by a broken-home background, or a high incidence of divorce among parents, or poor parental guidance.

But besides such socioeconomic or family factors, many specific cultural trends play an important role. In-group fads bring about new, and often poorly assessed, hazardous activities or multiply the risks of others: the hero image of the "hot-rodder" is but one such example. The "frontier" tradition supports the availability and use of firearms even under totally unwarranted conditions. The "drug

"This preparation may cause drowsiness. Do not drive or operate machinery while taking this medication."

Figure 27.3 (*right*) With technological advances comes increased danger due to high speeds, complex machinery, and greater availability of potentially harmful products, such as electric appliances, aerosol containers, and amplifiers capable of emitting sounds at dangerously high decibel levels.

culture" and the "pill culture" of today's American society promote the physiological hazards that the use of pharmacologic agents introduce needlessly into everyday activities. The pervasive, and early-fostered, worship of the automobile and mechanical contraptions in general expands unnecessarily what is today *the* most hazardous and most engaged-in risk activity.

The Agent

By far the greatest number of accidents involve the use by one or more individuals of a potentially dangerous "agent"—be it an automobile or sports gear or a poisonous paint or a tainted food. Any tool or material with which man extends his physical capacities is, of course, potentially dangerous

given the wrong circumstances and the wrong user. Yet, present technology could develop if properly directed, and oftentimes does develop, *safety devices* that reduce or block the injurious properties of such tools even in the face of most, if not all, potential misuses of them.

HOME ACCIDENTS   Home contents and the home itself are one category of accident-causative agents. Buildings, both private and public, can now be designed to withstand natural forces that would have brought disaster a few years ago. Building codes also are intended to impose precautions against fire, inadequate sanitation, and the use of poisonous materials—such as lead paints. Hazards in household equipment, such as light fixtures and appliances, have to some extent been looked into and corrected:

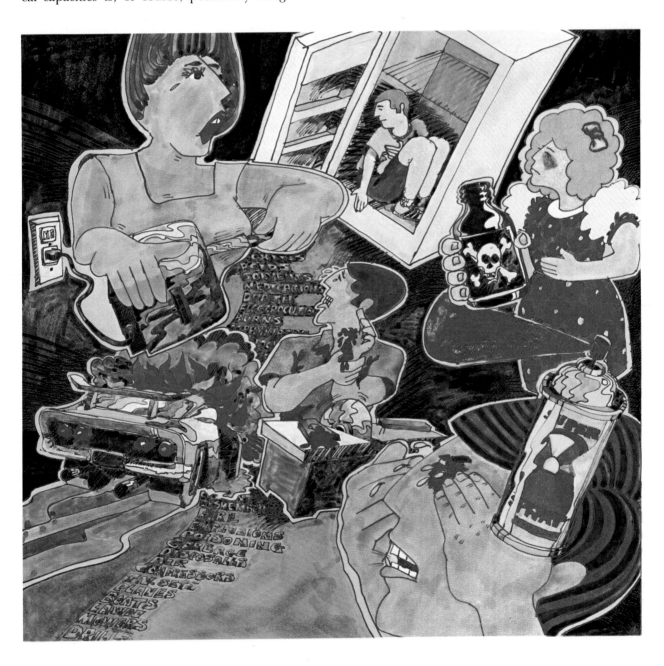

magnetic rather than latch hooks are now applied to refrigerator doors; three wire-grounded leads are used on all major appliances; nonslip throw rugs and floor wax are common; fire detector and alarm systems are increasingly installed in private homes.

On the negative side, however, dangerous toys are still prominently displayed for sale for children; TV radiation is imperfectly screened; high-speed rotary lawn mowers, hedge trimmers, snow blowers, and other machinery lie around for youngsters to operate without supervision. And the concern for poisonous or health-impairing properties of food or household materials is only barely beginning to bring about corrective measures.

OCCUPATIONAL AGENTS   Industrial safety, as was mentioned earlier, has considerably increased over the years. A number of elements are present in industry that do not exist in other accident-related areas and should operate not only to improve but actually to achieve on-the-job safety. Accidents in industry cost money and represent a dollar loss not only to the victims but to the operating concern as well. Supervisory personnel and safety engineers usually are present or quickly available to promptly investigate and identify the causes of an accident and the machinery that was its "agent." In an industrial setup, it is possible to take immediate steps against the future repetition of similar accidents in view of the recurring nature of the activities during which the accident took place.

In spite of these favorable elements, industrial safety remains an enormous problem, because of the number of people that are dependent on it and the diversity of the operations involved. Moreover, it is expected that the largest increase in the American labor force in the years ahead will come from two groups: women over thirty-five and young persons fourteen to twenty-five—the latter being the group already identified as the most susceptible to

accidents at present. Finally, the business philosophy permeating Western societies is such that private economic interests may prevail over the urgency of ensuring safety—witness the appalling current accident rate in the mining industry.

MOTOR VEHICLES   In the past few years there has been a marked increase in year-round use of recreational vehicles such as minibikes and snowmobiles, as well as an increase in power boating. Although they represent a source of potentially increasing hazards, the overwhelming accident-causative agent remains the automobile.

The automobile industry has identified and, under public pressure, modified a number of hazards: improved headlights now provide greater illumination of path of travel; side flashers indicate turns to operators of vehicles at an angle to the path of travel; windshields and side glass have been improved—tempered glass is now used to reduce jagged shards; recessed steering wheel hubs and knobs, padded surfaces, head rests, lap and shoulder belts, other passive-restraint devices, and improved side crash protection now protect the passenger in a crash. Engineering design has substantially reduced the possibility of a rollover following a collision, improved door latches make ejection after a crash less likely, emergency flashers warn other drivers if one is disabled on the road, and tires are now less likely to blow out and are able to absorb far greater punishment than was true just a few years ago.

However, the value of this identification and modification of hazards is tempered by the fact that various volunteer vehicle safety checks, conducted in states that do not require vehicle-certifying inspections, report that as high as 20 percent of the vehicles passing through their lanes exhibit at least one defect. Although problems with lights, both tail and head lamps, usually lead the list of defects, the

Figure 27.4 Governmental implementation of safety laws is one way to influence auto manufacturers to ensure highway safety, but safety is a behavioral concept and even the best-equipped vehicle is only as safe as the judgment and precautions taken by its driver.

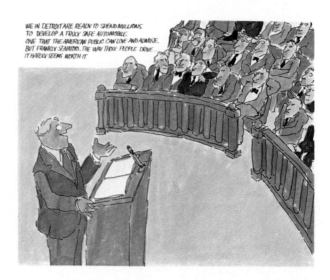

Connecticut Motor Vehicle Department reports that the rejection of tires increased from 5 percent in 1968 to 10 percent in 1969—a distressing finding in view of the dependence on the tire tread and pressure for safety on the road. One must add to that the increasing number of major defects that have been brought into the open by concerned investigators—for instance, "Nader's Raiders"—and that have forced car manufacturers to recall vast numbers of their products.

Roadways also are to be viewed as causative "agents" in car accidents rather than unsafe environmental conditions "happening" to exist at the scene of an accident. Slick surfaces, insufficient illumination, and blocked visibility are features that can be corrected through adequate technology. Similarly, solid objects adjacent to roadways can be removed, or guard rails can be installed to control the deflection of vehicles away from solid objects while

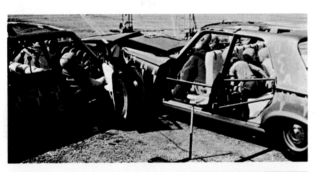

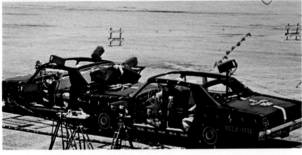

Figure 27.5 (*above*) At UCLA's school of automotive safety and engineering, cars are tested to determine ways in which future vehicles can be made more safe.

preventing them from bouncing back into lanes of moving traffic. Considerable reduction of car accident fatalities, for example, has been achieved through the expansion of the Interstate Highway System, a network of limited-access roadways where fatalities per 100 million vehicle-miles during 1970 were an impressive 2.7 compared to the 7.3 for all rural roads, or the 5.3 overall national average.

The Environment

Careful and responsible individuals living, working, or operating with technically sound agents still may not be safe in their activities if the environment in which they are carried out provides hazards.

Environmental hazards can be *natural* or *man-made*. Technology can learn to predict natural hazards so as to provide advance notice for escape—as is being done for hurricanes, and may be done in the near future for earthquakes—or it can develop ways to minimize their consequences without having to escape them—as the simple example of air-conditioning in homes, factories, or cars illustrates.

But it is with respect to the man-made environmental hazards that a society cannot be excused from the burden of removing them. It is a societal problem first and a technical one only secondarily. Safety engineers, urban planners, and other professionals are needed to design and implement the physical solutions, but it is for the people to demand the formulation and enactment of the necessary laws and ordinances, and to bring about the social climate, that will correct the existing hazards and avoid the generation of new ones.

For example, condemned school buildings are permitted to continue operating. Building codes are bent to favor the economic advantages of the developers. Pollution laws are knowingly going unenforced. Misleading or outright misrepresenting publicity is not taken to task. Alternatives to hazard-producing public activities are shelved to accommodate industrial or entrepreneurial interests. Agencies nominally set up to protect the consumer behave as camouflaged lobbies of special interests. Air transportation becomes increasingly hazardous not for lack of skilled pilots or safe aircraft but because of deficient airport facilities or faulty air-control regulations. Railroad passenger service, or public transportation systems in general, is neglected in deference to the car industry. And the future looks just as bleak. Labor-management negotiations already foretell shorter work-weeks and more leisure time, which means greater participation in a greater variety of activities and greater transportation needs. More than half of the labor force is manufacturing products that did not exist fifty years ago, and this phenomenon may be ex-

pected to repeat itself in less than twenty-five years—with a corresponding unprepared-for increase in potential hazards. The list is endless. And throughout the list, it is not the technological know-how but the will and the sense of social responsibility that are lacking. This is where the *social* environment shows up as the most critical of the accident causation components.

SAFETY AND CONSUMER PROTECTION

Many consumers are experiencing a growing awareness of environmental problems. Where once they blithely assumed that they were being protected by various local, state, and federal agencies, they now see evidence all around them of a lack of concern for their welfare: growing air, water, and land pollution, excessive noise, the presence of poten-

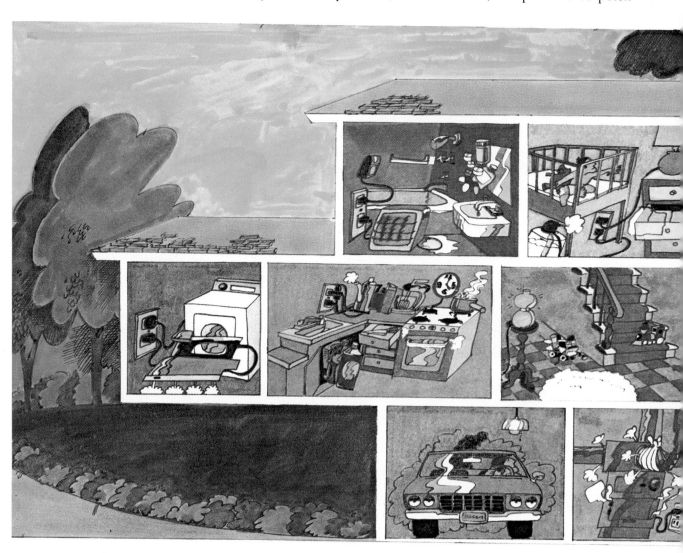

Figure 27.6   There are many areas in the home that can give rise to such accidents as fire or shock caused by electrical overload or faulty wiring, fire or asphyxiation caused by improper ventilation, poisoning due to harmful drugs and chemicals placed within easy reach of children, and injury due to falls.

tially dangerous chemicals in various foods, the hazards of unsafe toys and other products. Consumers have become more vocal in their discontent and their voices are being heard.

Many federal agencies have been given the responsibility for consumer protection, among them the Federal Communications Commission (FCC), the Federal Trade Commission (FTC), the Post Office Department, and the Department of Agriculture. However, it is the Food and Drug Administration (FDA) that plays the major role in attempting to protect the health of consumers.

The Food and Drug Administration

The FDA is literally the official food-taster to the nation. Approximately 4,500 FDA scientists, physicians, inspectors, technicians, and others attempt the almost impossible task of surveying the products of some 60,000 food, drug, and cosmetic companies that have annual sales of more than 130 billion dollars.

The main thrust of FDA activities is in four functional areas: the Bureau of Drugs, the Bureau of Foods and Pesticides, the Bureau of Veterinary Medicine, and the Office of Product Safety.

THE BUREAU OF DRUGS   The Bureau of Drugs makes certain that drugs and therapeutic devices are safe and effective. Before a drug can be sold it must live up to the therapeutic claims made for it. Safety is a relative term, and any drug, under certain conditions, can cause impairment, tissue damage, and even death. When a new drug is developed, a patent is immediately applied for to protect the

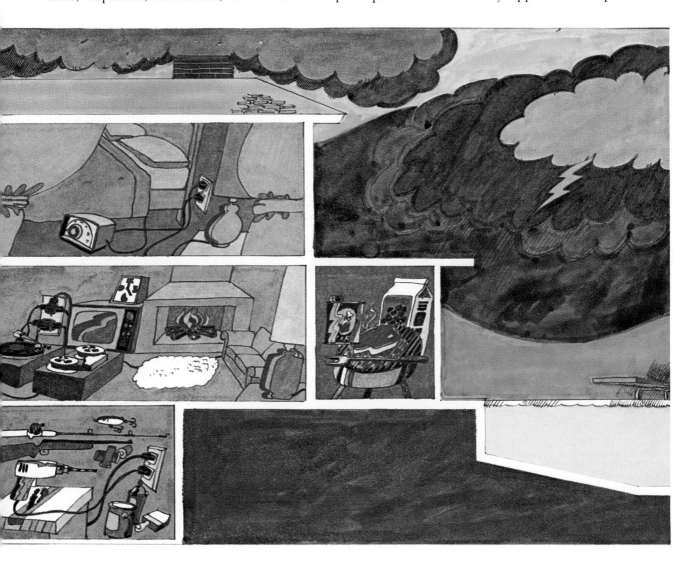

company against duplication by a competitor. The company has usually conducted considerable experimentation on animals prior to this application for a patent. It then submits an Investigational New Drug (I.N.D.) application to the FDA that must be approved before any human (clinical) trials can be done. The I.N.D. application must provide information about the properties of the drug, the manufacturing process, the animal trials, the proposed human trials, and the training and experience of the investigators. After approving the application, the FDA carefully monitors the testing on human subjects who must give their informed consent.

If the I.N.D. phase is successful, a New Drug Application (N.D.A.) is submitted to the FDA. Before it is approved, more detailed information about the drug and the manufacturing process is required. The manufacturing facility is usually inspected and proposed labeling approved. Large numbers of humans are involved at this phase, and the manufacturer must inform the FDA of any unexpected adverse reactions. The requirements are rigid. In a recent year, the FDA rejected five times as many N.D.A.'s as it approved. The new drugs may not reach the market for several years. Even after the drug is available to the public, the FDA has the power to recall it if undesirable side effects are observed, or if it is impure, adulterated, or mislabeled.

As part of its continuing surveillance program, the FDA regularly inspects drug manufacturing plants to test drug samples and assure proper manufacturing practices in those drugs already approved. In addition, the FDA tests and certifies every batch of insulin and antibiotics.

THE BUREAU OF FOODS AND PESTICIDES The Bureau of Foods and Pesticides works to insure safe, pure, and wholesome foods for the American public. The agency inspects processing and storage plants to make certain that they are sanitary. FDA inspectors also check the wholesomeness of ingredients and finished food products and the legality of the packages and labels.

The agency works with state and local health authorities to insure that shellfish are harvested from unpolluted waters. It also has an inspection service to assure safe food and water and good sanitary facilities for persons traveling between states by train, plane, ship, or bus.

The Bureau also is responsible for establishing safe levels for the use of chemical additives—such as preservatives, artificial flavors, and colors—and safe tolerances for residues of pesticides in foods.

Foods must be honestly and informatively labeled; ingredients must be listed (except for standardized foods such as catsup, mayonnaise, and margarine, where only added optional ingredients must be listed), and the net weight must be prominently stated. A food that is mislabeled, adulterated, improperly processed, or stored in an unsanitary establishment may be removed from the market by the FDA.

THE BUREAU OF VETERINARY MEDICINE The Bureau of Veterinary Medicine enforces the requirement that veterinary drugs, devices, and medicated feeds be safe and effective, in order to assure animal health and the safety and wholesomeness of food derived from treated animals. This bureau gives particular attention to residues of drugs found in tissues of slaughtered animals. Food derived from these animals cannot be marketed if the drug residue might transfer resistance or otherwise harm humans.

THE OFFICE OF PRODUCT SAFETY The Office of Product Safety enforces the Federal Hazardous Substances Act, which was enacted to protect American consumers, especially children, from accidents involving household chemicals. This Act requires that all

THE SAFETY-HAPPY FDA

by Paul H. Blachly

The thalidomide babies are almost ten years old. In early 1962, when the world learned that thousands of women who had taken thalidomide as a sedative/sleeping pill were giving birth to deformed infants, there was an anguished demand for safeguards against repetition of the tragedy.

Although thalidomide was almost entirely a European horror, there was in the United States an almost hysterical fear that someday, somehow, it might happen here. Congress hastily gave new powers to the Food and Drug Administration (FDA)—it became protector of the people and gatekeeper of the nation's drug market.

The FDA's powers have worked almost too well. It is true that no thalidomide-style tragedy has befallen the American public, but it also is true that the American public has been deprived of drugs of proven safety and effectiveness, drugs that it urgently needs. One of the FDA's own physicians has testified before a Senate subcommittee that with today's regulations and requirements even aspirin would never win the FDA's stamp of approval.

I spent almost six years trying to get approval for a drug that is highly effective for manic-depressive psychosis, a disorder in which patients have extreme swings in mood.

In 1949 an Australian physician, J. F. J. Cade, showed that lithium carbonate was highly successful in calming hyperactive, manic patients. Subsequently, many studies confirmed that this chemical was effective for mania—more effective than the tranquilizer and electric-shock therapies that already were in use. And some early research, later confirmed, suggested that regular use of the drug would be effective in relieving the depressive phase as well.

By 1964, when I was director of the Psychopharmacology Clinic at the University of Oregon, there were at least eighteen published studies that reported consistently beneficial results from the use of lithium carbonate with manic patients. No one reported that the drug was either ineffective or dangerous when it was used as directed. I decided that lithium carbonate was the best possible treatment for my manic-depressive patients. It was safe, effective, inexpensive, and it did not have the unfortunate side effect of dulling a patient's thought processes as the tranquilizers I had been prescribing did.

I had a local drug company make up some lithium-carbonate capsules for me and I arranged for our clinical laboratory to do the blood tests that are necessary when patients take the chemicals.

The thalidomide tragedy had struck only two years earlier and the public was touchy about all new drugs, so for my own protection I asked the FDA for a written statement that lithium carbonate was an approved drug.

To my surprise the FDA replied that lithium carbonate was still considered experimental. That meant I could use it only if I were doing research. And that meant writing up a formal research proposal and hiring a full-time staff to fill out the forms and carry out the research.

I wondered if the FDA knew something that I didn't—perhaps some unpublished research where someone had found new dangers or unreported side effects with lithium carbonate. The FDA wouldn't say—only that its panel of experts had not yet approved it. I asked who was on the panel, when they met, and what had been the subject of their deliberations. Again the FDA wouldn't say.

Perhaps their experts felt there were still unanswered questions about lithium carbonate and were waiting for the appropriate research to be done. I was willing to do the research—but the FDA wouldn't tell me what research was needed. All they said was that I was free to do any studies on lithium carbonate that I wanted—once I had completed

Adapted from Blachly, P. H. "They're Safety-Happy in the FDA and We're in Trouble," *Psychology Today* (May 1971), pp. 31–34, 98.

the appropriate forms. It was hypocritical—I would have been repeating research, taking time and resources away from research projects in which the answers were not yet known.

There had to be an easier way to get lithium carbonate to my patients, I thought. I tried to get around the law on a semantic formality. Since I had ordered the lithium carbonate from a Missouri chemical house, I argued, it had come across state lines as a chemical, not as a drug, and therefore was not under FDA control. They disagreed and said that if I followed this reasoning I would violate the intent of the law and would be prosecuted.

If I could have got lithium carbonate that had not crossed a state line, then I would have been out of the jurisdictional reach of the Food and Drug Administration. Unfortunately, there were in Oregon no primary sources of the pure type of lithium I wanted. Lithium is a salt that is mined in many states. Some of the salt in the Great Salt Lake is lithium—just the kind I needed.

I explained my plight to several of Oregon's congressmen, hoping they could help me through the red-tape barrier. They were sympathetic but powerless. Bernard Fensterwald Jr. who was chief counsel for the Senate Subcommittee on Administrative Practice and Procedure, sympathized with the frustrations of dealing with the FDA: "You ask the question: 'Can one conceive that the value of vaccination, digitalis, anesthesia, penicillin, or mass polio vaccination could have been discovered with present regulations of the Food and Drug Administration?' The answer most certainly is no. . . ."

When I suggested that there might be legal loopholes, Fensterwald cautioned me: ". . . Don't forget that the FDA is very vindictive. If they feel that you are trying to get around the Act, they are not above putting pressures on the University, financial or otherwise. They are not above using phony names to try to trap you into shipping the drug interstate."

O.K. It was a frustrating experience. I had bottles of lithium-carbonate capsules in my office, but I couldn't use them. I had manic patients who could have returned to their homes and jobs if they had had lithium-carbonate therapy. I had patients in deep depression who could have been brought out of their dark stupors. It occurred to me then that if a depressed patient committed suicide, a relative might seek damages on the ground that the government had withheld proven medication by an arbitrary and capricious decision.

I even considered prescribing the drug in defiance of the FDA, thinking that the publicity that would result from my arrest and trial would alert the public to the dilemma of the conscientious physician who wants to provide the best possible treatment for his patients.

Instead I planned an article that would condemn the FDA for the roadblocks it-had put in the path of lithium carbonate. I wrote the article in 1968, but for two years no journal would publish it. Then in the spring of 1970 the government suddenly announced that lithium carbonate was an approved drug, and *Psychiatric Opinion* published my paper four months later.

The battle for lithium carbonate is over now. The drug is legal—it can be prescribed for patients who need it. But the inefficiencies of the Food and Drug Administration persist and they continue to block the availability of needed drugs.

It costs millions to develop a new drug—or test out a new use—and send it through the FDA gauntlet. Large drug companies will pay the price—if they think they have a good chance of success and if there is the prospect of large profits.

In 1967 it was reported that L-dopa was remarkably effective in alleviating the symptoms of Parkinson's disease, the pitiful shaking palsy that afflicts many of the aged. L-dopa is a simple, naturally occurring amino acid. Because it offered little promise of profit, most drug companies were not interested. However, it was approved by the FDA recently, after Roche Laboratories pushed it through the mill.

In effect, the FDA has developed a licensing system that is geographically discriminatory. When L-dopa, methadone, and lithium carbonate are classed as experimental drugs, they are available only to patients who live near what the FDA calls a "clinical investigator." Physicians are forced to pose as "clinical investigators," hypocritically repeating research that has already been done, so that they can get supplies of a drug for their patients.

We are fortunate that other areas of medicine are not as dependent upon profit-potential as the development of drugs is—otherwise we might not now be benefiting from prosthetic heart valves, artificial kidneys, or organ transplants. Public fund drives and federal research grants financed these breakthroughs.

A significant drawback to using federal research grants to support drug research is that when the government pays for the research, the government gets the patent for the drug. And when they cannot have patents, pharmaceutical companies show little interest in manufacturing drugs even after they have been proven effective. This financial unattractiveness was one of the handicaps of lithium carbonate—it is an old and pure inorganic chemical that cannot be patented; it is not a big moneymaker.

The FDA's powers must be reexamined. The agency hamstrings physicians, frustrates researchers, cheats patients, slows the acquisition of scientific knowledge, and increases the cost of drugs for everyone.

The basis on which the FDA makes its decisions should be public information; scientists should be able to force the agency to show cause for its actions. At present the FDA may approve a new drug investigation and then cancel it at any time without saying why. A scientist should have the right to appeal when his research project is terminated, particularly when the termination is arbitrary.

Above all, the FDA must perpetually weigh the risk of using a new drug against the risk of not using it. Surely we can tolerate the risk that methadone may be found to have some subtle side effects if by doing so we can relieve the horror of heroin addiction that drives users to steal and kill to get money for fixes.

No one can quarrel with the FDA's concern with keeping dangerous drugs off the market. But I find it puzzling that some drugs are taken off the market when research shows they might be dangerous, while alcohol and tobacco, already known to be dangerous drugs, still are freely available.

One wishes that a rule of risk-taking could have been applied in the mid-1960s to lithium carbonate. More than 20,000 suicides are recorded in the United States every year; perhaps as many as half of these are associated with depressive states that can be alleviated with lithium carbonate. Such data should have influenced the length of time the drug remained on the unapproved list.

We need a new system of drug funding and patenting that will encourage research on drugs that have little profit-potential but are nonetheless desperately needed.

The FDA should say explicitly what it wants to know about a drug before any testing begins. It should set up reasonable descriptions of the experiments that must be run and the results that the experiments must show before the drug will be considered safe. The criteria should be made available to all interested physicians and researchers, so that they will know exactly what remains to be learned about a drug and so that they will not blindly duplicate each other's research. The drug should be made available immediately after the experiments have been done and the criteria have been met.

It is always possible that tomorrow someone will experience a negative reaction to a drug, so no drug can ever be proved absolutely harmless. But a person is considered innocent if there is any reasonable doubt as to his guilt; surely we would be wiser to consider a drug guilty only when there is a reasonable doubt about its innocence.

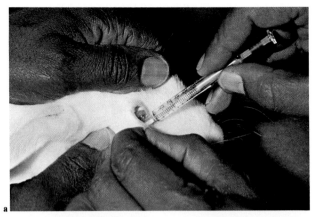

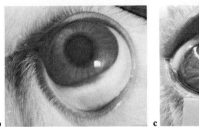
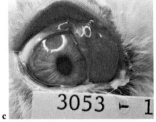

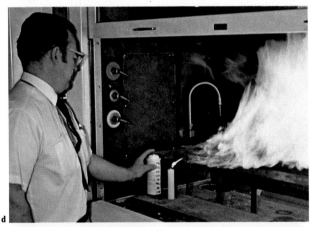

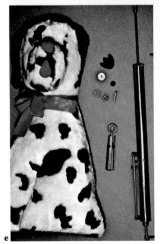
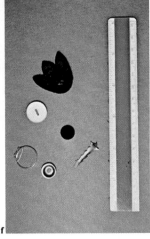

potentially dangerous substances intended or suitable for household use be conspicuously labeled to warn the user of the danger. The label must also provide safety and first-aid information and the warning: "Keep Out of Reach of Children." Products covered by the law include detergents and cleansers, waxes, polishes, bleaches, and paint thinners. If any product does not carry the required information on its label, the government may seize it.

State and Local Protection

As of 1969, nine states had some kind of consumer representation at the executive level of government, while approximately thirty states had some form of consumer fraud bureau or protection agency, usually functioning in the office of the attorney general. In some states, the staff of these bureaus follows up nearly every consumer complaint relating to mislabeling, false advertising, misrepresentation, and many other fraudulent promotions. The bureaus, because of their legal authority, are successful in providing restitution to consumers and also in initiating court action against offenders.

Private Organizations

Two private testing and rating agencies are active in providing consumers with unbiased information on a variety of products. Neither agency accepts advertising; they depend solely on funds realized from the sale of their publications. Consumers' Research, Inc. (CR) hires out most of its testing to well-known testing laboratories and to specialized consultants. It publishes the results in twelve monthly issues of *Consumers' Research Bulletin* and an *Annual Bulletin*. Consumers Union of U.S., Inc. (CU) tests more than 200 different consumer products each year. Testing results are published in the monthly *Consumer Reports* and the *Buying Guide*, issued in December.

Figure 27.7 Testing products for safety. (a) A rabbit's eye is washed with a liquid detergent. (b) Rabbit's eye prior to administration of detergent. (c) Eye twenty-four hours after receiving detergent wash. (d) A flame test using a common household aerosol. (e, f) Pressure tests for determining the amount of force necessary to remove loose items from toys. This stuffed animal's eye, consisting of six small parts, was pulled from place with only three pounds of pressure. Note that the eye was attached by a sharp, easily swallowed metal clip.

What Can Consumers Do?

The FDA, which has district offices and inspection stations throughout the country, welcomes consumer help in locating mislabeled, unsanitary, or otherwise harmful foods, drugs, or cosmetics. Persons who have a grievance should save whatever remains of the product or the empty container for use in case of investigation or for their doctor's information. They also should report the product to the manufacturer, packer, or distributor and to the store where it was purchased.

Anyone who experiences an unusual reaction after taking a prescription medicine should report it to his doctor immediately. The doctor, in addi-

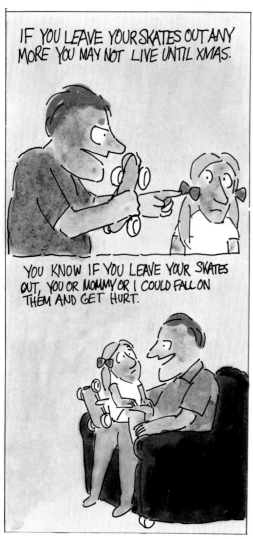

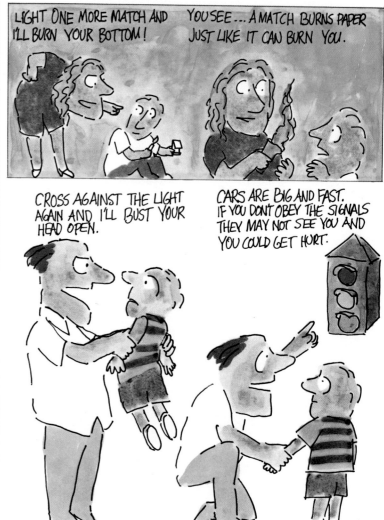

Figure 27.8 Parents and teachers should try to teach safety concepts rather than simply instilling fear in children.

tion to treating adverse reactions, will want to know of such problems for his own information and for reporting to the FDA or AMA.

For complaints about suspected false advertising one should notify the Federal Trade Commission. Complaints about meat and poultry products should be directed to the U.S. Department of Agriculture. One should notify his local health department about unsanitary restaurants and his state health department about problems with products made and sold exclusively within a state. He may also file complaints with some of the professional and private organizations discussed above.

FOR A FUTURE WITH SAFETY

In the epidemiological approach to accidents, only half of the task is the identification of the causative elements of the problem. The other half is their *prevention*. Just as the individual, the agent, and the environment are the three interacting causative components, prevention of accidents involves a blending of education, technological improvements, and societal action. However, technological improvements follow the commitment of will and resources of a society, and societal action depends on the values and the conscience of the nation. Thus, a future with safety lies with *education* of

people, both as operating individuals and as active members of their society.

Although it is laudable to teach a child in kindergarten the safest way to go to school, it is even more important that he learn time-space concepts applicable to crossing any street and not just a protected intersection. Whereas the elimination of hazardous agents—detergents, bleaches, sharp knives, firearms, and frayed electrical cords—from the reach of a young child is critical, it is even more critical that the child learn safe behavior from the example of the parent—shutting off a power mower when leaving it for even a few seconds, using safety devices while riding in a car, refraining from smoking, crossing streets only on "walk" signals, and so on. Furthermore, the establishment of behavioral objectives must be followed by learning activities where the "student," whatever his age, has the opportunity to demonstrate, practice, and perfect his ability to perform.

Education for prevention, however, involves more than simply teaching technique and process. Safe behavior comes with reasoned acceptance of risk and acceptance of risk when the value of what is to be gained outweighs that which may be lost. Education, then, must also provide perception, judgment attitudes, and decision-making abilities. It must help to clarify purpose, and to orient it.

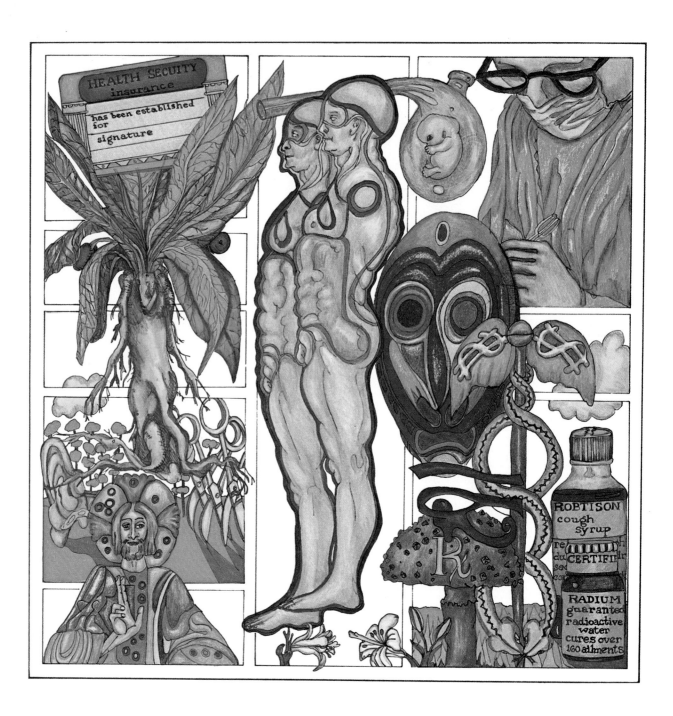

VII HEALTH CARE IN AMERICA

Individual knowledge, decisions, and actions for personal, family, and community health are vital in alleviating suffering and building health, but health problems and needs are often exceedingly complex and command the attentions of highly competent, efficient, and costly health professionals, equipment, and facilities. ¶ Historically, the United States has led the world in quality health care and community health programs. Tragically, however, quality health care has not always been available to all citizens and still is not available to many. The leading challenge today, then, is to continue the advancement of health science while simultaneously spreading its benefits to all human beings everywhere. Although health professionals can be expected to lead in this endeavor, it cannot become a reality without the understanding and support of all the people. ¶ This approach to health-care delivery in America is becoming increasingly heard from critics of the current health-care system, and it is the attitude taken by the authors of the chapters in this unit. Criticism of the health-care system is not meant to destroy it, but instead to help improve it and to provide the individual seeking health care with knowledge about the system's defects as well as its benefits ¶ But beyond the health-care system, man is concerned more basically with the question of meaning in life. As a species, man has demonstrated his ability to survive, sometimes at the peril of other species and to the detriment of his own best interests. Increasingly man is asking the question, "Survival for what?" and is concerned more fundamentally with the purpose of life. Virtually all human activities, however, ultimately hinge on both survival and health. Whether one's role is to be a scientist, artist, businessman(woman), soldier, minister, housewife, or citizen, the decisions and behaviors that facilitate health are prerequisite. Health science is not merely academic. It cries for application to alleviate suffering and to facilitate the well-being of mankind.

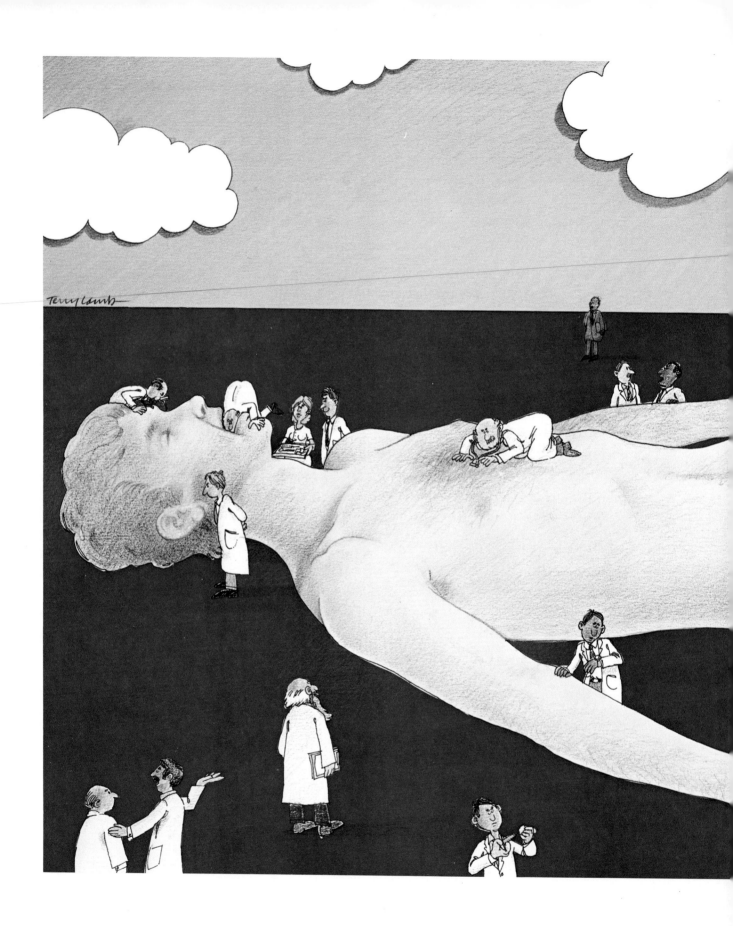

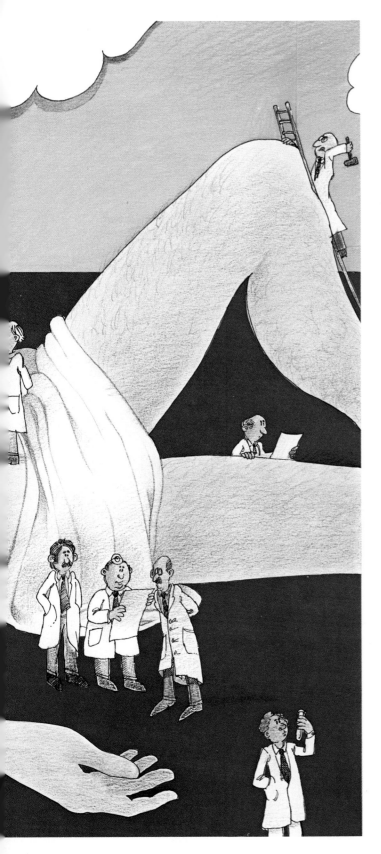

28

More and more people are accepting the definition of health recommended by the World Health Organization (WHO): "Health consists of a sense of physical, mental and social well-being, and not merely the absence of disease or infirmity," and are asking that society guarantee them the opportunity for this kind of health. This approach is reflected in the growing demand for government provision or sponsorship of such services as child care, family-planning clinics, and food programs for children and the elderly, in addition to making medical services more available. It also is reflected in demands for national health insurance and a guaranteed annual wage. A growing climate of opinion considers health care a right of all and not a privilege of just those people who can financially afford it. Health care for all the members of a community is seen as necessary to the well-being of the community as a whole.

CHANGING VIEWS OF COMMUNITY HEALTH

The view that health care is a right and that its provision is a responsibility of the society rather than the individual or his family has developed only within the last decade in this country. This view is partly a result of advances in medical technology and national affluence, the increased availability of effective health remedies and of evolving social organization, and the increasing awareness of how closely any one person depends on everyone else. The significance of these changes can be seen

Health Providers

in a brief examination of the evolution of community structure, health problems, and health-care provision since the beginning of this century in the United States.

1900 to 1945

During the first forty-five years of this century, acute infectious diseases, such as diphtheria, tuberculosis, and rheumatic fever, constituted the most serious health problems in the United States. The physician's arsenal against disease was severely limited before the age of modern medicine. Because antibiotics were unknown until the end of this period, the environmental and preventive approaches were the only real tools physicians had. DDT was used to eliminate the mosquitoes that carried yellow fever and malaria; rest was prescribed for tuberculosis; better water sanitation eliminated typhoid fever; and vaccinations stopped the scourge of diphtheria. Remedies, such as insulin for diabetes, that are commonly used today were unknown in 1900. The acute heart attack was only beginning

to be understood and treated in the 1920s. Surgery was extremely hazardous and hospitals were places where people went to die. It was only fifty years ago that Professor L. J. Henderson at Harvard observed that medical science had finally reached the point where "the average patient meeting the average doctor has more than a fifty-fifty chance of benefiting from the encounter."

Most Americans lived in small towns across the United States. Migration to urban and suburban areas had not yet begun in earnest. The majority of physicians were general practitioners, and most small towns had such a GP. The doctor's job was to provide support, understanding, and what limited therapeutic intervention he could for specific diseases. He provided support not only to patients but to their families. The structure of families at that time was conducive to this type of care. Large, extended families were not unusual, and the mobility of children was not great; many generations of the same family lived in close proximity, which meant that old people and sick members of the family could often be cared for at home.

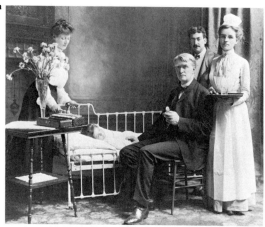

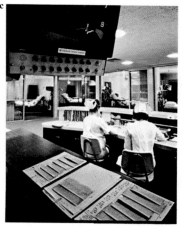

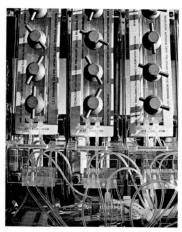

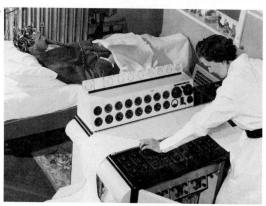

Figure 28.1   (a) The physician of the early twentieth century was hampered by limited technology: The x-ray machine was not yet perfected as a diagnostic tool; antibiotics had not yet been discovered; and heart disease, a major health problem even then, was poorly understood and treated only with bed rest. (b) Present medical knowledge is vast: diagnostic machinery, which includes the electrocardiograph, the electroencephalograph, the electron microscope, and so on, has aided the physician in the application of current therapeutic techniques. Today many of the body's organs can be replaced; there are machines that can do the work of the heart or the kidney; and current research daily makes inroads into the causes and treatment of cancer, heart disease, hereditary disorders, and so on. (c) With the addition of the computer to the ranks of diagnostic and therapeutic machinery, patients will benefit from the combined knowledge of many physicians and scientists. The application of the computer in health care has just begun—the future will see uses that are now within the realm of science fiction.

1945 to 1970

Drastic changes have taken place during the two and a half decades following World War II, in medicine as well as in the society. Increased medical research produced the knowledge and techniques to prevent most infectious disease by immunization, to cure infections when they were acquired, to make surgery safer, and to help body organs when injured or diseased (such as with the artificial pacemaker). As the average life span increased, chronic degenerative diseases and other health hazards became prevalent (see Unit VI), and new life styles contributed to illness in individuals and society by causing some diseases (for example, obesity, neurosis, lung cancer) and by making some bodily functions deteriorate until disease occurs (for example, ulcers, heart attacks).

Major changes in population size and distribution, and their consequences on family and community patterns, have contributed to the prevalence of socially aggravated ailments. Population growth, industrial expansion, and technological molding of life styles have built up pollution and ecological disruption into major problem areas. Population shifts have produced the giant urban sprawls of the megalopolis, with their accompanying transportation problems and hazards. The extended family has been fragmented into nuclear families—consisting only of the two parents and their own children—and the high divorce rate has meant that a sizable number of children live in homes where there is only one parent. Enhanced mobility has generated a diminishing sense of community for more people. The resulting social isolation, or *anomie*, and related anxieties have become a major sociopsychological health factor.

People have found themselves no longer able to look to other family members or within the small communities for help and care in time of illness and increasingly are faced with problems tran-

scending the individual, familial, or communal powers. Thus they have begun to look for new sources to provide and guarantee health care, all the more so because of the increasing costs of medical care. Current pressure on the government to institute programs like Medicare or some form of national health insurance is an example of the evolving view of the nature of health problems in the country.

A comparable, although not as rapid, evolution is detectable in world-wide health problems. Many countries have experienced a tremendous population growth under the shelter of the medical conquest of infectious diseases, but this growth has not been paralleled by a corresponding growth of life-sustaining conditions. Malnutrition remains the greatest immediate threat. In addition, contamination of the environment by the industrial societies, unrestricted by national boundaries, is increasingly becoming an earth-wide health hazard.

With such a rapid and all-encompassing evolution, and the even faster changes to be expected in the next decades, it is not surprising that organizations and individual practitioners dealing with health problems are encountering problems in trying to keep up with the demands on them.

HEALTH ORGANIZATIONS

The health-care organizations that have emerged to deal with infectious, chronic, and socially aggravated illness can be divided, for the sake of simplicity, into five major categories: *international organizations* dealing with world-wide problems through the cooperative efforts of several national governments, various *government agencies*, *corporate organizations*, *volunteer groups*, and *professional associations*. None of them constitutes a consumer organization, in the sense of having a participation or a representation of the people to whom health care is directed—a concept that will be examined in detail in Chapter

Figure 28.2 Mayor in Tilden, Ill., stands beside sign that tells the plight of his town.

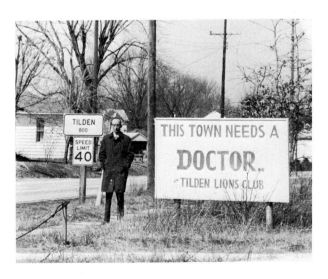

29. It must be understood that most sick people are cared for by physicians and nurses working in offices, clinics, and hospitals, and that the goals of most health-care organizations include research, fund raising, environmentally oriented preventive medicine, and education to raise the quality and effectiveness of health-care providers. Only rarely do they undertake to care for sick people directly.

International Health Efforts

Various national governments have joined forces in several instances during the past century to confront health problems on an international basis. Early efforts concentrated almost exclusively upon the eradication of infectious diseases, especially by the use of preventive measures such as mass vaccination, water sanitation, and quarantines. Unfortunately, even world-wide efforts at disease control will have little impact upon the great majority of the world's ill health until collective action is directed to the basic living conditions of much of earth's population.

The major international health agency is the *World Health Organization* (WHO), a specialized agency of the United Nations formed in 1948, following the precedents in world-wide disease control set by the League of Nations after World War I. Unlike its predecessor, which primarily collected statistics and traded information, WHO provides needy regions with practical aid—trained personnel, money, materials, equipment, and advice. WHO has operated primarily in underdeveloped countries, which suffer from the highest concentrations of disease and malnutrition, occasionally collaborating with other international organizations, such as the Red Cross, and national groups, such as CARE. Control of epidemics and alleviation of the effects of major disasters represent the main areas of WHO's activity. An example of international health cooperation in combating and restraining epidemics is the world-wide chain of influenza centers provided by the WHO to chart and monitor the spread of different strains of influenza, forewarn communities in the path of the epidemic, and

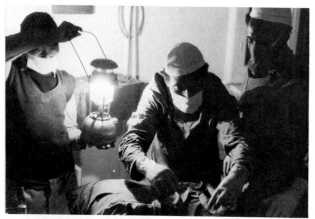
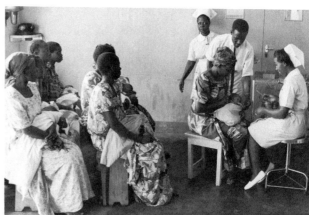
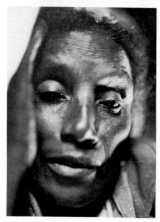
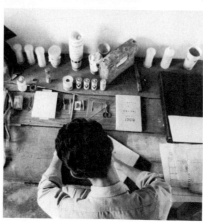

Figure 28.3 International health efforts. (*above left*) Health services are essential to improve health conditions in rural areas. Here, an African doctor performs a minor operation by the light of an oil lamp in a rural health unit. (*above right*) A health center for mothers and children in Uganda. (*far left*) The face of malaria. (*left*) A World Health Organization malaria field laboratory.

arm them with information on vaccines and immunization procedures.

Other undertakings of WHO include standardization of statistics on disease and mortality—which enable scientists to compare geographical health patterns—and the setting and publishing of standards for drug potencies and laboratory diagnoses. WHO also functions as a clearing house for health-related information and its distribution to health professionals, governments, and the public—in the belief that if all knowledge about disease prevention were fully utilized, 90 percent of the illness presently plaguing the earth's population could be eliminated.

Government Agencies

Governments have traditionally assumed some responsibility for the health of citizens. Now a consid-

erable shift is developing in what people take to be the responsibility of the government. Concurrent with this shift, increased urbanization has altered the extent to which concern and control about health problems is exhibited at federal, state, and local levels and has affected the resources available to each.

FEDERAL GOVERNMENT   At the end of the eighteenth century Congress created the *Public Health Service* to provide direct medical care to sailors and the merchant marine because these wanderers could not depend on family or community help. Soon the PHS had other responsibilities, such as establishing quarantines and supervision of water sanitation and food production and handling. During the depression comprehensive child care was added, and efforts were directed to the "social diseases" of tuber-

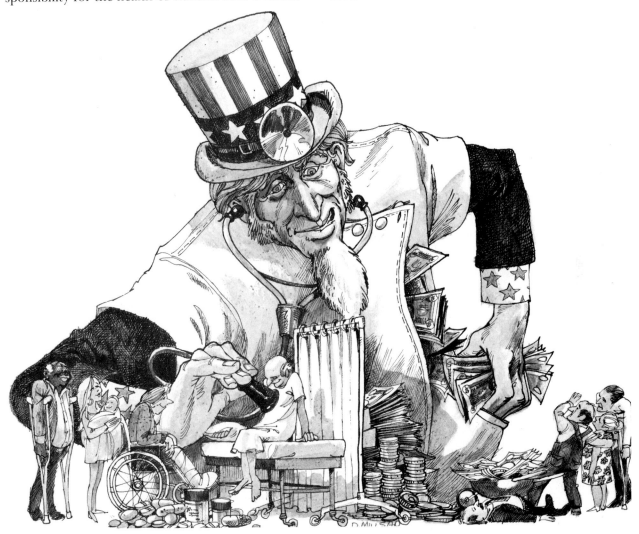

Figure 28.4   Government involvement in health care is seen by some as benevolent and necessary, by others as bureaucratic and socialistic.

culosis, gonorrhea, and syphilis. After World War II the PHS supervised the distribution of money for hospital construction and developed a huge program in medical research—the *National Institutes of Health* (NIH).

The federal government has assumed increasing responsibility for the support of health services over the years. This trend toward expanded federal responsibility and authority is evident not only in the field of medical care but in the financing of welfare services, education, and a variety of other activities. In 1953 these activities were consolidated by creating the cabinet level Department of Health, Education and Welfare (HEW), which absorbed the Public Health Service.

Within HEW, in addition to the old PHS programs there are many new ones (see Chapter 29) such as Health Planning, Neighborhood Health Center Development, Health Maintenance Organization Development, the Indian Health Service, the National Medical Library, Assistance for Education in the Health Professions, and the Food and Drug Administration (FDA). Consumer protection and some environmental surveillance activities have been brought together in the FDA and the Environmental Protection Agency, although the primary federal focus on the environment is elsewhere. On the whole, except for rare exceptions—the merchant marine and Indians—HEW does not provide medical care to sick people but concentrates on providing supportive assistance in the form of advice and funds (grants) for health-related activities to be carried out by others, both governmental and nongovernmental.

This approach is changing, as is evidenced by the many proposals for a National Health Insurance and the creation in 1970 of a National Health Service Corps in which the federal government will hire doctors and other personnel to be sent to medically deprived areas (see Chapter 29). As a first

---

NATIONAL INSTITUTES OF HEALTH APPROPRIATIONS FOR FISCAL YEAR 1970
$1,523,295,000

Bureau of Health Professions Education and Manpower

Grants and aid awarded to schools offering training in various aspects of health care

Development of curricula for training in current methods of health-care delivery

28%

National Cancer Institute

Research in cancer causes and prevention
Cancer therapy
Fundamental research in cell function

13%

National Heart and Lung Institute

Research in causes and prevention of:

Atherosclerotic heart disease
Congenital heart defects
Hypertension
Chronic lung disease
Restorative surgery and prosthetics
Basic research in cardiovascular physiology

11%

National Institute of General Medical Sciences

Research and development in automation of clinical procedures
Development of improved emergency care
Drug research

11%

National Institute of Arthritis and Metabolic Diseases

Research in causes and prevention of rheumatoid arthritis
Research in cause and prevention of diabetes; study of the mechanism of insulin

7%

Other NIH Subdivisions

National Institute of Allergy and Infectious Diseases 7%
National Institute of Neurological Diseases 7%
National Institute of Child Health and Human Development 5%
National Eye Institute 2%
National Institute of Dental Research 2%
National Institute of Environmental Health Sciences 1%
Division of Biologic Standards .5%
Other 5.5%

---

step toward National Health Insurance, in 1965 Congress passed Medicare and Medicaid, which also are run by HEW but are outside the PHS. *Medicare* is a *social insurance program* open to everybody over the age of sixty-five and is supported by payments by all employers and employees. The government then uses this money to pay enrollees' medical bills. This money covers about 50 percent of the bills and the patient pays the rest. *Medicaid* is a *welfare* program in which general tax money is distributed to the several states to help pay medical expenses for the indigent. In order to benefit from this program a person has to undergo a "demeaning means" test, in which he has to prove his poverty, and his family life is investigated by eligibility workers. Benefits are often limited and are being cut back further.

Other parts of the federal government besides HEW are involved in health-related activities: The Veterans Administration does research and provides medical care for the military and veterans, the Office of Economic Opportunity focuses on the poor, the Departments of Commerce and Interior monitor the environment, the Department of State sends medical assistance to foreign countries. The amount of money the federal government devotes to medical activities is truly impressive. In 1970 the total national health expenditure was 67.2 billion dollars, of which about 58 billion dollars was for personal health services. Federal expenditures totalled 18.8 billion dollars.

STATE HEALTH DEPARTMENTS Supported by local tax money as well as grants from HEW, each state has a health department that focuses primarily on backup services and preventive medicine. Each state has taken the responsibility for protecting the health of its citizens through activities that include recording of vital statistics (births and deaths) and reportable diseases (such as tuberculosis and illnesses associated with employment); provision of public health laboratory services (such as testing for syphilis and identifying infectious disease carriers); nutritional services; public health nursing services; surveys of hospital facilities and nursing homes; environmental sanitation programs; and food and drug control.

In addition, the state health (or in some cases the welfare) department runs its medicaid program, paying for direct health services to the indigent, and maintains certain special facilities, such as mental and tuberculosis hospitals. State health departments are facing serious challenges today. Most states are in the process of redistricting to reflect population changes. Governing bodies formerly composed of legislators representing rural areas are undergoing a transition to greater representation from urban centers. In particular, shortage of tax funds has affected state health department budgets. There also are new demands for health planning and for more control of the health system.

LOCAL AGENCIES Local health programs originally served specific political jurisdictions, that is, specific communities. A county was an identifiable political entity with a real source of income from property taxes. But the population has shifted from small towns to metropolitan areas that sometimes overlap several counties, and the tax base has shifted from

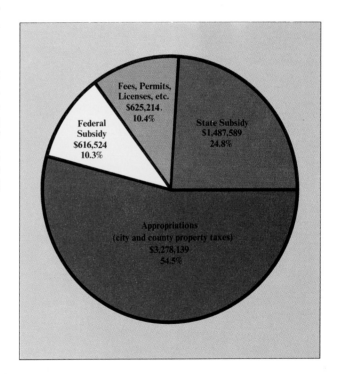

Figure 28.5 Breakdown of how local health-care programs are funded. Figures are for San Diego County, California.

a property assessment for support of local governments to an income assessment that supports the federal government. As a result, local health departments have had increasing difficulties acquiring funding and delineating political jurisdictions. Local welfare programs, for example, increasingly require federal support to remain viable.

Many community health problems also involve metropolitan, multicounty, and multistate areas that transcend paper boundaries. For example, polluted water that kills fish or livestock in one state may have been contaminated upstream in an entirely different state or community. In addition, population mobility and attitude has taxed the abilities of local health departments to trace the contacts of those infected with communicable diseases, such as tuberculosis or veneral disease.

It is at the local level that federal and state incentive money, mixed with local taxes, is used to provide services to people. Again, these services emphasize the preventive or are restricted to the indigent. Most cities, towns, or counties have a health department that administers vaccinations, treats venereal disease and tuberculosis, and inspects restaurants, sewage plants, and dairies, as well as running a hospital for the sick poor.

Corporate Organizations

Historically, industry has a long tradition of minimal concern for health matters, whether involving its own employees or the outside communities. The major corporate interest in these areas appears to have been for the costs or the adverse effects that health problems might impose on their own operations. Over the past several years, however, industry has reluctantly yielded to employee, governmental, and public pressures.

Unions and employee groups have been able to negotiate benefit packages, ranging from coverage for injury to workers on the job and workmen's

Figure 28.6 Hundreds of volunteer organizations exist that are supported solely by contributions. They are responsible for much of the research that has made possible the advances against such health problems as asthma, multiple sclerosis, cancer, and heart disease.

compensation claims to total health maintenance programs for the employee and, in some cases, his family. Generally these benefits are paid for by employer-employee contributions, but except for small infirmaries in some factories, the money is given to insurance companies or groups of doctors, and medical care is provided to employees by the health workers in the community. Perhaps the most critical aspect of industry-provided health benefits today is their erratic quality, being extremely comprehensive in some industries but rather meager in others. The nature and quality of health care received by an individual frequently remains determined by the place where he works and the type of work he does, and depends not on a sounder corporate perspective but on the attitudes of individual managements and the effectiveness with which an employee group can bargain.

Volunteer Groups and Private Foundations

Hundreds of organizations have evolved independently of governmental support to deal with specific problems at local, regional, and national levels. Most voluntary organizations focus on a specific disease or health problem; the best-known of these voluntary organizations are probably the American Heart Association and the American Cancer Society.

Almost all activities of voluntary agencies fall

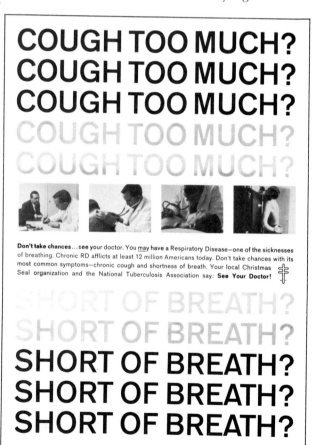

under three classifications—educating the public about the nature of a problem, providing such services as dressings, beds on loan, and wheelchairs to those who have the problem, or supplying money for research into the cause and solution of the problem. These organizations only rarely provide direct care. Money to fund these activities is raised either by individual drives or by united fund drives that collect for all agencies in a community.

Unlike volunteer groups, private *foundations* are exclusively financed by wealthy individuals or families or by an industry's endowment. Their objectives range from education for health and medical research to alleviation of rural community health problems.

Professional Organizations

While governmental and voluntary organizations aim at improving general health or fighting specific diseases, there are groups organized to represent individuals and institutions that *provide* health care or are involved with public health. These professional organizations include the American Medical Association, the American Hospital Association, the American Nurses Association, the American Public Health Association, groups of public health officers, environmental sanitation experts, and so on, and their numbers are increasing rapidly.

Almost all professional organizations state as their primary objective the protection of the public against unqualified practitioners, through the establishment and maintenance of standards for institutional and professional behavior. Although this self-policing function is vital, these associations—composed exclusively of established institutions (nursing homes or hospitals) and professionals (social workers, physicians)—gravitate toward activities that protect their own interests. This tendency has prompted accusations of their being tailored more toward protecting professional interests than serving actual community health needs.

Organizations of health professionals probably are no more guilty of inertia and resistance to change than are any other organizations, and self-interested behavior may be expected from any group of individuals who share common backgrounds, work experiences, and goals. This factor should not prevent approaches to community health problems from dealing with the tendencies toward monopoly and lack of accountability exhibited by professional organizations. For example, most groups of health specialists or institutions are reviewed and accredited only by members of similar organizations or professions. In all probability, increasing public awareness of this problem will force consumer representation on the boards of

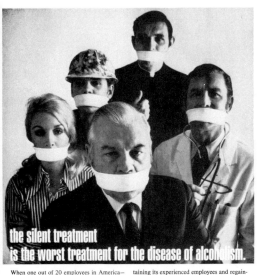

the silent treatment is the worst treatment for the disease of alcoholism.

When one out of 20 employees in America—including executives—has alcoholism, it's time for some plain talk about alcoholism. The alcoholic's family, friends and employer may mean well, but the silent treatment is no way to treat a disease. And alcoholism is a disease from which recovery is possible, rather than a moral weakness for which the alcoholic should be pitied—or fired. It's a disease which ranks with heart disease, cancer and severe mental disorders as a public health menace.

The National Council on Alcoholism has pioneered in setting up joint union-management alcoholism programs. In these programs, industry is achieving *recovery rates averaging 60 to 70 percent.* Management profits by re-taining its experienced employees and regaining lost productivity—estimated at six billion dollars. Unions profit by increasing health and welfare protection for members and keeping them in the active work force.

If you think alcoholism is affecting your business, **talk it over with the Director of Labor Management Services, National Council on Alcoholism, 2 Park Avenue, New York, N.Y. 10016.**

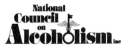

National Council on Alcoholism inc.

When you're 16 years old, you're never going to die.

That's something to think about, puff after puff after puff.

AMERICAN CANCER SOCIETY
THIS SPACE CONTRIBUTED BY THE PUBLISHER

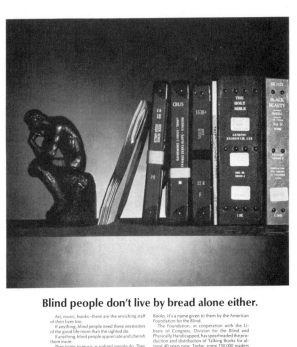

Blind people don't live by bread alone either.

Art, music, books—these are the enriching staff of their lives too.

If anything, blind people need these necessities of the good life more than the sighted do.

If anything, blind people appreciate and cherish them more.

They listen to music as sighted people do. They touch works of art to perceive them. They read books printed in braille.

Or they listen to them. They listen to books. On records and tape cassettes.

These books have a special name: Talking

Books. It's a name given to them by the American Foundation for the Blind.

The Foundation, in cooperation with the Library of Congress, Division for the Blind and Physically Handicapped, has spearheaded the production and distribution of Talking Books for almost 40 years now. Today, some 150,000 readers enjoy their benefits.

It's part of the Foundation's reason for being.

It's part of helping blind people become just people. Something we've been doing for more than 50 years.

The American Foundation for the Blind
More Than Fifty Years Of Helping Blind People Become Just People

professional organizations that perform such legal functions as licensing individuals to practice certain professions, inspecting and certifying institutions, and accrediting educational programs that prepare people for professional practice.

HEALTH PRACTITIONERS

As has been shown, there are many organizations that support the medical care system, but on the whole they do not concern themselves with taking care of individual sick patients. This function is left to the health practitioners. The present system of health care enables many types of professionals to practice the healing arts. Foremost, of course, is the physician. In the United States the vast majority of physicians are in individual private practice; that is, they see patients in their own office and charge a fee for each service rendered. However, there is a definite trend for physicians to gather together in groups, or to work for the various health-care organizations, or to become salaried employees of hospitals, neighborhood health centers, or clinics (see Chapter 29). Although only 10 percent of all

health workers are physicians, the vast majority of all the other health providers either work directly for physicians or receive their patients on referral from a physician.

Not all health practitioners are licensed to use medicine and surgery, even though some may still be legally and professionally entitled to use the term "doctor." Some may be unable or not allowed to use all therapeutic approaches in the treatment of their patients. Others have different philosophies of healing or different professional training. A prospective patient should understand these differences.

Health practitioners of many different types serve patients (see Table 28.1). The classifications in the table reflect each group's technical knowledge and degree of independence rather than an integral view of the health concept and may mislead laymen into assuming a quality ranking that is more appropriate *within* each category than among them. Furthermore, the present health education system provides little or no overlap in the preparation of different health practitioners even within

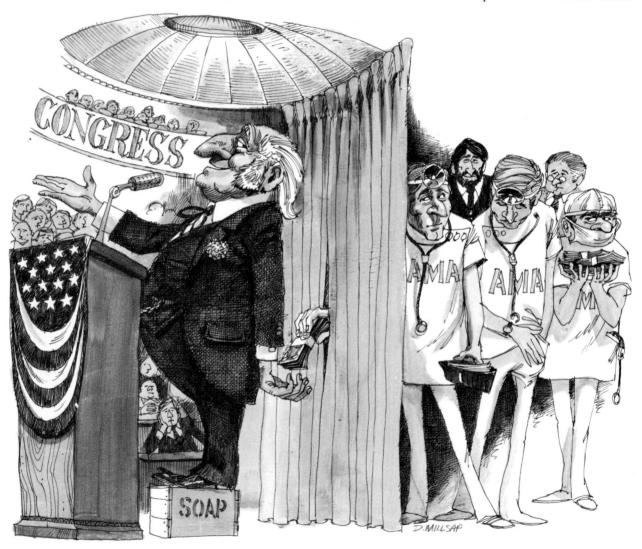

the same category. One of the most needed changes in the current health-care system—as will be discussed in Chapter 29—is the establishment of a main trunk of health education common to many health professions, with branching-out points for the training of different practitioners and re-entry points for the resumption of more advanced professional preparation.

Physicians

One type of physician that is slowly phasing out of the American health professions is the *Doctor of Osteopathy* (D.O.). Originally, osteopathy was based on the proper alignment of bones and the contention that spinal "lesions" were responsible for inadequate functioning of the nervous system and the circulation of blood to many parts of the body. Osteopathic treatment involved removal of such "lesions" by manipulation, and drugs were avoided. Today, however, the osteopathic approach to the treatment of disease is similar to that of the Medical Doctor (M.D.), and few osteopaths limit their practice to manipulation. Entrance requirements to, and education in, the osteopathic colleges are similar to those of the medical schools, and a one-year internship is required before taking licensure examinations. In fact, in some states, such as California and New York, M.D.'s and D.O.'s take the same licensure examination and may use either title.

By and large, however, the term "physician" today is identified with the *Medical Doctor*, or *M.D.* Becoming an M.D. in the present educational system involves a lengthy training with certain definite stages: premedical college education, medical school (including preclinical science and clinical science), hospital-based clinical experience including internship and residency, and finally, licensure. Additional residency training in a medical specialty is necessary to qualify to take the specialty board examinations.

Figure 28.7 (*left*) The AMA has come under fire for its lobbying practices and self-protective attitude toward criticism of and changes in the current state of medical care in the United States. Few people, however, realize the full powers and responsibilities of the organization, which include accreditation of medical schools, licensing boards that prepare and evaluate licensing examinations for medical-school graduates, establishing standards of medical ethics, and so on. Although the AMA is now a dominant force in establishing criteria for adequate medical care, it is interesting to note that a high percentage of young physicians are shunning the AMA and either joining other medical organizations or avoiding professional organizations entirely.

Table 28.1   Estimated Number of Persons Employed Within Each Health Field, 1968

HEALTH FIELD	*Number*
Administration of health services	39,000–45,000
Anthropology and sociology	1,400
Automatic data processing in the health field	700–1,000
Basic sciences in the health field	51,200
Biomedical engineering	9,000
Chiropractic and naturopathy	16,000–18,000
Clinical laboratory services	108,000
Dentistry and allied services	237,000
Dietetic and nutritional services	36,000
Economic research in the health field	500–600
Environmental control	217,500
Food and drug protective services	23,400
Health and vital statistics	1,500
Health education	20,000–21,000
Health information and communication	4,500–5,600
Library services in the health field	9,000
Medical records	38,500
Medicine and osteopathy (M.D. and D.O.)	313,000
Midwifery	4,400
Nursing and related services	1,825,000
Occupational therapy	11,200–12,200
Optometry, opticianry, and ocular services	53,450
Orthotic and prosthetic technology	3,600
Pharmacy	130,100
Physical therapy	19,500–21,500
Podiatry	8,000
Psychology	12,000
Radiologic technology	75,000–100,000
Secretarial and office services in the health field	250,000–275,000
Social work	24,200
Specialized rehabilitation services	8,900–10,100
Speech pathology and audiology	17,000
Veterinary medicine	25,000
Vocational rehabilitation counseling	11,100
Miscellaneous health services	35,000–37,000
Total	3,639,650–3,706,350

Source: Department of Health, Education and Welfare, Health Resources Statistics, 1969.

The present eight-year span of formal medical education (four years in college and four years in medical school) plus the now usual three or four years of internship and residency are increasingly being viewed by some medical educators as excessive and outdated. Many efforts are currently underway to explore curricular and institutional revisions that may considerably reduce the overall time it takes to become a physician, without affecting his final competence.

PREMEDICAL AND MEDICAL EDUCATION   Although the 107 medical schools in the nation require a minimum of three years of undergraduate study, most students have earned a bachelor's degree prior to entry—a plus point in the race for admission to the most sought-after schools. Premedical education has traditionally stressed laboratory sciences, but recently emphasis also has been placed on the social sciences.

During the first two years of medical school (*preclinical years*), the medical student continues to spend most of his time in the classroom, the library, and the laboratory. He studies the basic medical sciences—anatomy (the structure of the body), histology (the cellular organization of tissues), biochemistry (the chemical operations of living matter), physiology (the functions of body organs and systems), embryology (the development of the human fetus), pathology (the nature and effects of disease), as well as pharmacology and epidemiology.

In his second two years (*clinical years*), the medical student applies what he has learned in his first two. He enters the hospital wards and undertakes patient care under the supervision of a medical faculty member. He also gets introduced to many of the specialty areas of medicine and surgery. After successful completion of this training, the medical student receives the M.D. degree.

INTERNSHIP AND LICENSURE   Following graduation, the physician serves an internship of one year in an accredited hospital to prepare for licensure to practice. An intern generally spends the whole year in one area of medicine, usually pediatrics, surgery, or adult medicine; a few rotate through several areas in order to prepare for family practice. An intern gains experience by being an apprentice under the supervision of residents and practicing physicians and having day-to-day (interns may work 75 to 100 hours per week) responsibility for the care of acutely ill hospitalized patients. He or she will interview and examine the patient, evaluate laboratory tests to establish the diagnosis, and then order and direct therapy for a newly admitted patient. He or she will usually make daily "rounds" with the attending physician (a faculty member of the medical school or hospital) and so learn through consultation as well as actual doing. He also may receive formal lectures on various areas of medicine. Interns also are now caring for ambulatory (or walking) outpatients, so they can learn more about personal and community problems that affect health care. After internship, a physician usually takes the state licensing examination. If successful, he is licensed to practice medicine in that state only. In order to practice in other states, the physician is required to take additional examinations in each state where he wishes to practice. This policy has increased the shortage of physicians in some areas, and an organization known as the National Board of Medical Examiners is trying to develop an examination that will be acceptable to all states.

RESIDENCY AND SPECIALIZATION   Residency is a three- to five-year program, generally in a hospital, in which a physician receives his specialty training. Because the majority of his teachers in medical

Figure 28.8 Medical training. Each medical school sets its own standards for the years spent in the various stages of medical education. Current opinion among medical educators seems to indicate that the process should be compressed either by admitting students to medical school after the sophomore year or by shortening the time spent in preclinical study.

school were technical experts and specialists, the physician has been encouraged in subtle and not-so-subtle ways to choose a specialty. Given this background, and the fact that the general practitioner is usually accorded the lowest status, it is not surprising that approximately 90 percent of young physicians choose a speciality. Residency training is similar to internship training in that it is a master-apprenticeship approach. A list of the major specialties, and their definitions, appears in Table 28.2.

After his residency training, the completion of two years of full-time specialty practice, and the passage of a written and oral examination, the physician receives a diploma in his specialty and is called a "Diplomate." He is then considered to be "Board Certified" or "Boarded" in his specialty.

"Board Certified Specialist" and "Diplomate" are synonomous terms. "Board Eligible" describes a physician who has completed all the training requirements but not the examination. Diplomates are listed in the *Directory of Medical Specialists*, which is available in many libraries.

Other physicians take a different route of specialization, even though they will not qualify for inclusion in the Directory. Some complete fewer than the required years of residency training, others simply become interested in a specialty area and concentrate their practice in that area. While not "Board Certified" specialists, they may well acquire competence equal to that of their Diplomate colleagues. As is generally the case in the health professions, certification by a professional

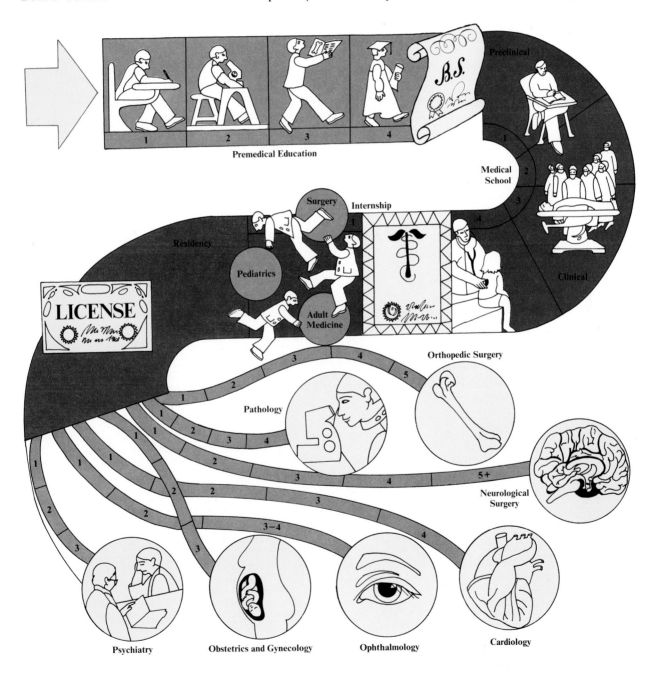

Table 28.2   Medical Specialties

SPECIALTY	*Definition*
Allergy	The study, diagnosis, and treatment of the altered reactions of the body to specific substances that produce allergic diseases in sensitive persons
Anesthesiology	The work of administering general and local anesthetics to reduce sensitivity to pain before an operation
Cardiovascular disease	The study of the structure and function of the heart and blood vessels and the diagnosis and and treatment of those diseases
Dermatology	The science of the skin: the structure, function, and diseases of the skin and the treatment of those diseases
Endocrinology	The study of the endocrine glands and their internal secretions and the treatment of their disorders
Gastroenterology	The study of the stomach and intestines and the treatment of their diseases
Hematology	The study of the nature, function, and diseases of the blood; the treatment of blood diseases
Internal medicine	Generally, that branch of medicine that is concerned with diseases that do not require surgery; specifically, the study and treatment of internal organs and body systems; it encompasses many of the subspecialties listed in this table; internists, the doctors who practice internal medicine, often serve as family physicians to supervise general medical care
Neurology	The science of the anatomy and physiology of the nervous system; the treatment of physical disorders of the system
Neurological surgery	A surgical specialty dealing with operations on the brain and nervous system
Obstetrics and gynecology	Obstetrics is concerned with the care of women during pregnancy, labor, and immediately after childbirth; gynecology is concerned with the diseases of the sexual and reproductive organs of women
Ophthalmology	The science of the structure, function, and diseases of the eye; the ophthalmologist diagnoses and treats problems of vision, including prescribing eyeglasses
Orthopedic surgery	The corrective treatment of deformities and diseases of the bones, muscles, and joints
Otology, laryngology, and rhinology (ear, nose, and throat)	The study of the anatomy and physiology of the ear, nose, and throat; the treatment of diseases affecting these organs
Pathology	Generally, the study of the nature, cause, and effects of disease, including changes in structure and function of the body; the pathologist does not see patients but works in a laboratory directing the work of technicians and examining body tissues and fluids
Pediatrics	The study and treatment of children's diseases; the pediatrician also supervises the maintenance of health care for children and coordinates any services a child needs from other specialists
Physical medicine (physiatry)	The application of treatments aiming toward the physical reconditioning and rehabilitation of diseased and disabled persons; coordination of physical and occupational therapy; supervision of the use of massage, exercise, heat, and other methods; closely akin to rehabilitation medicine
Plastic surgery	Surgical procedures used to reconstruct and reshape skin and bones; the repair of absent or defective tissue
Proctology	The science of the structure, function, and diseases of the anus and rectum; treatment of their diseases
Psychiatry	The study and treatment of mental disease and emotional disorder
Public health	The field of community or population health; the effort to undertake large-scale measures to prevent disease that individuals cannot perform for themselves; includes the study of environmental conditions that affect the cause and transmission of disease (epidemiology) and the provision of public services to maintain community health
Pulmonary disease	The diagnosis and treatment of diseases of the lungs
Radiology and roentgenology	The branch of medicine that deals with x-rays and other radioactive substances in the diagnosis and treatment of disease
Surgery (general)	The branch of medicine that deals with diseases that require operation or manipulation; general surgeons perform operations on any part of the body; surgical specialists limit themselves to particular organs or areas; upon receiving their M.D. degree and state license to practice, all doctors are considered "physicians and surgeons" and are allowed to do surgery
Thoracic surgery	Surgery of the chest
Urology	The study and treatment of diseases and abnormalities of the urogenital tract in men (the urine, kidney, bladder, male sex organs) and the urinary tract (excluding sex organs) in women

Source: Adapted from R. H. Blum. *The Commonsense Guide to Doctors, Hospitals, and Medical Care.* New York: Macmillan, 1964.

CAN DOCTORS CAUSE DISEASE?

by Norman Cousins

A cardinal rule for physicians, ancient even in the time of Hippocrates, is *primum non nocere* (first: do no harm). This admonition is the traditional opening lesson in the education of medical students. Dr. Oliver Wendell Holmes would seldom give a medical lecture without making some reference to the harm caused by doctors who followed the homeopathic ideas of Samuel Hahnemann, an eighteenth-century German physician who advocated giving patients more of whatever poison was supposed to be troubling them, along with a wide range of bizarre, gizzard-wrenching purgatives. To Dr. Holmes, the wonder was not that some human beings treated in this fashion should recover but that any should survive.

More recently, one of America's most accomplished diagnosticians, the late Dr. Emanuel Libman, was asked by a medical student to summarize the reasons for his success. Dr. Libman had a simple answer. Patients who came to him were never content unless they left clutching a prescription—whether they needed it or not. "So I give it to them," he said. "But mark this well: I am always damned sure that if what I prescribe doesn't help, at least it isn't going to hurt."

This advice may be simple and it is certainly traditional; but it hasn't been sufficiently observed—not through the centuries of recorded medical history and not even in our time. For the standard ideas of what constitutes safe and essential treatment haven't always turned out to be in the human interest. It wasn't so long ago that the routine way of combating illness—all the way from abdominal distress to a head cold—was to draw off a patient's blood. Generally, the incision for the blood-letting was made as close to the site of the pain as possible.

George Washington died shortly after such a procedure. He was suffering from heavy chest congestion and a high fever. Even before the physician arrived, a servant set about extracting blood from the General's veins. When the doctor arrived, the blood-letting was intensified. Washington became increasingly weak. This was apparently regarded by the doctor as an indication that the blood was not being drawn off in sufficient volume or swiftly enough, for the process was accelerated. The medical report doesn't specify the exact quantity that was extracted, but it does say that three separate blood-lettings were undertaken, the first of which yielded more than a pint. The General not only did not benefit from these strenuous efforts but went into shock and died.

Today's physicians would have no difficulty in recognizing that the profuse loss of blood, quite apart from its enfeebling effect, had resulted in a fatal loss of oxygen to Washington's brain. What is significant here is not just that General Washington was the victim of poor treatment but that eminent men of medicine of his time didn't know any better.

Today's doctors are appalled at the lethal ignorance represented by blood-letting and drastic purging, just as the physicians of Washington's day were appalled by the medical practices of a century or more earlier—and just as medical men a century from now will no doubt be appalled by much of what appears today to be enlightened medi-

Adapted from Cousins, N. "Can Doctors Cause Disease?" *Saturday Review* (August 22, 1970), pp. 30-32.

cal practice and procedure. Indeed, responsible leaders within the medical profession itself today are expressing growing concern over the quality of health care. A term that appears with increasing frequency in current medical literature is "iatrogenic" illness—that is, illness caused by physicians in the act of treating their patients.

A recent example of iatrogenic illness is the woman who was given potassium pills by her doctor. The pills had a protective coating, enabling them to resist the digestive acids of the stomach and dissolve in the lower intestine. Instead of dissolving properly, however, the pills lodged in the pleats of the intestines, where they caused severely painful symptoms. The correct diagnosis was not made until after three surgical operations in which the appendix and the gall bladder were mistakenly removed. Apart from the expense, which ran close to $50,000, the woman was hospitalized for almost five months before the correct correlation was made between the potassium pills and her abdominal symptoms. How many surgical operations in other cases have been performed because of these potassium pills no one knows.

Few medicines have produced as many iatrogenic illnesses as antibiotics; current medical literature is replete with examples of side effects that are often more serious or severe than the illnesses the antibiotics were supposed to combat. Cases have been recorded in which antibiotics have depressed the bone marrow, leading to anemia. Obviously, there are times when the physician has no choice except to use antibiotics. In the case of a child suffering from a serious infection of the inner ear, it would be unnecessarily hazardous not to administer antibiotics. But it is also true that antibiotics are prescribed in many cases when they are not absolutely indicated. In fairness to the physician, however, it should be pointed out that many patients do not feel they are being properly treated unless the doctor gives them antibiotics.

That is why it is so important for the public to be educated in the limitations and dangers of antibiotics. Perhaps more information about these drugs would make people a little more hesitant to put pressure on their doctors to prescribe antibiotics for everything from a sniffle to gastritis.

Ability of individuals to take drugs varies widely. Some people cannot tolerate aspirin, even in small doses. Most people are adversely affected by aspirin in very high doses. Yet the public has the impression that aspirin can be taken in virtually unlimited quantities without adverse effect. This is a dangerous misconception. In large doses, aspirin can damage the hearing or cause dangerous hemorrhages from the gastrointestinal tract. Yet some of the nation's best hospitals do not hesitate to administer two dozen aspirin tablets a day to a patient over a period of weeks. There is no question about the fact that pain can be held in check with such high dosages; the relevant question, however, is whether grave dangers are being courted.

Problems such as these come under the heading of iatrogenic illness. Unnecessary surgery or faulty surgery also comes under this heading. The promiscuous nature of surgery has been a matter of severe concern within the medical profession itself in recent years. Of sixty hysterectomy cases investigated in one study, only thirty-five showed clear-cut evidence calling for such surgery. Most of the other cases, the report said, could have been adequately treated by dilatation and curettage.

It is a serious error to suppose that any surgical operation is an inconsequential matter. To begin with, anytime a patient enters a hospital he runs a certain risk, whether from maltreatment by improperly (or even properly) trained personnel, or from infections caused by improper sterilization or handling of needles or other instruments, or from faulty sanitation, or from errors in filling prescriptions, or from overdoses of medication, or from errors in the administration of anesthesia, or from surgery, or even from falling on wet floors.

Almost by definition, a hospital is a collection center for diseases, infectious or otherwise. There is scarcely a hospital in the country in which patients have not contracted staphylococcus infections on the premises. Until recently, even the most severe hospital-bred infections could be combated effectively with high-potency antibiotics. Because of new resistant strains of microorganisms, however, doctors can no longer feel as confident as they once did about the use of antibiotics in hospital situations—or in any situation, for that matter.

To some extent, iatrogenic illnesses are directly related to the fact that there are too many patients and too few doctors, with the result that doctors are unable to provide the kind of attention that good practice requires.

According to professional surveys, the traffic has been built up to the point where many doctors have a daily case load of forty to fifty patients. Even if this number is averaged against a ten-hour day, it leaves about twelve minutes per patient. It may be said that the face-to-face time a doctor spends with a patient is not a matter of great consequence in view of all the diagnostic aids and assistants available to him. This is not sound comment. The time spent directly with a patient is not an inconsequential matter. The great Canadian physician-philosopher Sir William Osler declared that nothing a doctor can do is more essential to an accurate diagnosis and the welfare of his patient than providing ample time to hear him out. The modern practitioner, however, surrounded by electronic devices and laboratory tests, tends to become impatient with a patient's recital of his multiple symptoms and can hardly wait to get on with a blood count, sedimentation rate, electrocardiogram, or sundry other tests. Meanwhile, the key to the case may be submerged somewhere in the oral account, however rambling or disconnected.

Fortunately, there is an increasing disposition in many medical schools throughout the country to rethink the problems of "modern" medicine. The highly touted system of computerized medicine is being reconsidered. So is the tendency to make the patient's own story secondary to the battery of diagnostic tests. And there is increasing respect for the ability of the human body to prescribe for itself and to repair itself, given reasonable peace, a good diet, and an environment free of tension.

The good doctor brings all his natural and trained intelligence to bear on these vital questions: When to intervene, when not to intervene, and to what precise extent? To what degree, in any given case, should he attempt to enhance or augment the natural drive of the human body to prescribe effectively for itself? What are the factors—however elusive or complex—of individual variability that have a bearing on a precise diagnosis? Every patient, in a sense, puts his own and unique stamp on his disease.

Finally, the good doctor is not only a scientist but a philosopher. He knows that the facts of medicine will continue to change and that, therefore, his professional training can never be an absolute guide to good practice. It is his philosophy of medicine that has to serve as the solid base of his practice. The doctor's respect for life, his special qualities of compassion and tenderness—even under the most devilish of circumstances—these are the vital ingredients of his art. To such a doctor, the most exotic diagnostic machines are not more important than the simple act of sitting at the bedside of a patient. In this sense, the ultimate art of the good doctor is to make good patients. He does this by making the patient a full partner in his recovery. Such a doctor is worth all the recognition and reward a society is capable of offering.

association is more a guideline to choosing a physician with a competent base than a guarantee of individual excellence.

Selected Medical Practitioners

This category comprises those practitioners who function independently of physicians. Many, but not all, undergo a specified training leading to the granting of a degree.

Clinical psychologists are Ph.D.'s. They engage primarily in the diagnosis and treatment of mental illness in hospitals, clinics, and private practice. They also serve as consultants to community mental health programs and to school systems. Many are engaged in direct, basic, and applied research on problems related to their concerns. The training of a clinical psychologist, in addition to research training and experience, entails three to four years of post-baccalaureate graduate studies, including a year of supervised internship in an appropriate setting prior to the granting of the Ph.D. degree in clinical psychology.

Optometrists examine the eyes and related structures to determine the presence of visual abnormalities. They prescribe and adapt lenses or other optical aids and may use visual training aids to preserve or restore maximum efficiency of vision. They do not prescribe drugs, diagnose or treat eye diseases, or perform surgery. A license to practice optometry is required in all states. To qualify for a license, the applicant must be a graduate of a college of optometry that confers the Doctor of Optometry degree (O.D.) and pass a state board examination. A few states require a period of internship. Two years of preoptometry education at an accredited college is required before entry into the four-year curriculum at one of the eleven colleges of optometry in the nation.

Podiatry concerns itself with the examination, diagnosis, prevention, treatment, and care of conditions and functions of the human foot. The podiatrist may perform foot surgery, prescribe corrective devices, and prescribe and administer drugs and physical therapy. More than 8,000 podiatrists (Doctor of Podiatric Medicine, or D.P.M.) are in practice in the United States. To receive a license to practice, an applicant must have graduated from one of the five colleges of podiatry in the nation and passed a board examination.

Other types of practitioners, not adhering to orthodox medical concepts, are rapidly disappearing from the contemporary health scene. *Chiropractors* (Doctors of Chiropractic, or D.C.'s) and *naturopaths* (Doctors of Naturopathy, or D.N.'s) approach treatment in much the same way—through physical therapy, diet, and psychosomatic counseling—although from a different conceptual view of disease (chiropractors see it caused by minor displacements of the spine irritating the peripheral nerves, while naturopaths view it as upsets of the body balance due to interference with the natural forces that normally support it). Neither chiropractors nor naturopaths are granted hospital privileges and they must refer their patients to an M.D. or D.O. for hospitalization. *Christian Science practitioners* (selected church members with in-house training) view healing as a by-product of a way of life and provide spiritual ministry of prayer and help toward religious or moral problems, rather than medical diagnosis and treatment; in fact, the use of orthodox medicine and medication is not allowed by the church, except when required by law. *Lay-midwives*, women with limited education and apprenticeship training, are still found in low economic or rural areas where the delivery of a baby occurs usually in the home. They are licensed or registered practitioners in twenty-three states, while in others they may practice under annual permits.

Medical Allied Manpower

This category includes some sixty occupations or specialties that can be divided into two large categories based on time required for occupational training. The first category includes those occupations that require at least a baccalaureate degree, for example, clinical laboratory scientists and technologists, dietitians and nutritionists, health educators, medical record librarians, and occupational, speech, and rehabilitation therapists. The second group includes those occupations that require less than a baccalaureate degree, such as aides for each of the above categories, as well as physician assistants and radiologic technicians.

Figure 28.9 indicates projected employment for medicine and allied health services from 1950 to 1980. Even though personnel will triple during that time, serious shortages will still exist. Interest is rapidly developing in new educational programs geared to expand medical allied manpower, particularly in the post-baccalaureate category.

Doctor of Dental Surgery (D.D.S.)

Although the fifty-two dental schools in the nation require at least two and preferably three years of predental education, more than half of dental students have a bachelor's degree before entering dental school. The first two years of dental school emphasize the basic sciences; in some cases, medical and dental students take these courses together. During the second two years, students provide dental treatment to patients under the supervision of clinical instructors and learn to properly utilize the skills of the dental auxiliaries. Dental school graduates receive the degree of D.D.S. (Doctor of Dental Surgery) or its equivalent D.M.D. (Doctor of Medical Dentistry). To qualify for licensure in a state, dental school graduates must pass both a written and a clinical examination. A dentist may choose to specialize by limiting his practice to one of eight specialties listed in Table 28.3. He may make his specialty "official" by passing the American Board of Dental Examiners and becoming a Diplomate.

Dental Allied Manpower

The *Dental hygienist* is the only dental auxiliary who needs a license to practice. Licensure is necessary because the hygienist provides services directly to the patient. Some of his or her duties include scaling and polishing teeth, exposing and processing dental x-ray films, applying fluoride to children's teeth, and instructing patients in toothbrushing techniques and proper diet in relation to teeth. Most dental hygienists choose a two-year college program that leads to a certificate or diploma in dental hygiene or an Associate of Arts degree. Some choose a four-year bachelor's degree program that enables the dental hygienist to assume a leadership role in teaching and public health.

The *dental assistant* prepares the patient for treatment, mixes filling materials, passes instruments, handles the exposure and processing of x-ray films, sterilizes instruments, assists with laboratory work,

Table 28.3   Dental Specialties

SPECIALTY	Description
Endodontics	Treatment of interior tissues of the teeth such as pulp capping and root-canal therapy
Oral pathology	Diagnosis of mouth tissues, tumors, and injuries
Oral surgery	Surgical treatment of oral diseases, injuries, and defects of the jaw
Orthodontics	Straightening of teeth
Pedodontics	Dentistry for children
Periodontics	Treatment of gums and underlying bone
Prosthodontics	Providing artificial replacements for missing teeth
Public health dentistry	Prevention and control of dental diseases and promotion of dental health through public education

Figure 28.9   Projected employment for medicine and allied services 1950–1980.

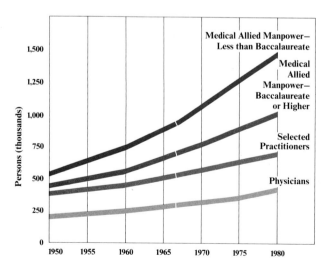

and keeps office records and accounts. In the past, dental assistants have been trained on-the-job by their dentist-employers. The trend is now toward a one-, and sometimes two-, year course in a community college.

Dental laboratory technicians are skilled craftsmen who perform many tasks involved in the construction of complete and partial dentures, fixed bridgework, crowns, and other dental restorations and appliances. Technicians do not have direct contact with patients but perform their work in accordance with instructions received from the dentist. Although a few dental laboratory technicians are employed in a dental office and work directly for a dentist, most are employed in commercial dental laboratories that serve the majority of the nation's dentists. Most dental laboratory technicians have received their training on-the-job in commercial laboratories or dental offices.

Figure 28.10 depicts projected employment for dentistry and allied services from 1950 to 1980. If the pressing demands for dental care are to be met in the future, dentists will have to utilize ever-increasing numbers of auxiliary personnel, especially dental hygienists and dental assistants.

Registered Nurses

Registered nurses are responsible for carrying out the physician's instructions. They supervise practical nurses and other auxiliary personnel who perform routine care and treatment of patients. Registered nurses provide nursing care to patients or perform specialized duties in a variety of settings from hospitals and clinics to schools and public health departments.

A license to practice nursing is required in all states. For licensure as a registered nurse (R.N.), an applicant must have graduated from a school of nursing approved by the state board for nursing and have passed a state board examination. Nurs-

ing schools provide three programs of nursing education, all of which prepare persons for licensure as R.N.'s and require at least graduation from high school prior to entry. The *associate-degree programs*, usually located in community colleges, are two years in length. *Diploma programs* are conducted by hospital schools and normally require three years of training. The third approach is the *baccalaureate* program, which usually requires four years of study in a college or university, although a few require five years.

The *nurse-midwife* is a registered nurse who has successfully completed a recognized six- to eight-month program, plus clinical experience leading to a certificate in nurse-midwifery. An alternate method for obtaining a certificate requires a master's degree in nursing and additional education in midwifery ranging from twelve to twenty-four months. The nurse-midwife cares for the mother during pregnancy and stays with her in labor, providing continuous physical and emotional support. She manages the labor and delivery, watchful for signs requiring the attention of a physician. She helps the mother to care for herself and her infant and to adjust the home situation to the new child. The nurse-midwife functions as a member of the obstetrical team in medical centers, institutions, universities, and community health projects with active programs of nurse-midwifery. The number of nurse-midwives has shown a steady increase in recent years, with most located in the eastern United States.

Nursing Allied Manpower

Practical nurses, also known as vocational nurses, provide nursing care and treatment of patients under the supervision of a licensed physician or registered nurse. Licensure as a licensed practical nurse (L.P.N.), or in California and Texas as a licensed vocational nurse (L.V.N.), is required by

Figure 28.10   Projected employment for dentistry and allied services 1950–1980.

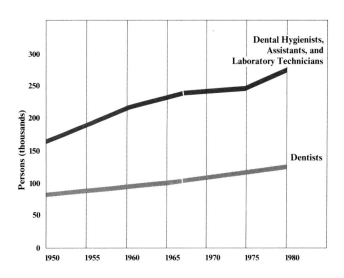

law in all states. To obtain it, an applicant must graduate from a state-approved school of practical nursing and pass a state board examination. Most states require at least two years of high school for admission to a practical nursing school program, which is usually twelve to eighteen months long.

Auxiliary nursing workers in hospitals and nursing homes function as assistants to nurses in providing many services related to the comfort and welfare of patients. *Nursing aides*, usually women, assist registered and practical nurses by performing less skilled tasks in the care of patients. *Orderlies* and *attendants*, usually men, assist by performing a variety of duties for male patients and certain heavy duties in the care of the physically ill, mentally ill, and mentally retarded. Although there are no definite educational requirements for these three classifications, on-the-job training programs provided by hospitals and clinics may include classroom instruction, demonstration, and practice taught by a registered nurse. The training program may last several months, depending on the hospital.

Figure 28.11 depicts projected employment of nursing and related personnel from 1950 to 1980. Severe shortages now exist and it is expected that these shortages will continue into the 1980s.

QUACKERY

A "quack" is a pretender to medical skill, a medical charlatan. "Quackery" is the practice of medicine by such a pretender. This definition is usually broadened to include all those who promote *false health information* for personal gain. Quackery in the United States is big business: it costs the public more than 2 billion dollars a year, not including the less obvious forms of quackery that may take place within the boundaries of certified medicine and medications. But worse than the financial waste, some forms of quackery cause injury, disability, or even—and not too infrequently—death. According to John Miner, Assistant District Attorney of Los Angeles County, quackery kills more people than all crimes of violence put together.

How do quacks get away with it? Some of their clients who survive and realize they have been duped are often too embarrassed to turn to the proper authorities. Others may be afraid or do not know where to turn for assistance. On the rare occasions when charlatans are convicted of quackery, the penalty is so slight in proportion to the huge profits they make that it does not act as a deterrant. In most states, the crime is considered a misdemeanor and is punishable by a few months in jail or by a small fine.

Why Quacks Succeed

Complete understanding of the success of quacks will probably have to await a better understanding of man himself. For now, their success is attributed to man's fear of pain, illness, aging, and death and, in recent times, sense of social isolation. Fear, hopelessness, and loneliness can drive even the intelligent, informed person to accept the panaceas offered by the quack.

As a nation, the United States has progressed rapidly in science and technology. It is difficult for people, proud and awed by these achievements, to accept an admission of ignorance on the part of the medical profession concerning the etiology and treatment of certain diseases. They have been conditioned to accept miracles and tend to gullibly accept the quack's promises. Interestingly, each achievement of legitimate medical research seems to open new and lucrative avenues to the enterprising charlatan. Many conditions from which man suffers are self-correcting: they will improve with or without competent treatment. This fact is a tremendous ally of the quack. He can call any condition "cancer," prescribe a miracle preparation, and when the patient recovers, the quack has a convert,

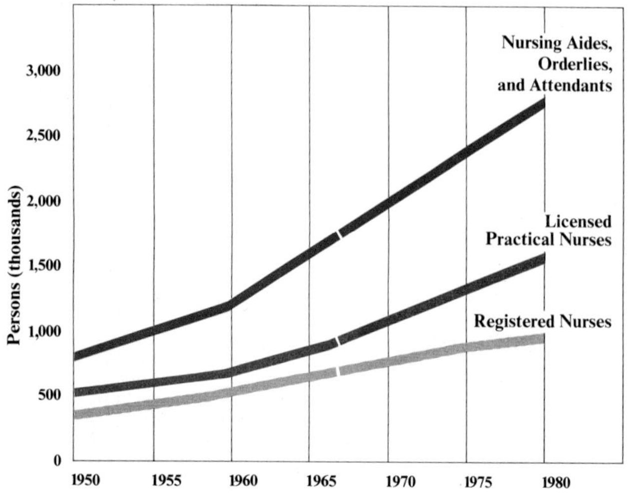

Figure 28.11 Projected employment for nursing and related services 1950–1980.

a person who will be happy to speak on his "doctor's" behalf or write testimonials in support of his treatment.

Whenever it is commonly known that physicians do not completely understand the cause or the cure for a particular disease, the field is wide open for quacks. Quacks have come up with "cures" for cancer, the common cold, obesity, and aging. Some of the worthless swindles in the health field include remedies for anemia or "tired blood" preparations, baldness cures, bust developers, treatments for diabetes, hemorrhoids (piles), impotency, psoriasis, pyorrhea, and ulcers. The list is virtually endless, and yet promoters reap rich rewards from an often unsuspecting public.

Arthritis quackery will serve as a good example. The number of worthless treatments is endless and continues to grow through the ingenuity of the

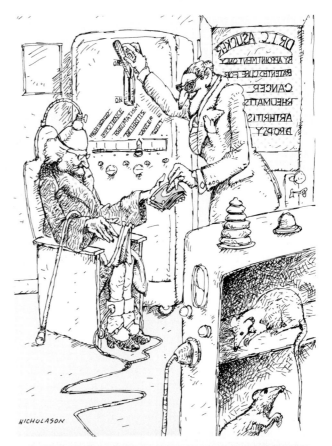

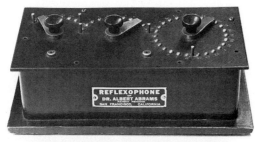

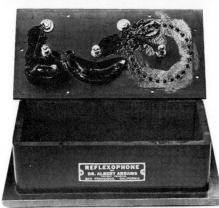

Figure 28.12 Medical quackery is one of the most lucrative and destructive aspects of the "con game." Each year millions of desperate people seek treatment that does nothing but allow the ailment to become more severe. One of the most valuable aids to proper treatment is the educated patient who seeks early treatment and recognizes the inflated rhetoric and claims of the "medical" charlatan. (*above*) The "Reflexophone" was touted as a miraculous discovery—disease was cancelled out by matching its "disease frequency" with the same frequency on the machine. (*right*) The elaborate machinery pictured here typifies the facade of technological complexity displayed by quacks to their "victims."

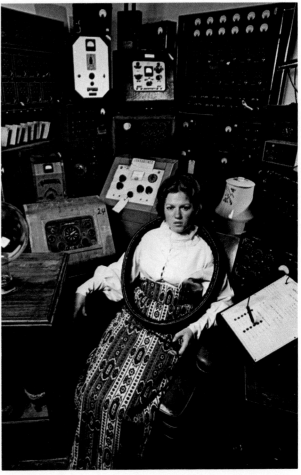

charlatan. "Therapeutic" devices such as vibrators, copper bracelets, magnetic rings, colored lights, and so-called radioactive materials have always enjoyed brisk sales. Arthritis quackery is so successful that it amounts to nearly half a billion dollars a year. For every dollar spent on legitimate research on the cause and cure of arthritis, more than 25 dollars will be spent on useless quack "cures" and remedies.

Another psychosocial factor that plays in favor of quackery is the belief by many that the greater the cost of a treatment, the more effective it must be. Plain aspirin is helpful in reducing the pain from which arthritics or other ailing persons suffer. Capitalizing on this fact, fraudulent promoters have included the basic ingredient, acetylsalicylic acid, in a variety of pills and capsules and made fantastic claims for them. Analysis has shown these products to be no more than glorified aspirin—but they do not sell at aspirin prices.

Health Advertising

The modern version of the tribal "medicine man," promoting unnecessary and often harmful "health" products and devices, prospers today as never before. Through the use of the printed word, radio, and television, he has found new and effective ways to mislead more victims and misrepresent more "medical" wares.

Professional medical societies prohibit personal advertising and patient solicitation as unethical. However, the practitioner may, with the blessing of his society, list his name, degree, and specialty in the telephone directory, in the directory of his office building and on his office door, and announce in the local newspaper that he is establishing a practice or moving it to another location. Yet there are more subtle promotions that are not frowned on. Although the American Medical Association will extend membership to any licensed physician who

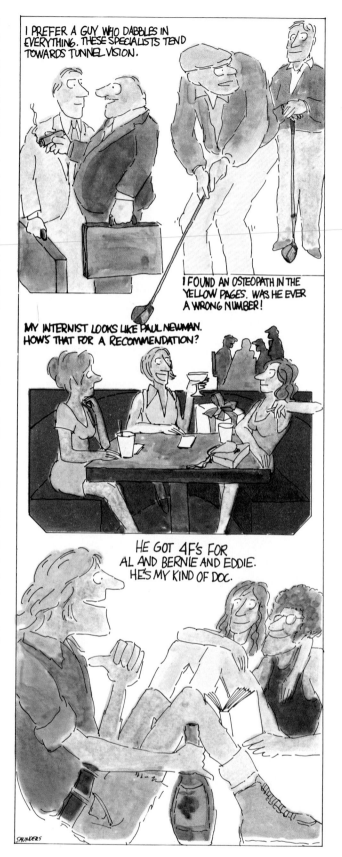

Figure 28.13 A few of the wrong ways to choose a doctor.

is a member of his local medical society, many patients assume that AMA membership is a warranty of some extra competence. It is difficult for someone without a family doctor—for example, a new arrival in town—to find a good physician. People may depend on the opinions of friends, but it is difficult to evaluate the technical competence of medical practitioners. Social exposure—the cocktail party or the club routes—a reputable office address, or an elaborate decor are accepted ways of enhancing the practitioner's prestige. But one must remember that the gain of additional patients and financial success through such "advertising" does not automatically contribute to the practitioner's professional competence.

Much of today's "health" advertising encourages people to prescribe medication or treatment for themselves. Commercials may list common symptoms of fatigue, aches, inability to sleep, or tension and then suggest that if one has any of these, he may be suffering from———. Then, they suggest a product with the hope that the person will prescribe it for himself.

The "legitimate" drug industry itself plays similar games. Over-the-counter, or OTC, drugs (that can be sold without medical prescriptions), as well as prescription drugs themselves, are approved by the Federal Drug Administration after sometimes a less than complete examination. But both are frequently advertised with misleading statements or presented as great improvements, at a greater cost, over their less elaborately touted but no less effective main active ingredient.

Recognizing Quackery

Although many agencies and laws are supposedly designed to protect the consumer from quackery and fraud, the best line of defense is an informed public. Quackery, of one kind or another, often fol-lows certain patterns. The following questions were designed to guide their recognition.

1. Does the sponsor claim that he is battling the medical profession, which is attempting to suppress his wonderful discovery? Does he maintain that surgery, x-ray, or medication prescribed by a reputable physician will do more harm than good?
2. Is the remedy sold from door to door by a self-styled "health adviser" or promoted from town to town in lectures to the public? Is it promoted in a sensational magazine, by a faith healer's group, or by a crusading organization of laymen?
3. Does the sponsor use scare techniques, predicting all sorts of harmful consequences if the product is not used?
4. Is the product or service offered as a "secret" remedy or a heavily camouflaged one?
5. Does the promoter show people "testimonials"—or use medically associated cue words or images—to demonstrate the wonders that his product or service has performed for others?
6. Is the product or service claimed to be good for a vast array of illnesses or guaranteed to provide a quick cure?

The more crass forms of quackery could be readily recognized through some of the above criteria. Others, however, may be subtle enough to demand more detailed knowledge on the part of the consumer. Unfortunately, the buyer is generally left to rely on the seller for most information about health, a problem in this society, where many sellers are not only neglecting to provide information upon which the consumer can make a decision but are in fact trying to obscure relevant information. At present, the protection of the individual must focus on better consumer and health education, providing the base for sound, independent decisions about one's health choices and purchases. Hopefully, the day will come when "caveat venditor" (let the seller beware) will be the cry of the health marketplace; until that time, the buyer had better beware.

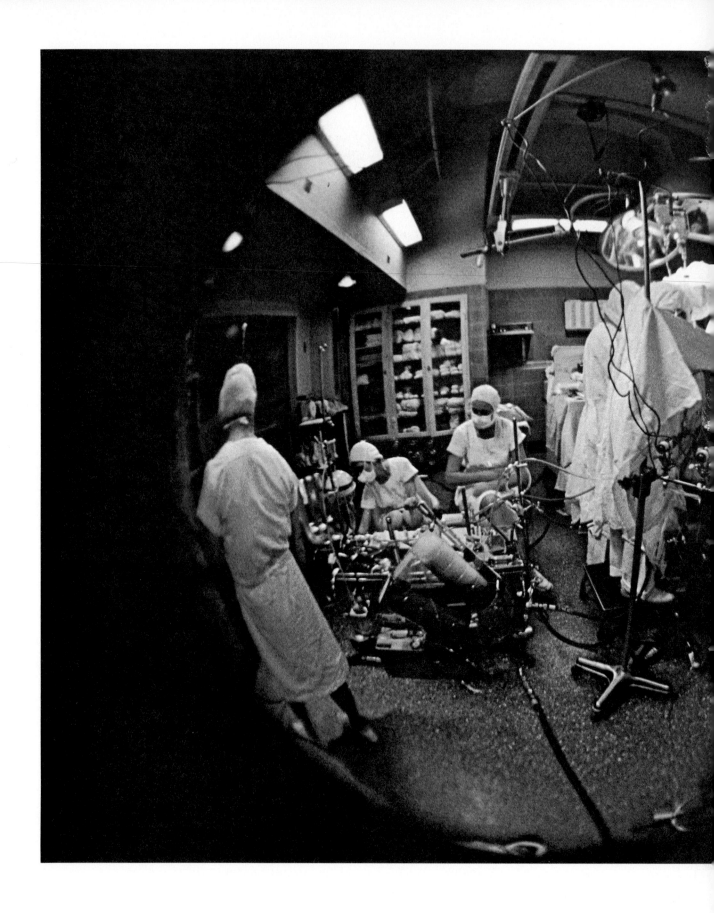

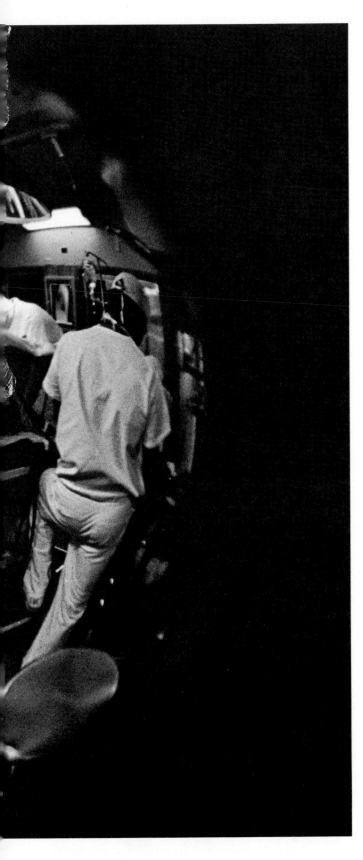

29

Chapter 28 provided some information on the organizations and the people who handle the health care of the nation. It discussed some of the deficiencies and some of the pitfalls of the present system but also noted the extensive training provided to the reputable professionals and the concern for the public health that institutions are increasingly developing. Where does the United States stand in comparison to other nations with respect to medical care?

There is agreement among public health authorities that infant mortality and life expectancy are among the best and most sensitive indices of the true level of health in a population even though these factors also depend upon nonmedical health conditions. By such criteria, it becomes clear that this nation is not doing as well as it should. Each year, the United States loses twenty-two out of every 1,000 babies born alive; as many as eighteen countries lose fewer babies, yet in 1953 only seven countries had lower infant mortality rates. Furthermore, American men have lower life expectancies than those in seventeen other countries, while women in nine other countries have longer life expectancies than American women. And yet, each year the United States spends more money per person and a greater percentage of its Gross National Product on health care than does any other nation.

The deficiency in the American medical care system is not one of quality; the United States has the finest facilities anywhere in the world, and American medical research is second to none. The

Health Care Delivery

deficiency area is the *delivery system* — the inability to bring this excellent medical care equally to *all* the people. A close look at the present system reveals that this inability stems from a whole set of problems, ranging from manpower shortages to skyrocketing costs.

PROBLEM AREAS

The rapid evolution in medical technology, social structures, and public concern over the past three decades has not been paralleled by a corresponding evolution of its health education and health-care systems.

Health Manpower

There are more than two hundred careers involved in caring for the health of Americans, including medical scientists, architects, sociologists, economists, pharmacists, and administrators. More than 3.5 million people, or about 5 percent of the total civilian labor force, are employed in the health-services field. Health workers now outnumber construction and agricultural workers, who once had the largest representation in the work force. Obviously, health manpower comprises many people other than the health practitioners described in Chapter 28. If there are deficiencies in today's health manpower, they can hardly be in terms of the overall numbers. In fact, the most readily detectable manpower problems lie in the health practitioner category and involve the number and distribution of physicians and an inadequate involvement of other professionals.

SHORTAGE OF PHYSICIANS   There are about 150 practicing physicians (which includes interns, residents, and military physicians) for every 100,000 persons in the United States, or about one physician for every 670 people. Although this relationship seems barely tolerable, the situation would be even worse were it not for foreign medical graduates working in the United States, who comprise about 14 percent of the nation's practicing physicians and about 28 percent of its interns and residents.

Distressing as these figures may be, they still fail to convey the true situation in terms of real availability of physicians to the average patient. The fact is that among today's medical doctors specialists outnumber general practitioners by two to one. This ratio has increased markedly over the years: In 1931, 125,000 of the 150,000 practicing physicians (83 percent) were family doctors; in 1967 115,000 of 303,000 (40 percent) were family doctors. Physician specialization has been encouraged in many forms but has not been channeled in any way whatsoever: the patients' needs have never been considered in the development of specialists. Specialists tend to focus on a particular area (dermatology, cardiology, obstetrics, and so on) and are hardly in a position to care for the whole patient. Clearly, specialists do not service as many patients as the same number of general practitioners could. The ratio of specialists to general practitioners will, if anything, get worse, because only 12 percent of medical school graduates in recent years have been entering general practice. In order to correct this trend, general practice was elevated to the specialty of Family Medicine in 1969 in hopes of providing more status and encouraging more doctors to choose the field.

In 1970, America's 107 medical schools accepted 10,000 freshman students but had to turn down another 15,000 well-qualified applicants. Medical schools are experiencing severe financial problems at the time when they are being pressed to take in more students. In a recent year, forty-three medical schools had to receive special financial distress grants from the government so that they could continue operations. Experts in the fields of public health, medical economics, and government have been sounding the alarm for years. Yet, from 1930

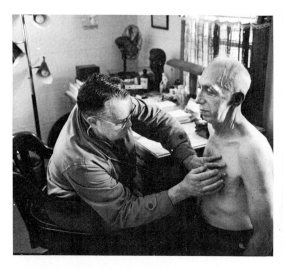
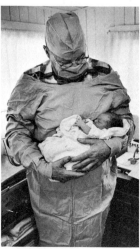
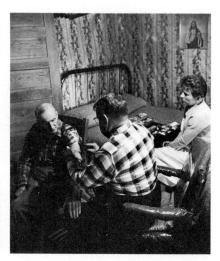

until recently the American Medical Association (AMA) has lobbied against attempts to increase physician output. Although this pressure was initially an important method of quality control, the AMA has been accused of keeping the supply of physicians down so that doctors would be assured of high demand and excellent incomes. On the AMA's side, it is clear that the current numbers of physicians would be adequate if they could be utilized more effectively.

DISTRIBUTION OF PHYSICIANS Traditionally, the development of American medicine has been permissive; Americans have allowed and, in a sense, even encouraged physicians to practice where they want, what they want, and for the people they want. Physician availability varies greatly from state to state and among different areas within a state's boundary. Therefore, average figures—on the national, state, or even county level—often hide gross inadequacies and inefficient manpower utilization. Mississippi, for example, has about one-third as many physicians, relative to its population, as has New York state—69 for every 100,000 people as compared to 203 per 100,000. One study of four upper-midwest states disclosed that over 1,000 remote towns, because of their small size and declining economic condition, did not have a single physician. One area in Los Angeles County has a physician-population ratio of a low 9 per 100,000, compared with about 1,800 per 100,000 in Beverly Hills and 125 per 100,000 for the whole county.

Given the societal premises of free enterprise, this haphazard and spotty development of medical service cannot be blamed solely on the physicians. Being in business for themselves, physicians have tended to establish their practices where they most want to live and are assured of patients who can pay their bills. As in any decision, economic as well as professional considerations were important in determining the *establishment* of health services and naturally were perpetuated in *delivering* them. Unless incentives, monetary or other, are provided for physicians to practice in underserviced areas, the present maldistribution of health services must be expected to continue—and even worsen. The shocking truth today is that some 20 million Americans are receiving inadequate health care or no care at all.

The Cost of Health Care

In 1969, the United States was spending approximately 60 billion dollars on health care—6.7 percent of its GNP (Gross National Product)—more than 290 dollars for every person in the country. In 1970, although the cost of living rose by 6.2 percent, the cost of medical services rose 7.3 percent and total health care expenditures rose 11 percent to 67 billion dollars. Of these expenditures, about 23 billion dollars was spent on physicians, dentists, and other professional services; some 30 billion for hospital and nursing-home care; 7 billion for drugs; 5.5 billion for health activities and supplies; and 4.5 billion for construction of research and medical facilities.

PROBLEMS OF HEALTH INSURANCE More people than ever before are covered by some form of health insurance, but there are still 20 to 30 million Americans without any coverage, and most policies have severe limitations—many cover only hospital care and not visits to a doctor in his office. Income seems to be a major factor in determining how much and what kind of health-insurance protection a family is provided with. Almost all persons in families with incomes of 10,000 dollars or more carry some insurance, but only 57 percent in families with incomes between 3,000 and 5,000 dollars and 36 percent in families with incomes under 3,000 dollars have any health coverage. In 1969, omitting all government outlays, insurance met

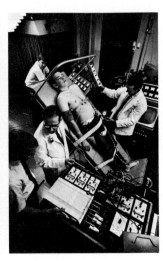

Figure 29.1 In the group of three photos on the far left are pictured the diverse tasks of the rural doctor. The rural doctor must, by necessity, practice general medicine, whereas the urban doctor (*near left*) can focus his practice on a specialized area of medicine.

about 30 percent of consumer expenditures for health care. When government programs such as Medicare are added, nearly 50 percent of expenditures were covered. Thus, out-of-pocket payments by consumers amount to approximately one-half of their health expenditures.

There are more than 1,700 different insurance carriers, offering a bewildering array of health-insurance policies that are beyond the comprehension of most Americans. The result is that millions have serious gaps in their health protection—even though they may believe to be covered—while others have double (overlapping) coverage. More than 22 million have double coverage for hospital expenses, more than 20 million have double coverage for surgical expenses, and nearly 11 million have double coverage for regular medical expenses. At the other end of the spectrum, Medicare, which was designed to help people sixty-five years old or older, covers only 45 percent of the basic

	La Jolla, Calif.	Eupora, Miss.	South Bend, Ind.
TONSILLECTOMY			
Hospital Costs			
Semiprivate Room (per day)	$ 53.00	$ 18.00	$ 39.00
Operating Room (per hour)	55.00	50.00	40.00
Lab	12.00	30.00	15.00
Miscellaneous	5.00	27.00	5.00
Surgeon's Fee	160.00	75.00	115.00
Anesthesiologist's Fee	85.00	55.00	35.00
	(per hour)	(per hour)	(25 mins.)
Total	$370.00	$255.00	$249.00
APPENDECTOMY			
Hospital Costs			
Semiprivate Room	265.00	72.00	195.00
	(five days)	(four days)	(five days)
Operating Room	90.00	50.00	61.00
Lab	12.00	21.00	20.00
Miscellaneous	5.00	27.00	8.00
Surgeon's Fee	350.00	160.00	200.00
Anesthesiologist's Fee	85.00	50.00	70.00
Total	$807.00	$330.00	$484.00
CHILDBIRTH (uncomplicated delivery)			
Hospital Costs			
Semiprivate Room	159.00	54.00	180.00
	(three days)	(three days)	(five days)
Delivery Room	85.00	25.00	100.00
			(includes anesthesia)
Lab	14.00	3.00	11.00
Nursery	81.00	22.50	72.00
Miscellaneous	——	11.50	5.00
Obstetrician's Fee	350.00	100.00	250.00
Anesthesiologist's Fee	65.00	——	——
Total	$754.00	$215.00	$618.00

health-care costs of the elderly. Medicaid, designed to subsidize health care for low-income citizens, has been underfinanced, has placed an added burden on the poorly distributed and disorganized health-care system, and has led to rising costs, causing many states to cut back on services offered.

Clearly, the haphazard approach to health insurance in the United States is not fulfilling individual needs, and there is little indication that it is capable of doing so.

RISING HEALTH-CARE EXPENDITURES Many factors are involved in the escalation of health-care expenditures. Some of them parallel escalation factors operating in other national activities—such as inflationary cost-of-living increases and overall population growth—while others are specific to the health-care activities.

When the *expansion* of health-care expenditures has been accounted for, one still finds that *costs* have gone up, apparently faster than the cost-of-living rise. Overhead costs have risen more sharply than the average. So have wages of hospital personnel, reflecting redressing of previous disparities, quality upgrading, and the shortage of trained manpower to meet an increasing demand. To the consumer, all this leads up to the cost of physicians' services going up almost twice as fast, and the cost of hospitalization going up four times as fast as the general cost-of-living (see Figure 29.3).

This expensive health care has important implications. It means that many people cannot afford it. It also means that many decisions about health care—like those about physicians' choices of a career—are being made on financial grounds rather than on the basis of medical needs.

AREAS OF POTENTIAL WASTE *Hospitalization* accounts for the largest chunk of health expenditures, and its

costs are among the fastest rising ones. It is, therefore, an area of health care where the most careful scrutiny is needed to assess potential waste or misuse. Certainly, the hospital is the best place for the very ill, but why should it be so expensive? One critical factor is that hospitals charge, and are paid, on a cost-plus basis; that is, the more they spend, the more they receive. Such a system does not encourage efficiency or economies, whether in the construction or in the operation of a hospital.

Another important factor is hospitalization practices. Hospitals traditionally have been built without careful regard to need. It is a generally accepted fact that hospital beds tend to fill up as they become available. Yet, many patients in acute hospitals today do not need to be there. Although estimates vary, it is believed that approximately 30 percent of patients in acute hospitals could be adequately cared for in a less expensive type of facility, or even at home. Furthermore, because most health-insurance policies do not cover out-of-hospital expenses, physicians may often admit their

Figure 29.2 *(left)* Costs of various medical-surgical procedures. The purpose of these figures is not to suggest that one gets more for his money if he lives in a rural area—it is impossible to compare medical services on a purely economic level. It is of paramount importance, however, for any health consumer to know that fees differ from doctor to doctor and that when a patient pays a hospital bill he has not only paid for a room or a bed in that hospital but might have "rented" an operating room or paid for a surgical draping.

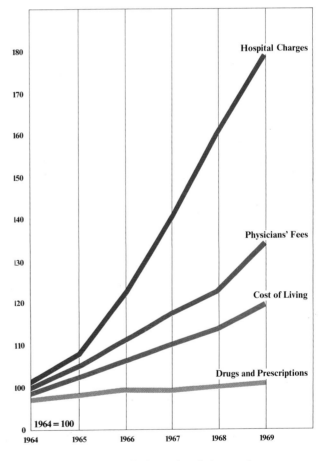

Figure 29.3 Rising medical costs in relation to what they were in 1964. Note that while drugs and prescriptions have stayed fairly constant and below cost-of-living increases, physicians' fees have slowly risen and hospital charges have soared.

patients to the hospital for routine tests that could otherwise be performed on an out-patient basis. And acute, or short-term, hospital care is the most expensive type of health care available, currently about 90 dollars a day, but charges of 200 dollars per day are not unusual. There are reasons, however, why hospital charges are so high: they must be ready for rare emergencies, which require expensive equipment twenty-four hours each day; they must be staffed by highly qualified personnel; and the number of personnel required averages three to five employees per patient.

Another area of potential waste is surgery. To say that the present system of health care encourages surgery would probably be viewed as heresy. However, if one examines current practices, he may see reasons for such a statement. As mentioned earlier, most insurance policies do not pay for services that are provided outside the hospital. On the other hand, most insurance policies do provide dollar allowances for surgery. Surgeons are held in high esteem by the public, but their financial rewards are generally dependent on whether they operate. Thus, the system provides more incentives to operate than not to operate. Also, many patients feel more satisfied (and healthier) if something is done to them.

There is considerable documentation to support the contention that much unnecessary surgery is occurring in the United States. When surgeons are on salary and only medical incentives enter the decision to operate, incidence of surgery has been seen to drop by 50 percent as compared to that involving physicians paid on a fee-for-operation base. Tonsillectomies, for example, amount to 6 or 7 percent of all operations in the United States, yet the same operation accounts for only 1 percent of total surgery in Sweden, where surgeons are on salary—and life expectancy (for males) ranks sixteen places ahead of the United States. Unneces-

sary surgery means not only unnecessary surgeon's fees, but unnecessary hospitalization and unnecessary risk of further health expenditures in case of post-operative complications—not to mention the risk to the patient.

A third area of misplaced expenditures concerns *physician manpower*. Having to resort to specialists because of the lack of available general practitioners may at times involve greater expenses than the actual needs of the patient would warrant. But, more generally, there are many tasks now necessarily performed by physicians that could be carried out by less expensively trained professionals, as will be discussed in more detail in the next section.

IMPROVING THE SYSTEM

There is certainly no simple answer to these problems. Health-care expenditures will continue to move upward during the 1970s, probably to over 100 billion dollars by 1975 and in the 200 billion range in the early 1980s. Under the present system, this staggering increase will continue to mean a dominance of financial over medical considerations whenever health decisions will be made, whether by the patients, the doctors, or the institutions. The only hope of reversing this trend is to increase the effectiveness of the health system. Virtually everyone agrees that the system needs to be changed, but few agree on the method. Some favor evolutionary change, others revolutionary change. Some call for drastic governmental actions, others hope for action by the private sectors of the nation. Some propose a selective curtailing of health services, others point to the magnitude of unprovided-for health problems. Many of the current debates, however, have some common aspects, which will now be discussed.

Personnel Reforms

The first step toward increasing the effectiveness of the health system must be to reorganize the

Figure 29.4 Paramedics are being employed in increasing numbers to perform routine functions, freeing the physician for the more complex tasks of medical evaluation and treatment.

use of health manpower. By 1975, medical schools expect to graduate approximately 10,000 physicians each year compared to the present 8,000. Even if the physician output were increased by 50 percent—an increase that would require more than 1 billion dollars and a considerable expansion of trained medical faculty—there would still be a doctor shortage under the present system. And the cost of training physicians would still continue to rise, as medical knowledge and technology increase. Clearly, it will be less and less economical to have such highly trained professionals perform tasks that could be handled by properly but less expensively trained medical personnel. By having them take over some of the routine aspects of patient care, not only will the cost to the patient be reduced but physicians will be free to concentrate on the more involved medical problems and the "physician crunch" will be minimized.

NEW EDUCATIONAL PROGRAMS *Physician Assistants* already are being prepared in a number of colleges and other institutions across the nation. In some programs their preparation—usually a two-year training period—does not require a bachelor's degree: many of these programs build on competences already acquired while serving as medical corpsmen in the military services. Other programs, requiring at least a bachelor's degree, also are being used for the training of more advanced allied medical personnel, usually with a nursing background. It is in this second direction that the next decade may see more detailed definition of new categories of *medical* "associates" or "masters" who could relieve the physician of more complex routine responsibilities.

A successful and efficient program for recruiting and training these new medical professionals, at whatever rank, must provide them with the opportunity for *upward mobility*. The need for such provision involves a common knowledge base for all health professions, so that a person at a given level of competence could reenter the common knowledge area, acquire additional medical education, and work his way up the ladder as far as his will and abilities could take him, including the physician level. The full use of such a program would require changes in the licensing laws and regulations. America still applies a rigid guild system to nurse's aides, nurses, physician assistants, and other allied health personnel that does not permit them to count prior education and training toward the requirements for advancement and therefore leaves little or no room for upward mobility.

NEW PRACTICE HABITS The present system does not encourage the equitable *distribution* of physicians and certain other health personnel. Most physicians have avoided practicing in poverty and rural areas for a variety of reasons. The main one used to be economic, but it is no longer. It is certainly

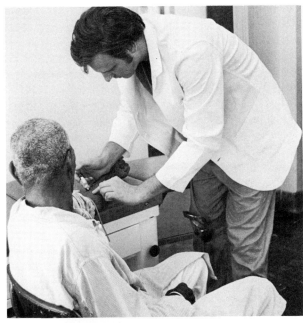

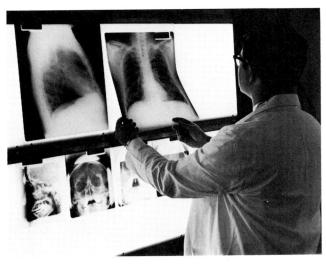

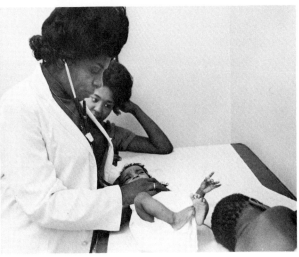

now possible for a physician to earn as much money in these areas as he can in an urban or well-to-do setting. The primary barrier to a better distribution of physicians is *sociocultural*. Urban areas provide better facilities and more opportunities to mingle with colleagues who provide intellectual stimulation. There are more satisfying activities for the physician's spouse, and the education system for his children is usually better. In addition, it is easier for an urban physician to arrange for free time because there are doctors who can take over the responsibility of his patients for short periods.

One temporary solution to the problem is to offer young physicians and dentists the opportunity to practice in understaffed health areas—such as poverty areas—as an alternative to military service. Another proposal is the granting of special scholarships and fellowships to students who agree to future service in underserviced areas; or perhaps the government could repay educational debts of physicians and dentists serving in such areas. A third possibility is to make it more financially rewarding for physicians and others to set up practice in areas of need. The Canadian province of Ontario, for example, has a program that provides financial assistance to doctors and dentists to establish and maintain a practice in areas designated as underserviced. The province guarantees them an annual net income when assigned to a designated area; the practitioner practices on a normal basis, with the province making up any deficit in the guaranteed income and the practitioner retaining any income from the practice in excess of the guarantee.

These various suggestions try to cope with the problem without dealing with the additional consideration that medical or dental practice is a business in which financial reward is prominent. It may be that a change in perspective, as well as practice habits, will go much farther toward solving the health problems. One step in that direction is the concept of group practice.

Group practice is an organization of full-time physicians and other health professionals who act as a team, sharing their skills and knowledge and using the same buildings, equipment, laboratory, and technicians. They divide the total group income according to a prearranged plan, which may vary from the solo doctor's fee-for-service system to having all the doctors on salary. Group practice is cooperative rather than competitive medicine. It is a method of organization already used by a number of leading clinics and medical centers associated with educational or charitable institutions. Some advantages of group practice for the *patient* are that: (1) most services are provided under one roof; (2) the consumer can be assured of having a physician who has been selected by other doctors and performs under the watchful eyes of his colleagues, an effective promoter of good quality care; (3) physicians may be on salary, so medical decisions are made less dependent on monetary considerations; (4) services are available on a twenty-four hour basis every day of the year; (5) if one's personal physician is not available—or moves to another locality—a competent doctor from the same team will be at hand, with direct access to the patient's medical records; (6) referral for consultation is easily arranged, usually with minimal stress to the patient. An expanded version of group practice is discussed in the next section.

Health Coverage Reforms

One major debate about health coverage is whether health care, at least in its traditional sense, is a right or a privilege of the citizen. The practical translation of the debate is who should pay for it, the individual, the employer, the community, or the government. Regardless of *who* should pay, the ques-

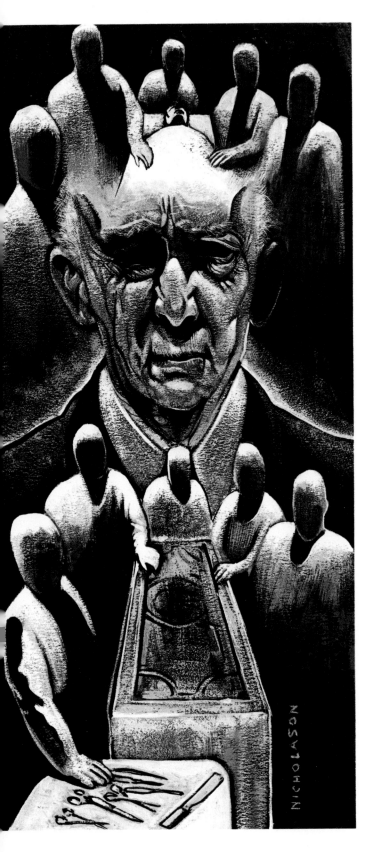

tion must also be resolved as to *how best* the health coverage can be carried out. An approach that may combine improved medical practice and improved financial coverage is the *Group Practice Prepayment Plan,* or *GPPP.*

GPPPs are group practices whose patients receive their health care in return for a monthly fee paid in advance. Three well-known examples of GPPPs are the Health Insurance Plan of Greater New York, the Group Health Cooperative of Puget Sound (Seattle area), and the Kaiser Foundation Medical Care Program. Together, these three groups already care for about 4.5 million patients.

For the *consumer,* GPPPs offer additional advantages besides those already listed for any group practice. Administrative red tape such as claim forms and bills are almost eliminated. The consumer knows what his medical care and hospitalization costs are going to be because they are on a fixed monthly base, and he can budget for them—the same advantage would work for whomever is responsible for his financial coverage. More importantly, prepayment encourages early entry into the health-care system; that is, the patient will not delay to see the doctor until he no longer can avoid it, which means that preventive care can be more effectively applied.

For the *physician* involved in a GPPP, there also exist a number of advantages:

1. He will be practicing in a setting with which he is familiar. During medical school, internship, residency, and his duty in the Armed Forces, he functioned within a type of group practice.
2. After spending so many years to become a doctor, he is usually married, has a family, and is deeply in debt. Entry into group practice allows him to avoid the additional expense of equipping an office.
3. Even after his long period of training, there is still much for him to learn; the group approach is a

Figure 29.5 In this age of youth-oriented culture, the problems associated with old age are often ignored. Medical science works tirelessly to lengthen the life span, but for many the question becomes one of quality and not just quantity of that life. The problems of the elderly—both physical and psychological—are enormous, yet geriatrics (specialization in problems of the elderly) remains one of the least-sought-after specialties in medicine.

cooperative one and encourages the sharing of knowledge.

4. He will have regular time off to partake of self-renewal through additional study or merely to enjoy a more normal and wholesome family life. Solo practitioners find it difficult to free themselves for even short periods of time without incurring the anger of their patients.

5. Group practice offers a doctor the chance to concentrate his efforts on the practice of medicine as he was taught to do. The financial aspects are handled by capable administrators trained to handle such matters. Group practice earnings are competitive with those of solo practice because of three factors: they begin at a higher level; they are more predictable; and they do not fall off as rapidly in later years.

6. Doctors in GPPPs can plan for treatment based on their medical judgment, knowing that their patients will not suffer financially as a result.

GPPPs appear to improve on the *general cost* problems of health care as well. For one thing, the exercise of preventive medicine is as much to the financial advantage of the group as it is to the patient, which means it constitutes a practical advance toward a lessening of health-care costs.

With prepayment each potential patient contributes to a fund in advance. Caring for illness takes money out of that fund, so that each case *prevented* or hospitalization *avoided*, allows more money to remain in the fund for the doctors and the patients to share. The physician may earn more money by promoting health, whereas under the fee-for-service system he only had income when the patient was sick; conversely, the patient can benefit from more extensive and expensive treatment when needed, without exhorbitant payments.

Studies have shown that patients under GPPPs have less frequent hospitalization, shorter hospitalization, and less surgery than those under solo practitioners. One example is illustrated in Table 29.1. In another study, the rate of appendectomies

dropped 59 percent when teams of salaried physicians replaced solo practitioners paid on a fee-for-service base. A third study compared utilization rates under Blue Cross/Blue Shield coverage with those of GPPPs; the GPPPs had 40 percent less hospitalization, while the other beneficiaries had 2.5 times higher rates of tonsillectomies, twice the rate of appendectomies, and 1.5 times the rate for female surgery (particularly on breast and uterus).

Given all these advantages of GPPPs, why are they not more widely adopted? Some consumers worry that they may have to wait weeks for an appointment with their personal physicians; but most GPPPs allow patients to "drop in" and be taken care of in order of arrival by the physician on duty—emergencies, of course, are handled immediately. Another objection is that group plans encourage assembly-line medicine; but the way a physician practices depends on the physician, not the plan—some physicians will practice assembly-line medicine whether in group or solo practice. Other consumers object to being limited to only those doctors in the plan, although most plans have several physicians in each specialty area and their competence is constantly tested by the peer group interaction.

Physicians, too, voice reservations. Some object

Table 29.1   Comparison of Patient Care Under a GPPP and Solo Practitioners

COST ITEM	Rates per 1,000 Beneficiaries per Year	
	GPPP	Solo Practitioners
Hospitalization	90	135
Hospital days	570	1,032
Major surgical procedures	33	69

Source: U.S. Department of Health, Education, and Welfare. *Public Health Service-Labor Seminar on Consumer Health Services,* 1968, p. 39.

that no one physician takes responsibility for the whole patient—the same objection to be raised in the present system of outnumbered general practitioners. To overcome this objection, most groups encourage patients to select a personal physician who assumes responsibility for guiding them to needed care. Other physicians fear that group practice destroys incentive and that a doctor under these conditions may not do his best for a patient—or possibly for himself. Some others merely do not like to submit to the regulations, intragroup medical audits, limitation to certain formularies (drug lists), and other procedures that must be followed in any well-run group.

Most objections, from consumers or physicians alike, appear to reflect more their own individual preferences or habits than any deep-seated flaw in the GPPP approach—even though undoubtedly many imperfections remain to be corrected. And it is true that membership in a GPPP requires cooperation on the part of both patient and participating physician and the willingness to accept the disadvantages. It is perhaps in this respect that this approach to health care comes closest to a needed new perspective: cooperation and willingness, by both the professional and the cared-for, to produce together a better health system.

The federal government, concerned over the skyrocketing cost and inadequate effectiveness of current health care, has become interested in GPPPs and is now encouraging more of this kind of practice. It is distressing, but perhaps not altogether unexpected in view of the many interests to which such approaches may pose a threat, that today seventeen states still prohibit by law medical care corporations such as GPPPs. Even if not everyone may want to utilize GPPP care, a free society should at least make available in all states an alternative to the traditional, fee-for-service care.

The Delivery System

Reorganization of health manpower, new practice habits, and health-coverage reforms merge into an opportunity to modify another component of health care, the delivery system.

The traditional medical care delivery system has evolved slowly over the years with little planning. In spite of remarkable medical advances in recent years, it has remained virtually unchanged. Patients who enter this system may be characterized into four major groups: the well, the "worried well," the "early sick," and the sick. Everyone falls into one category or another and even though the population has increased and the problems changed over the years, the point of entry into the medical care system has not changed—it is still the physician. Also under the traditional fee-for-service system, the patient has to pay for each visit to his doctor. This is a kind of "entry fee." This fee has been an effective regulator and has caused most people to put off seeing their doctor until they are really sick. It has effectively discouraged early entry into the system, which is essential for early treatment and preventive care.

If the entry fee is replaced by a monthly payment, as it is in the GPPPs, there is no immediate barrier to access, and the physician is likely to be overwhelmed by the above four kinds of patients. Highly trained doctors then spend much of their time trying to find something wrong with healthy people. Seeing the well and worried well is frustrating to the doctor because he feels he should be doing what he was taught to do in medical school—curing the sick.

One part of a proposed answer to this dilemma is *multiphasic screening*, a type of health testing that combines a detailed computerized medical history and a series of diagnostic tests administered by paramedical personnel. Tests include a variety of

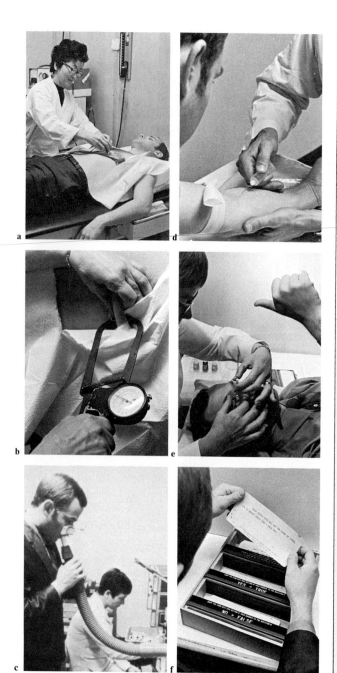

Figure 29.6 Several steps of the multiphasic screening test. (a) an electrocardiogram is taken; (b) skin-fold test measures body fat; (c) lung capacity is measured; (d) blood sample is taken for analysis; (e) the eyes are checked for glaucoma; (f) patient receives set of cards for psychological evaluation. (*right*) A sample of a computer printout shows the results of diagnostic tests of a fifty-year-old female who underwent tests similar to ones pictured above.

```
                    PERMANENTE MEDICAL GROUP — OAKLAND
        DUPLICATE REPORT — MULTIPHASIC HEALTH CHECKUP (MHC)  —  5/20/69

     TEST,PATIENT                RETIRED                    S.F. DR. SMITH
     MR: 225859C J1    AGE 50    FEMALE      WIDOWED          LAST MHC  6/16/68

                             SUMMARY OF REPORT
           ***********************************************

             (TEST)                 (NORMAL)   (THIS EXAM)
          CIRCULATORY:
     **   B.P.SUPINE(GODART): 90-159/ 50- 89    164/100
          HEMATOLOGY:
     **   HEMOGLOBIN GM.:         12.0- 16.0      9.2
     **   MHC MCMCG:              26.0- 34.0     20.6
     **   MCHC %:                 32.0- 38.0     25.6
     ¬  BLOOD CHEMISTRY:
     **   GLUCOSE 1 HR MG%:       UNDER-  263     332
     **   GLUCOSE 2 HR MG%:       UNDER-  150     164
     **   VDRL:                      NEG          POS
     **   QUANTITATIVE VDRL:                    RRWWWN
          URINE:
     **   GLUCOSE:                   NEG          MED
     **   CLINITEST:                 NEG          3+
     **   ACETONE:                   NEG          POS

     **  BREAST X-RAY:  FIBROCYSTIC DIFFUSE CHANGES
     **  HEARING:       CLINICALLY IMPAIRED HEARING LEFT

         PATIENT RECEIVED FOLLOWING (ADVICE RULE) DIRECTIONS:
         700-REQUEST PT.RET. AMS LAB FOR 2-HR SERUM SUGAR
         801-NOTICE SENT TO PHYSICIAN: CONSIDER EARLY APPTMT.

     *      IN PAST YEAR SPELLS OF WEAKNESS OR PARALYSIS OF ARMS OR LEGS
     *      IN PAST YEAR BLURRING OF EYESIGHT LASTING OVER A FEW MINUTES
     *      IN PAST YEAR ANY LOSS OF HEARING WHICH IS STILL PRESENT
     *      IN PAST 6 MONTHS OFTEN HAD PAIN IN THE EAR
     *      IN PAST 6 MONTHS 2 OR MORE NOSE BLEEDS NOT FROM INJURY OR A COLD
     *      IN PAST YEAR COUGHED UP ANY BLOOD




     TND = TEST NOT DONE    PRT = PAT. REFUSED TEST    TNI = TEST NOT INDICATED
     BND = BLOOD NOT DRAWN    UNSAT = TEST UNSATISFACTORY    - = DATA NOT AVAILABLE
     NSA = NO SIGNIFICANT ABNORMALITY
     * = PATIENT ANSWERED YES ON THIS MHC AND NO ON LAST MHC
     ** = CONSIDER POSSIBLE ABNORMAL          ¬ = NOTE           242-11:57:21
```

measures, from heart and thyroid function to neuromuscular and hearing checks. X-rays are taken, as well as a series of twenty blood-chemistry measurements. A computer indicates if additional tests are needed or if an immediate appointment with a doctor is advisable. All of the patient's results are stored by the computer for future reference. This screening serves as an entry regulator, separates the well from the sick, and establishes entry priorities. Officials proposing the method point out that it also serves to detect symptomless and early illness, provides the doctors with a preliminary survey and a basic health profile for future reference, permits maximal utilization of paramedical personnel, and considerably reduces doctor and hospital costs. Figure 29.7 illustrates a delivery system that makes use of health testing as the entry point.

In addition to health testing, three distinct areas are proposed to take care of the particular needs of the patient. The well and the worried well are channeled to the *health-care center*, staffed primarily by paramedical personnel under medical supervision. This center would be a separate facility and would provide health information through a variety of approaches such as health exhibits, lectures, and films. Immunizations, clinics of various kinds, and counseling would also be available in the health-care center. The emphasis in this center would be on prevention—attempting to keep people well—a facet almost completely neglected in the traditional approach (notable exceptions are pediatrics and public health programs).

A *preventive-maintenance service* would provide care for the chronic diseases that make up an in-

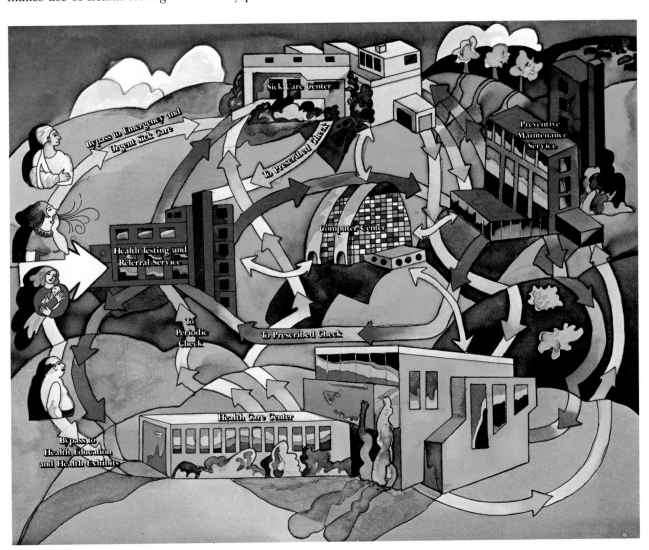

Figure 29.7 A model health-care system. This system would establish a new method of entry into the health system, the health-testing service. After health testing the patient would be referred for sick care, health care, or preventive maintenance as required and would be transferred among the services as his condition changed. The computer center would regulate the flow of patients and information to other units, coordinating the entire system, which would depend heavily on paramedical personnel to save doctors' time. (After Sidney R. Garfield, "The Delivery of Medical Care," *Scientific American*, 222, April 1970, 22. Copyright © 1970 by Scientific American, Inc. All rights reserved.)

creasing proportion of the patient load. Generally, patients with chronic conditions such as obesity, diabetes, arthritis, and so on require routine treatment, observation, and follow-up. Again, paramedical personnel, under physician supervision, are able to improve the patient's condition or at least prevent progression of the illness and guard against further complications.

Paramedical personnel will be able to take primary responsibility in health testing services, health-care services, and preventive-maintenance services. This system leaves the *sick-care center* to the physician where he can perform the diagnosis and treatment for which his medical education prepared him. This system would relieve him of the necessity of working with well patients and those who require fairly standard treatment. It would, hopefully, mean that he could spend more time with the patients who really need his sick care and may improve the patient-doctor relationship, which has become strained under the pressure of such great numbers.

THE ROLE OF COMMUNITIES

Many of the current health problems unquestionably can be corrected by more far-sighted planning with respect to personnel, financial coverage, and delivery systems. However, countries that exercise central planning still fall short of disposing of all health problems. Air pollution, chronic disease, and social disorders also exist in the Soviet Union, Sweden, and Great Britain, where planned economy and health planning have not succeeded in eliminating the problems that plague the least-planned societies. Central restructuring of a society's health-care apparatus, then, does not by itself solve individual or community health problems.

Early Attempts at Community Involvement

The Regional Medical Programs Act, which created regional advisory groups for heart disease, cancer, and stroke, required consumer representation in these groups. However, a survey in the late 1960s revealed that most of these consumers were bankers, insurance brokers, and prominent civic leaders; only one man who might have qualified as disadvantaged—a laborer—was a representative in such groups as late as 1967.

The Regional Medical Programs Act was accompanied by legislation creating the Partnership for Health program, intended to turn back to regional and local areas the responsibility for planning for health and for determining fund-allocation priorities. The primary reason for this move was that federal matching funds had been distributed to state and local health departments on the basis of federal rather than local priorities. For example, if the federal government appropriated "X" million dollars for control of heart disease, a state health department had to invest in the same direction in order to qualify for federal matching funds. Thus, federal appropriations dictated the size and the goal of state appropriations. Under the Partnership for Health Act, a comprehensive health planning group reviewed and approved state plans. Local planning bodies also reviewed all proposals for community health activities in their areas, including the building of hospitals and other health-care facilities. The Partnership for Health Act recognized the importance of broad community involvement and therefore required all these state and local planning groups to be composed of 51 percent consumers, the rest to be professional providers. Thus, local communities could approve or reject community projects in accordance with priorities generated by that community.

Although the intent was admirable, the actual operational results, as with earlier legislation, were less satisfactory than had been hoped for. Two major problems resulted when this legislation was converted into operation. In the first place, the actual amount of funds available to local and state

Figure 29.8   Community health projects such as those sponsored by the "Young Lords" help to further health goals by providing hot breakfasts and recreational activities for children.

planning bodies was deficient. The second major problem was how to define "consumer." Could a bank president represent people on welfare? Is an insurance-company executive a consumer or provider? The appointment of consumers often was followed by demands for representation from other groups. As a result, some regional advisory groups doubled in size every two or three meetings, and eventually became totally unmanageable.

The same basic philosophy of participation underlaid the Great Society programs of the Johnson Administration in the mid-1960s. The Office of Economic Opportunity (OEO) generated programs that would provide the poor with "vehicles for social change" in which they exercised primary roles in decision making. The disadvantaged were to have "maximum feasible participation" in the rehabilitation of their communities. Although these programs were noble in intent, many of them resulted in frustration and failure. Critics, for example, have accused these programs of attempting to reinstate the kind of political machine based on personal influence—eliminated in the late 1930s and 1940s—that allowed the poor a voice in local government. The communities themselves were unable to form stable partnerships with government agencies or educational institutions. Major problems arose—as in the case of the Partnership for Health Act—from endless debates about what factions represented a community and how funds were spent.

The Health Rights Program was developed and funded over 50 neighborhood health centers in communities where lack of health care was only one index of their poverty. In each center, policy was controlled or influenced by a true consumer board comprising representatives of the community it served. In addition to attracting health practitioners to areas where there were shortages, the centers invested much effort in training community people, usually previously unemployed, in health activities. These family health workers help to bridge the language and cultural gap between the professionals and the patient. The neighborhood health centers from the start took the broadest view of health. For instance, one center in Mississippi found malnutrition to be a major problem. For a while they stocked food in the pharmacy but then went on to develop an agricultural cooperative so the "patients" could grow their own food. These centers are helping to establish a model for the changes in health delivery described previously.

Community-Generated Action

In contrast with such earlier *outside* efforts to involve communities and individuals into working out health problems with preexisting health institutions, a new kind of health *activism* is growing in communities all over the country. One example is the current furor over abortion laws. Prompted by the recent medical advances in birth-control techniques and the changing sexual mores of today's society, feminists and other activists claim free abortion as the right of every woman and press with increasing effectiveness for appropriate institutional reforms.

Another example is perhaps even more illustrative. In New York City, thousands of children in poorly kept buildings suffer lead poisoning from eating the lead-based paint that has peeled off cracked walls and window sills. There was pressure on the city government to provide free testing for slum children so that the poisoning could be detected early, before brain damage occurred. This testing was promised but was slow in being established, until a group of young Puerto Rican activists, called the "Young Lords," took matters into their own hands. They found ways to put mobile units on the streets to test children for poisoning. This action aroused enough publicity to insure that the city's program would be made more effective and more promptly instituted.

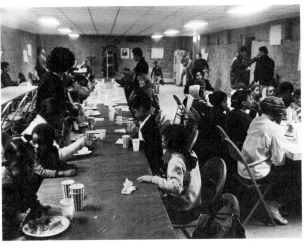

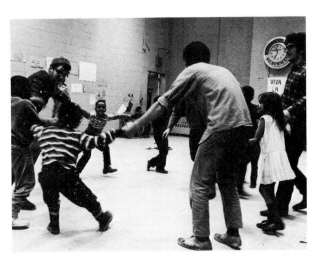

One of the most promising expressions of this new self-generated community involvement is the "free clinics" program. Free clinics have sprung up in most major cities, both in poverty areas and where there are large numbers of young people seeking to loose their dependence from the "establishment." These clinics are largely community run, in many cases with the aid of volunteer doctors and nurses, and much of the record-keeping work is done by local, nonprofessional people who are known and trusted by the community. These clinics, therefore, are often more successful than the large, impersonal, urban hospital clinics in bringing people in before their problems are acute. The full

effectiveness of free clinics has yet to be evaluated, but they undoubtedly demonstrate the changing attitude of the community toward the health care of its members.

Prospective Roles of the Community

From the various examples discussed in the preceding two sections, it appears clear that communal health efforts are developing in two main directions, both needed and virtually complementary. *Consumer representation* in decision-making bodies will grow, with particular regard to the identification of the community health problems and the allocation of resources to deal with them. The effec-

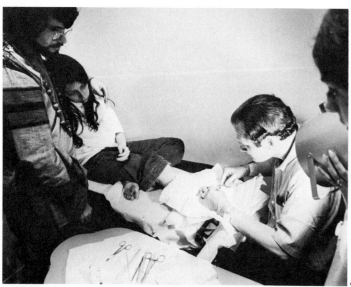

a

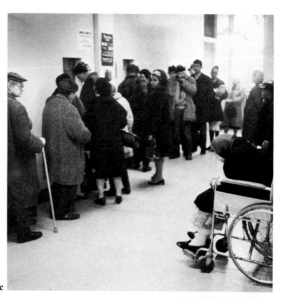

c

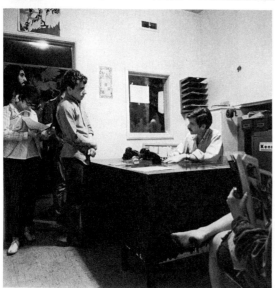

b

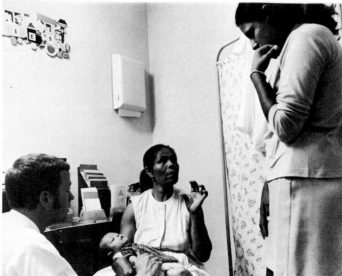

d

tiveness of health institutions requires a restored cooperation between communities and providers and the demise of bureaucratic features that tend to transform organizations into "establishments" that are unresponsive to people. On the other hand, organizational changes are slow and painful processes and the problems at hand are too urgent; additional study or further precision in defining such problems only postpone coping with them. Hence the need for the other type of communal involvement, the self-generated *communal organization* of individuals sharing similar concerns.

HEALTH CARE AND MEDICAL CARE

The 7 percent of the Gross National Product now being spent on health probably approaches the limit of American investment. There already is a serious reduction in funds appropriated by the federal government for biomedical research and a reluctance to expand medical school facilities. There is a need to reconsider the relative efficacy of different forms of care and the "returns" on investments in community health services. The advent of some form of national health insurance will undoubtedly transform the financing and organization of medical care services, and even greater changes will presumably occur in the nature and the practicing philosophy of the health manpower. But the effects of medical care reorganization on the actual health status of a population are limited.

The question has been asked: "Is maximum medical care a first priority for a nation where millions of people still have not enough to eat?" The point is well taken. In the United States over the last twenty years, there has been little change in traditional indicators, such as infant mortality and longevity, in spite of great scientific studies and considerable increase in per capita medical expenditures. Perhaps those indicators do not tell the whole story; perhaps one should apply them separately to two nations within the nation, the nation of the affluent Americans and the nation of the poor Americans. And, indeed, infant mortality is much lower among middle-class whites, for example, than it is among low-income blacks. True, one group generally has comprehensive medical care while the other does not, but it also has a higher standard of living, including better housing and sanitation and more and better food for expectant mothers. Perhaps, then, greater gains would be made for the nation as a whole by insuring better nutrition for expectant mothers than by providing them with maximum, comprehensive medical care.

The point, in more general terms, is that it is important to distinguish between *medical* care and *health* care. Health, as has been shown, is a comprehensive concept that goes beyond "not being unwell." A majority of health problems are rooted in the social and economic structure of a community. The prerequisite of the improvement of health in America may thus be seen as the improvement of quality of life for all Americans. Even in strict medical and economic terms, *preventive* care will go a long way toward decreasing the load on *treatment* care. Rather than increasing hospital beds, physicians, health centers, or even health insurance, the object should be to reduce the number of potential patients who may need them.

Figure 29.9 (a, b) Free clinics have gained support as important promulgators of health care. (c) One of the basic protests of the medical students' organization, Student Health Organization, is that "patients who cannot afford to pay receive inferior treatment under depressing conditions and that many of the poor receive almost no health care at all." This photo, taken at the out-patient clinic at Bellevue Hospital, shows patients waiting hours for prescribed medication. (d) A mother at the free clinic for migrant workers in the San Joaquin Valley, California describes her health problem with the aid of an interpreter.

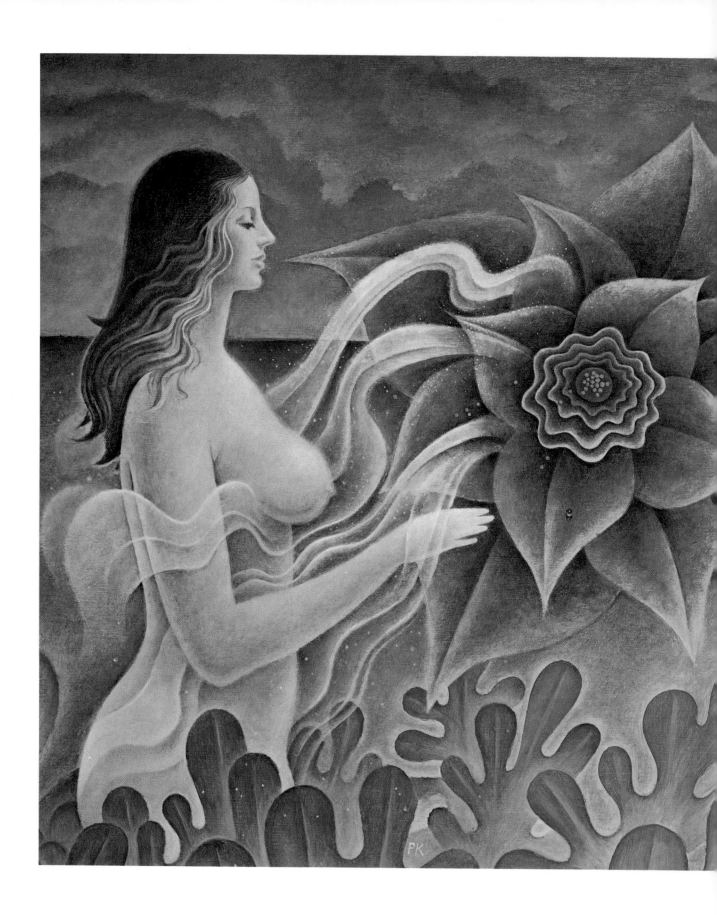

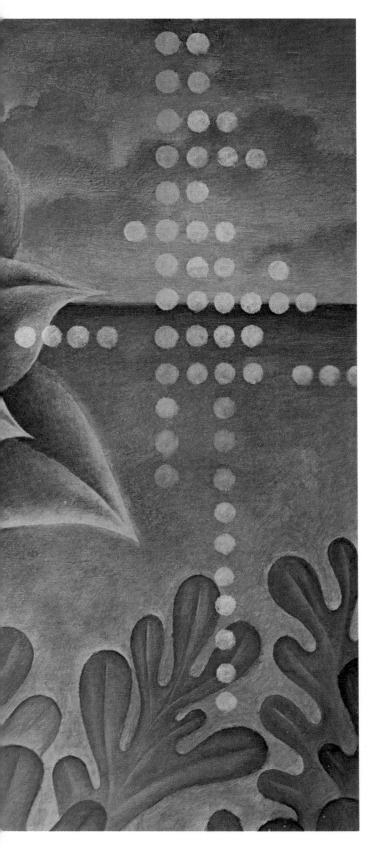

30

The examination of health presented in this book has ranged very widely, from molecules to human institutions, from the hopeful beginning of life to its sometimes dreary end. It has not touched on all problems and it certainly has not revealed all of man's knowledge. From what this book has been able to cover, what is the "take-home" message? No two people will give the same answer, and you as the reader should formulate your own. But there are a few threads woven through all these pages, and it may be helpful to pull them out and take one last look at them.

BASIC CONCEPTS OF HEALTH

The central concept learned from the science of genetics is that each man and woman is a *unique* person: not in a million years nor among billions of people will one human being be identical to another. Unique individuals will have unique feelings, thoughts, needs, aspirations, and ways through which they try to fulfill their needs, desires, and goals. Health, too, becomes an individual, exquisitely personal thing, precious to each man as it can never be precious to anyone but himself, because health means the capacity to optimize conditions for his achievement of his happiness.

A second central concept of health is that the human body projects beyond its physical contour and contents to blend with everything around it. The human body *plus* its environment, and the interaction between the two, are the true dimensions

Health and the Individual

of the human being. Just as the individual human being is unique, so is the blend of his body with his environment. Genetic versus developmental factors; body growth and sustenance versus air, water, and food; internal versus external stimuli to the mind; muscle movement versus action that changes the surrounding world—all such appositions stress that there is no discontinuity between body and environment. It follows that health can only be achieved if one takes care of his body and his environment both.

It also has been shown that the *way* to health involves two components: knowledge and implementation. Each component, then, must apply both to one's body and to one's environment. Health science must learn about both, and health care must act to improve both. In trying to do so, the world of the individual begins to merge with those of others. One begins with his own self-interest, his own desires for a full life. In seeking knowledge and the discipline to apply it, one discovers he must deal with his environment and with the people who contribute to making or changing it.

One is thus drawn to include among his desires and interests other persons whom he loves—his parents, spouse, children, relatives, friends. The knowledge one seeks and the use to which he puts it now aim at protecting these persons as well as himself and strive to fulfill their as well as his own desires. Soon one realizes that the health of his small circle is intimately related to that of his community, to the health of people whom he does not individually know but whose lives affect his own. Many health matters, one eventually learns, transcend even this concept of community health and expand to a state, national, or international level. And, throughout, the "social" view of man's environment blends with the "physical" and the "biological" views into an *ecological* perspective of the full human immersion in nature's world.

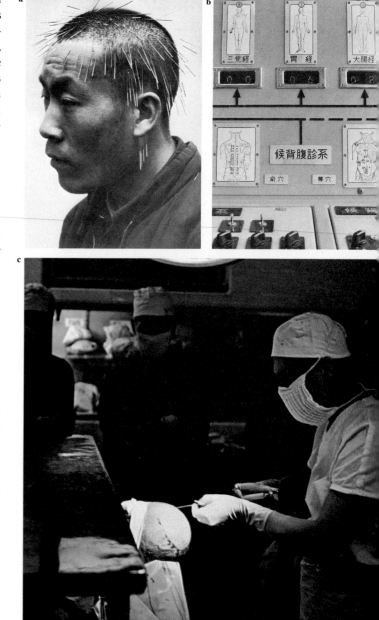

Figure 30.1 The dissemination of health information and the application of medical technology as seen in various nations and areas of the world. (a) Acupuncture, an ancient therapeutic technique that seeks to alleviate pain by the removal of pressure, is currently enjoying great popularity. While in China, James Reston, the political analyst for the *New York Times*, suffered a gastrointestinal attack and was treated with this method, which proved to be highly successful. (b) A Chinese computer programmed to analyze and prescribe various aspects of acupunctural therapy. (c) Brain operation in Taiwan hospital. (d) Egyptian child receiving fluoride treatment in a mobile dental unit. (e) Nigerian man receiving smallpox vaccination with hypo-spray jet gun. (f) Nurse attending aboriginal patient enroute to hospital.

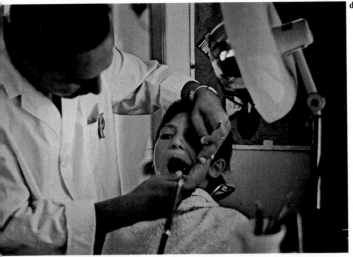

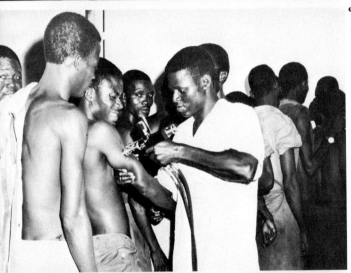

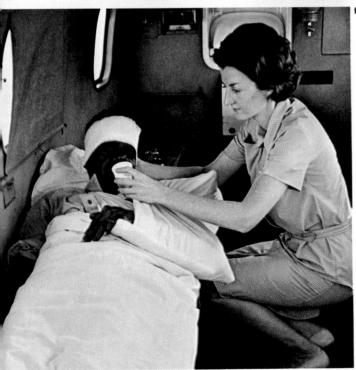

One *acquires* knowledge through personal observation and experience with his own body. He extends it through sharing in the observations and experience of others. He seeks beyond the available knowledge through his own personal effort and by teaming up with others to probe even further.

One *uses* knowledge to take care of his own body through its daily activities and through being alert for signs of danger to it. He applies it to select "healthy" conditions for his loved ones and to seek help from others when it appears needed. He shares it with others to identify the current hazards or imminent threats to all, so that they can jointly find avenues to combat them. He also uses his knowledge to evaluate the quality and effectiveness of those on whom he depends for the specialized services necessary to insure his health.

He also *implements* knowledge at various levels. As an individual, one can choose to devote his lifetime activities to the service of health and become a health professional. In the family, one provides the other members with what physical, emotional, or mental health care can be given without specialized, professional knowledge—a function second to none in the provider and model roles of a dedicated parent. As members of a community, one may develop, or help develop, new modes of collective and individual health care, as alternatives or complements to established, professional services. And as a responsible citizen one works to ensure that what responsibilities are delegated to others, professional or governmental, will not be misused or abused.

CHALLENGES FOR THE FUTURE

What is likely to happen as the health scene of today projects into the future? Whatever one's own personal view and plans for his own involvement, it is an exciting picture. It is a picture in motion, not a static one. It is a picture of action for everyone,

not of passivity. It is full of challenges and responsibilities.

For the health *scientist*, the enormous studies
made over the past few decades are but a base and
a promise for even more dramatic progress in the
years ahead. Doors have been opened, but hardly
entered, to a number of momentous questions,
from "What are the precise mechanisms underlying
genetic and developmental regulations of the human body?" to "How does the brain mediate emotions and intelligence in the human mind?" The
more powerful that science grows in its mastery
over the human body, the more critical become the
decisions on when and how to apply it: genetic engineering and manipulation of the mind may be
just beyond today's horizon, but the wisdom to
use these awesome powers has progressed little
over the thousands of years of human civilization.
Partly in anticipation of such problems and partly
because of an increasing encroachment into today's
health scene, a new field is slowly emerging for the
health scientist to attack, namely that of psychosocial disease and health. More and more scientists
are coming to recognize that the kinds of health
hazards and the risks of exposure to them depend
on the individual's life style and the structure of the
society he lives in.

For the *health-care professional*, the future offers
at least as many exciting challenges as it does for the
scientist. The profile of community health problems
during the last quarter of this century probably
will be as different from that of the past three decades as they were from the preceding ones. The
challenges that will shape this profile are many,
and most of them involve the patterns of life, social
values, and the structure and governance of communities.

The rising health-care expectations of the disadvantaged segments of society and their recognition
by everyone else have already added pressure for

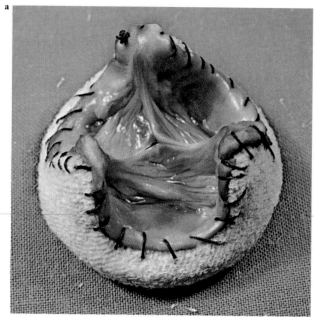

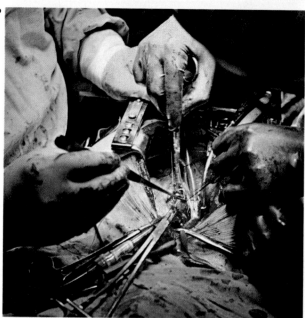

Figure 30.2 The advances made in medical science in the
twentieth century have included diagnostic machines that measure the electrical activity of the heart and brain, drugs that
have afforded normal lives to diabetics and epileptics, and
surgical techniques that boggle the imagination. (a) A human
heart valve taken from the heart of an accident victim has been
sutured to a teflon collar. This type of valve has been found to
be the least damaging to the blood. When a human heart valve
is not available, totally fabricated "ball-type" valves (which work
like a ping pong ball in a snorkel) are used. The metal that is
used in this valve, unlike the human-teflon valve, causes the
blood to clot, and patients with ball-type valve replacements
must be medicated with anticoagulant drugs. (b) The valve is
sutured into place. The whitish tissue to the left of the instruments is the heart. The large plastic tube leads to a heart-lung
(coronary bypass) machine.

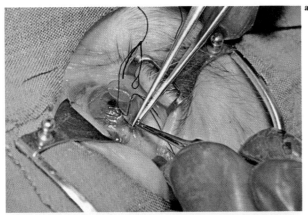

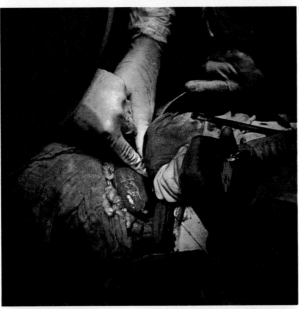

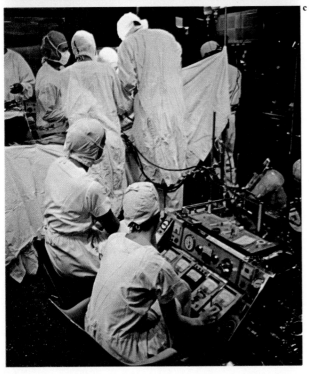

more comprehensive services. Statistics reveal the painful extent to which the poor have not had access to care, and it is becoming increasingly apparent that the health problems faced by a community do not follow a course separate from its other social problems. A growing health hazard of the next decades will be the continuing pollution of air and water. Other mushrooming problems that threaten mental and social well-being revolve around the use of drugs by large numbers of people, including alcoholism, and the rising rates of suicide, alienation, and mental distress.

At least some of these problems are a consequence of the incredibly rapid changes that have been taking place in American society and of the tremendous pressures contained within it. Many health problems will be responsive to *education*, and one can expect that the coming years will see more and better health education programs devised for both the layman and the professional. Frank information about dangerous drugs will be important, as will sex education and knowledge to deal with individual health hazards—whether they involve the spread of venereal disease, cigarette smoking and lung cancer, diet and exercise and coronary disease, or control and prevention of "accidents."

Much of the past effort of health professionals has been directed to the *correction* of diseases, and this approach will continue, although with the emphasis shifted to new groups of ailments. Major developments are to be expected toward *prevention* of disease, which has only been barely attacked until now, except through the epidemiology of infections. But a third avenue concerning health is *looking beyond* the absence of disease to the attainment of optimal health, a concept that has only recently been recognized. This is where the health professional will have to join in a global attack on what constitutes the political, economic, and social dimensions of an optimal community of man. Such a

Figure 30.3 (a) A human cornea is transplanted from the eye of a deceased donor to the previously sightless eye of the recipient. (b) A kidney transplant. The most successful of organ-transplant surgery is that of the kidney. The reasons for its success are: (1) the transplanted organ is from a living donor who is usually related to the patient so that tissue rejection is less likely: (2) there are two kidneys so that unless both are diseased, the body can maintain itself on the functioning kidney or on a hemodialysis (kidney-filtration) machine until a compatible replacement kidney can be obtained: and (3) drugs that assist the body in accepting the transplanted kidney have been highly successful. (c) Open-heart surgery is performed using the heart-lung machine. This machine, invented in the United States, was used for the first time in 1953. Prior to the application of this machine, heart surgery was limited to sewing up wounds or holes in the heart. Now a patient's heart can be relieved of its normal function for as long as four and one-half hours while surgeons replace valves, arteries, and, occasionally, the entire organ.

goal, even more than the others, can only be realized at the price of important organizational changes and a rearrangement of society's priorities. Nevertheless, the behavior of the individual remains crucial. Institutions may be restructured but little will be accomplished until their members go beyond the demonstration of individual concern to assume collective responsibility.

INDIVIDUAL ACTION

These, then, are the challenges the future holds for the health *consumer*. Each individual has an inner "thrust" to maintain or promote his own health and no one can be more concerned with or more reliably responsible for it. Professional care represents enormous, and costly, expertise and should certainly be brought to bear when necessary, but it is the individual who must make the move by the intelligent use of adequate knowledge of self, of health, and of the available supportive resources. He should make judgments as to how and where he should enter the health-care system and how he is treated within it—a far cry from the current reality, where the patient enters the health-care system at a designated point, is passively processed through it, and emerges at the other end to pay the bill, with minimal questions.

Health care is *not* the exclusive business of health professionals, physicians, or others. Tradition in this regard is being challenged ever more widely on several grounds. Especially significant has been the reaction of population groups who find themselves without adequate care, as in low-density (rural) areas or in high-density but economically deprived ones (ghettos). From such challenges emerges the concept of "consumer-oriented" health care, to which concept the immediate future hopefully will have much to contribute. The informed, health-conscious person thus is likely to find himself not only well prepared to deal with his own health problems but to function more effec-

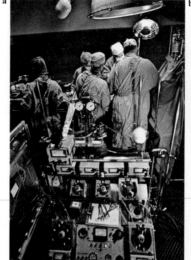
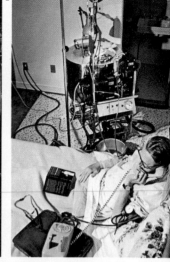
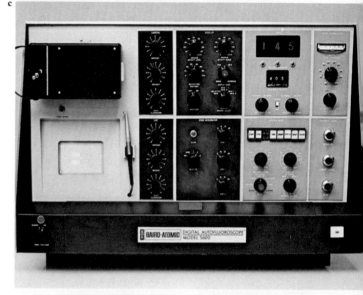
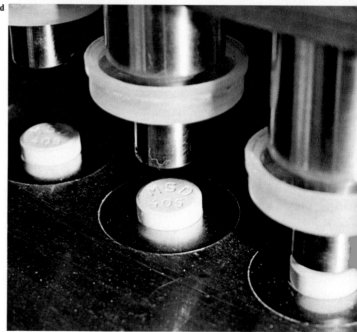

tively as a citizen. As the focus of health care expands from the individual afflicted with disease to the prevention of disease to the search toward the optimal conditions for health, the problems of health care merge with the problems of ensuring the quality of life. The thrust to move effectively to achieve individual desires becomes the driving force toward more satisfactory social living.

Perhaps this expanding focus of health care is nowhere better illustrated than in the area of human sexuality. The healthy individual engaging in sexual activity with a healthy partner finds enormous gratification for himself, while bestowing gratification on another. This primitive "social" act, which not only goes back through the generations of man but is shared in some form with most of life, also is the fundamental step in biological procreation. Associated with it may be a series of pathologies, departures from healthy sexuality, ranging from venereal disease—which is a medical and public health problem—to child molestation and rape—which are problems for both the psychiatrist and the law. Also associated is the problem of overpopulation, with its attendant problems of malnutrition, environmental despoliation, and man's future on a planet of finite resources.

On the highest level, the focus of health science is *man* and the overwhelming global challenge of health as it relates to the future of man and his place on earth. Health becomes a matter of ideology and philosophy, but also a compelling reality involving each individual, each member of every community and institution, in the United States and throughout the world. Mankind has more health knowledge than ever before. The technology to implement it across all health problems, wherever they are or however great is their scale, is either at hand or within human reach. The task now is to develop, with the high priority they deserve, the social understanding and the social organization necessary not only to conquer disease but to achieve universal health.

Figure 30.4 (a) Open-heart surgery. The blood is drained from the heart with tubes and fed into the heart-lung machine, where it is mixed with oxygen and then fed back into the circulatory system through a tube attached to an artery in the leg. (b) The hemodialysis machine. When one kidney (or both) ceases to perform its normal function and a kidney transplantation is inadvisable, the patient must check into the hospital twice a week and be connected to the kidney machine in which the blood is filtered. This lifesaving procedure is completely painless—the cost of maintaining someone on hemodialysis, however, is approximately $25,000 a year. (c) Nuclear medicine. This machine, often used in diagnosing brain conditions, is a radioisotope scanning device. Isotopes are injected into the patient's bloodstream. Organs are delineated on pictures that appear on the black screen on the upper-left panel of the machine. The physician then "reads" these pictures for "hot" or "cold" spots. A "hot" spot is an area of increased blood flow, which indicates the presence of a tumor. A "cold" spot is indicative of an abscess in which there is fluid or pus but little blood. (d) A modern machine used in the manufacturing of pharmaceutical products.

A

acne vulgaris *See* text, Chapter 20.

Addison's disease A disease produced by underactivity of the adrenal glands and the insufficient supply of the adrenal hormones aldosterone or hydrocortisone in the body. It is caused by destruction of the adrenal cortex by unknown factors or by an infective process such as tuberculosis. Aldosterone deficiency is characterized by the inability of the body to retain the salts necessary to maintain blood pressure. When hydrocortisone is deficient, symptoms include weakness, loss of appetite, and low blood sugar. There also is a characteristic pigmentation of the skin. The disease can be fatal if an "adrenal crisis" occurs and the patient enters a state of shock and general collapse. The presence of Addison's disease is confirmed through blood and urine analyses, and treatment consists of the administration of supplementary amounts of the deficient hormone. *See also* text, Chapter 25.

amebiasis Better known as amoebic dysentery, a protozoan infection of the lower intestine resulting in abdominal pain and diarrhea. It is transmitted through food contaminated by infected insects or persons or through water contaminated by sewage, it has an incubation period of from five days to three months, and it can last for many years. Symptoms range from mild discomfort and loose bowel movements to acute diarrhea and dehydration, sometimes resulting in death. Amebiasis confers no immunity, and there is no vaccination process. Preventive measures consist mainly of attempts to decrease the modes of transmission.

amoebic dysentery *See* amebiasis.

angina pectoris *See* text, Chapter 24.

appendicitis *See* text, Chapter 25.

arthritis *See* text, Chapter 25.

asthma A symptom of severe irritation of the lungs and bronchial tubes resulting from an allergic reaction, particle irritation, or microbe infection. It is characterized by coughing, wheezing, and shortness of breath. The causes of asthma are unknown, but allergic asthma can be precipitated by several substances, including pollen, dust, and animal hair. Treatment of asthma involves inhalation or injection of adrenalin. Asthma attacks are best prevented by avoiding substances that will precipitate a reaction. *See also* text, Chapter 25.

atherosclerosis *See* text, Chapter 24.

athlete's foot The common name for ringworm of the foot. It is a fungal infection characterized by blistering, scaling, and cracking of the skin between the toes. It is a common, universally occurring disease, more prevalent in men than in women or children. Athlete's foot is usually transmitted indirectly through contact with contaminated clothing, shower stalls, or gymnasium floors; it has an incubation period of from ten to fourteen days; and it may never disappear completely. Thorough washing and drying of the skin around the toes and prolonged exposure of the feet to the drying effects of air by not wearing shoes or by wearing sandals will usually eliminate the fungus. In extreme cases an antifungal drug, griseofulvin, may be used to fight the infection. *See also* ringworm.

B

bacillary dysentery *See* shigellosis.

bacterial endocarditis An infection of the inner heart lining that can be either acute or subacute and that creates growths on the heart valves. It is usually a complication of minor surgery or of respiratory infections such as pneumonia, and it is most common in persons with congenital heart valve defects or with valves otherwise damaged by such childhood diseases as rheumatic fever. Symptoms of the acute form include high fever and chills eventually leading to death; symptoms of the subacute form, which is more common, include fatigue, weakness, anemia, and mild fever. As the disease advances, emboli composed of portions of the growths on the valves begin to occlude arteries throughout the body. Treatment consists of the administration of antibiotic drugs such as penicillin, and prevention of the disease in susceptible persons is accomplished by the administration of antibiotics prior to and after minor surgery.

bacterial pneumonia An acute infection and vasocongestion of the lung characterized by fever, coughing, chest pain, and difficult breathing. In most cases it is caused by the pneumococcal bacteria and is better known as pneumococcal pneumonia, but other common types of bacteria from the mouth and throat can produce pneumonia as a complication of other diseases. Pneumonia is transmitted through the mouth or nasal discharges associated with coughing or nose-blowing; it has an incubation period of from one to three days; and it usually lasts from seven to ten days if untreated. Medical treatment consists of isolation and rest for the patient and treatment with antibiotics. *See also* text, Chapter 22.

botulism A deadly food poisoning produced by an anaerobic bacterium that grows in the soil and in the intestines of some animals. It is contracted by the ingestion of a toxin produced by bacterial spores sealed inside improperly canned food and allowed to multiply. Symptoms, which occur within eighteen hours and vary in severity depending on the amount of toxin ingested, include headache, weakness, and paralysis; death can be rapid due to the inability to breathe. Treatment consists of the administration of a specific antitoxin. The poison can be avoided by boiling canned foods, which destroys the toxin.

Bright's disease *See* nephritis.

bronchitis *See* text, Chapter 25.

brucellosis *See* undulant fever.

bubonic fever *See* plague.

C

cancer *See* text, Chapter 23.

cat-scratch fever A mild viral infection usually transmitted through the lick, bite, or scratch of a cat. It has an incubation time of from one to two weeks and usually lasts no longer than forty-eight hours. Symptoms include slight fever and headache, and a rash or outbreak of boillike eruptions occasionally will occur at the site of the scratch. The disease cannot be contracted from infected persons. No vaccination procedures exist for cat-scratch fever.

cerebral palsy The name for a wide variety of physical defects that result from brain damage occurring before or shortly after birth. Exact cause of the damage is often unknown, but such conditions as Rh-blood factor clash between mother and fetus, maternal kidney disease, or high-fever infections of an infant may lead to cerebral palsy. Symptoms of the disease depend on the degree of brain damage and range from partial weakening of one limb to general loss of motor ability and mental retardation. The most common manifestation of the disease is loss of coordination due to imbalance of opposing muscular groups. Cerebral palsy is noncontagious and noncurable. Treatment consists of lessening the severity of the muscular defects through supportive bracing and physical therapy.

chancroid A venereal disease characterized by the presence of a soft chancre (an open sore) on the genitalia and severe, painful swelling of the lymph nodes of the groin. The disease is transmitted through sexual intercourse with infected persons, has an incubation period of from one to three days, and is contagious until healed. Treatment consists of administration of antibiotics, and prevention is best accomplished, but not assured, by thorough washing immediately following intercourse

with an infected person. No immunity is conferred, and no artificial immunity is available.

chickenpox A viral disease found throughout the world and endemic to almost all large urban areas. Symptoms include moderate fever, headache, and a characteristic rash, which develops first on the trunk and spreads to the extremities. The rash is composed of blisterlike eruptions in the outermost layer of skin that break, form a crusty scab, and finally fall off. Chickenpox is transmitted by droplet infection, is communicable from one day before to six days after the first appearance of the rash, has an incubation period of from two to three weeks, and usually lasts about five days. Because the disease confers a lifetime immunity against reinfection, it is most prevalent in children. Treatment is symptomatic, and secondary infections are prevented through washing and restricting unnecessary movement. Prevention of the spread of chickenpox is accomplished by isolation of infected persons; artificial immunization is unavailable.

cholera A severe bacterial infection of the small intestine found most often in temperate underdeveloped countries such as India. Symptoms of the disease include unceasing diarrhea, vomiting, loss of kidney function, and extreme thirst. Cholera is transmitted through contaminated food or water, has an incubation time of from five to six days, and usually results in death through dehydration and uric acid poisoning. When death does not occur, recovery usually takes place within two weeks. Immunization is achieved through inoculation. Cholera is no longer a problem in the United States.

cirrhosis *See* text, Chapter 25.

Clostridium perfringens A bacterium, from the same family as those responsible for botulism and tetanus, that causes a mild food poisoning through spoiled meat dishes. Symptoms of the disease include abdominal pain and diarrhea occurring within six

hours after ingestion of the toxin. The disease usually lasts less than one day and is nonfatal. Ingestion of the toxin can be avoided by heating and cooling meat dishes as rapidly as possible and by not eating meat that has been long at room temperature.

colitis *See* ulcerative colitis.

Colorado tick fever A mild viral disease that occurs only in the northwestern United States. Symptoms include moderate fever and a rash. The disease is common in squirrels and is transmitted to man by the bite of ticks that have fed on an infected animal. The disease has an incubation time of from four to five days. Colorado tick fever confers a lifetime immunity against reinfection, but no artificial immunity is available, and no means is available to treat the disease. Prevention is accomplished through insect-eradication programs.

common cold *See* text, Chapter 22.

conjunctivitis An acute, usually bacterial, infection of the conjunctiva characterized by dilation of the blood vessels of the sclera, secretion of pus from the eyes, swelling of the eyelids, and light sensitivity of the eyes. The disease is highly contagious and is transmitted by direct contact or indirect contact with soiled articles such as towels, handkerchiefs, or bed linen. The incubation time is from one to three days, and conjunctivitis is communicable until symptoms disappear. Applications of tetracycline ointment quickly relieve the symptoms, but the disease may remain infectious for several days.

coronary heart disease *See* text, Chapter 24.

Cushing's syndrome *See* text, Chapter 25.

cystic fibrosis A chronic hereditary disease characterized by malformation or absence of the excretory duct of any of several glands. The organs most commonly affected are the pancreas, liver, sweat glands, mucus-producing glands of the lung and throat, and the testicles. Symptoms depend on the gland affected, but the

Appendix A
Common Diseases of Man

usual course of the disease is chronic and progressive respiratory infection resulting in early death. Antibiotics can prolong the life of the patient and decrease the severity of lung infections. Special diets are often necessary to assure the normal development of affected children.

D

diabetes   *See* text, Chapter 25.

diphtheria   An acute bacterial infection characterized by mild fever, sore throat, and a running nose; it sometimes lasts several weeks. It has an incubation period of from one to six days, is usually contagious for about two weeks beginning three days before the onset of symptoms, is fatal 5 to 10 percent of the time, and is transmitted through contact with nasal or throat discharges of an infected person. Though the symptoms are not severe, the toxin released by the bacterium can permanently damage the heart or nervous system. Diphtheria usually confers a lasting immunity, and children born to immune mothers retain a passive immunity for about six months. Active immunization can also be induced through vaccination.

diverticulosis   A fairly common condition characterized by patchy weakening and outward ballooning of the intestinal wall in the descending colon; the inflammation of this condition is known as diverticulitis. Diverticulosis is not a dangerous condition by itself, but because inflammation of the intestinal wall can lead to rupture and peritonitis, diverticulitis is serious. When inflammation occurs, symptoms include fever, abdominal pain, and either constipation or diarrhea. If rupture does occur, the inflamed portion of the intestine must be surgically removed.

Down's syndrome   *See* text, Chapter 14.

dysentery   *See* amebiasis; shigellosis.

E

eczema   A term used to lump together all skin irritations of unknown origin characterized by redness, itching, blisters, or scales. If the conditions persist, the skin will eventually become tough and leathery. The application of creams and ointments containing cortisone or the oral administration or injection of cortisone can usually improve the condition.

emphysema   *See* text, Chapter 25.

endocarditis   *See* bacterial endocarditis.

enterobiasis (pinworms)   An infection of the intestinal tract characterized by disturbed sleep, irritability, and itching of the anal area. It is common among children and affects about 20 percent of the United States population. Pinworms are transmitted by the ingestion of eggs laid on the perianal skin and transferred to clothing or hands and eventually to food. The disease is communicable for two to eight weeks after infection and disappears spontaneously. The spread of pinworms is best prevented by strict cleanliness and good toilet habits.

epilepsy   *See* text, Chapter 25.

G

gallstones   Accumulation in the gall bladder of stones composed of cholesterol, bile pigment, and calcium. They often are painless and do no harm. They occur in about a quarter of the older people in the United States and cause chronic inflammation of the gall bladder. Occasionally a stone will pass out of the gall bladder into the common bile duct and obstruct the flow of bile into the duodenum. Severe pain in the lower right chest, nausea, and often vomiting follow; jaundice is present in some cases. When these symptoms occur, the presence of gallstones is confirmed by x-ray. Treatment consists of the surgical removal of the gall bladder and stones; preventive measures are unknown.

gastritis   Inflammation of the stomach accompanied by gastric indigestion. Gastritis is a catchall term for chronic or acute afflictions caused by many different and sometimes unknown agents. It is most common in older people and is characterized by irritation and reddening of the stomach lining. Symptoms of acute gastritis are nausea, headache, temperature increase, and finally vomiting to remove the irritant, followed by fatigue. Treatment consists of avoidance of irritating substances. Symptoms of the chronic condition, which often indicates a developing ulcer, are similar to those of acute gastritis but are less severe. The causes of chronic gastritis are difficult to identify, but it has been attributed to various vitamin deficiencies, secretory malfunctions, and the mild abuse of alcohol. Treatment of the chronic form consists of bed rest, a bland diet, and medication to reduce the acid level of the stomach. *See also* text, Chapter 25.

gastroenteritis   A catchall term for a variety of severe gastrointestinal inflammations that may be symptoms of another disease or independent infection by a number of bacterial and viral agents. Symptoms include nausea, vomiting, diarrhea, and abdominal cramps, and treatment usually consists of a change of diet and in severe cases, surgery. Gastroenteritis may result from food poisoning, chronic alcoholism, hepatitis, or malaria, among others. When it results from infection by a microbial agent, the disease usually lasts from one to two days and is more likely to be fatal among infants than among other age groups. It is endemic in many underdeveloped areas of the world and is primarily transmitted by fecal contamination of food.

German measles   *See* rubella.

glaucoma   *See* text, Chapter 19.

gonorrhea   *See* text, Chapter 22.

ground itch   *See* hookworm.

H

hay fever   *See* text, Chapter 25.

hemophilia   *See* text, Chapter 14.

hemorrhoids (piles)   Varicose veins of the rectum. They can be caused by prolonged constipation, excess straining at defecation, diarrhea, or pregnancy. Hemorrhoids are characterized by small folds of swollen skin around the anus; these folds are often painful or itchy. Because hemorrhoids are more annoying than dangerous, treatment usually consists of measures to prevent their irritation through stool-softening medication or soothing ointments and suppositories. In extreme cases hemorrhoids can be removed surgically.

hepatitis   Inflammation of the liver. It can occur in two forms, acute, or serum hepatitis, and chronic, or infectious hepatitis. Serum hepatitis is caused by a virus and is transmitted by intravenous or intramuscular injection with surgical equipment contaminated with the blood, serum, or plasma of an infected person. Infectious hepatitis, which also is viral, is transmitted through food or water contaminated by feces of an infected person; it is communicable from several days before until a week after the onset of symptoms. The incubation period of serum hepatitis is from forty days to one year; for the infectious form it is from two to six weeks. Symptoms of the two types are indistinguishable and include low appetite, high fever, and jaundice that can last for several weeks or months. Treatment includes bed rest and a diet high in proteins and carbohydrates. The administration of gamma globulin to exposed persons often prevents the occurrence of the disease or lessens its impact. *See also* text, Chapter 25.

hernia The protrusion of any organ beyond the space it normally occupies. The term is most often associated with protrusions of an abdominal organ through the abdominal wall. The abdominal wall is weak in the areas of the groin, the navel, and the center of the diaphram where the esophagus enters the abdomen. If undue strain is put on these weak areas by coughing or lifting heavy objects, there is a possibility that the wall will rupture and a portion if the intestines or stomach will protrude through the muscle layer. If the hernia is inguinal (groin) or umbilical, a portion of the small intestine will protrude, causing swelling at the site; the swelling will often disappear when the patient lies on his back. In the case of an esophagial hernia, the stomach or a portion of it will protrude into the chest cavity, interfering with the functioning of the heart or lungs. Esophagial hernias are characterized by heartburn and indigestion after meals or when lying down. The danger of a hernia is the possibility that the protruding organ will be strangulated and die due to the lack of an adequate blood supply. Treatment of hernias consists of trussing to hold in the protruding organ or surgery to close the hole in the abdominal wall.

herpes simplex *See* text, Chapter 20.

herpes zoster Better known as shingles, a viral infection of a cutaneous nerve root characterized by pain, redness, and blisters along the nerve. It usually affects a nerve of the trunk of the body, and the rash and blisters follow the nerve around the body in a beltlike manner; it can also affect the eyes. Herpes zoster usually affects adults and is caused by the same virus that produces chickenpox in children. Because the disease is self-limiting, pain-relieving measures usually are the only treatment, but cortisone is occasionally used to arrest the progress and antibiotics are used to treat secondary infections of the blisters. The disease confers a lasting immunity against reinfection and is extremely rare in persons who have had chickenpox during childhood.

histoplasmosis A common fungal infection of the lungs characterized by weakness, mild fever, mild chest pains, and cough; the disease often passes unnoticed. The histoplasmosis mold grows in soil and animal excrement and is transmitted to man through inhalation or ingestion of the fungal spores; it is not communicable from man to man. The incubation period is from five to eighteen days after exposure, and excessively high doses of the spores can result in a rare and fatal form of the disease. Susceptibility to the disease is general, and the best means of prevention is avoidance of contaminated areas or adequate sanitary precautions when near such areas. Treatment is symptomatic, and the disease confers an immunity against serious reinfection.

hookworm A serious intestinal infection resulting in anemia and malnutrition. The disease is contracted through the skin, usually the feet, and initially produces a severe local irritation called ground itch. The hookworm larvae, which live in the soil, penetrate to the lymphatic system or to a blood vessel and travel to the lungs. From within the lungs they migrate to the throat and are swallowed. Once in the digestive tract the larvae mature into worms and fasten themselves to the intestinal wall. The worms feed on the blood of their host. Eggs appear in the stools of the host about six weeks after infection and continue to be present as long as the infection continues. Administration of specific drugs eliminates the worms. The best means of prevention is adequate sanitation and sewer facilities.

hypertension *See* text, Chapter 24.

I

influenza *See* text, Chapter 22.

K

kidney stones *See* urolithiasis.

Klinefelter's syndrome *See* text, Chapter 14.

kwashiorkor *See* text, Chapter 17.

L

leprosy An infectious bacterial disease that affects the skin, the mucous membranes of the mouth, and the testes. The disease is universal but is most prevalent in Asia, Africa, and South America. It is characterized by ulcerous lesions of the skin in which the cutaneous nerves are destroyed, leading to eventual death of the tissue. Only moderately infectious, the disease is transmitted by direct contact with an infected person and has an incubation time of from a few months to twenty years. Lepers cannot be cured, but the progress of their disease can be slowed through the use of sulfa drugs and antibiotics. Isolation of diseased persons is essential to prevent the spread of leprosy.

leukemia A cancer of the white blood cells that can be either chronic or acute. Early symptoms of the chronic condition, which develops slowly and has a long duration, include loss of appetite, weakness, general atrophy, and night sweats. As the chronic condition progresses, symptoms become acute and include high fever, sores and bleeding of the gums, and severe weakness. The number of white blood cells can be from fifteen to one-hundred times that found in normal blood, and anemia and an enlarged spleen usually accompany the disease. The cause of leukemia is unknown, as is any cure, but it is possible to prolong the life of the patient through the use of cortisone, therapy with radioactive substances, and blood transfusions. *See also* text, Chapter 23.

liver-fluke disease *See* schistosomiasis.

lockjaw *See* tetanus.

lousiness *See* pediculosis.

lymphogranuloma venereum An acute infectious venereal disease primarily affecting the lymphatic system of the groin. Symptoms include fever, abdominal pain, loss of appetite, swelling of the lymph nodes of the groin, swelling of the genitalia, and lesions and ulcerations of the skin of the groin and genitalia. The disease is transmitted by sexual intercourse or by contact with contaminated clothing. Lymphogranuloma venereum has an incubation period of from five days to a month and is infectious until lesions disappear. Antibiotics or sulfa drugs are used to treat the disease, and the best means of prevention is avoidance of sexual intercourse with known infected persons.

M

malaria An infectious protozoan disease characterized by remittent fever alternating with chills. Because the disease is transmitted by the bite of a mosquito, it is most prevalent in tropical areas. The incubation time is two weeks. Symptoms begin with general muscular aches and fever, rapidly progressing to chills accompanied by violent shaking and cyanosis. Administration of quinine or a similar drug eliminates the symptoms, but patients can usually recover without medication. Prevention of malaria is best accomplished through eradication of the vector mosquito; daily small doses of quinine in infested areas will also prevent the disease.

measles (rubeola) An infectious viral disease common in children and characterized by severe rash. It is transmitted through contact with discharges from the nose or throat of an infected person, who can spread germs by sneezing or coughing. It is infectious from a week to eleven days after it is contracted. Early symptoms, which appear about ten days after exposure, include fever, coughing, and swelling and congestion of the mucous membranes of the nose and throat. White spots appear in the mouth and the following day a rash begins to develop on the scalp and forehead, gradually spreading over the entire body in about four days. As the rash, which is composed of red blisterlike eruptions, progresses, the fever begins to subside. The rash disappears after five days. Treatment consists of isolating the patient and guarding against secondary infection. Measles confers a lifetime immunity, and injections of gamma globulin will provide an artificial immunity for two to six weeks.

meningitis An acute inflammation of the meninges, the membranes enclosing the brain and spinal cord. The disease usually results from a bacterial infection following an injury to the head or as a complication of several infectious diseases. Incubation time for the disease is two to ten days, and symptoms include fever and general aching and pain in the entire body, progressing to severe headaches, vomiting, and intense pain. Treatment of meningitis includes hospitalization and the administration of antibiotic drugs. The disease can usually be prevented or diagnosed early by careful attention to infections of the nose and throat and by the administration of antibiotic drugs to anyone exposed to the disease. Meningitis is rarely fatal if treated properly. *See also* text, Chapter 25.

migraine Headaches caused by vasodilation of the arteries of the brain; they are usually severe. Migraine attacks affect a specific area of the head and progress in a characteristic sequence. Headaches begin with a dull building pain and progress to symptoms of confusion, depression, temporary blindness, abdominal pain, or nausea. Treatment of migraine consists of immobilizing the patient in a darkened room and making him as comfortable as possible. There is no known way to prevent a migraine headache, but an early awareness and treatment of an impending attack can lessen the severity.

mononucleosis *See* text, Chapter 22.

multiple sclerosis A chronic degenerative disease of the central nervous system, usually affecting people between the ages of twenty and forty. Symptoms of the disease can include weakness and loss of coordination in the legs and hands, problems with speech and vision, or loss of certain autonomous functions, such as digestion. Symptoms result from the destruction of the myelin sheaths that cover nerve fibers in the brain and spinal cord. The patient usually retains complete mental facility, but because nervous impulses cannot be properly transmitted, he loses muscular control. Multiple sclerosis is marked by long periods of seemingly good health alternating with the manifestations of symptoms that usually become more severe with each occurrence. Because the causes of the myelin sheath destruction are unknown, there is no cure or method of prevention for multiple sclerosis, but proper care and otherwise good health can reduce the frequency of attacks. *See also* text, Chapter 25.

mumps An acute viral infection of the parotid and salivary glands located beneath the angle of the jaw bone. It is common and mild during childhood and usually confers a lifelong immunity. Symptoms include swollen glands, puffiness in the side of the face, difficulty opening the mouth, and mild to moderate fever. The disease is transmitted by direct contact with the nasal or throat discharges of an infected person and has an incubation period of from two to three weeks. Complications are rare in children, but mature males often develop a secondary infection in the testicles that can lead to sterility; the disease may also affect the ovaries and breasts of women. For this reason adults who have not had mumps as children should be vaccinated.

muscular dystrophy A chronic condition characterized by gradual weakening, atrophy, or paralysis of a muscle, muscular group, or entire limb. The condition usually results from a disorder of the nerves controlling the affected area. There are several forms of muscular dystrophy affecting different age groups and different areas of the body. There is no known cure for muscular dystrophy.

myasthenia gravis A chronic nervous-system disease of unknown cause. It primarily affects the voluntary muscles of the face, mouth, and eyes and results in slack facial expression, difficulty in eating and talking, and strained vision. Muscles become extremely weak and tire quickly. The disease usually affects adults and develops slowly, but it can affect children or be acute. The administration of specific drugs can lessen the severity of the disease, and facial exercises can strengthen the muscles involved. Occasionally the thymus gland is removed surgically or treated with x-rays with some beneficial effect.

mycoplasmal pneumonia An acute infection and vasocongestion of the upper respiratory tract characterized by fever and coughing. It is caused by the Eaton agent, a viruslike organism. Mycoplasmal pneumonia is transmitted through the mouth or nasal discharges of an infected person, has an incubation period of from one to three weeks, and can last from three days to several weeks. Treatment consists of isolation and rest for the patient, and maintenance of general good health is the best means of prevention.

N

nephritis A general term for any condition marked by inadequate excretory functioning of the kidney due to inflammation of the blood vessels in the nephrons. Common symptoms include the presence of the protein albumin in the urine, swollen ankles, fatigue, and headaches. If the condition becomes severe it can include such symptoms as nausea and vomiting, swelling of the abdomen, and unconsciousness. Acute nephritis is most commonly called Bright's disease and can become chronic if not treated promptly. Treatment consists of bed rest and limitations on fluid and protein consumption. *See also* text, Chapter 25.

nephrosis A chronic childhood disease of unknown cause characterized by degeneration of a noninflamed kidney. Symptoms include remittent edema alternating with periods during which the child seems perfectly normal. During the periods of edema, severe swelling occurs in the face, abdomen, and feet. Swelling subsides quickly with the excretion of large amounts of urine, and the symptom-free periods can last from a few days to months or be permanent. Nephrosis usually affects a child for several years and disappears spontaneously. Treatment consists of a special diet and the administration of certain adrenal hormones.

O

otitis media *See* text, Chapter 19.
otosclerosis *See* text, Chapter 19.

P

paralysis agitans *See* Parkinson's disease.

paratyphoid fever An acute bacterial infection of the intestines similar to typhoid fever. Symptoms include sudden and continuing fever, diarrhea, and the appearance of red spots on the body. The disease is transmitted by direct contact with an infected person or carrier or by contact with food contaminated by an infected person. Paratyphoid has an incubation period of from one to ten days and is communicable from the onset of symptoms to several days after recovery. Susceptibility is general, and the disease usually confers a lasting immunity against reinfection. Treatment consists of isolation and the administration of antibiotic drugs.

Parkinson's disease (paralysis agitans) A chronic condition of old age characterized by progressive paralysis and eventual death. Symptoms begin with a palsy or rigidity of a single limb that spreads to both limbs on one side, all the limbs, and finally to the muscles of the trunk and face. The disease seems to originate in the brain, and surgery to reduce the activity of concerned areas of the brain often is performed. Specific chemotherapy can reduce the severity of symptoms and in some instances improve the patient's condition.

pediculosis Infestation with lice. Two common species of lice attack man, the body louse and the crab louse; men are not bothered by animal lice. The body louse infests only the head, beard, and body, and the crab louse infests the pubic region. Lice are transmitted by direct contact with an infested person or by contact with the clothes of an infested person. Symptoms of pediculosis include extreme irritation and itching of the infested area. Eradication of lice is usually accomplished through bathing and applications of poison dusting powder.

peptic ulcer *See* text, Chapter 25.

pertussis *See* whooping cough.

phenylketonuria (PKU) *See* text, Chapter 14.

piles *See* hemorrhoids.

pink-eye *See* conjunctivitis.

pinworm *See* enterobiasis.

plague An acute, bacterial infection of two types, bubonic fever and pneumonic plague. If untreated, one-quarter to one-half of the cases are fatal. Symptoms of both types include fever, low blood pressure, delirium, and coma. Bubonic plague is further characterized by swelling of the lymph nodes of the groin. The disease exists in wild rodents in several areas of the world and is transmitted to man through the bite of an infected rat flea; pneumonic plague also can be spread by droplet infection. The incubation period is from two to six days, and susceptibility is general. The disease confers a temporary immunity, and a temporary artificial immunity is available through vaccination. Treat-

ment of plague involves the administration of antibiotics. The best means of prevention is the eradication of urban rat populations.

pneumonia *See* bacterial pneumonia; mycoplasmal pneumonia; viral pneumonia; text, Chapter 22.

pneumonic plague *See* plague.

poliomyelitis An acute viral infection of a part of the spinal cord. It can vary in severity from mild to severe, but it usually strikes in one of three recognizable forms. Symptoms of the most mild form include fever, headache, diarrhea, and aching muscles; this form often is not recognized as polio. The second form of the disease is known as nonparalytic and is characterized by temporary paralysis of the limbs. A final form, known as paralytic, can be permanently disabling or cause death. The disease is usually transmitted through droplet infection or contact with the feces of a person infected with the mild form of the disease. The incubation period is from one to three weeks, and the disease is communicable from two days to six weeks after infection. Polio cannot be treated, but vaccination provides a lifetime immunity against infection.

polycythemia A chronic disease of unknown cause characterized by the overproduction of red blood cells by the bone marrow. Because the blood becomes viscous, it cannot be pumped to the brain or other organs with maximum efficiency, and symptoms of headache, dizziness, blurred vision, and hearing disorders result. Loss of sensation in the limbs and amnesia also can occur. The disease is usually treated with intravenous injections of radioactive phosphorus, which slows the production of red blood cells. Occasionally blood will be extracted from the patient at periodic intervals. Polycythemia is conducive to several complications, including thromboembolism, gout, and anemia.

psoriasis A chronic skin disease of unknown cause characterized by recurrent eruptions of local inflammation. Eruptions are composed of patches or red spots that increase in size until they resemble a thick scaly welt. As the welt heals the skin is temporarily discolored and the scales begin to fall off the eruption. Psoriasis is usually found on the feet, hands, and knees, but it also can occur on the scalp and chest. Treatment of the disease is aimed at reducing the severity of the skin eruptions and includes special low-fat or low-alcohol diets, hormone injections, radiation therapy, administration of sedatives or tranquilizers, and the application of special ointments. Psoriasis cannot be spread from

one person to another, but little else is known about its cause or the means to prevent it.

puerperal fever. *See* streptococcal puerperal fever.

pyorrhea *See* text, Chapter 20.

R

rabies (hydrophobia) *See* text, Chapter 25.

rheumatic fever *See* text, Chapter 24.

ringworm A fungal infection of the skin characterized by blistering, scaling, and loss of hair. It is highly contagious and exists in several different forms. The disease is most prevalent in children and persons living in warm, damp climates. Ringworm can be transmitted directly or indirectly through contact with an infected person's clothing, and it has an incubation period of from ten to fourteen days. A common source of transmission is an infected household pet. Thorough washing and drying of the affected areas and the application of antifungal ointments eliminate the infection. Where hairy parts of the body are involved the hair is usually clipped short or removed. *See also* athlete's foot.

Rocky Mountain spotted fever A tick-borne rickettsial infection most prevalent in the Rocky Mountain states but also occurring infrequently throughout the United States and parts of Canada and Mexico. Symptoms include fever, a rash starting on the wrists and ankles and spreading over the entire body, headache, and infection of the conjunctiva. The disease is common in wild rodents and is transmitted to man by the bite of an infected wood or dog tick. The incubation time is from two to ten days. If untreated, spotted fever lasts for about two weeks and is fatal 20 percent of the time. The administration of tetracycline until the fever disappears usually assures recovery. The best prevention is avoidance of tick-infested areas and careful and prompt removal of any ticks from one's person or pets.

Rubella (German measles) A mild, highly contagious viral infection common between the ages of four and nineteen. Symptoms include fever, rash, and swollen glands in the throat and neck. The disease is transmitted by direct contact or by droplet infection and has an incubation period of from two to three weeks. Rubella is infectious from seven days before until about ten days after the appearance of the rash. Treatment consists of isolating the patient and guarding against secondary infection. Rubella confers a lifetime immunity, and vaccination is available but rarely administered. If contracted during the first trimester of pregnancy, the adult form of the disease can cause serious birth defects. Vaccination of susceptible pregnant women is often advised. *See also* text, Chapter 14.

rubeola *See* measles.

S

salmonellosis   An acute food poisoning produced by several types of salmonella bacteria. Symptoms include fever, sudden pain of the abdomen, diarrhea, loss of appetite, nausea, and vomiting. A common disease, the infection is usually contracted through ingestion of contaminated meat or poultry, but it can be spread from person to person by direct contact. The incubation period is from six hours to two days. Salmonellosis is rarely fatal, and treatment usually consists of keeping the patient as comfortable as possible while the disease runs its course. The best means of prevention is thorough cooking of all meat dishes and eggs.

scabies   An infection of the skin by a small mite. Symptoms include intense itching along small lesions at the base of the fingers and toes, in the armpits, on the breasts of women, and on the genitalia of men. The female mites burrow under the skin, creating tunnels about a quarter of an inch long in which eggs are laid. As the eggs hatch, the burrow opens to the surface and the mites escape. The disease is transmitted by direct contact and has an incubation time of from one to two weeks. It is communicable until the mites are eradicated. Treatment consists of frequent bathing in hot water followed by applications of a special ointment to the affected areas.

scarlet fever   A streptococcal infection characterized by fever, sore throat resembling tonsillitis, rash, and swelling of the glands of the neck and tongue (strawberry tongue). The disease is transmitted by direct contact, droplet spread, or contact with clothing of an infected person. It has an incubation period of from one to three days and usually is communicable for two to three weeks after infection. If untreated the disease can have serious complications, including nephritis, scarring of the valves of the heart, and severe arthritis. The administration of penicillin decreases the severity of the symptoms and usually prevents complications. Scarlet fever confers a lifetime immunity.

schistosomiasis   Liver-fluke disease. It is common in most underdeveloped areas of the world. The worms deposit eggs in various organs of the body, and as each egg matures it produces a small scar in the tissue. The long-term effect of this process is gradual deterioration of any organ involved. The disease is contracted by contact with water containing the worm larvae, which enter the body through the skin. The larvae migrate to the liver and mature before entering the veins of the abdomen as adult worms. Eggs discharged in the urine and feces hatch into larvae, which must invade a fresh-water snail. After living within the snail for several weeks, the larvae become free-swimming and can attack man. Symptoms appear from four to six weeks after infection, and the disease is communicable as long as eggs are discharged from the body, sometimes for twenty-five years. The worms and eggs are killed by the injection of a specific drug. The best means of prevention is avoidance of endemic areas.

shigellosis (bacillary dysentery)   An acute bacterial infection of the intestine. Symptoms include fever, vomiting, abdominal cramps, diarrhea, and often the passing of blood. The disease occurs throughout the world but is more severe in warmer climates. It is transmitted by contact with food, water, or objects contaminated by the feces of an infected person, and it has an incubation period of from one to seven days. Shigellosis is infectious as long as bacteria are present in the feces, usually two weeks. Water and salt are given to replace that lost by diarrhea, and the patient is made as comfortable as possible; in severe cases antibacterial drugs can be used to combat the infection. The best prevention consists of adequate disposal of feces and purification of water supplies.

shingles   *See* herpes zoster.

smallpox   A highly contagious viral disease known for the disfiguring pockmarks that it produces. Symptoms of the disease include fever, headache, and pain of the abdomen lasting from three to four days. As these symptoms pass and temperature returns to normal, a rash of small red blisters forms over the body. The blisters form scabs and fall off in about three weeks, leaving characteristic scars. Smallpox is transmitted by direct contact with an infected person, by contact with the scab of a smallpox blister, or by droplet infection. The incubation

period is from seven to sixteen days, and the disease is infectious from the time symptoms appear and until all the scabs have fallen off. The disease is fatal about 30 percent of the time but confers a lifetime immunity to survivors. Artificial immunity is available through repeated vaccination at five- to seven-year intervals.

staphylococcal disease   A general term referring to infection of any of several parts of the body by staphylococcus bacteria. The disease is universal but more prevalent in crowded living areas, infant nurseries, and hospital wards. Symptoms depend upon where the disease occurs: in the community, staphylococcal disease is usually characterized by fever, headache, and widespread skin lesions that can lead to conjunctivitis or pneumonia; in infant nurseries, skin lesions are common and such complications as abscess of the breast or brain, pneumonia, and septicemia occur; in hospital wards, the elderly are usually victims and suffer from lesions that may develop into pneumonia, septicemia, or death. The disease is transmitted by direct contact with an infected person or a carrier or by contact with the clothing or bed linen of an infected person, and it has an incubation period of from two days to several weeks. It is contagious until all lesions disappear. The administration of appropriate antibiotic drugs hastens recovery and decreases the severity of symptoms. Prevention is best accomplished by personal hygiene and avoidance of infected persons.

staphylococcal food poisoning   An acute reaction to toxins produced by several strains of staphylococcus; it is not an infection. Symptoms include abdominal pain, diarrhea, nausea, and vomiting. It is contracted by eating foods in which staphylococci have grown and produced toxic wastes; such foods are commonly pastries, salads, and sliced meat products. The incubation period is from two to four hours, and the disease usually lasts less than two days. It is rarely fatal, and treatment consists of making the patient as comfortable as possible.

strep throat   *See* tonsillitis.

streptococcal puerperal fever   An acute bacterial infection of the genital tract of women who have recently given birth or undergone an abortion. Symptoms include fever, headache, and pain in the lower abdomen. The disease is transmitted by direct contact with a streptococcal carrier or infected person or by contact with contaminated clothing or bed linen.

Incubation time is from one to three days, and the infection is communicable for about three weeks. Penicillin is used to treat puerperal fever. Fatal cases are now rare.

syphilis *See* text, Chapter 22.

T

tapeworm   A parasitic infection of the digestive tract characterized by the presence of worm segments, or proglottides, in the feces. Symptoms may be absent or may include abdominal pain, diarrhea, constipation, anemia, or weight loss. The disease is contracted by eating inadequately cooked beef or pork containing the worm larvae. The proglottides first appear in the feces from eight to ten weeks after infection and may continue to appear for as long as forty years. Tapeworm eggs are passed with the proglottides and hatch into larvae after being eaten by cows or hogs. A major complication of pork tapeworm is invasion of the larvae into the muscles or nervous system of the host. Drugs are available that can kill the intestinal worms, but no therapy is available to eliminate the larvae. The best means of prevention is avoidance of raw meats.

Tay-Sachs disease   *See* text, Chapter 14.

tetanus (lockjaw)   An acute bacterial infection of the central nervous system with a fatality rate of about 35 percent. The bacteria responsible for the disease live in the intestines of horses, cattle, and men, in animal feces, and in soil. The bacterial spores enter the body through a cut or puncture wound and incubate from four days to three weeks. Tetanus symptoms include infection at the site of entry, painful muscular spasms, fever, headache, stiffening of the muscles of the neck and jaw, and eventual stiffening of the entire body. The best prevention is through vaccination and the administration of a booster injection when danger of infection is suspected. In unvaccinated individuals antitoxin serum is available. Tetanus does not always confer an immunity against reinfection.

tonsillitis (strep throat)   Usually a streptococcal infection of the tonsils, the spongy lymph glands located in the back of the mouth on either side of the throat. Symptoms include fever, headache, nausea, pain and redness of the throat, and swelling of the lymph glands of the neck. The disease is transmitted by direct contact with a carrier or an infected person, by contact with the clothing of bed linen of an infected person, or by

droplet infection. The incubation time is from one to three days, and the disease is communicable for ten days after infection. Tonsillitis is rarely serious unless it becomes chronic, and in the absence of treatment symptoms usually disappear within nine days. The administration of penicillin shortens the course of the disease and reduces the potential for spread. The best means of prevention is avoidance of infected persons.

trachoma   A chronic viral eye disease characterized by inflammation of the eyes, excessive tearing, small scarring, blisters on the eyelids that eventually cause it to become deformed, light sensitivity, and the growth of blood vessels into the cornea leading to possible blindness. The disease is highly contagious and is transmitted by direct contact with the tears of an infected person or indirectly through contact with soiled articles. The incubation time is from five to twelve days, and trachoma is infectious until symptoms disappear. Applications of tetracycline ointment usually eliminates the infection. No immunity is conferred, and the best prevention is avoidance of infected persons.

trichinosis   A roundworm infection of the muscles characterized by abdominal pain, nausea, fever, muscular pain, and sometimes swelling of the eyelids. The disease is usually contracted by eating larvae-infested pork. The ingested larvae develop into worms in the small intestine. As the adult worms reproduce, second-generation larvae penetrate the intestinal wall and migrate in the blood and lymphatic systems to various muscles, where they form small painful cysts. As the cysts become imbedded in the muscles, they are surrounded by scar tissue and the symptoms disappear. The parasite is most common in the United States and eastern Europe, and susceptibility is general. No treatment exists, and no immunity is conferred against reinfection. Adequate cooking or freezing of all pork products is the best way to avoid the disease.

trichomoniasis   A chronic protozoan disease of the genitourinary tracts of both men and women. Symptoms are sometimes absent in men, but in women they are inflammation of the vagina accompanied by yellowish discharges. The disease is transmitted by sexual intercourse and is most common among women from sixteen to thirty-five years of age. The incubation period is from four to twenty days, and the disease is communicable until treated. Chemotherapy usually eliminates the disease. Avoiding sexual

intercourse with infected persons is the best way to prevent trichomoniasis.

tuberculosis   *See* text, Chapter 22.

tularemia   An acute bacterial disease common in wild animals and sometimes transmitted to man. Rabbits are the chief source of infection, and incidence of the disease in the United States fluctuates with the rabbit-hunting seasons. The disease is contracted by contact with infected animals and occasionally through the bite of an infected fly or tick; the bacteria are destroyed by cooking. Symptoms include ulcerous inflammation at the site of infection, regional swollen lymph glands, fever, and chills. The incubation time is from one to ten days. If untreated, tularemia is fatal in 5 percent of the cases, but administration of antibiotics assures recovery. Permanent immunity is conferred upon the victim, and vaccination is available. The use of disposable rubber gloves when handling wild rabbits may prevent the occurrence of the disease.

Turner's syndrome   *See* text, Chapter 14.

typhoid fever   An acute bacterial infection characterized by fever, headache, slow pulse, bodily rash, constipation or diarrhea, and enlargement of the spleen. The disease is transmitted by direct contact with an infected person or through water contaminated by infected feces or urine. The incubation period is from one to three weeks, and susceptibility is general. If untreated, typhoid fever lasts for about three weeks, is infectious throughout its course, and is fatal about 10 percent of the time. Specific antibiotic chemotherapy reduces the fatality rate to 2 percent and relieves the severity of the symptoms. Typhoid fever confers a high immunity against reinfection, and artificial immunity is available through vaccination.

typhus fever   An acute rickettsial infection characterized by fever, headache, and a rash that spreads from the inside of the thighs and armpits over the entire body. Two major types of typhus fever exist, epidemic louse-borne and endemic flea-borne, differing in the severity of their symptoms and mode of transmission. The disease is transmitted from rats, which are the reservoir of infection, to men via the feces of feeding lice or fleas. The incubation time is from one to three weeks. The fatality rate for untreated epidemic typhus is from 10 to 40 percent; for untreated endemic typhus it is about 2 percent. Tetracycline reduces the fatality rate of both types and relieves the severity of the symptoms. Typhus fever confers a limited immunity for several years, and artificial immunization is available through vaccination. Additional preventive measures consist of attempts to eliminate rats, lice, and fleas from crowded residential areas.

U

ulcer *See* peptic ulcer.

ulcerative colitis A catchall term describing any condition in which the large intestine is inflamed and extensively ulcerated and the cause is unknown. Symptoms include severe, often bloody, diarrhea, moderate fever, and general atrophy of the body and weight loss. A bland diet accompanied by medication to slow the diarrhea is the usual treatment in mild cases. If inflammation persists and becomes severe, the colon is surgically removed.

undulant fever (brucellosis) An acute bacterial infection characterized by remittent fever, sweating, headache, constipation, and pain and weakness of the entire body. The disease is common among domestic farm animals and is transmitted to man by contact with an infected animal or by drinking unpasteurized milk from an infected goat, sheep, or cow. Incubation period is from five days to three weeks, and although the fatality rate is only 2 percent, the infection and symptoms can persist for several years. Antibiotics are used to combat the disease, but the relapse rate is high. The degree of immunity conferred by undulant fever is unknown, and no means of artificial immunity exists.

urolithiasis (kidney stones) The formation of stones in any part of the urinary tract. Stone formation is thought to result from the precipitation of urinary sediment from too highly concentrated urine and is promoted by urinary infection and infrequent urination. Symptoms of kidney stones include pain in the lower abdomen and progressive uric acid poisoning. The disease is treated by drinking great amounts of water and administering drugs to dissolve the stones or by surgery to remove the stones.

V

viral pneumonia An acute infection and vasocongestion of the lung characterized by fever, headache, chest pain, and coughing. The disease can be caused by several different viruses and is often a complication of such viral diseases as influenza, chickenpox, measles, or the common cold. Viral pneumonia is transmitted by direct contact with an infected person, by indirect contact with mouth or nasal discharges, or by droplet infection. The incubation period is from two to eight days, and the disease is infectious until symptoms disappear. No specific treatment is available, and the best means of prevention is avoidance of infected persons and maintenance of resistance through good health.

W

whooping cough (pertussis) An acute bacterial infection of the throat and lungs that primarily affects children. Symptoms include mild fever and a characteristic violent cough that can last as long as two months. Whooping cough is transmitted by direct contact, droplet infection, or indirect contact with mouth or nasal discharges of an infected person. It has an incubation period of from one to three weeks and is contagious during the early stages. Antibiotics reduce the period of communicability but do little to relieve the symptoms. Whooping cough confers a lasting immunity, and artificial immunization is available through vaccination.

Y

yellow fever An acute viral disease characterized by early fever, headache, and vomiting, followed by subnormal temperatures, intestinal bleeding, and jaundice. The disease is transmitted by the bite of an infected mosquito, and the incubation period is from three to six days. The fatality rate of yellow fever can be as high as 40 percent during an epidemic, and no method of treatment is known. In nonfatal cases recovery takes place in about ten days, and the patient is immune for life. Artificial immunization is available through vaccination.

The information contained in the following pages surveys the current range of laws regarding drug violations in the United States, using heroin, marijuana, pills, and alcohol as representative drugs. Arranged for easy comparison, this table will be of benefit in understanding the variety and complexity of current drug laws, as of 1971. Many of the states are presently examining their drug laws, and some are making extensive changes.

In comparing the penalties in the various states, one should note that violations with regard to alcohol usually carry much less severe penalties than those for other drugs, including marijuana. Also of interest is that although marijuana is sometimes treated as a dangerous drug along with amphetamines and barbiturates, it is more often regarded as a narcotic along with heroin.

It should be noted that prosecution to the limit is rare and is reserved for flagrant cases. In addition, the ways in which individual judges and counties interpret and apply these laws vary widely.

Appendix B
A Survey of Drug Laws
in the United States

A SURVEY OF DRUG LAWS IN THE UNITED STATES

STATE OR AREA	Heroin	Marijuana	Amphetamines or Barbiturates	Alcohol

Alabama	*sale:*
	1st offense: 2–5 yrs
	2nd offense: 5–10 yrs
	subsequent offenses:
	  10–20 yrs
	
	possession:
	1st offense: 2–5 yrs
	2nd offense: 5–10 yrs
	subsequent offenses:
	  10–20 yrs
	
	sale to a minor:
	maximum sentence
		sale:
		1st offense: 2–5 yrs
		2nd offense: 5–10 yrs
		subsequent offenses:
		  10–20 yrs
		
		possession:
		1st offense: 2–5 yrs
		2nd offense: 5–10 yrs
		subsequent offenses:
		  10–20 yrs
		
		sale to a minor:
		maximum sentence
			barbiturate sale:
			nmt 1 yr, nmt $500, ob
			subsequent:
			  nmt 2 yrs, nlt $1,000, ob
				legal age—21
				sale to a minor:
				1st offense: nmt 6
				  months and
				  $50–$500
				2nd offense:
				  3–6 months and
				  $50–$500
				3rd offense:
				  6–12 months and
				  $50–$500
				Intoxication level:
				.10% of blood content
				drunkenness:
				$5–$100

Alaska	*sale:*
	1st offense: 2–10 yrs and
	  nmt $5,000
	2nd offense: 10–20 yrs
	  and nmt $7,500
	subsequent offenses:
	  20–40 yrs and nmt
	  $10,000
	
	possession:
	1st offense: 2–10 yrs
	  and nmt $5,000
	2nd offense: 10–20 yrs
	  and nmt $7,500
	subsequent offenses:
	  20–40 yrs and nmt
	  $10,000
	
	sale to a minor:
	1st offense: 10–20 yrs
	  and $5,000–$10,000
	2nd offense: 15–30 yrs
	  and nmt $2,500
	3rd offense: life
		sale:
		1st offense: 2–10 yrs and
		  nmt $5,000
		2nd offense: 10–20 yrs
		  and nmt $7,500
		subsequent offenses:
		  20–40 yrs and nmt
		  $10,000
		
		possession:
		1st offense: up to 1 yr a/o
		  up to $1,000
		2nd offense: 10–20 yrs
		  and nmt $7,500
		subsequent offenses:
		  20–40 yrs and nmt
		  $10,000
		
		sale to a minor:
		1st offense: 10–20 yrs
		  and $5,000–$10,000
		2nd offense: 15–30 yrs
		  and nmt $2,500
		3rd offense: life
			sale:
			$100–$500, nmt 180
			  days, ob
				legal age—21
				sale to a minor:
				nmt 1 yr, nmt $500, ob
				Intoxication level:
				.10% of blood content
				drunkenness:
				nmt $300, nmt
				  6 months, ob

Arizona	*sale:*
	1st offense: 2–10 yrs
	2nd offense: 5–20 yrs
	subsequent offenses:
	  nlt 15 yrs
	
	possession:
	1st offense: 2–10 yrs
	2nd offense: 5–20 yrs
	subsequent offenses:
	  nlt 15 yrs
		sale:
		1st offense: 2–10 yrs
		2nd offense: 5–15 yrs
		subsequent offenses:
		  10 yrs–life
		
		possession:
		1st offense: 1 yr and
		  $1,000
		2nd offense: 2–20 yrs
		subsequent offenses:
		  5 yrs–life
			sale:
			1 yr–life
			
			*possession without
			prescription:*
			nmt 1 yr, nmt $1,000, ob
				legal age—21
				sale to a minor:
				1st offense: $100–
				  $300, 30 days–6
				  months, ob
				subsequent offenses:
				  $100–$1,000,
				  30 days–1 yr, ob
				Intoxication level:
				.15% of blood content
				drunkenness:
				nmt $200 or nmt 2
				  months

Code: a/o—and/or g—grams poss.—possible nmt—not more than nlt—not less than ob—or both

STATE OR AREA	Heroin	Marijuana	Amphetamines or Barbiturates	Alcohol
Arkansas	*sale:* 1st offense: nmt $2,000 and 2–5 yrs 2nd offense: nmt $2,000 and 5–10 yrs subsequent offenses: nmt $2,000 and 10–20 yrs *possession:* 1st offense: nmt $2,000 and 2–5 yrs 2nd offense: nmt $2,000 and 5–10 yrs subsequent offenses: nmt $2,000 and 10–20 yrs	*sale:* 1st offense: nmt $2,000 and 2–5 yrs 2nd offense: nmt $2,000 and 5–10 yrs subsequent offenses: nmt $2,000 and 10–20 yrs *possession:* 1st offense: nmt $2,000 and 2–5 yrs 2nd offense: nmt $2,000 and 5–10 yrs subsequent offenses: nmt $2,000 and 10–20 yrs	*sale:* $100–$1,000 (per bottle, package, or container)	*legal age*—21 *sale to a minor:* 1st offense: $100–$250 2nd offense: $250–$500, 6 months–1 yr, ob *Intoxication level:* .10% of blood content *drunkenness:* $5–$100, 5–30 days, ob
California	*sale:* 1st offense: 5–15 yrs 2nd offense: nlt 10 yrs subsequent offenses: nlt 15 yrs *possession:* 1st offense: 2–10 yrs 2nd offense: 5–20 yrs subsequent offenses: 15 yrs–life	*sale:* 1st offense: 2–10 yrs 2nd offense: 5–15 yrs subsequent offenses: 10 yrs–life *possession:* 1st offense: 1 yr in county jail or 1–10 yrs in state prison 2nd offense: 2–20 yrs subsequent offenses: 5 yrs–life	*sale:* 1st offense: 5 yrs–life 2nd offense: 5 yrs–life subsequent offenses: 10 yrs–life *possession for sale:* 1st offense: 2–10 yrs 2nd offense: 5–15 yrs subsequent offenses: 10 yrs–life *possession without prescription:* 1st offense: nmt 1 yr in county jail or 1–10 yrs in state prison subsequent offenses: 2–20 yrs	*legal age*—21 *sale to a minor:* nmt 6 months, nmt $500, ob *Intoxication level:* no codified presumptions *drunkenness:* nmt 6 months, nmt $500, ob
Colorado	*sale:* 1st offense: 10–20 yrs 2nd offense: 15–30 yrs 3rd offense: 20–40 yrs *possession:* 1st offense: 10–20 yrs 2nd offense: 15–30 yrs 3rd offense: 20–40 yrs	*sale:* 1st offense: 10–20 yrs 2nd offense: 15–30 yrs 3rd offense: 20–40 yrs *possession:* 1st offense: 10–20 yrs 2nd offense: 15–30 yrs 3rd offense: 20–40 yrs	*sale:* 1st offense: 1–14 yrs and nmt $1,000 subsequent offenses: 5–30 yrs and nmt $5,000 *possession:* nmt $500, nmt 1 yr, ob	*legal age*—21 3.2 *beer*—18 *sale to a minor:* $10–300, nmt 90 days, ob *Intoxication level:* .10% of blood content *drunkenness:* public intoxication in itself not a crime
Connecticut	*sale:* 1st offense: 5–10 yrs and nmt $3,000 2nd offense: 10–15 yrs and nmt $5,000 subsequent offenses: nmt 25 yrs *possession:* 1st offense: nmt 10 yrs and $3,000 2nd offense: nmt 15 yrs and $5,000 subsequent offenses: nmt 25 yrs	*sale:* 1st offense: 5–10 yrs and nmt $3,000 2nd offense: 10–15 yrs and nmt $5,000 subsequent offenses: nmt 25 yrs *possession:* 1st offense: nmt 1 yr and nmt $1,000 2nd offense: nmt 15 yrs and $5,000 subsequent offenses: nmt 25 yrs	*sale:* 1st offense: 5–10 yrs and nmt $3,000 2nd offense: 10–15 yrs and nmt $5,000 subsequent offenses: 25 yrs *or* 1st offense: nmt $1,000, nmt 2 yrs, ob subsequent offenses: nmt $5,000, nmt 10 yrs, ob *or* nmt 3 yrs or max. term (whichever is less) in the custody of the commissioner of correction	*legal age*—21 *sale to a minor:* nmt $1,000, nmt 1 year, ob *Intoxication level:* .15% of blood content *drunkenness:* nmt $20 or nmt 30 days

STATE OR AREA	Heroin	Marijuana	Amphetamines or Barbiturates	Alcohol
Delaware	*sale:* 1st offense: $5,000 – $50,000 and 10 – 25 yrs 2nd offense: 15 – 30 yrs *possession:* 1st offense: nmt $3,000 and nmt 5 yrs 2nd offense: 3 – 10 yrs *sale to a minor:* 1st offense: 15 – 30 yrs 2nd offense: 25 – 50 yrs	*sale:* 1st offense: $1,000 – $10,000 and 5 – 10 yrs 2nd offense: 7 – 15 yrs *possession:* 1st offense: $500 and nmt 2 yrs 2nd offense: 2 – 7 yrs *sale to a minor:* 1st offense: 7 – 15 yrs fine at discretion of court 2nd offense: 15 – 25 yrs	*sale:* 1st offense: $1,000 – $10,000 and 5 – 10 yrs 2nd offense: 15 – 25 yrs *use, possession:* 1st offense: nmt $500 and nmt 2 yrs 2nd offense: 2 – 7 yrs *sale to a minor:* 1st offense: 7 – 15 yrs fine at discretion of court 2nd offense: 15 – 25 yrs	*legal age* – 21 *sale to a minor:* nmt $100 and up to 30 days *Intoxication level:* .15% of blood content *drunkenness:* nmt 5 days or nmt $10
Florida	*sale:* 1st offense: nmt 10 yrs and nmt $10,000 2nd offense: 10 – 20 yrs and nmt $20,000 subsequent offenses: nlt 20 yrs and nmt $20,000 *possession:* 1st offense: nmt 5 yrs and nmt $5,000 2nd offense: 10 yrs – life and nmt $10,000 subsequent offenses: nmt 20 yrs and nmt $20,000	*sale:* 1st offense: nmt 10 yrs and nmt $10,000 2nd offense: 10 – 20 yrs and nmt $20,000 subsequent offenses: nlt 20 yrs and nmt $20,000 *possession:* 1st offense: nmt 5 yrs and nmt $5,000 2nd offense: 10 yrs – life and nmt $10,000 subsequent offenses: nmt 20 yrs and nmt $20,000	*sale:* 1 – 5 yrs	*legal age* – 21 *sale to a minor:* nmt 6 months or nmt $500 *Intoxication level:* .10% of blood content *drunkenness:* nmt $25 or nmt 3 months
Georgia	*sale:* 1st offense: 5 – 10 yrs subsequent offenses: 10 – 20 yrs, poss. life *possession:* 1st offense: 2 – 5 yrs and nmt $2,000 2nd offense: 5 – 10 yrs and nmt $3,000 subsequent offenses: 10 – 20 yrs and nmt $5,000	*sale:* 1st offense: 5 – 10 yrs subsequent offenses: 10 – 20 yrs, poss. life *possession:* 1st offense: 2 – 5 yrs and nmt $2,000 2nd offense: 5 – 10 yrs and nmt $3,000 subsequent offenses: 10 – 20 yrs and nmt $5,000	*sale:* 1st offense: nmt 2 yrs and nmt $2,000	*legal age* – 21 *sale to a minor:* nmt $1,000, nmt 12 months on chain gang, ob *Intoxication level:* .10% of blood content *drunkenness:* nmt $1,000, nmt 1 yr, ob
Hawaii	*sale:* 1st offense: nmt $1,000 and nmt 10 yrs subsequent offenses: nmt $2,000 and nmt 20 yrs *possession:* 1st offense: nmt 5 yrs 2nd offense: nmt 10 yrs *sale to under 20:* 1st offense: nmt $1,000 and nmt 20 yrs subsequent offenses: nmt $2,000 and nmt life	*sale:* 1st offense: nmt $1,000 and nmt 10 yrs subsequent offenses: nmt $2,000 and nmt 20 yrs *possession:* 1st offense: nmt 5 yrs 2nd offense: nmt 10 yrs *sale to under 20:* 1st offense: nmt $1,000 and nmt 20 yrs subsequent offenses: nmt $2,000 and nmt life	*sale:* 1st offense: nmt $1,000 and nmt 10 yrs 2nd offense: nmt $2,000 and nmt 20 yrs *possession:* 1st offense: nmt $1,000 and nmt 10 yrs 2nd offense: nmt $2,000 and nmt 20 yrs *sale to under 20:* 1st offense: nmt $1,000 and nmt 20 yrs 2nd offense: nmt $2,000 and nmt life	*legal age* – 20 *sale to a minor:* nmt $500, nmt 6 months, ob *Intoxication level:* .15% of blood content *drunkenness:* $100 – $1,000, nmt 1 yr, ob

Code: a/o – and/or   g – grams   poss. – possible   nmt – not more than   nlt – not less than   ob – or both

STATE OR AREA	Heroin	Marijuana	Amphetamines or Barbiturates	Alcohol
Idaho	*sale:* nmt 15 yrs *possession:* nmt 10 yrs *sale to a minor:* nmt 15 yrs	*sale:* nmt 15 yrs *possession:* nmt 10 yrs *sale to a minor:* nmt 15 yrs	*sale:* nmt 5 yrs and nmt $5,000	*legal age* — 21 *beer* — 20 *sale to a minor:* 3 months – 1 yr, $300 – $1,000, ob *Intoxication level:* .15% of blood content *drunkenness:* 3 months – 1 yr, $300 – $1,000, ob
Illinois	*sale:* 1st offense: $5,000 and 2 – 10 yrs 2nd offense: 5 yrs – life *possession:* 1st offense: $5,000 and 2 – 10 yrs 2nd offense: 5 yrs – life *sale to a minor:* 10 yrs – life, no probation	*sale:* 1st offense: nmt 1 yr, nmt $1,500, ob subsequent offenses: 2 – 10 yrs a/o $5,000 *possession:* 1st offense: nmt 1 yr, nmt $1,500, ob subsequent offenses: 2 – 10 yrs a/o $5,000 *sale to a minor:* 10 yrs – life, no probation	*sale:* 1st offense: $100 – $1,000, nmt 1 yr, ob subsequent offenses: $500 – $2,500, nmt 5 yrs, ob *sale to a minor:* 1st offense: nlt $500, nmt 2 yrs, ob subsequent offenses: nlt $1,500, 5 – 6 yrs, ob	*Legal age* — 21 *sale to a minor:* 1st offense: nmt $100, nmt 6 months, ob subsequent offenses: $50 – 100, nmt 6 months, ob *Intoxication level:* .10% of blood content *drunkenness:* nmt $500
Indiana	*sale:* 1st offense: $2,000 a/o 5 – 20 yrs subsequent offenses: $5,000 a/o 20 yrs – life *possession:* 1st offense: $1,000 a/o 2 – 10 yrs subsequent offenses: $2,000 a/o 5 – 20 yrs	*sale:* 1st offense: $2,000 a/o 5 – 20 yrs subsequent offenses: $5,000 a/o 20 yrs – life *possession:* 1st offense: $1,000 a/o 2 – 10 yrs subsequent offenses: $2,000 a/o 5 – 20 yrs	*sale:* 1st offense 1 – 10 yrs in state prison and nmt $1,000 *or* nmt 1 yr in county jail or state penal farm and nmt $500 2nd offense: nmt $3,000 and 2 – 15 yrs *possession:* 1st offense: 1 – 10 yrs in state prison and nmt $1,000 *or* nmt 1 yr in county jail or state penal farm and nmt $500 2nd offense: nmt $3,000 and 2 – 15 yrs	*legal age* — 21 *sale to a minor:* nmt $500 and up to 6 months *Intoxication level:* .15% of blood content *drunkenness:* $1 – $100 and up to 6 months
Iowa	*sale:* 1st offense: $2,000 and 2 – 5 yrs 2nd offense: $2,000 and 5 – 10 yrs subsequent offenses: $2,000 and 10 – 20 yrs *possession:* 1st offense: $2,000 and 2 – 5 yrs 2nd offense: $2,000 and 5 – 10 yrs subsequent offenses: $2,000 and 10 – 20 yrs *sale to a minor:* 5 – 20 yrs	*sale:* 1st offense: $2,000 and 2 – 5 yrs 2nd offense: $2,000 and 5 – 10 yrs subsequent offenses: $2,000 and 10 – 20 yrs *possession:* 1st offense: $2,000 and 2 – 5 yrs 2nd offense: $2,000 and 5 – 10 yrs subsequent offenses: $2,000 and 10 – 20 yrs *sale to a minor:* 5 – 20 yrs	*sale:* 1st offense: $1,000 and nmt 1 yr 2nd offense: $2,000 and nmt 5 yrs *sale to a minor:* 1st offense: nmt $2,000 and nmt 5 yrs 2nd offense: nmt $5,000 and nmt 20 yrs	*legal age* — 21 *sale to a minor:* nmt $100, nmt 30 days, ob *Intoxication level:* no codified presump- tions *drunkenness:* nmt $100 or nmt 30 days

STATE OR AREA	Heroin	Marijuana	Amphetamines or Barbiturates	Alcohol

Kansas	*sale:*
	1–3 yrs
	possession:
	1–3 yrs
		sale:
		1–3 yrs
		possession:
		nmt 1 yr in county jail
			sale:
			1st offense: 1–5 yrs
			2nd offense: 5–15 yrs
			3rd offense: life
			possession:
			1st offense: nmt 1 yr
			subsequent offenses:
			  1–3 yrs
				legal age—21
				sale to a minor:
				nmt $100 or nmt
				  30 days
				Intoxication level:
				.15% of blood content
				drunkenness:
				nmt $100 or nmt
				  30 days

Kentucky	*sale:*
	1st offense: 5–20 yrs
	  and nmt $2,000
	2nd offense: 10–40 yrs
	  and nmt $2,000
	possession:
	1st offense: 2–10 yrs and
	  nmt $2,000
	subsequent offenses:
	  5–20 yrs and nmt
	  $2,000
	sale to a minor:
	$2,000 and 20 yrs–life
		sale:
		1st offense: 5–20 yrs
		  and nmt $2,000
		2nd offense: 10–40 yrs
		  and nmt $2,000
		possession:
		1st offense: 2–10 yrs and
		  nmt $2,000
		subsequent offenses:
		  5–20 yrs and nmt
		  $2,000
		sale to a minor:
		$2,000 and 20 yrs–life
			amphetamine sale:
			6 months–1 yr,
			  $300–$500, ob
			barbiturate sale:
			nmt 1 yr, $300–$500,
			  ob
				legal age—21
				sale to a minor:
				revocation of license
				Intoxication level:
				.10% of blood content
				drunkenness:
				$10–$100, 5–30 days, ob

Louisiana	*sale:*
	30 yrs, $1,500, ob
	possession:
	30 yrs, $1,500, ob
		sale:
		1st offense: $500 a/o 1 yr
		2nd offense: $2,000 a/o
		  5 yrs
		subsequent offenses:
		  20 yrs
		possession:
		1st offense: $500 a/o 1 yr
		2nd offense: $2,000 a/o
		  5 yrs
		subsequent offenses:
		  20 yrs
			sale:
			5 yrs, $5,000, ob
				legal age—18
				sale to a minor:
				nmt $300, nmt 6 months,
				  ob
				Intoxication level:
				.10% of blood content
				drunkenness:
				nmt $100, nmt 90 days,
				  ob

Maine	*sale:*
	1st offense: $1,000 and
	  2–8 yrs
	2nd offense: $2,000 and
	  5–15 yrs
	subsequent offenses:
	  10–20 yrs and $5,000
	possession:
	1st offense: $1,000 and
	  2–8 yrs
	2nd offense: $2,000 and
	  5–15 yrs
	subsequent offenses:
	  10–20 yrs and $5,000
		sale:
		1–5 yrs if both parties
		  over 21
		2–6 yrs if buyer 18–20,
		  seller over 21
		if buyer under 18, seller
		  over 21:
		  1st offense: 3–8 yrs
		  2nd offense: 4–10 yrs
		1–5 yrs if seller under 21
		possession:
		1st offense: $1,000 and
		  11 months
		2nd offense: $2,000
		  and 2 yrs
			sale:
			$1,000 and 2 yrs
			possession:
			$1,000 and 2 yrs
				legal age—20
				sale to a minor:
				nmt $100 or nmt
				  60 days
				Intoxication level:
				.10% of blood
				  content
				drunkenness:
				1st offense: nmt $20,
				  nmt 30 days, ob
				2nd offense: nmt $60,
				  nmt 90 days, ob

Maryland	*sale:*
	1st offense: 20 yrs and
	  nmt $25,000
	2nd offense: 40 yrs and
	  nmt $50,000
	possession:
	1st offense: 4 yrs and
	  nmt $25,000
	2nd offense: 10 yrs and
	  nmt $50,000
		sale:
		1st offense: 5 yrs and
		  nmt $1,500
		2nd offense: 10 yrs and
		  nmt $3,000
		possession:
		1st offense: nmt $1,000
		2nd offense: nmt $2,000
			sale:
			1st offense: 5 yrs and nmt
			  $1,500
			2nd offense: 10 yrs and
			  nmt $3,000
				legal age—21
				sale to a minor:
				nmt $1,000, nmt 2 yrs,
				  ob
				Intoxication level:
				.15% of blood
				  content
				drunkenness:
				nmt $50, nmt 60
				  days, ob

Code: a/o—and/or   g—grams   poss.—possible   nmt—not more than   nlt—not less than   ob—or both

STATE OR AREA	Heroin	Marijuana	Amphetamines or Barbiturates	Alcohol
Massachusetts	*sale:* 1st offense: 3 – 10 yrs 2nd offense: 10 – 25 yrs *possession:* 1st offense: $5,000, 2½ yrs in house of correction, or 5 yrs in state prison 2nd offense: 5 – 15 yrs	*sale:* 1st offense: $500 – $1,000 and 6 months – 2 yrs 2nd offense: $500 – $2,000 and 5 – 10 yrs subsequent offenses: $2,000 and 10 – 20 yrs *possession:* 3½ yrs in state prison and $1,000, or 2½ yrs in jail, house of correction	*sale:* nmt $2,000, nmt 6 months, ob	*legal age* – 21 *sale to a minor:* nmt $200, nmt 6 months, ob *Intoxication level:* .15% of blood content *drunkenness:* nmt 30 days and nmt $15
Michigan	*sale:* 20 yrs – life *possession:* 1st offense: nmt $5,000 and nmt 10 yrs 2nd offense: nmt $5,000 and nmt 20 yrs subsequent offenses: nmt $5,000 and nmt 20 – 40 yrs	*sale:* 20 yrs – life *possession:* 1st offense: nmt $5,000 and nmt 10 yrs 2nd offense: nmt $5,000 and nmt 20 yrs subsequent offenses: nmt $5,000 and nmt 20 – 40 yrs	*possession:* $500, 1 yr, ob	*legal age* – 21 *sale to a minor:* nmt 1 yr, nmt $1,000, ob *Intoxication level:* .15% of blood content *drunkenness:* nmt $50 or 30 days
Minnesota	*sale:* nmt $1,000 and 5 – 20 yrs *possession:* nmt $1,000 and 5 – 20 yrs *sale to a minor:* $2,000 and 10 – 40 yrs	*sale:* nmt $1,000 and 5 – 20 yrs *possession:* nmt $1,000 and 5 – 20 yrs *sale to a minor:* $2,000 and 10 – 40 yrs	*sale:* $1,000 and 1 yr	*legal age* – 21 *sale to a minor:* nmt 1 yr, nmt $1,000, ob *Intoxication level:* .10% of blood content *drunkenness:* $10 – $100 and 20 – 90 days
Mississippi	*sale:* nmt 6 yrs, nmt $2,000, ob *possession:* nmt 6 yrs and nmt $2,000	*sale:* nmt 6 yrs, nmt $2,000, ob *possession:* nmt 6 months, nmt $500, ob	*amphetamine sale:* nmt 4 yrs, nmt $2,000, ob *barbiturate sale:* nmt 2 yrs, nmt $1,000, ob	*legal age* – 21 *Beer not over 4% by weight* – 18 *sale to a minor:* 1st offense: $500 – $1,000 2nd offense: $1,000 – $2,000, 1 yr, ob *Intoxication level:* .15% of blood content *drunkenness:* 6 months, $500, ob
Missouri	*sale:* 1st offense: 5 yrs – life subsequent offenses: 10 yrs – life *possession:* 1st offense: nmt 20 yrs in state prison or 6 months – 1 yr in county jail 2nd offense: 5 yrs – life subsequent offenses: 10 yrs – life *sale to a minor:* poss. death penalty	*sale:* 1st offense: 5 yrs – life subsequent offenses: 10 yrs – life *possession* – less than 25 g: 1st offense: nmt 1 yr, nmt $1,000, ob 2nd offense: nmt 5 yrs in state prison or nmt 1 yr in county jail, $1,000, ob *sale to a minor:* poss. death penalty	*sale:* 2 – 10 yrs in state prison or 1 yr in county jail, nmt $1,000, ob *possession:* 2 – 10 yrs in state prison or 1 yr in county jail, nmt $1,000, ob	*legal age* – 21 *sale to a minor:* $1,000, 1 yr, ob *Intoxication level:* .15% of blood content *drunkenness:* $5 – $25

A SURVEY OF DRUG LAWS IN THE UNITED STATES (continued)

STATE OR AREA	Heroin	Marijuana	Amphetamines or Barbiturates	Alcohol
Montana	*sale:* 1 yr–life *possession:* 5 yrs	*sale:* 1 yr–life *possession (6 oz):* 1st offense: $1,000, or 1 yr, ob 2nd offense: $1,000, or 1 yr, ob in county jail *or* 3 yrs in state prison	*sale:* 1 yr–life *possession:* nmt 5 yrs	*legal age*—21 *sale to a minor:* 1st offense: $500, 6 months, ob 2nd offense: $500–$2,000, 1–5 yrs, ob *Intoxication level:* .15% of blood content *drunkenness:* nmt 90 days
Nebraska	*sale:* 5–20 yrs *possession:* 1–2 yrs and $500 or 6 months in county jail	*sale:* 5–20 yrs *possession—* *less than 1 lb:* $500 and 7 days rehabilitation program	*sale:* 1–5 yrs and $2,000 or 6 months in county jail	*legal age*—20 *sale to a minor:* $250–$500 and 15 days *Intoxication level:* .10% of blood content *drunkenness:* 1st offense: nmt $50 or 30 days 2nd offense: 60 days
Nevada	*sale:* 1st offense: 1–20 yrs and $5,000 2nd offense: life and $5,000 *possession:* 1st offense: 1–6 yrs and $2,000 2nd offense: 1–10 yrs and $2,000 subsequent offenses: 1–20 yrs and $5,000 under 21: 1–6 yrs in state prison and $2,000 *or* nmt 1 yr in county jail and $1,000 *sale to a minor:* 1st offense: life and $5,000 2nd offense: life (no parole)	*sale:* 1st offense: 1–20 yrs and $5,000 2nd offense: life and $5,000 *possession:* 1st offense: 1–6 yrs and $2,000 2nd offense: 1–10 yrs and $2,000 subsequent offenses: 1–20 yrs and $5,000 under 21: 1–6 yrs in state prison and $2,000 *or* nmt 1 yr in county jail and $1,000 *sale to a minor:* 1st offense: life and $5,000 2nd offense: life (no parole)	*sale:* 1st offense: 1–6 yrs and $2,000 2nd offense: 1–10 yrs and $2,000 subsequent offenses: 1–20 yrs and $5,000 *possession:* 1st offense: 1–6 yrs and $2,000 2nd offense: 1–10 yrs and $2,000 subsequent offenses: 1–20 yrs and $5,000 under 21: 1–6 yrs in state prison and $2,000 *or* nmt 1 yr in county jail and $1,000 *sale to a minor:* 1st offense: 1–20 yrs subsequent offenses: 1–20 yrs (no probation)	*legal age*—21 *sale to a minor:* nmt 6 months, nmt $500, ob *Intoxication level:* .15% of blood content *drunkenness:* nmt 6 months, nmt $500, ob
New Hampshire	*sale:* 1st offense: nmt 20 yrs, nmt $5,000, ob subsequent offenses: nmt 25 yrs *possession:* 1st offense: 5 yrs, $2,000, ob 2nd offense: 10 yrs, $5,000, ob	*sale:* 1st offense: nmt 10 yrs, $2,000, ob 2nd offense: nmt 15 yrs, $5,000, ob *possession:* 1st offense: 1 yr, $500, ob 2nd offense: 3 yrs, $1,000, ob	*sale:* 1st offense: nmt 10 yrs, $2,000, ob 2nd offense: nmt 15 yrs, $5,000, ob *possession:* 1st offense: 1 yr, $500, ob 2nd offense: 3 yrs, $1,000, ob	*legal age*—21 *sale to a minor:* nmt $500, nmt 6 months, ob *Intoxication level:* .15% of blood content *drunkenness:* nmt $25, nmt 6 months, ob

Code: a/o—and/or   g—grams   poss.—possible   nmt—not more than   nlt—not less than   ob—or both

STATE OR AREA	Heroin	Marijuana	Amphetamines or Barbiturates	Alcohol
New Jersey	*sale:* nmt 12 yrs, nmt $2,500, ob *possession:* nmt 5 yrs, nmt $1,500, ob	*sale:* nmt 5 yrs, nmt $1,500, ob *possession (more than 25 g):* nmt 5 yrs, nmt $1,500, ob *possession (less than 25 g):* nmt 6 months, nmt $500, ob	*sale:* nmt 5 yrs, nmt $1,500, ob *possession:* nmt 5 yrs, nmt $1,500, ob	*legal age—21* *sale to a minor:* nmt $1,000, nmt 3 yrs, ob *Intoxication level:* .10% of blood content *drunkenness:* nmt 6 months, nmt $500, ob
New Mexico	*sale:* 1st offense: nmt $5,000 and 10–20 yrs 2nd offense: nmt $10,000 and 20–40 yrs subsequent offenses: nmt $20,000 and life *possession:* 1st offense: nmt $2,000 and 2–10 yrs 2nd offense: nmt $2,000 and 5–20 yrs subsequent offenses: nlt $2,000 and 10–40 yrs	*sale:* 1st offense: nmt $5,000 and 10–20 yrs 2nd offense: nmt $10,000 and 20–40 yrs subsequent offenses: nmt $20,000 and life *possession (more than 1 oz):* 1st offense: nmt $2,000 and 2–10 yrs 2nd offense: nmt $2,000 and 5–20 yrs subsequent offenses: nlt $2,000 and 10–40 yrs *possession (1 oz):* 1st offense: less than 1 yr and $1,000 2nd offense: $5,000, 1–5 yrs, ob subsequent offenses: $5,000 and 2–10 yrs	*sale:* 1st offense: nmt $1,000 and 1 yr subsequent offenses: nmt $3,000 and 3 yrs *sale to a minor:* 1st offense: nmt $5,000 and 2 yrs subsequent offenses: nmt $5,000 and 6 yrs	*legal age—21* *sale to a minor:* $25–$100, nmt 6 months, ob *Intoxication level:* no codified presumptions *drunkenness:* 6 months or less
New York	*sale:* 1st offense: 1–3 yrs 2nd offense: 5–15 yrs *possession:* nmt 1 yr or $1,000 *sale to a minor:* 1st offense: 1–3 yrs 2nd offense: $8\frac{1}{3}$–25 yrs	*sale:* 1st offense: 1–3 yrs 2nd offense: 5–15 yrs *possession:* nmt 1 yr or $1,000 *sale to a minor:* 1st offense: 1–3 yrs 2nd offense: $8\frac{1}{3}$–25 yrs	*sale:* 1st offense: 1–3 yrs subsequent offenses: $2\frac{1}{2}$–7 yrs	*legal age—18* *sale to a minor:* nmt 3 months *Intoxication level:* .15% of blood content *drunkenness:* nmt 15 days
North Carolina	*sale:* 1st offense: nmt $1,000 a/o nmt 5 yrs 2nd offense: nmt $2,000 and 5–10 yrs subsequent offenses: nmt $3,000 and 15 yrs–life *possession:* 1st offense: nmt $1,000 a/o nmt 5 yrs 2nd offense: nmt $2,000 and 5–10 yrs subsequent offenses: nmt $3,000 and 15 yrs–life	*sale:* 1st offense: nmt $1,000 a/o nmt 5 yrs 2nd offense: nmt $2,000 and 5–10 yrs subsequent offenses: nmt $3,000 and 15 yrs–life *possession:* 1st offense: nmt $1,000 a/o nmt 5 yrs 2nd offense: nmt $2,000 and 5–10 yrs subsequent offenses: nmt $3,000 and 15 yrs–life	*sale:* 1st offense: 6 months–5 yrs subsequent offenses: 1 yr–10 yrs *possession:* 1st offense: 6 months–5 yrs subsequent offenses: 1 yr–10 yrs	*legal age—21* *light wine, beer—18* *sale to a minor:* nmt $50 and nmt 30 days *Intoxication level:* .10% of blood content *drunkenness:* nmt $50 or nmt 20 days

A SURVEY OF DRUG LAWS IN THE UNITED STATES (continued)

STATE OR AREA	Heroin	Marijuana	Amphetamines or Barbiturates	Alcohol
North Dakota	*sale:* nmt $10,000 nmt 20 yrs, ob *possession:* nmt $2,500, nmt 5 yrs, ob	*sale:* nmt $5,000 nmt 10 yrs, ob *possession:* nmt $500, nmt 1 yr, ob	*sale:* nmt $5,000 nmt 10 yrs, ob	*legal age* — 21 *sale to a minor:* nmt 1 yr, nmt $500, ob *Intoxication level:* .10% of blood content *drunkenness:* no penalty for intoxication solely
Ohio	*sale:* 20 – 40 yrs *possession:* 1st offense: 10 – 20 yrs 2nd offense: 15 – 30 yrs subsequent offenses: 20 – 40 yrs	*sale:* 20 – 40 yrs *possession:* 1st offense: 10 – 20 yrs 2nd offense: 15 – 20 yrs subsequent offenses: 20 – 40 yrs	*sale:* nmt $1,000, nmt 1 yr, ob *possession:* nmt $1,000, nmt 1 yr, ob	*legal age* — 21 *3.2 beer* — 18 *sale to a minor:* $25 – $300, 6 months, ob *Intoxication level:* .15% of blood content *drunkenness:* at the discretion of justice of peace
Oklahoma	*sale:* 1st offense: nmt $1,000, nmt 5 yrs, ob 2nd offense: nmt $3,000, 3 – 10 yrs, ob subsequent offenses: nmt $5,000, 10 – 20 yrs, ob *possession:* 1st offense: nmt $1,000, nmt 5 yrs, ob 2nd offense: nmt $3,000, 3 – 10 yrs, ob subsequent offenses: nmt $5,000, 10 – 20 yrs, ob *sale to a minor:* 10 yrs – death in electric chair	*sale:* nmt $5,000, nmt 7 yrs, ob *possession:* nmt $5,000, nmt 7 yrs, ob *sale to a minor:* 1st offense: nmt 20 yrs subsequent offenses: 5 yrs – life	*sale:* 1st offense: nmt 1 yr, nmt $500, ob subsequent offenses: nmt 2 yrs, nmt $1,000, ob	*legal age* — 21 *sale to a minor:* $50 – $200 and 30 days – 5 yrs *Intoxication level:* .15% of blood content *drunkenness:* $10 – $100 or 5 – 30 days
Oregon	*sale:* nmt 10 yrs and $2,500 *possession:* nmt 10 yrs and $2,500	*sale:* nmt 10 yrs and $2,500 *possession:* $1,000 and 1 yr	*sale:* nmt 10 yrs and $2,500	*legal age* — 21 *sale to a minor:* nmt 1 yr, nmt $500, ob *Intoxication level:* .15% of blood content *drunkenness:* no penalty for intoxi- cation solely
Pennsylvania	*sale:* 1st offense: $5,000 and 5 – 20 yrs 2nd offense: nmt $15,000 and 10 – 30 yrs subsequent offenses: nmt $30,000 and life *possession:* 1st offense: nmt $2,000 and 2 – 5 yrs 2nd offense: nmt $5,000 and 5 – 10 yrs subsequent offenses: nmt $30,000 and life	*sale:* 1st offense: $5,000 and 5 – 20 yrs 2nd offense: nmt $15,000 and 10 – 30 yrs subsequent offenses: nmt $30,000 and life *possession:* 1st offense: nmt $2,000 and 2 – 5 yrs 2nd offense: nmt $5,000 and 5 – 10 yrs subsequent offenses: nmt $30,000 and life	*sale:* 1 yr, $5,000, ob	*legal age* — 21 *sale to a minor:* 1st offense: $100 – $300 and 1 – 3 months on failure to pay fine subsequent offenses: $300 – $500 and 3 months – 1 yr *Intoxication level:* .10% of blood content *drunkenness:* nmt $5

Code:　a/o — and/or　g — grams　poss. — possible　nmt — not more than　nlt — not less than　ob — or both

STATE OR AREA	Heroin	Marijuana	Amphetamines or Barbiturates	Alcohol
Rhode Island	*sale* 20–40 yrs *possession:* 1st offense: 2–15 yrs and nmt $10,000 2nd offense: 5–20 yrs and nmt $10,000 subsequent offenses: 10–30 yrs and nmt $10,000 *sale to a minor:* 30 yrs–life	*sale:* 20–40 yrs *possession:* 1st offense: 2–15 yrs and nmt $10,000 2nd offense: 5–20 yrs and nmt $10,000 subsequent offenses: 10–30 yrs and nmt $10,000 *sale to a minor:* 30 yrs–life	*sale:* 1st offense: $1,000 a/o 2 yrs subsequent offenses: $5,000 a/o 5 yrs	*legal age*—21 *sale to a minor:* 1st offense: $50 2nd offense: nmt $100 *Intoxication level:* .10% of blood content *drunkenness:* 60 days–3 yrs (for treatment)
South Carolina	*sale:* 1st offense: $3,000 and 3½ yrs 2nd offense: 5 yrs subsequent offenses: 10 yrs *possession:* 1st offense: nmt $2,000, nmt 2 yrs, ob 2nd offense: $2,000–$5,000, 2–5 yrs, ob subsequent offenses: 5–10 yrs *sale to a minor:* 1st offense: $5,000 and 5 yrs 2nd offense: 10 yrs	*sale:* 1st offense: $3,000 and 3½ yrs 2nd offense: 5 yrs subsequent offenses: 10 yrs *possession:* 1st offense: $2,000 and 2 yrs 2nd offense: $2,000 and 2–5 yrs subsequent offenses: 5–10 yrs *sale to a minor:* 1st offense: $5,000 and 5 yrs 2nd offense: 10 yrs	*sale:* 1st offense: $2,000 and 2 yrs 2nd offense: $2,000 and 2–5 yrs 3rd offense: 5–10 yrs	*legal age*—21 *beer and wine*—18 *sale to a minor:* at discretion of court *Intoxication level:* .10% of blood content *drunkenness:* nmt 60 days or nmt $200
South Dakota	*sale:* 1st offense: nmt 10 yrs a/o $5,000 2nd offense: nmt 15 yrs a/o $10,000 subsequent offenses: 40 yrs a/o $20,000 *possession:* 1st offense: nmt 5 yrs a/o $5,000 2nd offense: nmt 15 yrs a/o $10,000 subsequent offenses: nmt 40 yrs a/o $20,000	*sale:* 1st offense: nmt 10 yrs a/o $5,000 2nd offense: nmt 15 yrs a/o $10,000 subsequent offenses: 40 yrs a/o $20,000 *possession (1 oz or less):* 1st offense: nmt 1 yr a/o $500	*sale:* 1st offense: nmt 5 yrs a/o $5,000 2nd offense: nmt 15 yrs a/o $10,000 subsequent offenses: nmt 40 yrs a/o $20,000 *sale to a minor:* twice above sentences	*legal age*—21 *3.2 beer*—19 *sale to a minor:* $100, nmt 30 days, ob *Intoxication level:* .15% of blood content *drunkenness:* nmt $100, nmt 30 days, ob
Tennessee	*sale:* 5–15 yrs and $18,000 *possession:* 5–15 yrs and $18,000 *sale to minors:* twice above sentence	*sale:* 1–5 yrs and $3,000 *possession:* 1st offense: 11 months, 29 days, a/o $1,000 2nd offense: 2 yrs and treatment *sale to minors:* twice above sentence	*sale:* 3–8 yrs and $10,000 *possession:* 3–8 yrs and $10,000 *sale to minors:* twice above sentence	*legal age*—21 *sale to a minor:* nmt 1 yr, nmt $10,000, ob *Intoxication level:* .15% of blood content *drunkenness:* nmt 1 yr, nmt $1,000, ob

STATE OR AREA	Heroin	Marijuana	Amphetamines or Barbiturates	Alcohol
Texas	sale: 1st offense: 2 yrs –life subsequent offenses: 10 yrs –life possession: 1st offense: 2 yrs –life subsequent offenses: 10 yrs –life sale to under 19: 1st offense: 5 yrs –life subsequent offenses: 10 yrs –life	sale: 1st offense: 2 yrs –life subsequent offenses: 10 yrs –life possession: 1st offense: 2 yrs –life subsequent offenses: 10 yrs –life sale to under 19: 1st offense: 5 yrs –life subsequent offenses: 10 yrs –life	sale: 1st offense: $3,000 or 30 days –2 yrs 2nd offense: 2 – 10 yrs	legal age –21 sale to a minor: $100 –$1,000, nmt 1 yr, ob Intoxication level: no codified presumptions drunkenness: nmt $100
Utah	sale: nmt 15 yrs a/o $15,000 possession: 1st offense: $299 a/o 6 months 2nd offense: $1,000 a/o 1 yr subsequent offenses: nmt 5 yrs	sale: nmt 15 yrs a/o $5,000 possession: 1st offense: $299 a/o 6 months 2nd offense: $1,000 a/o 1 yr subsequent offenses: nmt 5 yrs	amphetamine sale: nmt 10 yrs a/o $10,000 barbiturate sale: nmt 5 yrs a/o $5,000 possession: 1st offense: $299 a/o 6 months 2nd offense: $1,000 a/o 1 yr subsequent offenses: nmt 5 yrs	legal age –21 sale to a minor: 30 days –1 yr, $100 – $1,000, ob Intoxication level: .08% of blood content drunkenness: nmt 6 months
Vermont	sale: 1st offense: nmt 5 yrs and nmt $10,000 2nd offense: nmt 10 –25 yrs and nmt $25,000 possession: 1st offense: nmt 1 yr, nmt $1,000, ob 2nd offense: nmt 2 yrs nmt $2,000, ob sale to a minor: 1st offense: nmt 5 yrs and nmt $10,000 subsequent offenses: nmt 25 yrs and nmt $25,000	sale: 1st offense: nmt 5 yrs and nmt $10,000 2nd offense: nmt 10 –25 yrs and nmt $25,000 possession: nmt 6 months, nmt $500, ob sale to a minor: 1st offense: nmt 5 yrs and nmt $10,000 subsequent offenses: nmt 25 yrs and nmt $25,000	sale: 1st offense: nmt 5 yrs and nmt $10,000 2nd offense: nmt 10 –25 yrs and nmt $25,000 possession: nmt 6 month, nmt $500, ob sale to a minor: 1st offense: nmt 5 yrs and nmt $10,000 subsequent offenses: nmt 25 yrs and nmt $25,000	legal age –21 sale to a minor: nmt $200, nmt 1 yr, ob Intoxication level: .10% of blood content drunkenness: no penalty for intoxication solely
Virginia	sale: 1st offense: 1 –40 yrs, nmt $25,000, ob 2nd offense: 10 yrs –life, nmt $50,000, ob possession: 1st offense: 1 –10 yrs, or nmt 12 months and nmt $5,000 2nd offense: 2 –20 yrs or nmt 12 months and nmt $10,000	sale: 1st offense: 1 –40 yrs, nmt $25,000, ob 2nd offense: 10 yrs –life, nmt $50,000, ob possession: 1st offense: nmt $1,000, nmt 1 yr, ob 2nd offense: 2 –20 yrs or nmt 12 months and nmt $10,000	sale: 1st offense: nmt 1 yr, nmt $1,000, ob 2nd offense: 1 –5 yrs or nmt 12 months and nmt $10,000	legal age –21 3.2 beer –18 sale to a minor: nmt $1,000, nmt 1 yr, ob Intoxication level: .15% of blood content drunkenness: $1 –$25
Washington	sale: nmt 10 yrs a/o $25,000 possession: nmt 10 yrs a/o $25,000	sale: nmt 5 yrs a/o $10,000 possession (4 oz or less): 90 days a/o $250	sale: nmt 5 yrs a/o $10,000 possession: nmt 5 yrs a/o $10,000	legal age –21 sale to a minor: nmt $5,000, nmt 10 yrs, ob Intoxication level: .10% of blood content drunkenness: nmt 90 days or nmt $250

Code: a/o –and/or   g –grams   poss. –possible   nmt –not more than   nlt –not less than   ob –or both

STATE OR AREA	Heroin	Marijuana	Amphetamines or Barbiturates	Alcohol

West Virginia	*sale:*
	1st offense: nmt $1,000
	2nd offense: nmt $5,000
	subsequent offenses:
	  10–20 yrs and nmt
	  $10,000
	
	possession:
	1st offense: nmt $1,000
	2nd offense: nmt $5,000
	subsequent offenses:
	  10–20 yrs and nmt
	  $10,000
		sale:
		1st offense: nmt $1,000
		2nd offense: nmt $5,000
		subsequent offenses:
		  10–20 yrs and nmt
		  $10,000
		
		possession:
		1st offense: nmt $1,000
		2nd offense: nmt $5,000
		subsequent offenses:
		  10–20 yrs and nmt
		  $10,000
			sale:
			1st offense: nmt $1,000,
			  1–5 yrs, ob
			subsequent offenses:
			  nmt $10,000, 2–10
			  yrs, ob
			
			possession:
			1st offense: nmt $1,000,
			  1–5 yrs, ob
			subsequent offenses:
			  nmt $10,000, 2–10
			  yrs, ob
				legal age—21
				3.2 beer—18
				sale to a minor:
				at discretion of court
				Intoxication level:
				.10% of blood
				  content
				drunkenness:
				$1

Wisconsin	*sale:*
	1st offense: 2–10 yrs
	2nd offense: 5–10 yrs
	subsequent offenses:
	  10–20 yrs
	possession:
	1st offense: 2–10 yrs
	2nd offense: 5–10 yrs
	subsequent offenses:
	  10–20 yrs
	sale to a minor:
	1st offense: 3–25 yrs
	2nd offense: 20 yrs–life
		sale:
		1st offense: 5 yrs
		  a/o $5,000
		2nd offense: 10 yrs a/o
		  $5,000
		possession:
		1st offense: 1 yr a/o $500
		2nd offense: 2 yrs a/o
		  $1,000
		sale to a minor:
		1st offense: nmt 15 yrs
		subsequent offenses:
		  30 yrs–life
			sale:
			1st offense: nmt 5 yrs,
			  nmt $5,000, ob
			2nd offense: nmt 10 yrs,
			  nmt $5,000, ob
				legal age—21
				beer—18
				sale to a minor:
				$100–$500, 60 days,
				  ob
				Intoxication level:
				.15% of blood
				  content
				drunkenness:
				nmt $50 or nmt
				  30 days

Wyoming	*sale:*
	20 yrs a/o $25,000
	possession:
	1st offense: 6 months,
	  $1,000, ob
	2nd offense: 6 months,
	  $1,000, ob
	subsequent offenses:
	  5 yrs, $5,000, ob
		sale:
		20 yrs a/o $25,000
		possession:
		1st offense: 6 months,
		  $1,000, ob
		2nd offense: 6 months,
		  $1,000, ob
		subsequent offenses:
		  5 yrs, $5,000, ob
			amphetamine sale:
			10 yrs a/o $10,000
			barbiturate sale:
			2 yrs a/o $2,500
				legal age—21
				sale to a minor:
				nmt $100, nmt 6
				  months, ob
				Intoxication level:
				.15% of blood
				  content
				drunkenness:
				no penalty for intoxica-
				  tion solely

District of Columbia	*sale:*
	1st offense: $100–
	  $1,000 a/o nmt 1 yr
	2nd offense: $500–
	  $5,000 a/o nmt 10 yrs
	possession:
	1st offense: $100–
	  $1,000 a/o nmt 1 yr
	2nd offense: $500–
	  $5,000 a/o nmt 10 yrs
		sale:
		1st offense: $100–
		  $1,000 a/o nmt 1 yr
		2nd offense: $500–
		  $5,000 a/o nmt 10 yrs
		possession:
		1st offense: $100–
		  $1,000 a/o nmt 1 yr
		2nd offense: $500–
		  $5,000 a/o nmt 10 yrs
			sale:
			1st offense: $100–
			  $1,000 a/o nmt 1 yr
			2nd offense: $500–
			  $5,000 a/o nmt 10 yrs
			possession:
			1st offense: $100–
			  $1,000 a/o nmt 1 yr
			2nd offense: $500–
			  $5,000 a/o nmt 10 yrs
				legal age—21
				light wine, beer—18
				sale to a minor:
				nmt 1 yr, nmt $1,000,
				  ob
				Intoxication level:
				.15% of blood
				  content
				drunkenness:
				nmt $100, nmt 90 days,
				  ob

Federal	*sale:*
	1st offense: 15 yrs a/o
	  $25,000
	subsequent offenses:
	  30 yrs a/o $50,000
	possession:
	1st offense: $5,000 a/o
	  1 yr
	2nd offense: $10,000 a/o
	  2 yrs
		sale:
		1st offense: 1 yr a/o
		  $5,000
		subsequent offenses:
		  2 yrs a/o $10,000
		possession:
		1st offense: $5,000 a/o
		  1 yr
		2nd offense: $10,000 a/o
		  2 yrs
			amphetamine sale:
			1st offense: 5 yrs a/o
			  $15,000
			subsequent offenses:
			  10 yrs a/o $30,000
			barbiturate sale:
			1st offense: 3 yrs a/o
			  $10,000
			subsequent offenses:
			  6 yrs a/o $20,000
			possession:
			1st offense: $5,000 a/o
			  1 yr
			2nd offense: $10,000 a/o
			  2 yrs	

I FOUNDATIONS OF HEALTH SCIENCE

1 Introduction to Health Science

Dubos, R. *Man Adapting.* New Haven, Conn.: Yale University Press, 1965.
Dubos considers health and disease to be expressions of an organism's success or failure to adapt to a changing environment. Health thus means more than merely reacting through passive mechanisms to physiochemical conditions; rather, human health requires the ability of creatively responding to one's environment.

Jones, B. (ed.). *The Health of Americans.* Englewood Cliffs, N.J.: Prentice-Hall, 1970.
Suggestions for the improvement of health and health care in the United States are outlined in this book.

Kosa, J., A. Antonovsky, and **I. K. Zola** (eds.). *Poverty and Health.* Cambridge, Mass.: Harvard University Press, 1969.
The authors contend that present-day health care is a middle-class luxury, but poverty and medical discrimination can be eliminated with the advanced state of American technology.

Warshofsky, F. *Twenty-First Century: The Control of Life.* New York: Viking Press, 1969.
This highly readable book traces life from its beginning in the womb up to the problems of overpopulation and the latest experiments on the heart and brain.

2 The Body in Action

Canon, W. B. *The Wisdom of the Body.* New York: Norton, 1963.
The human body is an unstable physiological matrix of separate parts requiring a complex system of autonomous controls to maintain the coordination and life of the whole. A discussion of the interrelationships and interactions of parts of the body with one another form the bulk of Canon's discussion.

Fisher, S., and **S. E. Cleveland.** *Body Image and Personality.* New York: Dover, 1968.
The authors argue that a person's self-image, his attitudes about his body, and the manner in which he integrates tactile stimulation all influence his characteristic behavior and mental health.

Gamow, G., and **M. Ycas.** *Mr. Tompkins Inside Himself.* New York: Viking, 1967.
This is a lighthearted but interesting discussion of the internal functioning of the human body. Far-fetched fictional situations are used to explain the complex physiology of the body.

Nourse, A. E. *The Body.* New York: Time-Life Books, 1970.
This beautiful book contains a discussion of man's past beliefs about his body, a general account of the body's needs and functions, and examples of recent medical research.

O'Malley, C. D., and **J. B. de C. M. Saunders.** *Leonardo da Vinci on the Human Body.* New York: Henry Schuman, 1952.
This is a collection of the anatomical works of Leonardo da Vinci. The text and illustrations give an interesting insight into development of the science of anatomy at the end of the fifteenth century.

Singer, C. *A Short History of Anatomy and Physiology.* New York: Dover, 1957.
This book provides a detailed historical account of advances in the science of anatomy from ancient times to the present. It is heavily illustrated with original drawings.

II MENTAL AND EMOTIONAL FUNCTIONING

3 Physiological Basis of Behavior

Calder N. *The Mind of Man.* New York: Viking, 1970.
A profusely illustrated, fascinating presentation of current research on the brain and human nature.

Delgado, J. M. R. "Brain Research and Behavioral Activity," *Endeavor*, 26 (1967), 149–154.
This article describes how physiological mechanisms in various segments of the brain can be triggered by electrical stimulation.

Isaacson, R. L. "When Brains are Damaged," *Psychology Today*, 3 (January 1970), 38, 40–42.
The author discusses the changes that take place in infant and adult animals when damage is done to the hippocampal region of the brain.

Levi, L. *Stress, Sources, Management and Prevention.* New York: Liveright, 1967.
In this fascinating book the author discusses the relationship between body and mind. Special attention is paid to the physiological and behavioral effects of stress and to the treatment of psychosomatic illnesses.

McGaugh, J., N. M. Weinberger, and **R. L. Whalen** (eds.). *Psychobiology.* San Francisco: Freeman, 1967.
This is a volume of readings from *Scientific American* on the biological basis of behavior. Research in numerous disciplines is included in this comprehensive book.

"Probing the Brain," *Newsweek*, 77 (June 21, 1971), 60–67.
This excellent article surveys brain functioning and the most recent experiments and surgical procedures being done on the brain.

Rorvick, D. M. "Brain Waves," *Look*, 34 (October 6, 1970), 88–94.
The prospect of controlling one's own brain waves is discussed in this fascinating article on the new field of biofeedback training.

4 Psychological Development

Ardrey, R. *African Genesis.* New York: Atheneum, 1961.
In this controversial book Robert Ardrey argues that man is an innately violent and aggressive animal.

Adler, A. *What Life Should Mean to You.* New York: Putnam, 1959.
In this informative book Alfred Adler discusses such aspects of the human personality as feelings of inferiority and rejection, the significance of dreams, early memories, the influences affecting the child and adolescent, and the basic necessities for a happy marriage and successful adjustment to life.

Branden, N. *The Psychology of Self-Esteem.* Los Angeles: Nash, 1969.
Psychologist Nathaniel Branden contends that the person who has a rational self-interest and self-value will be better able to cope with and change his world and to achieve his goals. He provides a philosophical basis for his theory and them explores factors involved in developing self-esteem.

Erikson, E. H. *Childhood and Society.* 2nd ed. New York: Norton, 1963.
In this classic work, Erik Erikson discusses his eight stages of psychological development in the light of Freud's theory of infantile sexuality. Also included are fascinating chapters on American Indian societies, Adolf Hitler, and Maxim Gorky.

Farson, R. E. (ed.). *Science and Human Affairs.* Palo Alto, Calif: Science and Behavior Books, 1965.
This book is a collection of lectures by such men as Carl Rogers, Abraham Maslow, and Gordon Allport on the theme that science can and will affect human nature. The basic conclusion is that the behavioral sciences must evaluate the directions in which they are headed if they are going to treat men as human beings in human environments rather than as animals in laboratory situations.

Maslow, A. *Toward a Psychology of Being.* 2nd ed. Princeton, N.Y.: Van Nostrand, 1968.
The fundamental concepts of Maslow's humanistic psychology are contained in this classic work.

Sanford, N. *Issues in Personality Theory.* San Francisco: Jossey-Bass, 1970.
The author avoids the traditional methods of dealing with personality theory and presents instead a thoughtful discussion of some underlying premises of the study of personality. This book is an attempt to transcend behavioral models and arrive at an image of man as an autonomous creature free from the restraints of behavioristic control.

Saul, L. J. *Emotional Maturity.* Philadelphia: Lippincott, 1960.
Saul stresses childhood environment as the major contributing factor to emotional development. The book is filled with interesting histories and examples of such facets of emotional maturity as independence, love and sex, hostility, self-control, and the dynamics of personality.

White, R. W. *Lives in Progress.* New York: Holt, Rinehart & Winston, 1966.
White examines three case histories to provide the backdrop for a larger discussion of the development of human personality.

5 Mental Health and Mental Illness

Chessick, R. D. *How Psychotherapy Heals.* New York: Science House, 1969.
Chessick discusses the complex methods of long-term psychotherapy. Although intended primarily for specialists, this book also will aid the general reader in understanding the work of psychoanalysts and psychotherapists.

Freud, S. *Psychopathology of Everyday Life.* New York: Macmillan, 1917.
This book is the famous study of so-called "Freudian slips." According to Freud, forgetfulness and errors in speaking, reading, or writing often are the result of subconscious repression rather than simple mistakes.

Green, H. *I Never Promised You a Rose Garden.* New York: Holt, Rinehart & Winston, 1964.
This sensitive and powerful novel of a brilliant and schizophrenic young girl and her struggle with reality is an often-frightening account of life in a mental institution.

Halleck, S. *The Politics of Therapy.* New York: Science House, 1971.
Halleck argues that the practice of psychiatry in the United States is politically biased in favor of the *status quo.*

Stein, J. *Neurosis in Contemporary Society: Process and Treatment.* Belmont, Calif.: Wadsworth, 1970.
Stein presents traditional and modern approaches to the study of neurosis and surveys the origin of neurosis, neurotic behavior, and the various schools of psychotherapy that treat neuroses.

Szasz, T. S. *Ideology and Insanity.* Garden City, N.Y.: Doubleday, 1970.
A collection of essays by a controversial psychiatrist, this book presents a case for removing mental and emotional problems from the area of medicine and treating them instead as "problems in living." The essays cover a variety of related topics, from involuntary commitment to community psychiatry.
_____. *The Manufacture of Madness.* New York: Harper & Row, 1970.
This important study challenges traditional notions of psychiatry and mental illness. The author compares present-day institutional psychiatry to the Inquisition of the sixteenth century.

Wolf, A., *et al. Beyond the Couch.* New York: Science House, 1970.
This book is a collection of conversations between four psychoanalysts who discuss possible approaches to group therapy.

III CHEMICAL ALTERATION OF BEHAVIOR

6 The Role of Drugs in the Good Life

Blum, R. H., and **associates.** *Society and Drugs.* San Francisco: Jossey-Bass, 1969.
The history and sociology of drugs are explored in this well-informed work.

Smith, A. E. W. *The Drug Users.* Wheaton, Ill.: Harold Shaw, 1969.
Smith analyzes the phenomenon of drug taking, including the physical benefits and dangers of various drugs. He presents a philosophical view of the social and spiritual conditions that are responsible for the current drug epidemic.

Snyder, S. H. "What We Have Forgotton About Pot—A Pharmacologist's History," *New York Times Magazine* (December 13, 1970), pp. 26–27, 121–126, 129–131, 134.
Historically, the cannabis plant has been used throughout the world for various medical ills. This article presents a history of this use, with particular attention to the Western world and the way in which marijuana came to be outlawed in the United States.

Further Readings

7   Common Drugs of Misuse and Abuse

Black, J. "The Speed That Kills," *New York Times Magazine* (June 21, 1970), pp. 14–18, 22–28.
Black vividly describes the physiological and resultant social changes that take place with the abuse of amphetamines.

DeBold, R. C., and **R. C. Leaf** (eds.). *LSD, Man and Society.* Middletown, Conn.: Wesleyan University Press, 1967. These papers, discussing the use and abuse of LSD, were presented at a symposium at Wesleyan University in 1967. Sociological and scientific viewpoints are included.

"The Drug Revolution," *Playboy,* 17 (February 1970), 53–74, 200–201.
This article is an informative and lively conversation gathering together disparate perspectives on the controversial issues of drug use. Panelists range from Joel Fort to Baba Ram Dass to a government official.

Edson, L. "$C_{21}H_{23}NO_3$—The Primer for Parents and Children," *New York Times Magazine* (May 24, 1970), pp. 92–93, 95.
The physiological aspects and complications of heroin addiction are explained in this article.

Grinspoon, L. "Marihuana," *Scientific American,* 221 (December 1969), 17–25.
This excellent summary of research into the effects of marijuana attributes the controversy surrounding the drug to the social circumstances of this era rather than to the results of scientific experimentation.

Hollister, L. E. *Chemical Psychoses.* Springfield, Ill.: Charles C Thomas, 1968.
This study covers the history and physiological and psychological effects of various consciousness-altering drugs. It also presents various chemical theories of psychosis, possible therapeutic uses of psychotomimetic drugs, and a brief examination of the social implications of drug use today.

Kaplan, J. *Marijuana—The New Prohibition.* New York: World, 1970.
Kaplan believes that the destructiveness of anti-marijuana laws far outweighs the benefits obtained to society and advocates radical changes in the structure of present drug laws.

Schoenfeld, E. *Dear Dr. Hip Pocrates.* New York: Grove, 1968.
This book is a collection of informative and amusing excerpts from Dr. Hip Pocrates' weekly "underground" column.

Snyder, S. W. "Work with Marijuana: 1, Effects," *Psychology Today,* 5 (May 1971), 37–40, 64–65.
In this brief article Snyder discusses the results of recent experiments on the physiological and behavioral effects of marijuana.

Tart, C. T. "Work with Marijuana: 2, Sensations," *Psychology Today,* 5 (May 1971), 41–43.
This report presents the responses of experienced marijuana users to a questionnaire on the effects of marijuana. The questions were concerned with such common sensations as touch and smell, physical movement, interpersonal relations, thought processes, and sexuality.

8   Alcohol Abuse

Cahalan, D. *Problem Drinkers.* San Francisco: Jossey-Bass, 1970.
This book is the result of a national survey involving 1,359 respondants. The social and personality characteristics that distinguish problem drinkers from alcoholics and the means to predict problem drinking are among topics discussed in this well-documented book.

————, **I. H. Cisin,** and **H. M. Crossley.** *American Drinking Practices.* New Brunswick, N.J.: Rutgers Center of Alcohol Studies, 1969.
This extensive book is a series of discussions on such specific correlates of alcohol use as age and social status.

McCarthy, R. D. (ed.). *Drinking and Intoxication.* New York: Free Press, 1959.
Ancient and modern social drinking practices are described in this collection of essays.

McClelland, D. C. "The Power of Positive Drinking." *Psychology Today,* 4 (January 1971), 40–41, 78–79.
In this article the author discusses the possible relationship between alcoholism and the need for a sense of power.

Pittman, D. J., and **C. R. Snyder** (eds.). *Society, Culture and Drinking Patterns.* New York: Wiley, 1962.
This collection of articles contains discussions of the anthropological and sociological aspects of alcohol use and abuse.

Plant, T. F. (ed.). *Alcohol Problems: A Report to the Nation.* New York: Oxford University Press, 1967.
This readable book, written by a commission of experts on alcoholism and noted men in relevant disciplines, surveys contemporary alcohol use and abuse and offers specific suggestions for future treatment and study.

Roueche, B. *The Neutral Spirit.* Boston: Little, Brown, 1960.
Roueche provides an interesting nontechnical discussion of the most widely used intoxicant known to man. He discusses the history of the development of alcoholic beverages, as well as the physical and emotional effects of moderate and excessive drinking.

9   Smoking and Health

Borgatta, E. F., and **R. R. Evans** (eds.). *Smoking, Health and Behavior.* Chicago: Aldine, 1968.
This collection of essays outlines some of the pertinent factors involved in the controversy over the relationship between smoking and health.

Eysenck, H. J. *Smoking, Health and Personality.* New York: Basic Books, 1965.
The author is concerned with the relationships between smoking, personality, and such diseases as lung cancer and coronary thrombosis.

Hunt, W. A. (ed.). *Learning Mechanisms in Smoking.* Chicago: Aldine, 1970.
This book is the edited proceedings of a conference sponsored by the American Cancer Society. Several aspects of habituation, tolerance, and the roles of psychological, social, and pharmacological factors in cigarette smoking are discussed.

Lichtenstein, E. "How to Quit Smoking," *Psychology Today,* 4 (January 1971), 42, 44–45.
Lichtenstein examines the effectiveness of aversive conditioning, group therapy, emotional role playing, and "cold turkey" as approaches to helping people quit smoking.

Magnuson, W. G., and **J. Carper.** "Toward a Safer Cigarette," in W. G. Magnuson and J. Carper, *The Dark Side of the Market Place.* Englewood Cliffs, N.J.: Prentice-Hall, 1968, pp. 185–207.
This article deals with cigarette advertising and the reluctance of cigarette manufacturers to produce a safer product.

U.S. Department of Health, Education and Welfare. *Smoking and Health.* Washington, D.C.: U.S. Government Printing Office, 1964.
This report contains a wealth of statistical information about the relationship between smoking and health.

10   Controlling Drug Use and Abuse

Blum, S. "Marijuana Clouds the Generation Gap," *New York Times Magazine* (August 23, 1970), pp. 28–29, 45, 48, 55–58.
Marijuana use is increasing not only among teen-agers but among adults as well. This article explains why more and more adults are turning on with pot.

Goodman, W. "The Choice for Thousands: Heroin or Methadone?" *New York Times Magazine* (June 13, 1971), pp. 14–15, 81–84.
In New York City various methadone maintenance programs have been set up to help heroin addicts return to normal living. This article primarily discusses the positive effects of such programs.

Institute on New Developments in the Rehabilitation of the Narcotic Addict. *Rehabilitating the Narcotic Addict.* New York: Arno Press, 1966.
This volume contains brief descriptions of several different programs for the treatment of drug addicts. The readable summaries provide good reference material for anyone interested in the programs offered addicts.

Solomon, D. (ed.). *The Marihuana Papers.* New York: Bobbs, Merrill, 1966.
A comprehensive selection of writings from many perspectives, this book surveys scholarly, literary, and scientific aspects of marijuana use.

Yablonsky, L. *The Tunnel Back: Synanon.* New York: Macmillan, 1965.
The history of Synanon and its controversial methods of narcotic rehabilitation are given a thoughtful and sympathetic account in this well-written book.

11 Drugs in Perspective

Cohen, S. *The Drug Dilemma.* New York: McGraw-Hill, 1969.
Beginning with the assumption that youthful drug taking in society is undersirable, this book distinguishes itself by its calm, unmoralistic attitude toward the problem. Drug taking is presented as a recurrent historical phenomenon precipitated by social and psychological problems, which are themselves the real threat to society. The author outlines the dangers of drug taking and describes the role of parents and teachers in providing youth with a clearer sense of the meaning of life.

Fort, J. *The Pleasure Seekers.* Indianapolis, Ind.: Bobbs-Merrill, 1969.
Fort explores the history of drug use and abuse in America, describes the nature and effects of the various mind-altering substances, and reveals the hypocrisy of drug legislation. The noted drug expert also discusses the various factors involved in both use and abuse of drugs and offers solutions and alternatives to the drug problem.

IV FAMILY HEALTH
12 Human Sexuality

Broderick, C. B., and **J. Bernard.** *The Individual, Sex, and Society.* Baltimore: Johns Hopkins, 1968.
Intended as a handbook for teachers and counselors, this anthology provides valuable, clearly written information on human sexuality. Topics include sex education, sex in society, normal sexual functioning, and controversial sexual behavior.

Ford, C. S., and **F. Beach.** *Patterns of Sexual Behavior.* New York: Harper & Row, 1951.
This classic book analyzes changing societal attitudes toward sexual behavior.

Herschberger, R. *Adam's Rib.* New York: Harper & Row, 1970.
This book, first published in 1948, has seen a rebirth with the women's liberation movement. In such chapters as: "Is Rape a Myth?" "Society Writes Biology," and "Education for Frigidity," the author analyzes antifeminine sex-role stereotypes.

Hoffman, M. *The Gay World.* New York: Basic Books, 1968.
Hoffman combines the insights of psychiatry and the social sciences in his thoughtful and intelligent probing of the social and individual roots of homosexuality.

Kinsey, A. C., W. B. Pomeroy, C. E. Martin, and **P. H. Gebhard.** *Sexual Behavior in the Human Female.* Philadelphia: Saunders, 1953.
This is Kinsey's classic study of the patterns of sexual behavior of the American female.

_____, **W. B. Pomeroy,** and **C. E. Martin.** *Sexual Behavior in the Human Male.* Philadelphia: Saunders, 1948.
The patterns of sexual behavior of the American male are explored in this important work.

Marshall, D. S., and **R. C. Suggs** (eds.). *Human Sexual Behavior.* New York: Basic Books, 1971.
This anthropological survey presents aspects of human sexuality in various remote areas of the world and provides a wealth of data on sex practices and mores among primitive cultures.

Masters, W. H., and **V. E. Johnson.** *Human Sexual Inadequacy.* Boston: Little, Brown, 1970.
Experiences in the clinical treatment of human sexual dysfunction are described.

_____. *Human Sexual Response.* Boston: Little, Brown, 1966.
This classic work in the anatomy and physiology of sexual response details the processes of sexual expression in clinical terms.

Roszack, B., and **T. Roszack.** *Masculine/Feminine.* New York: Harper & Row, 1971.
This book contains differing viewpoints on the subject of female subjugation. Included are articles by Friedrich Nietzsche, G. B. Shaw, Simone de Beauvoir, Marlene Dixon, and Robin Morgan.

West, D. J. *Homosexuality.* Chicago: Aldine, 1968.
West utilizes the results of physiological and psychological research in his examination of the causes, social significance, and treatment of homosexuality.

Winick, C. W., and **P. M. Kinsie.** *The Lively Commerce: Prostitution in the United States.* Chicago: Quadrangle Books, 1971.
The authors present a psychosocial view of prostitution in the United States during the last half-century, drawing upon previous studies and more than 2,000 interviews with persons directly or indirectly involved with prostitution.

13 Reproduction and Birth Control

Berrill, L. J. *The Person in the Womb.* New York: Dodd, Mead, 1968.
In this beautifully written book, Dr. Berrill describes what takes place in the womb as a new individual develops. Aspects of human development from ovulation and genetic complications to the significance of prenatal individuality are discussed from both the scientific and humanistic perspectives.

Dunbar, E. "Foolproof Birth Control," *Look,* 35 (March 9, 1971), 45–46, 48.
It is estimated that more than 100,000 men had vasectomies in 1970. In this article the author cites the major reasons for the recent increased demand for the operation.

Greenhouse, L. J. "Constitutional Question: Is There a Right to Abortion?" *New York Times Magazine* (January 25, 1970), pp. 30–31, 88–91.
Greenhouse summarizes various legal arguments for the liberalization of abortion laws.

Guttmacher, A. F. *Birth Control and Love.* New York: Macmillan, 1969.
Unwanted pregnancy can bring disharmony to an already-crowded family or disaster to a woman who will seek an illegal abortion. The author believes that pregnancy should result from decision rather than be a risk of sexual expression. This readable book details methods of contraception, discusses abortion, and covers the problem of infertility.

Markham, M., "Even Before You Know the Baby is There," *Family Health,* 2 (June 1970), 45–47.
The foundations for embryonic growth are laid during the first two months of pregnancy. Yet it is at this most important stage that most women, perhaps unaware of their condition, are the least careful about their nutrition. In this concise article Markham discusses the needs of the growing embryo and offers suggestions for the mother-to-be to meet those needs.

Newton, N. A. "Childbirth and Culture," *Psychology Today,* 4 (November 1970), 75.
In this brief article on childbirth, the

author provides evidence from cross-cultural and animal studies for a psychophysiological mechanism that regulates birth.

Raphael, D. "When Mothers Need Mothering," *New York Times Magazine* (February 8, 1970), pp. 67–70.
After dispelling myths about breast-feeding, Dr. Raphael discusses some of the difficulties that may arise. Her main argument is that continued care of a new mother, thus allowing her to relax, leads to success in breast-feeding, whereas the chemistry of anxiety inhibits the flow of milk.

Rugh, R., and **L. Shettles.** *From Conception to Birth: The Drama of Life's Beginnings.* New York: Harper & Row, 1971.
This book is a detailed account of embryonic and fetal development, including more than a dozen remarkable color photographs of the developing human fetus.

Witt, L. "The Male Contraceptive: A Bitter Pill?" *Today's Health,* 48 (June 1970), 17–19, 60–63.
With the continuing controversy over birth-control pills for women, more and more research is being done on contraceptives for males. This article contains brief discussions of the means of male contraception that are presently being tested.

14   Heredity and Health

Asimov, I. *The Genetic Code.* New York: Orion, 1962.
This readable book describes the chemical properties of the genetic code and the history of genetic research.

Edelson, E. "Improving on Heredity," *Family Health,* 2 (December 1970), 17–20.
It is estimated that one out of every four infant deaths is attributable to genetic disease. This article discusses the new methods used to avoid or soften these tragedies; primary attention is given to genetic counseling.

Glass, D. C. (ed.). *Genetics.* New York: Rockefeller University Press, 1968.
This volume contains a series of papers delivered at a conference of geneticists and social scientists. The social, ethical, and legal consequences of recent advances in genetics are discussed.

Moody, P. A. *Genetics of Man.* New York: Norton, 1967.
The author attempts to provide an understanding of the basic principles of human genetics. Aimed at the lay reader, this book covers such topics as genetic inheritance, twin studies, and the origins of human individuality.

Stent, G. S. *Molecular Genetics.* San Francisco: Freeman, 1971.

Stent presents a thorough treatment of the concepts of molecular genetics.

Watson, J. D. *Molecular Biology of the Gene.* 2nd ed. New York: Benjamin, 1970.
This work, written by the noted winner of the 1962 Nobel Prize for discovering the structure of DNA, has become a classic in the field of biology.

15   Marriage in American Society

Farber, S., and **R. H. L. Wilson** (eds.). *Teen-age Marriage and Divorce.* Berkeley: Diablo Press, 1967.
Farber and Wilson compiled this short book from a symposium attended by experts from a wide variety of fields related to marriage. The book contains discussions on why teen-agers marry and the conflicts and difficulties involved.

Hunt, M. M. *The World of the Formerly Married.* New York: McGraw-Hill, 1966.
One out of every three contemporary marriages will end in divorce. The author surveyed the middle-class divorced population, and his account of their lives is interesting and informative.

Kanter, R. M. "Communes," *Psychology Today,* 4 (July 1970), 53–57, 78.
Kanter describes several kinds of present-day communes and compares them with those that were "successful" in the nineteenth century. Based on these comparisons, Kanter makes predictions as to which will survive.

Leslie, G. R. *The Family in Social Context.* New York: Oxford University Press, 1967.
This book is a monumental analysis of the family in terms of its structure and significance as a social institution and as a social group. Cross-cultural and historical information is included.

Nimkoff, M. F. *Comparative Family Systems.* Boston: Houghton Mifflin, 1965.
Nimkoff describes and compares twelve family systems from around the world.

Otto, H. A. "Has Monogamy Failed?" *Saturday Review,* 53 (November 21, 1970), 23–25, 62.
Never before have so many people questioned the validity of marriage. The growth of communes and a "new marriage" explicitly providing the optimum conditions for development of each partner's personal potential are discussed in this article.

Westermarck, E. *A Short History of Marriage.* New York: Humanities Press, 1968.
More than a simple history of marriage, this book explores the variety of marriage contracts and rituals across time and cultures.

16   Parenthood

Bronfenbrenner, U. "Parents Bring up Your Children," *Look,* 35 (January 26, 1971), 45–46.
Professor Bronfenbrenner contends that as parents spend less time with their children, the task of socialization is assumed by peer groups and television. If this trend continues, the author writes, more alienation, indifference, and antagonism can be expected from youth.

CRM Books. *Developmental Psychology Today.* Del Mar, Calif.: CRM Books, 1971.
Although intended as a college textbook, this fully illustrated volume is good general reading not only about child development but adolescence, youth, adulthood, and old age. The sections on perceptual and intellectual development in infancy are of particular interest.

Despert, J. L. *Children of Divorce.* New York: Doubleday, 1962.
The effects divorce has upon children and the legal aspects of divorce are discussed by Dr. Despert, along with suggestions for parents to best prepare their children for their new way of life.

Dodson, F. *How to Parent.* Los Angeles: Nash, 1970.
This book is a complete guide to the emotional and intellectual development of children to six years of age. Avoiding generalities, the author offers specific advice for handling all phases of the development of the preschool child.

Ginott, H. *Between Parent and Child.* New York: Macmillan, 1965.
This excellent book emphasizes the importance of regarding a child's behavior as a special way of communicating ideas he may not be able to verbalize.

Gordon, T. *Parent Effectiveness Training.* New York: Peter Wyden, 1970.
The author proposes in this book a "no-lose" method of solving conflicts. Both parents and child take part in the decision-making process so that neither "wins" or "loses."

Holt, J. *How Children Fail.* New York: Pitman, 1964.
This book is an important critique of American education. Holt is an advocate of the open-classroom situation.
———. *How Children Learn.* New York: Pitman, 1967.
A sequel to *How Children Fail,* Holt shows how some children are able to learn on their own, experimentally or as a game.

Kramer, R. "You've Come a Long Way, Baby, in Three Centuries," *New York Times Magazine* (March 15, 1970), pp. 99–102, 109, 112.
The differences in child-care practices in

the seventeenth and twentieth centuries are described in this article.

Vincent, C. E. *Unmarried Mothers*. New York: Macmillan, 1961.
According to the author, society implicitly condones illicit sex but condemns the consequences: pregnancy out of wedlock. Although cultural attitudes of the American public seem to be changing at an accelerating rate, this book remains an interesting inquiry into the problems of unwed motherhood.

V PERSONAL HEALTH CARE

17 Nutrition

Bailey, H. *The Vitamin Pioneers*. New York: Pyramid, 1970.
This fascinating book records the discovery of various vitamins and describes their function in maintaining health.

Council on Foods and Nutrition to the A.M.A. Board of Trustees. "Malnutrition and Hunger in the United States," *Journal of the American Medical Association*, 213 (July 13, 1970), 272–275.
Malnutrition is a critical problem in segments of America. This article discusses the nature of malnutrition and the implications it has for American society.

Dobbing, J. "Food for Thinking," *New Scientist*, 46 (June 25, 1970), 636–637.
In this brief, well-written article, the author discusses the possibility of permanent brain damage resulting from malnutrition early in life. His hypothesis is that the brain is most vulnerable, as are other parts of the body, during "growth spurts." He says that the brain's major growth begins in the last trimester of gestation and ends approximately eighteen months after birth.

Mayer, J. *Overweight: Causes, Cost, and Control*. Englewood Cliffs, N.J.: Prentice-Hall, 1968.
Mayer attempts to dispell misconceptions about obesity and presents physiological causes and effects of this condition. He takes a nutritional approach to weight control and provides information on the variety of medicinal treatments in current use.

Pyke, M. *Food and Society*. New York: Transatlantic Arts, 1970.
People do not eat nutrients; they eat food. The foods people eat are determined by their culture, history, and dominant religious beliefs; this book explains why.

Simeons, A. T. W. *Food: Facts, Foibles, and Fables*. New York: Funk & Wagnalls, 1968.
Part fact and part fiction, this book traces the evolution of human nutrition

and speculates on the reasons why people eat what they do today.

Takton, M. D. *The Great Vitamin Hoax*. New York: Macmillan, 1968.
The average American family eats varied enough foods to provide the vitamins, minerals, and other essential nutrients to sustain a healthy life, but many people still insist on supplementing their diet with chemically manufactured vitamins. The author contends that the American public has been duped by profit-hungry businessmen into over-estimating the daily need for vitamins.

Wyden, B. "Overweight? – A Fresh Look at the Problem," *Reader's Digest*, 97 (December 1970), 129–132.
Based on a study of rats, this article contends that overfeeding in childhood may lead to a continuous weight problem in later life. The premise is that if overfed when young, the body produces extra fat cells that may shrink with weight loss but are always there, ready to fill out again when normal eating is resumed.

18 Physical Fitness

Bowerman, W. J., and **W. E. Harris.** *Jogging*. New York: Grosset & Dunlop, 1967.
In this short book the authors provide the novice jogger with all the information he may need on how and why he should jog. The final part of the book consists of a series of jogging plans developed at the University of Oregon.

Cooper, K. H. *Aerobics*. New York: M. Evans, 1968.
This book is the result of a comprehensive four-year study on exercise. Various exercises and programs are suggested.
———. *The New Aerobics*. New York: Bantam, 1970. This book, a sequel to *Aerobics*, outlines a more complete program of vigorous aerobic exercise.

Kohler, M. *The Secrets of Relaxation*. New York: Stein & Day, 1969.
Fatigue, mental and physical, is discussed in this helpful book. Illustrations of exercises that help achieve relaxation and a discussion on the importance of relaxation are provided.

Krippner, S., and **W. Hughes.** "Genius at Work," *Psychology Today*, 4 (June 1970), 40–43.
This interesting article discusses the possible relationship between dreaming and creativity. Several examples are given of famous people whose dreams have provided creative experiences.

Luce, G., and **J Segal.** *Insomnia*. New York: Doubleday, 1969.
The meaning of sleep and the many facets of insomnia, its causes and

prevention, are discussed in this fascinating book. The authors also explore the nature of each individual's unique sleeping needs and habits.
———. *Sleep*. New York: Lancer, 1966.
In the well-documented book the authors discuss all aspects of sleep and its relation to one's health, sanity, and sexuality.

Shepherd, R. J. (ed.). *Frontiers of Fitness*. Springfield, Ill.: Charles C Thomas, 1971.
Shepherd has collected the results of recent research in the physiology of exercise.

Steincrohn, P. J. *How to Get a Good Night's Sleep*. Chicago: Henry Regnery, 1968.
In this highly readable book Dr. Steincrohn discusses the nature of sleep and dreams, the conditions that can prevent sleep, and in the final chapter, some practical methods for overcoming insomnia.

Ward, R. R. *The Living Clocks*. New York: Knopf, 1971.
This fascinating study of biological clocks explores how living organisms respond to the cyclic movement of the earth, the ocean, the moon, and the sun.

19 The Eyes and Ears

Baker, J. *The Truth About Contact Lenses*. New York: Putnam, 1970.
Beginning with a brief but thorough explanation of eye function, the author procedes to explain how contact lenses work, who can wear them, how they should be worn and cared for, and whom a prospective wearer should consult for his individual needs.

Gregory, R. L. *Eye and Brain*. New York: McGraw-Hill, 1966.
This book analyses the physiology and psychology of perception.

Mueller, C. B., and **M. Rudolph.** *Light and Vision*. New York: Time-Life Books, 1970.
This beautifully illustrated book is an excellent introduction to eye function as well as to the nature of light and the photographic process.

O'Neill, J. J. *The Hard of Hearing*. Englewood Cliffs, N.J.: Prentice-Hall, 1964.
The physiology of the ear and the physics of sound are explained as background material for this study of the diagnosis and treatment of hearing disorders.

Rushton, W. A. H. "O Say Can You See?" *Psychology Today*, 3 (October 1969), 46–53.
This detailed article provides ample background material for the study of color vision and color blindness.

Stevens, K. M., and **W. A. Hemenway.** "Beethoven's Deafness," *Journal of the American Medical Association*, 213 (July 20, 1970), 434–437.
In this detailed medical account, the authors discuss the possible causes of Beethoven's deafness.

Stevens, S. S., and **F. Warshofsky.** *Sound and Hearing.* New York: Time-Life Books, 1970.
Typical of the Time-Life series, this is a highly readable and well-illustrated book. It explores the nature of sound and the physiology of hearing by using data from numerous disciplines.

Trevor-Roper, P. *The World through Blunted Sight.* Indianapolis, Ind.: Bobbs-Merrill, 1970.
An intelligent study of the interaction of psychology and art, this book traces the influence of defective vision on art and personality.

20 The Teeth, Skin, and Hair

Berland, T. "Periodontal Disease: Hidden Threat to Grown-ups' Teeth." *Today's Health,* 47 (August 1969), 28–30.
Most adults are aware of the basic steps necessary to prevent tooth decay. This article stresses the often unknown importance of proper gum care to prevent periodontal disease.

Brown, W. E. *Cosmetic Surgery.* New York: Stein & Day, 1970.
In nontechnical terms, the author examines the procedures, benefits, price ranges, and psychological repercussions of all forms of cosmetic surgery from silicone treatment to face and body lifts.

Kuno, Y. A. S. *Human Perspiration.* Springfield, Ill.: Charles C Thomas, 1956.
This detailed book provides a complete discussion of human perspiration. It includes a physiological description of the skin and glands as well as a discussion of the importance of perspiration as a temperature- and fluid-regulating mechanism for the body.

Lambert, C. L., and **H. Freeman.** *The Clinic Habit.* New Haven, Conn.: College and University Press, 1967.
The health practices and dental health of 800 families are analyzed in this study. The concluding implication is that the use of public dental clinics in childhood sets a pattern of "medical dependency" that discourages the patient from seeking other means of preventive dental care.

Lufkin, A. W. *A History of Dentistry.* Philadelphia: Lea & Febiger, 1948.
Evidence of tooth decay and periodontal disease has been found in the fossil remains of ancient man. This book traces the growth of dentistry

from early history to the middle of the twentieth century.

Marples, M. J., *The Ecology of the Human Skin.* Springfield, Ill.: Charles C Thomas, 1965.
This book is a techical reference work covering most aspects of skin physiology and disease.

McClure, F. J. *Water Fluoridation: The Search and the Victory.* Bethesda: National Institutes of Health, 1970.
McClure documents the events leading to the fluoridation of public water supplies in the United States. He describes the beneficial effects of fluoridated water, its extensive testing, and the legal and political debate that continues to exist over the prospect of fluoridating public water supplies.

Revere, P. *Dentistry and Its Victims.* New York: St. Martin's Press, 1970.
The author goes beyond descriptions of the care and problems of teeth and discusses the patient-dentist relationship: how to tell a good dentist from a bad one, what to expect from a dentist, what is wrong with the current dental-care delivery system. In an entertaining manner this "anonymous" dentist makes one realize the importance of his teeth and of good dental care.

"Toothpaste, Without the Sex and Nonsense," *Changing Times,* 22 (December 1968), 15.
Toothpastes can be useful agents in the prevention of dental caries, but not all the claims made in advertisements are valid. This article prescribes sensible outlines for choosing an effective toothpaste.

Woodforde, J. *The Strange Story of False Teeth.* London: Routledge & Kegan Paul, 1968.
Woodforde discusses the social significance of the development of false teeth.

VI HEALTH AND DISEASE

21 The Conquest of Disease

Dale, P. M. *Medical Biographies, The Ailments of Thirty-three Famous Persons.* Norman, Okla.: University of Oklahoma Press, 1952.
This is a collection of nontechnical medical biographies of selected famous persons from Buddha to Grover Cleveland. Interesting but possibly inaccurate, these vignettes illustrate the importance of health and medicine throughout history.

De Kruif, P. *Microbe Hunters.* New York: Harcourt Brace Jovanovich, 1926.
The author presents an interesting historical account of advances in microbiology from the time of Leeuwenhoek. Biographical sketches reveal the manner in which certain

diseases were conquered through the discovery of microbes.

King, L. S. *The Growth of Medical Thought.* Chicago: The University of Chicago Press, 1963.
This comprehensive book surveys the intellectual history of medicine. Emphasis is placed on the achievements of ancient Greek medicine, Paracelsus, Vesalius, Harvey, and the formulators of the cell theory.

Lynch, L. R. (ed.). *The Cross-Cultural Approach to Health Behavior.* Cranbury, N. J.: Associated University Presses, 1969.
This book is a collection of anthropological writings dealing with health practices in a variety of societies.

Sigerist, H. E. *Civilization and Disease.* Ithaca, N.Y.: Cornell University Press, 1945.
Disease affects the religion, philosophy, laws, literature, and technology of a civilization. This book attempts to delineate the major aspects of the relationship between disease and the cultures of mankind.

Zimmerman, L., and **I. Veith.** *Great Ideas in the History of Surgery.* New York: Dover, 1967.
This book is a synopsis of the great ideas in surgery and the men who proposed them from the time of the Egyptians to the present day. Excerpts and illustrations from the original studies are included.

Zinsser, H. *Rats, Lice, and History.* Boston: Little, Brown, 1935.
Supposedly concerned with the life history of typhus fever, this book becomes an interesting digression on the historical significance of disease and the impact of rats and lice on mankind.

22 Infectious Diseases

Anderson, G. W., *et al. Communicable Disease Control.* New York: Macmillan, 1962.
This is a detailed book dealing with community medicine and the epidemiology of infectious diseases common in the United States.

Cockburn, A. *The Evolution and Eradication of Infectious Diseases.* Baltimore, Md.: Johns Hopkins, 1963.
This book provides valuable background material for the study of epidemiology. It covers such aspects as the role of speculation in research, the evolution of infectious diseases, and the basic principles of disease eradication. Several diseases are discussed as examples of the principles presented in the first half of the book.

Dennie, D. C. *A History of Syphilis.* Springfield, Ill.: Charles C Thomas, 1962.
This book primarily consists of biographies of researchers and great physicians who dealt with syphilis from the time of Columbus. The final chapters of the book are concerned with the breakthroughs in syphilis research and a survey of modern treatments.

Dubos, R., and J. Dubos. *The White Plague: Tuberculosis, Man and Society.* Boston: Little, Brown, 1952.
The nature of tuberculosis and preventive and therapeutic procedures are discussed in this book. The authors conclude that man must incorporate what he knows about biology into his social system and the workings of everyday life before he can seriously consider eradicating social diseases.

Gallagher, R. *Diseases that Plague Modern Man.* Dobbs Ferry, N. Y.: Oceana, 1969.
This fascinating book contains brief histories of ten communicable diseases, along with profiles of the diseases and how they can be prevented. The international efforts that have been created to control cholera, influenza, leprosy, plague, syphilis, and tuberculosis are among those discussed.

Leff, S., amd V. Leff. *From Witchcraft to World Health.* New York: Macmillan, 1958.
This intriguing book is a social history of medical practice from primitive to modern times.

Rosebury, T. *Life on Man.* New York: Viking, 1969.
This book is a fascinating account of man's aversion to "germs" and to his own excrement and of his concomitant obsession with cleanliness. Rosebury, a bacteriologist, underscores the importance of the symbiotic relationship between man and his microbes by citing the hapless fate of laboratory animals kept in a germfree state. The presentation is witty and charming, yet scholarly.
———. *Microbes and Morals.* New York: Viking, 1971.
This book is an interesting discussion of the history of venereal disease. It also traces the development of societal attitudes toward VD and offers an explanation for the present epidemic proportions of the disease.

23 Cancer

Berenblum, I. *Cancer Research Today.* London: Pergamon Press, 1967.
This account of recent cancer research presents the results of biochemical experimentation in clear and understandable language.

Edson, L. " 'C Particle': A Unified Theory of Cancer," *New York Times Magazine* (March 7, 1971), pp. 29, 69–70. 76–79.
This comprehensive article focuses on Robert Huebner's theory that cancer is caused by a single noncontagious virus. The various studies that led Dr. Huebner to this hypothesis are discussed, as well as the major arguments against it.

Garb, S. *Cure for Cancer, A National Goal.* New York: Springer, 1968.
Originally written for health professionals, this study argues that the search for a cancer cure is being retarded by inefficient organization in the current research program and lack of sufficient funds. This is a good source of information on the political and financial aspects of health research.

Glemser, B. *Man Against Cancer.* New York: Funk & Wagnalls, 1969.
Glemser describes the progress made and the problems yet unsolved in the fight against cancer.

Shimkin, M. B. *Science and Cancer.* Washington, D.C.: U.S. Government Printing Office, 1969.
This illustrated Public Health Service publication was written to inform the general public about the medical and biological aspects of cancer. It also discusses some recent research developments in the cause and treatment of cancer.

Star, J. "How Silastic Transformed Breast Surgery," *Look,* 35 (July 27, 1971), 12.
The author discusses the advantages of silastic implants in women who have had to have cancerous breast tissue removed.

24 Cardiovascular Diseases

Amosoff, N. *The Open Heart.* G. St. George (tr.). New York: Simon and Schuster, 1966.
This book is a compassionate account of the emotional turmoil experienced by cardiovascular surgeons. The author explains in personal terms the processes involved in such operations as heart-valve transplants and other open-heart surgery.

Blakeslee, A., and J. Stamler. *Your Heart Has Nine Lives.* Englewood Cliffs, N.J.: Prentice-Hall, 1963.
This book is a highly readable yet academically sound presentation of the nine contributing factors to coronary artery disease (the basis of most heart attacks) and the steps an individual can take to prevent a heart attack. It is mandatory reading for those who smoke, are overweight, eat rich foods, or get little exercise.

Boyland, B. R. *The New Heart.* Philadelphia: Chilton, 1969.
This book presents the history of treatment of heart dysfunctions and carries the discussion to the present with a prognosis for the future. All of the surgical procedures are described in simple terms, making this book a good source for quick reference.

Hurst, J. W., and R. B. Logue (eds.). *The Heart.* New York: McGraw-Hill, 1966.
This book is a comprehensive textbook of cardiovascular physiology.

Lamb, L. E. *Your Heart and How to Live with It.* New York: Viking, 1967.
After clearly describing the functioning of the heart and the processes through which it becomes diseased, Dr. Lamb outlines in practical terms how heart disease can be prevented through proper exercise and diet.

Selzer, A. *The Heart: Its Function in Health and Disease.* Berkeley: University of California Press, 1966.
Written in technical but well-defined terms, this book fills the gap between the scientific journals and the often unreliable popular accounts of heart function and disease.

"Sugar and the Heart," *Medical World News,* 12 (February 12, 1971), 39–47.
The average American consumes two pounds of sugar each week. The undesirable effects of such consumption, particularly in relation to heart disorders, are only now coming to light.

25 Systemic Diseases

Burnet, F. M. *The Integrity of the Body.* Cambridge, Mass.: Harvard University Press, 1963.
The fundamentals of immunology and autoimmune disease are discussed in this short work.

Nathan, P. *The Nervous System.* New York: Lippincott, 1969.
The basic physiological and psychological aspects of neurology are clearly explained in this book.

di Sant'Agnese, P. A. "Unmasking the Great Impersonator—Cystic Fibrosis," *Today's Health,* 48 (February 1969), 38–41, 68.
This brief article contains valuable information on the nature and treatment of cystic fibrosis, as well as a general discussion of lung and glandular functioning.

Ubell, E. "Do Allergy Shots Really Help?" *Family Health,* 3 (June 1971), 18–19.
The theory behind allergy shots and their effectiveness is clearly explained in this brief article.

de Wardener, H. E. *The Kidney*. Boston: Little, Brown, 1967.
Intended for medical school students, this is a good reference book on the functioning and diseases of the kidney.

Wolf, S. *The Stomach*. New York: Oxford University Press, 1965.
The physiology of the stomach and its disorders are described in detail in this text.

26 Ecology and Pollution

Bernarde, M. A. *Our Precarious Habitat*. New York: Norton, 1970.
Bernarde discusses the various ways in which technological society affects the environment. He also is concerned with the political aspects of pollution.

Burns, W. *Noise and Man*. New York: Lippincott, 1968.
After a careful analysis of the nature of sound and the mechanism of hearing, Burns probes the physiological and emotional consequences of noise.

Bugg, R. "The Junk We Breathe," *Today's Health*, 47 (September 1969), 28–30, 83–84.
This article is a discussion of the possible relationship between pollution and respiratory disease.

Cailliet, G., P. Setzer, and M. Love. *Everyman's Guide to Ecological Living*. New York: Macmillan, 1971.
The authors provide advice and suggestions about activities that concerned people can undertake to relieve the impending environmental crises.

Commoner, B. *Science and Survival*. New York: Viking, 1967.
Is science creating a technology that will overrun rather than be ruled by mankind? How long can people continue to let technology advance unchecked without evaluating the consequences of a massive failure such as occurred in the 1965 blackout? The author poses these and other questions and calls for scientists and citizens to undertake social action to assure the beneficence of technology.

De Bell, G. (ed.). *Environmental Handbook*. New York: Ballantine, 1970.
This book contains articles on all aspects of pollution and the environment. Among the contributors are Rene Dubos, Paul Ehrlich, and Lewis Mumford. Also included is a section of suggestions for community action.

Ehrlich, P., and A. Ehrlich. *Population, Resources, Environment*. San Francisco: Freeman, 1970.
A comprehensive, detailed analysis of the world-wide crisis of overpopulation and the resulting demands on food, resources, and environment.

Heer, D. M. *Society and Population*. Englewood Cliffs, N.J.: Prentice-Hall, 1968.
Heer discusses the sociological significance of population studies. He is primarily interested in explaining the "population explosion."

McCleary, E. "How to Live With Air Pollution," *Family Health*, 3 (August 1971), 20–22.
McCleary provides valuable suggestions for anyone interested in learning to cope with the 215 million tons of pollution produced each year in America.

Shepard, P., and D. McKinley (eds.). *The Subversive Science*. Boston: Houghton Mifflin, 1969.
A collection of essays from a variety of fields, this book surveys the perspectives of ecological investigations. The editors have included stimulating papers written by eminent authorities from the fields of biology, psychology, philosophy, anthropology, and history.

27 Accidents and Safety

Garb, S., and E. Eng. *Disaster Handbook*. New York: Singer, 1964.
Natural and man-made disasters usually catch victims unprepared. This book is an attempt to forewarn doctors, nurses, and the general public of the effects of disasters and provide a mode of effective action during a disaster.

Halsey, M. N. *Accident Prevention*. New York: McGraw-Hill, 1961.
The study of accident prevention is based on the premise that accidents are caused by the actions (or lack of actions) of people in certain environmental situations and that both people and environments are capable of being manipulated to reduce the chance of accidents. Halsey examines ways to prevent accidents in many areas of human activity and discusses the role of physicians and public health workers in instituting these safety procedures.

Hartley, J. *New Ways in First Aid*. New York: Hart, 1971.
This well-illustrated and easy-to-read book could be a valuable guide to anyone in an emergency situation.

Henderson, J. *Emergency Medical Guide*. New York: McGraw-Hill, 1963.
This emergency first-aid book is complete with detailed descriptions of symptoms and treatment and helpful illustrations.

Magnuson, W. L. "200,000,000 Guinea Pigs," in W. L. Magnuson and J. Carper, *The Dark Side of the Market Place*. Englewood Cliffs, N.J.: Prentice-Hall, 1968, pp. 123–155.
Written by the Chairman of the Senate Commerce Committee, this article is a

vivid exposé on needlessly dangerous products sold to the unknowing consumer.

Nader, R. *Unsafe at any Speed*. New York: Grossman, 1965.
Nader details the unsafe construction of most automobiles and explores possible safety improvements.

"The Tools Are Here—Who's Going to Pick Them Up?" *Medical World News*, 12 (April 16, 1971), 41–48.
Based on the premise that the majority of emergency-care centers are drastically inadequate, this article discusses the various components that would constitute an efficient emergency service.

VII HEALTH CARE IN AMERICA

28 Health Providers

Brenner, J. "Medical Care Without a Hassle," *New York Times Magazine* (October 11, 1970), pp. 30–31, 107–118.
Dr. Brenner discusses the medical and social implications of the free clinic he founded and directs in Cambridge, Massachusetts. Dealing primarily with alienated and often penniless youth has led Dr. Brenner to various conclusions about the reinforcing nature of street life and the kind of doctor-patient relationship that is necessary in such a situation.

Garfield, S. R. "The Delivery of Medical Care," *Scientific American*, 222 (April 1970), 15–23.
Extensive use of paramedical personnel is proposed in this article as part of a highly innovative plan for improving the present methods of medical care delivery.

Magnuson, W. L., and J. Carper. "The New Quackery," in W. L. Magnuson and J. Carper, *The Dark Side of the Market Place*. Englewood Cliffs, N.J.: Prentice-Hall, 1968, pp. 156–184.
The new quacks wear white medical gowns, surround themselves with diplomas and electronic machinery, and are taking in more money per year than is spent in research on all diseases. This article discusses exploitation by phony practitioners.

Pappworth, M. H. *Human Guinea Pigs*. Boston: Beacon Press, 1968.
In this revealing book, Dr. Pappworth discusses the increasing tendency among physicians to use their patients in experiments, with or without their consent. After citing examples, he suggests principles and legislative changes that should apply to such situations.

"The Plight of the U.S. Patient," *Time*, 93 (February 21, 1969), 53–58.
The plight of the American patient is

aptly described in this article, which includes information on hospital mismanagement, the need for doctors to keep up-to-date, the trend toward group practice, and the government's responsibility to the sick.

Ribicoff, A. "The 'Healthiest Nation' Myth," *Saturday Review*, 53 (August 22, 1970), 18–20.
Senator Ribicoff argues that the high cost of American medical care is not commensurate with its quality.

Schwartz, J. L. *Medical Plans and Health Care*. Springfield, Ill.: Charles C Thomas, 1968.
The author has made a comparative analysis of twelve prepaid health plans in order to determine the effect of consumer participation in the policy making of each plan.

Young, J. H. *The Medical Messiahs*. Princeton, N.J.: Princeton University Press, 1967.
This book is a thoroughly fascinating history of medical quackery in the United States during the past century.

29 Health Care Delivery

Blum, R. H. *The Commonsense Guide to Doctors, Hospitals, and Medical Care*. New York: Macmillan, 1964.
Many people have no criteria with which to judge the quality of their doctors, hospitals, and related health-care facilites. The author presents a guide from which the nonmedical person can secure adequate health care.

Cobb, C. M. "Solving the Doctor Shortage," *Saturday Review*, 53 (August 22, 1970), 24–26.
Cobb provides a brief survey of the various facets of the medical and paramedical fields that are open to the student.

Crichton, M. *Five Patients, The Hospital Explained*. New York: Knopf, 1970.
Using the experiences of five patients at Massachusetts General Hospital, the author explains the benefits and drawbacks of the large teaching hospital, which has become the focal point for innovation in medical care. He examines the development of modern diagnostic and surgical techniques, takes a critical look at current teaching methods and rising hospital costs, and looks hopefully at some of the ways in which hospital services are being extended and improved through the use of television and computers.

"Dealing with the Dying Patient," *Medical World News*, 12 (May 21, 1971), 30–36.
Doctors are faced daily with death. This article contends that many are inadequately trained to deal with it, thus causing undue stress and anxiety for their patients. In an attempt to clarify the problem, Dr. Elizabeth Kubler-Ross has plotted the various stages she believes a dying patient goes through.

DeGroot, L. J. (ed.). *Medical Care*. Springfield, Ill.: Charles C Thomas, 1969.
This comprehensive anthology provides an excellent overview of American health care. All aspects of medical care from a physician's education to hospital services, public medical care, and insurance policies are discussed in detail. This book could be a valuable aid to the student seeking reference on almost any aspect of health-care delivery.

Ehrenreich, B., and **J. Ehrenreich.** *The American Health Empire*. New York: Random House, 1970.
The need to improve the health care of many people is emphasized in this controversial book. In an attempt to find the direction of change that the American medical system must take, the authors compare American health-care delivery with that provided by other nations.

Kadish, J., and **J. W. Long.** "The Training of Physician Assistants, Status and Issues," *Journal of the American Medical Association*, 212 (May 11, 1970), 1047–1051.
As the doctor shortage becomes increasingly apparent, more avenues are being opened for the training of physician assistants. This article lists and discusses developing assistant programs.

Scott, B. "When a Doctor Needs a Doctor," *Today's Health*, 48 (May 1970), 54–55, 64.
Scott discusses the various ways in which the medical field regulates the quality of its practitioners.

30 Health and the Individual

Dubos, R. *Mirage of Health*. Garden City, N.Y.: Doubleday, 1959.
Because all life is interdependent, no organism, including man, can completely dominate the world. Throughout history societies have sought to define healthful living and all have reached the conclusion that the coexistence of living organisms, men, and dangerous microbes is a necessity.

Wallin, S. S. (ed.). *Toward Century 21*. New York: Basic Books, 1970.
The noted contributors to this book discuss a wide assortment of prospects and possibilities for the future. Biopsychological, humanistic, political, and technological perspectives are all treated.

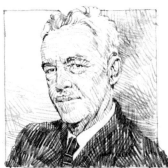

S. Howard Bartley, a professor of psychology at Michigan State University since 1947, was educated at the University of Kansas, where he received his Ph.D. in 1931, and at Washington University Medical School, where he was a member of the Department of Ophthalmology and a research associate in the Laboratory of Neurophysiology. His major concerns are the neuro-physiology of the visual system, an area in which he pioneered modern research, and the study of fatigue. Dr. Bartley has written more than 200 articles appearing in scientific and professional journals and six books, including *The Mechanism and Management of Fatigue* (Charles C Thomas, 1965) and *Fatigue and Impairment in Man* (McGraw-Hill, 1947, reprinted by Johnson Reprint Corporation, 1969), which he coauthored.

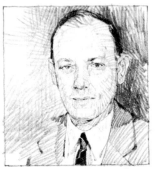

Abraham I. Braude, a professor of medicine and pathology at the University of California at San Diego Medical School, also is director of the microbiology laboratory of the University Hospital. He received his M.D. from the University of Chicago (Rush Medical College) in 1940 and was awarded a Ph.D. from the University of Minnesota in 1950. Since then Dr. Braude has taught in the medical schools of the University of Michigan, the University of Texas, and the University of Pittsburgh. He is a member of several professional societies and the author or co-author of more than eighty journal articles.

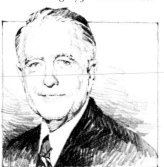

George M. Briggs received his Ph.D. in biochemistry from the University of Wisconsin in 1944. He then taught poultry nutrition at the University of Maryland and the University of Minnesota, and he subsequently spent ten years on the staff of the National Institutes of Health, first as chief of the Nutrition Unit in the Laboratory of Nutrition and Endocrinology, and later as executive secretary of the Biochemistry and Pharmacology Training Committees. He is presently a professor of nutrition at the University of California, Berkeley, and a biochemist in the Agricultural Experiment Station. Dr. Briggs is past president of the American Institute of Nutrition and of the Society for Nutrition Education. His publications include more than one hundred articles and a book he co-authored, *Nutrition and Physical Fitness* (Saunders, 1966).

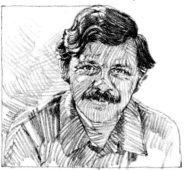

G. A. DeLaria, a resident in general and thoracic surgery at the University Hospital of the University of California at San Deigo, was educated at Tufts University where he received a B.S. in biology in 1964 and an M.D. in 1968. Presently on a National Institutes of Health training grant in cardiac physiology and bioengineering, he is working on the development of an artificial heart. After obtaining his doctorate in bioengineering, Dr. DeLaria plans to return to clinical medicine and complete a program in cardiovascular surgery.

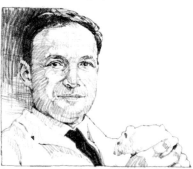

J. Anthony Deutsch was educated at Oxford University in England where he received his Ph.D. in 1956. Since then he has taught and done research at Oxford University, Stanford University, the University of California at Los Angeles, New York University, and the University of California at San Diego, where he currently is located. His research interests involve such physiological aspects of psychology as the mechanisms of hunger and satiety, intercranial self-stimulation, and the cholinergic mechanisms of learning and memory. Dr. Deutsch is a member of several professional societies, including the American Psychological Association. He is the author of almost one hundred articles appearing in technical journals and of the book *Physiological Psychology* (Dorsey Press, 1966).

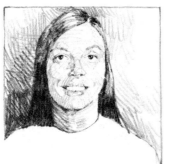

Joyce A. F. Diener, articles editor for *Psychology Today* magazine, graduated from Ohio Wesleyan University with honors in psychology in 1965. She received her doctorate from the University of California at Berkeley in 1970. Her graduate research centered around reproductive behavior. She completed studies of maternal behavior in beagles and copulatory behavior in rats under the direction of Frank A. Beach.

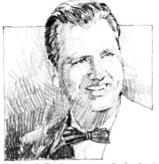

Fitzhugh Dodson, a psychologist in private practice in Redondo Beach, California, received his Ph.D. from the

University of Southern California. He has taught at Lewis and Clark College, Clarement College, El Camino College, and California State College at Long Beach. Dr. Dodson is co-founder with his wife of the La Primera Preschool in Torrance, California and the author of the book *How To Parent* (Nash, 1970).

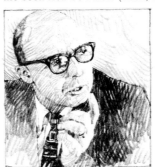

Joel Fort, a physician, author, lecturer, and consultant, specializes in public health, drug abuse, human sexuality, youth problems, and social reform. He is the founder and leader of the Center for Solving Special Social and Health Problems—Fort Help—in San Francisco, and he has held teaching positions at San Francisco State College and at the University of California at Berkeley. Dr. Fort has been a consultant on drug abuse to the World Health Organization and social affairs officer for the United Nations as well as a consultant to the Office of Economic Opportunity and to health departments in both San Diego and Minneapolis. He is the author of more than thirty magazine and journal articles and several books, including *The Pleasure Seekers: The Drug Crisis, Youth and Society* (Bobbs-Merrill, 1969) and *Alcohol: Our Biggest Drug Problem* (McGraw-Hill, 1971).

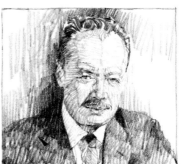

Paul Gebhard is a professor of anthropology and the director of the Institute for Sex Research at Indiana University. Educated at Harvard University in the field of anthropology, he received a B.S. in 1940 and a Ph.D. in 1947. Dr. Gebhard was a co-author with Alfred Kinsey of *Sexual Behavior in the Human Female* (Saunders, 1953) and was the senior author of *Pregnancy, Birth and Abortion* (Harper & Row, 1958), *Sex Offenders: An Analysis of Types* (Harper & Row, 1965), and *The Sexuality of Women* (Stein and Day, 1970).

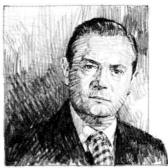

Luigi Giacometti is the scientific director of the Oregon Zoology Research Center, where he currently is studying the comparative histology and physiology of skin. Dr. Giacometti, a naturalized American citizen, was educated at University Medical School in Rome, Italy and received his Ph.D. in biology from Brown University in 1964. Since then he has done research for the Department of Cutaneous Biology of

Contributing Consultants

the Oregon Regional Primate Research Center and is an associate professor of dermatology at the University of Oregon Medical School. Dr. Giacometti has published a number of articles on the histology and physiology of skin, many of them concerning the skin of nonhuman primates.

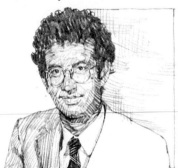

Jeoffry B. Gordon is a clinical instructor in the Department of Community Medicine at the University of California at San Diego and acting director of ambulatory services of the University Hospital as well as director of their OEO Comprehensive Health Services Project. He received an M.D. from Western Reserve University in 1967 and an M.P.H. from Tulane University. His interests are in the restructuring of medicine to promote compassionate, community-oriented health-care delivery. He is a member of several professional and medical associations including the Medical Committee for Human Rights and the Medical Care Section of the American Public Health Association.

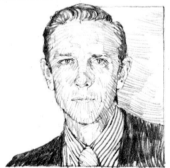

Ralph M. Grawunder, a professor of health science and safety at San Diego State College, received his Ed.D. from Columbia University in 1955. Since then he has served on the boards of directors of the San Diego County Heart

Association and the San Diego Council on Smoking and Health. Dr. Grawunder's major interests are in the areas of health in later maturity, the behavioral bases of health instruction, adult physical fitness, and education for control of drug use and abuse. He is a member of several professional assocations including the Society for Public Health Education and the California Association for Health, Physical Education and Recreation.

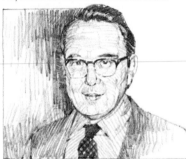

Clifford Grobstein, vice chancellor for Health Sciences and dean of the School of Medicine at the University of California at San Diego, received his Ph.D. in zoology from the University of California at Los Angeles. He has taught at Oregon State College, Stanford University, and the University of California. Dr. Grobstein's major field of interest is developmental biology, and he served as president of both the Society for the Study of Development and Growth and the American Society of Zoologists. He has been a member of the editorial boards of the *Journal of Experimental Zoology* and the *Journal of Developmental Biology* and has published more than fifty articles in numerous scientific journals.

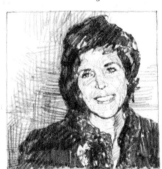

Ruth Grobstein received her B.A. from New York University and a Ph.D. from the Department of Biology at Yale University. She was formerly associated with the medical school of Yale and is presently an assistant research biologist and lecturer at the University of California at San Diego, where her husband also is located.

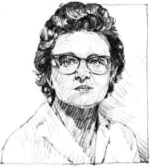

Barbara E. Gunning is an associate professor in the School of Family Studies and Consumer Sciences at San Diego State College. She was granted a Ph.D. in human nutrition from the University of California at Berkeley in 1961. Her previous teaching experience was at the University of Arizona. Dr. Gunning also has held research positions in nutrition and biochemistry at Highland General Hospital in Oakland and the Veterans Administration Hospital in Tucson. Her research interests are primarily related to atherosclerosis and alcoholism. Dr. Gunning is a member of many professional organizations and has had more than fifty articles published in various scientific journals.

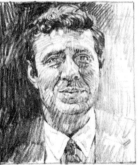

Seymour L. Halleck received his M.D. from the University of Chicago in 1952 and took his psychiatric residency at the Menninger Foundation from 1955 through 1958. He is now a professor of psychiatry at the University of Wisconsin, as well as the chief of psychiatric services for the Wisconsin Division of Corrections, chairman of the section of legal psychiatry of the American Psychiatric Association, and a member of many other medical and psychiatric associations. In addition, he has been a psychiatric consultant to both the Wisconsin Diagnostic Center and the Wisconsin School for Girls and the coordinator of the psychiatric services for the Wisconsin Division of

Corrections. Dr. Halleck is the author of numerous articles in both technical journals and trade magazines and of the books *Psychiatry and the Dilemmas of Crime* (Harper & Row, 1967) and *The Politics of Therapy* (Science House, 1971).

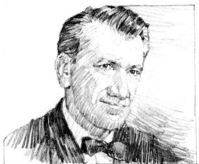

Daniel Horn, director of the Public Health Service's National Clearinghouse for Smoking and Health, attended Northeastern and Harvard Universities and earned a Ph.D. in psychology from Harvard in 1943. Before joining the Public Health Service, Dr. Horn was director of program evaluation for the American Cancer Society and was a pioneer in establishing the relationship of cigarette smoking with lung cancer. Since coming to Washington in 1962, Dr. Horn has helped develop and is now directing the federal government's program of education and behavioral research to reduce the hazards of cigarette smoking. Dr. Horn is a Fellow of the American Public Health Association and the American Association for the Advancement of Science and is a member of the Board of Trustees of the American Cancer Society.

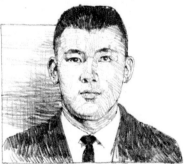

Michael C. Hosokawa, an assistant professor of health education at the University of Oregon, also serves as a research consultant to the Psychiatric Education Research Team on that campus. He was educated at Northern Colorado University, where he received a B.A. in biology in 1962; Oregon State University, where he received an M.Ed. in health education in 1963; and the

University of Oregon, where he received an Ed.D. in health education in 1969. Dr. Hosokawa has been a member of the Health Education Committee of the Oregon Tuberculosis and Respiratory Disease Association; is a member of the local Comprehensive Health Planning Agency and of the Committee for Continuing Education in Public Health for the Oregon Public Health Association; and currently serves on the board of directors of the west central region of the Oregon Tuberculosis and Respiratory Disease Association. He is the author and co-author of several articles in various health-related journals.

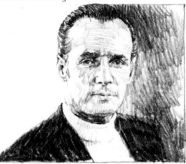

Morton Hunt received his education at Temple University and the University of Pennsylvania, where he majored in English. He became a free-lance writer in 1949 and since then has written some 300 articles, many of them on the psychology and sociology of love, sex, and marriage, that have appeared in *The New Yorker, Harper's,* and other prominent magazines. He also has written a number of books, among them *The World of the Formerly Married, The Natural History of Love,* and *Her Infinite Variety: The American Woman as Lover, Mate and Rival.*

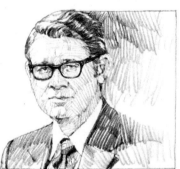

J. Willis Hurst, professor and chairman of the Department of Medicine at Emory University School of Medicine, was educated at the University of Georgia, where he received his B.S. in 1941 and M.D. in 1944. In 1947 he moved to Massachusetts General Hospital to take special cardiovascular training under Paul Dudley White. Dr.

Hurst is a member of the National Heart and Lung Council and currently is president of the American Heart Association. He is the author of more than 120 scientific articles and five textbooks on heart disease, of which his most well-known is *The Heart* (McGraw-Hill, 1966).

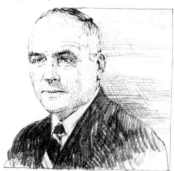

Warren R. Johnson is a professor of health education and director of the Children's Physical Developmental Clinic at the University of Maryland. Educated at the University of Denver, Boston University, and Harvard University, Dr. Johnson has degrees in both English and education. He has served as a director on the Board of Sex Information and Education Council of the United States, and was president of the American Association of Sex Educators and Counselors. He also has been a consultant on sex-related matters for the National Association for Independent Schools, the National Institutes of Health, and the Maryland State Department of Education. Currently a Fellow of the Society for the Scientific Study of Sex, Dr. Johnson's publications include numerous articles dealing with human sexuality and a critically acclaimed book, *Human Sexual Behavior and Sex Education* (Lea and Febiger, 2nd. ed., 1968).

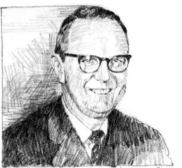

Francis C. Kenel, an associate professor of health and safety at the University of Maryland, was educated at Michigan State University where he received his

B.S. in 1955 and his Ed.D. in 1967. His major fields of interest are traffic and safety education, industrial accident prevention, driver improvement, and police traffic administration. Dr. Kenel has been an educational consultant to the Allstate Foundation, the Human Research Resources Organization, the Illinois Office of Public Instruction, and numerous other state and national agencies. He is the author or co-author of several articles, pamphlets, and books dealing with driving task analysis and traffic safety.

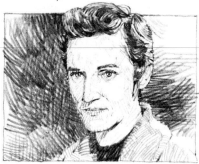

Lois P. Kessler is an assistant professor in the Department of Health Science and Safety at San Diego State College in California. She received a B.S. from the University of Rochester in New York and an M.A. from San Diego State College. Mrs. Kessler's academic interests in the field of human sexuality and the patterns of sexual behavior carry over into the community, where she is a member of the executive board of the San Diego chapter of Planned Parenthood. She also is a faculty member of the Women's Studies Program at San Diego State College, which was the first school to adopt such a program.

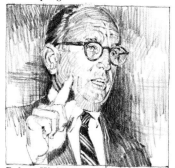

Robert W. Kistner was educated at the University of Cincinnati, where he received his B.A. in Liberal Arts in 1938 and his M.D. in 1942. After a tour of duty in the U.S. Army Air Force as a

flight surgeon, he took further training in pathology and gynecology at Johns Hopkins Hostital and at Boston Lying-in Hospital (now the Boston Hospital for Women). Dr. Kistner has held teaching appointments at Harvard Medical School and at New York State Medical School and is a member of many medical socieites including the American Fertility Society. In addition, he is the author of more than 150 medical articles and several books, of which the best known is *The Pill* (Hutchinson, 1970). At present, Dr. Kistner is assistant professor of obstetrics and gynecology at Harvard Medical School and senior gynecologist, Boston Hospital for Women.

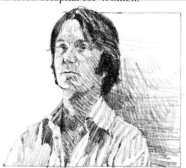

Dennis Krebs is an assistant professor of psychology and chairman of the undergraduate program in the Department of Social Relations at Harvard University. He was born in British Columbia, Canada and attended the University of British Columbia from which he graduated with honors in psychology. He was awarded a Woodrow Wilson Fellowship in 1967 and came to Harvard with his wife to do graduate work in clinical psychology. He received his M.A. in 1968. He then went into the field of personality and social psychology, which has become his field of specialization, and received his Ph.D. in 1970 after completing a thesis on the relationship between empathy and altruism. Dr. Krebs currently is conducting research on altruism, empathy, role-taking, moral development, the effect of a number of variables such as physical attractiveness on self-conception and social interaction, and psychophysiological differences between criminal psychopaths and normals.

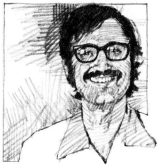

Fred Leavitt is an assistant professor of psychology at California State College at Hayward. He received a B.A. in psychology from Eastern New Mexico University in 1964 and was awarded a Ph.D. in psychology from the University of Michigan in 1968. The following year he did post-doctorate fellowship work at the University of California at Berkeley. Dr. Leavitt's major teaching and research interests are in the fields of comparative psychology and psychopharmacology.

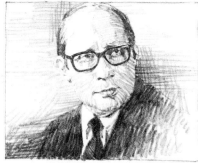

Charles E. Lewis, a professor and head of the division of health administration in the School of Public Health at the University of California at Los Angeles, received an M.D. degree from Harvard Medical School in 1953 and a Doctor of Science degree from the University of Cincinnati in 1959. Since then he has had teaching appointments in the medical schools of Baylor University, the University of Kansas, Harvard University, and UCLA. Dr. Lewis is a member of a number of task forces and committees related to community health, preventive medicine, and health services research. He is the author of many technical articles on toxicology, epidemiology, and research in the fields of health services and manpower.

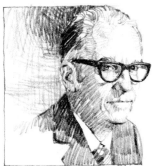

Purvis L. Martin, associate clinical professor in the Department of Obstetrics and Gynecology at the School of Medicine, University of California at San Diego, received his M.D. from the University of California at San Francisco in 1937. Dr. Martin is a member of many civic organizations and medical societies; he is a past president of the San Diego Academy of Medicine, past president of the San Diego Gynecological Society, and president-elect of the Pacific Coast Obstetrical and Gynecological Society. In addition, Dr. Martin is the author of many medical articles dealing with cervical carcinoma and other concerns of obstetrics and gynecology.

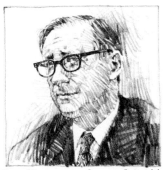

Jean Mayer, a professor of nutrition at Harvard University, is recognized as one of the world's leading nutritionists. Dr. Mayer was educated at the University of Paris, which in 1950 awarded him a D.Sc., summa cum laude, and at Yale University, where he received his Ph.D. in 1948. Since 1950, Dr. Mayer has taught nutrition at Harvard. Dr. Mayer is most noted for his pioneering research on the problems of obesity and the physiological regulation of appetite. He also has done exten- sive work on malnutrition in Africa and Asia, and in 1966 he helped found the National Council on Hunger and

Malnutrition in the United States. As special consultant on nutrition to President Nixon, Dr. Mayer was responsible for organizing and directing a three-day White House Conference on Food, Nutrition and Health, and it was he who persuaded Nixon to include a food stamp program for the poor in his welfare reform plan. Dr. Mayer has been on the editorial boards of several scientific journals, and has published over 500 articles on nutrition in scientific and popular journals. He has contributed to more than fifty books, and is the author of *Overweight: Causes, Cost, and Control* (Prentice-Hall, 1966).

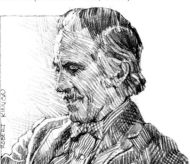

David C. McClelland was educated at Wesleyan University, the University of Missouri, and Yale University, where he received his Ph.D. in psychology in 1941. For the past thirty years, he has been teaching psychology at the college level, and since 1956, he has been a professor of psychology in Harvard University's Department of Social Relations. Dr. McClelland's research interests include the human need for achievement, methods of improving early identification of talent, and the effects of critical life experiences on fantasy. He has received honorary degrees from five universities and was awarded the Guggenheim Fellowship for study abroad in 1958. Dr. McClelland is the author of three books and numerous articles on psychology and has co-authored several books dealing with various aspects of human motivation. He is currently a consulting editor for the D. Van Nostrand Company (psychology series) and three psychology journals.

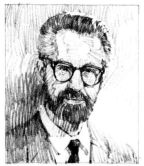

Aubrey C. McTaggart is a professor of health science and safety at San Diego State College. He received a bachelor's degree from the University of British Columbia in 1951 and an M.S. and Ph.D. from the University of Illinois in 1956 and 1962. Dr. McTaggart has held teaching positions in Canadian junior and senior high schools and at the University of Illinois, as well as San Diego State. He is the author of several journal articles and has written one book, *The Health Care Dilemma* (Holbrook Press, 1971).

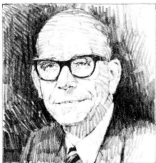

William Montagna has been director of the Oregon Regional Primate Research Center since 1963. He also is professor and head of the Divison of Experimental Biology and professor of dermatology at the University of Oregon Medical School. Dr. Montagna attended Bethany College and received his Ph.D. in zoology from Cornell University. He has taught at the Long Island College of Medicine and at Cornell and Brown Universities. His research interests include the biology of skin, the biology of nonhuman primates, and the male reproductive system. Dr. Montagna has published more than 200 research papers and is the author and editor of several books on skin. He also has written a textbook titled *Comparative Anatomy* and a book called *Man*, which currently is being used as a text for sociology, anthropology, biology, and physical education courses. Dr. Montagna is a former president of the Society for Investigative Dermatology and is a consultant to several national organizations and journals.

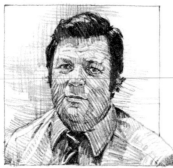

William D. Ross, an associate professor in the Department of Physical Development Studies at Simon Fraser University, received his Ph.D. from the University of Oregon in 1962. His major interests are in the areas of physical growth and development, including anthropometry, studies of body composition and skeletal age, and other assessments of structure and function in relation to normal growth. Dr. Ross has been a field representative for the fitness and recreation division of the Saskatchewan Department of Education and an instructor in the Peace Corps training programs for Peru, Colombia, and Jamaica. He is the author of more than eighty journal articles and five movie scripts.

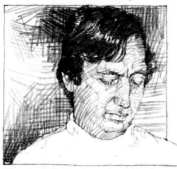

Marvin J. Schissel received his doctorate of dentistry from New York University in 1955. After a tour of duty in Korea as a member of the U.S. Army Dental Corps, he returned to the New York area where he established a practice and affiliated with Triboro Hospital as a clinical assistant visiting dentist. Dr. Schissel is the author of several

magazine articles and one book, *Dentistry and Its Victims* (St. Martin's Press, 1970), under the *nom de plume* "Paul Revere." His book is outspokenly critical of the practice, traditions, and organizational ethics of American dentistry and attempts to expose the faulty practice and shoddy work of some American dentists.

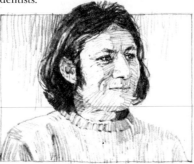

Eugene Schoenfeld, better known as Dr. Hip Pocrates, received a B.A. in history from the University of California at Berkeley in 1955 but remained on that campus for two additional years studying pre-med. In 1957 he entered medical school at the University of Miami, and in 1961, after two summers externship at the Schweitzer Hospital in Lambarene, Gabon, he was awarded an M.D. Continuing his education in Yale's School of Public Health and later as a research physician in the Schweitzer Hospital, Dr. Schoenfeld developed a major interest in community health. One of the products of this interest is his syndicated column, "Dear Dr. Hip Pocrates," which answers medical questions about drugs, sex, and nutrition in frank terms. A collection of the questions and answers from this column appear in his book. *Dear Dr. Hip Pocrates* (Grove Press, 1968). In addition, Dr. Schoenfeld is a consulting editor of *Psychedelic Review*, contributing editor to *Modern Medicine*, and the author of a number of journal articles.

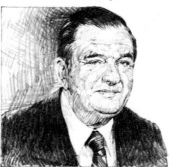

Michael B. Shimkin, professor of community medicine and oncology (the study of tumors) at the University of California at San Diego School of Medicine, is a renowned authority in the field of cancer research. He received

his M.D. in 1937 from the University of California at San Francisco Medical School. Dr. Shimkin was affiliated with the National Cancer Institute for twenty-five years. He has been editor of the *Journal of the National Cancer Institute* and of *Cancer Research*. He has contributed more than 250 articles on various aspects of cancer research to the scientific literature and is the author of the book *Science and Cancer* (U.S. Government Printing Office, 1969).

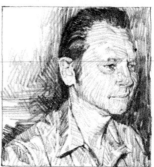

William C. Sloan is a professor of biology at San Diego State College. He received his Ph.D. from the University of Florida in 1958 and has since taught at that institution as well as at Vanderbilt University. Dr. Sloan was a National Institutes of Health postdoctoral fellow at the University of California at Berkeley. His major research interest is in comparative physiology, especially excretory mechanisms. Dr. Sloan is a co-author of *Central Concepts of Biology* (Macmillan, 1971).

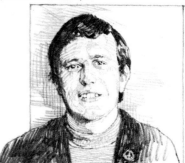

David E. Smith was educated at the University of California, where he received a B.A. in Zoology from Berkeley in 1960 and an M.S. and M.D. from San Francisco in 1964. Since then his interest has been in the fields of neurotoxicology and psychopharmacology, and he has founded the Haight-Ashbury Medical Clinic in San Francisco, where he deals with a number of drug-related maladies. Dr. Smith also is a consultant on drug abuse to the Department of Psychiatry at San Francisco

General Hospital; a member of the U.S. Office of Education, Drug Education Project Advisory Committee; and an assistant clinical professor of toxicology at the Medical Center in San Francisco. He is the author of *The New Social Drug: Cultural, Legal, and Medical Perspectives on Marijuana* (Prentice-Hall, 1970) and *Love Needs Care: The History of San Francisco's Haight-Ashbury Free Clinic* (Little, Brown, 1971), and he edits the *Journal of Psychedelic Drugs*.

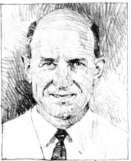

Walter D. Sorochan is an associate professor of health science and safety at San Diego State College. He was educated at the University of British Columbia, the University of Oregon, and Indiana University, where he received his Ph.D. in health and safety in 1969. Dr. Sorochan has completed research in many areas related to health education, including the attitudes of health instructors and students toward various aspects of health and the effectiveness of secondary and college-level health education techniques. In addition to his health education studies, Dr. Sorochan is currently conducting research on student drug use and air quality in public establishments in San Diego. He also is writing a textbook titled *Orthobiosis* (right style of living), and will begin a textbook of elementary school health education in the near future.

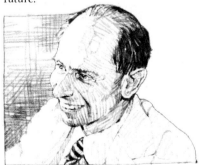

Curt Stern was born in Hamburg, Germany and received a Ph.D. in Zoology from the University of Berlin in

1923. He served on the faculty of the University of Rochester, New York, from 1933 to 1947, and since 1947 he has been on the faculty of the University of California at Berkeley. His research has been largely on the chromosomal and developmental genetics of the Drosophila fruit fly. In addition, his interest in teaching genetics to health science students has led him to write *Principles of Human Genetics* (Freeman, 1960). He is now preparing a third edition of the book.

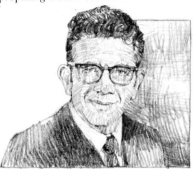

Robert Straus received his Ph.D. in sociology from Yale in 1947 and has since taught at Yale, the State University of New York Upstate Medical Center, and the University of Kentucky at Lexington. He helped plan and develop a new medical center at Lexington beginning in 1956 and served as chairman of the National Advisory Committee on Alcoholism from 1966 to 1969. Dr. Straus is currently chairman of the Department of Behavioral Science in the University of Kentucky College of Medicine. He has done research on drinking behavior and alcohol problems, institutional dependency, and processes of hospital patient care. His writings on alcohol and alcoholism cover a span of twenty-five years and include the co-authored book *Drinking in College* (Yale University Press, 1953).

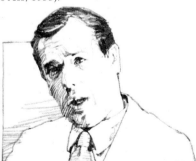

Jared R. Tinklenberg, an instructor of psychiatry at Stanford University received his M.D. at the University of Iowa and his psychiatric training at Stanford. In addition to his teaching post Dr. Tinklenberg is the assistant

director of Stanford University In-patient Psychiatric Service and the residency coordinator in the Department of Psychiatry. His research interests lie in the field of clinical psychopharmacology, especially the effects of tetrahydrocannabinol (the active ingredient of marijuana) on the mind; in accord with this interest Dr. Tinklenberg serves as consultant on drug abuse to numerous public and private agencies. His other research interests include the study of thought and perception disorders in psychotic individuals.

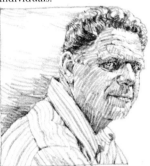

Silvio S. Varon was educated in Europe and received a B.S. from Gymnase Scientifique of Lausanne, Switzerland in 1941, a doctorate of engineering from the Federal Polytechnical School of Lausanne, Switzerland in 1945, a B.A. from the Classical Lyceum in Milan, Italy in 1946, and an M.D. from the University of Milan Medical School in 1959. Since then he has held several research and teaching positions in hospitals and universities in both Europe and the United States. At present he is an associate professor in the Department of Biology and the School of Medicine of the University of California at San Diego. Dr. Varon's major research interests are in neurobiology and neurochemistry, and he is a member of several professional societies including the Society for Neuroscience and the International Society for Neurochemistry.

A

abdomen The lower half of the body trunk.

abortion The termination of a pregnancy before the fetus is capable of living outside the mother's body.

abscess A pus-filled cavity formed by the destruction of tissue from a severe infection.

accommodation The ability to focus on near or far objects by controlling the contraction of the ciliary muscles to alter the shape of the lenses of the eyes.

acetylcholine The chemical neurotransmitter used mainly in the sensory and voluntary motor pathways of the nervous system.

acromegaly A condition characterized by excessive growth of hands, feet, and jaw during adulthood; it is caused by the overproduction of growth-stimulating hormone (GSH).

action potential The reversal of the electrical charge on the surface of a nerve membrane, enabling it to transmit nerve impulses.

active immunity The immunity acquired through the production of antibodies after contact with live pathogens or vaccines. See also *immunity; passive immunity.*

addiction Physical dependence on a drug; it is produced by an altered physiological state in the body of the user. See also *habituation.*

adenocarcinoma A form of cancer that originates in the glands of the body.

adenoids The lymph glands located in the back of the nose, above the throat.

adenosinetriphosphate (ATP) A compound with a high-energy phosphate bond that is broken down to release the energy necessary for muscular contractions, maintenance of body heat, the synthesis of various proteins, and several other energy-requiring chemical reactions.

ADH See *antidiuretic hormone.*

adrenal glands The endocrine glands that produce the hormones cortisone, adrenalin, and noradrenalin, among others; also called the suprarenal glands.

adrenalin The hormone secreted by the adrenal glands that affects the heart and muscles; also known as epinephrine.

aerobic exercise Any form of exercise in which the demands of the body for oxygen are met by a sufficient delivered supply; usually an extended exercise that does not involve extreme physical exertion. See also *anaerobic exercise.*

affective appraisal The cognitive awareness of an emotion.

affective psychoses A group of psychoses characterized by a disorder of mood. See also *manic-depressive psychosis.*

albinism The absence of the tissue pigment melanin.

alcoholism The chronic use of alcohol to the extent that its use contributes to sickness, accidents, or dependency on the drug to avoid withdrawal symptoms.

aldosterone A hormone produced by the adrenal cortex that helps maintain the fluid and salt balances of the body.

alleles Pairs of genes on homologous chromosomes that affect the same traits. When two alleles are identical, a person is said to be *homozygous* for that trait; when the alleles carry differing instructions, he is said to be *heterozygous.*

allergen Any substance capable of producing an allergic condition.

allergy An overreaction of the immune response characterized by the release of excess histamine; also called hypersensitivity.

alpha rhythm A characteristic brain-wave pattern occurring just prior to falling asleep and in certain meditational trances.

aleveolar jawbone The bone sockets in which the teeth are anchored.

alveoli The small air sacs of the lungs in which the exchange of gases between air and blood takes place.

amino acids The basic constituents of all proteins; the end products of protein fragmentation.

amniocentesis The process by which cells are removed for examination from the amniotic fluid surrounding a fetus during pregnancy.

amniotic sac The fluid-filled sac that encloses the fetus during prenatal development.

amphetamines Stimulant drugs used to combat fatigue and reduce appetite; known to users as "uppers."

amygdalae Structures located in the rear portion of the limbic system of the brain that contain switch-on and switch-off controls for certain stereotyped behaviors.

anaerobic exercise Any form of exercise in which the body develops an oxygen deficiency; usually an extreme exertion over a short time period. See also *aerobic exercise.*

analgesic A drug that relieves pain.

anaphylactic shock A state of shock produced by an allergic reaction to drugs (such as antibiotics).

anaplastic The term for a cancer in which the cellular structure is so altered that it no longer resembles the cellular structure of the tissue from which it originated.

anatomy The study of the structure of the body.

anemia A condition characterized by a deficiency of hemoglobin in the blood or by an insufficient quality or quantity of red corpuscles.

anesthesia A state characterized by a general or local loss of sensation, induced by drugs (anesthetics).

angina pectoris Chest pains resulting from an insufficient supply of blood to the heart muscle.

anomie The loss of social roots or feelings of social isolation.

Antabuse A drug used in the treatment of alcoholism that causes a toxic reaction if alcohol is consumed; also called disulfiram.

antagonism The arrangement of muscular groups in opposing pairs that work against one another to permit fluidity and precision of movement.

antechamber The fluid-filled space in the eye between the front of the lens and the cornea; also called anterior chamber.

antibiotics Organic drugs, usually

produced by fungi, that inhibit the growth of bacteria.

antibody A class of proteins manufactured by the body to specifically destroy an invading bacterium, virus, or other such agent. See also *antigen*.

anticoagulants Drugs that reduce the ability of the blood to clot.

antidepressants Mood-elevating drugs that increase activity and drive. See also *monoamine oxidase* (MAO) *inhibitor*.

antidiuretic hormone (ADH) A pituitary hormone necessary to maintain proper fluid balances in the body.

antigen Any agent that provokes the production of a specific antibody.

antihistamine A chemical substance that inhibits the production of histamine by the body.

anxiety A feeling of uneasiness, fear, or distress that arises when a person is faced with possible or imagined danger or misfortune.

aorta The artery that carries oxygenated blood from the left ventricle to the body; the largest artery in the body.

apocrine glands The scent-producing sweat glands found primarily in the armpits and pubic regions. See also *eccrine glands*.

appendix A narrow, closed tube protruding from the beginning of the large intestine.

aqueous humor The fluid filling the anterior and posterior chambers of the eye and secreted by the ciliary body.

ariboflavinosis A disease caused by a deficiency of the vitamin riboflavin and characterized by cracking of the corners of the mouth, sore skin, and bloodshot eyes.

arteries Vessels carrying blood away from the heart.

arterioles The smallest arteries leading to the capillaries.

arteriosclerosis A general hardening and thickening of the walls of the arteries. See also *atherosclerosis*.

astigmatism A visual abnormality produced by an unevenly curved cornea.

atherosclerosis The deposit of fat on the inside of the arteries and the subsequent hardening of the inner linings. See also *arteriosclerosis*.

ATP See *adenosinetriphosphate*.

atria The chambers of the heart that receive blood from the veins. See also *ventricles*.

atrophy Withering of tissue from disuse.

audiometer An instrument used to detect the degree and type of a hearing loss.

auditory canal A large open canal extending from the outer ear to the eardrum.

auditory nerve The nerve that transmits acoustic impulses from the inner ear to the auditory portions of the brain.

autograft The transplant of skin tissue from one site to another on the same individual. See also *homograft*.

autoimmune response The production of antibodies directed against the body's own cells or tissues.

autonomic nervous system The subsystem of the motor branch of the nervous system that regulates the glands and the smooth and cardiac muscles. See also *voluntary nervous system*.

autosome Any chromosome other than the sex chromosomes. See also *sex chromosomes*.

avoidance A form of defense mechanism in which a person consciously seeks to avoid stressful situations.

axon The cablelike portion of a nerve cell that carries electrical impulses away from the cell body.

B

bacilli Rod-shaped bacteria.

bacteria Unicellular, plantlike microorganisms; the main groups are bacilli, cocci, and spirilla.

bactericide Any chemical that kills bacteria.

barbiturates Sedative-hypnotic drugs that act as central-nervous-system depressants; known to abusers as "downers."

basal cells Cells that underlie the surface cells of a tissue.

basal layer See *stratum germinativum*.

basal metabolism The minimum amount of energy that must be expended to maintain life.

basilar membrane One of the two membranes that divide the cochlea of the ear into three chambers. See also *Reissner membrane*.

behavior The sum of an organism's responses to any internal or external situation.

behavior therapy A type of therapy based on conditioning methods; its purpose is to eliminate maladaptive behavior (symptoms) and promote adaptive behavior.

benign Mild in character; not cancerous or malignant. See also *malignant*.

beriberi A disease caused by a dietary deficiency of the vitamin thiamin and characterized by weakness and eventually heart failure.

bile A yellow or greenish fluid secreted by the liver into the small intestine; it is used in the emulsification of fats.

biodegradable Capable of being broken into smaller parts by the action of microorganisms.

biological succession The gradual changes in an ecosystem in both the plant and animal life forms that populate it.

biomagnification The accumulation of certain chemicals from one trophic level to the next.

biopsy The microscopic examination of surgically removed tissue to aid in diagnosis.

bipolar cells A layer of nerve cells in the neural retina that covers the photoreceptor cells and transmits impulses to the ganglion cells.

bipolar neurons Nerve cells in the inner ear connected to the hair cells, whose axons bundle together to form the auditory nerve.

blood pressure The pressure exerted by the blood on the walls of arteries.

bone marrow The pulpy center of bones in which red blood cells, granulocytes, and monocytes are manufactured.

bromides Nonbarbiturate sedative-hypnotic drugs that have been used to alleviate severe anxiety.

Glossary

bronchi The large passageways in the lungs that transport air between the alveoli and the trachea.

bubo An abscesslike swelling of lymph nodes resulting from the assimilation of infectious agents in those areas; often located in the groin in connection with venereal disease.

bulbourethral glands Two small glands, located at the outlet of the urinary bladder, that secrete a clear mucous lubricant that makes up much of the fluid portion of semen.

C

Caesarean Delivery of a baby through an incision in the abdomen when normal delivery is impossible or inadvisable.

caffeine A mild stimulant that promotes wakefulness.

calories A measure of the energy produced by a given amount of food when it is eaten and burned in the body.

canal of Schlemm A duct that drains the eye's antechamber of excess fluid.

Cannabis sativa The Indian hemp plant from which hashish and marijuana are derived.

capillaries The smallest blood-carrying vessels linking arterial and venous blood systems; they permeate all tissues, providing oxygen and nutrients and eliminating waste products.

carbohydrates Chemicals produced by living organisms from carbon, oxygen, and hydrogen; used as the main currency for the distribution of chemically stored energy among living organisms, or within the body. Common carbohydrates include cellulose, starch, glycogen, and the simpler sugars.

carcinogenic Cancer-inducing.

carcinomas Cancers that arise from epithelial cells such as those in skin, glands, and the lining membranes of organs.

cardiac Pertaining to the heart.

cardiac arrest Any complete stoppage of the heart.

cardiovascular Relating to the heart and circulatory system.

caries The gradual destruction of tooth enamel and the underlying structures eventually leading to infection of the pulp and tooth loss.

carrier An individual who harbors and gives off disease-causing organisms or genes without showing any symptoms.

cataract Cloudiness or opacity of the lens of the eye, resulting in blindness.

cell The basic unit of all living things; it is surrounded by a membrane and contains gel-like cytoplasm and various membrane-encased structures. See also *cytoplasm; membrane; mitochondria; nucleus; protoplasm.*

cellular antibodies Antibodies that adhere to tissue cells and remain fixed to these tissues. See also *humoral antibodies.*

cementum A bonelike substance that covers the root of a tooth.

central nervous system (CNS) The brain and spinal cord; it is enveloped by membranous sheaths (meninges) and encased in bony structures (skull and vertebral column).

cervix The narrow, necklike end of the uterus opening into the vagina.

chancre A lesion or open sore that appears at the site of a syphilitic infection.

chemotherapy The use of drugs in the selective inhibition of agents of disease.

cholesterol A chemical compound found in the fatty parts of animal tissue; it is thought to be involved in atherosclerosis.

choroid The layer of tissue in the eye wall that contains the blood vessels.

chromosomes Chainlike assemblies of nucleic acids and proteins located in the cell nucleus; they contain the program for all the inheritable properties of a cell and enable it to reproduce itself.

cilia Minute, hairlike structures found in the bronchi and other passages of the body that serve to move fluids through wavelike oscillations.

ciliary body An extension of the choroid layer of the eye; it surrounds the lens and contains the muscles responsible for accommodation.

ciliary muscles The muscles that control the shape of the lens of the eye.

classical conditioning An experimental method in which a conditioned stimulus and an unconditioned stimulus are paired. See also *operant conditioning.*

climacteric See *menopause.*

clitoris The female structure corresponding to the male penis; it is the focal point of sexual response in the female.

clostridia The family of bacteria to which the organisms that cause tetanus and botulism belong.

clot The transformation of blood into a fibrous jelly that seals broken or cut blood vessels.

CNS See *central nervous system.*

cocci Round or spherical bacteria.

cochlea A spiral-shaped structure within the inner ear. See also *organ of Corti.*

codominance A relationship in which each allele of a gene in a heterozygote is phenotypically expressed. See also *dominant gene; recessive gene.*

codon A group of three consecutive bases within the DNA strand that codes a specific piece of genetic information.

cognitive Relating to knowledge acquired through one's sensual, perceptual, and conceptual abilities.

coitus Sexual intercourse involving insertion of the penis into the vagina.

coitus interruptus Withdrawal of the penis from the vagina prior to ejaculation.

colic Cramping abdominal pain; often a symptom of colitis or enteritis.

colitis A general term for inflammatory diseases of the large intestine.

collagen A protein found in the bones and connective tissues of the body.

collagenous fibers The fibers within the dermis that give strength to the skin.

collateral circulation An increased number of utilized capillaries, enabling the blood to reach a tissue through many different routes.

communicable Capable of being passed from one individual to another through direct contact or through intermediary agents such as insects or foul water.

community psychiatry The psychiatric movement toward prevention of emotional disorders; mental-health care provided by the community through public funds.

compensation The defense mechanism by which one counterbalances failure in one area by excelling in another.

conchus The visible portion of the outer ear.

conditioning See *classical conditioning; operant conditioning.*

condom A thin rubber covering for the penis used as a contraceptive device and a prophylactic against venereal disease.

conduction loss The loss of hearing due to interference with the transmission of sound waves through the outer or middle ear. See also *sensorineural loss.*

cones The light-receptor cells of the retina that distinguish color and bright light. See also *rods.*

congeners Toxic substances that are by-products of fermentation or processing and are found in minute amounts in most alcoholic beverages.

congenital Present at birth.

conjunctiva A transparent membrane covering the exposed portions of the sclera, the inner surface of the eyelid, and the cornea.

connective tissue Supportive tissue such as bone, cartilage, muscle sheaths, and so on.

contagious Capable of being passed from one individual to another through direct contact; directly communicable.

cornea The exposed and transparent portion of the eye, separated from the iris and the pupil by the anterior chamber.

coronary Referring to the heart vessels.

coronary artery disease The degeneration of the arteries that supply blood to the heart muscle.

coronary thrombosis Formation of a blood-obstructing clot within a coronary artery, leading to a heart attack.

corpus luteum An area within the ovary that has evolved from the residual material of a Graafian follicle and that produces the hormone progesterone.

cortex The outer portion of a gland or organ.

cortisone A hormone secreted by the cortical (outer) layers of the adrenal glands and prepared synthetically as an antiinflammatory drug.

crossing over The process that occurs during meiosis in which chromosomes break and recombine with corresponding segments of their homologues; also called gene recombination.

crown The visible portion of a tooth; also, the dental restoration of the visible portion of a damaged tooth by completely covering the natural crown with a gold or plastic veneer.

cunnilingus Oral stimulation of the vagina, vulva, clitoris, or anus. See also *fellatio.*

curettage The scraping of the interior of an organ or cavity. See also *D and C.*

cyanosis The characteristic blue color of skin resulting from oxygen deprivation.

Cyclozocine A long-acting opiate antagonist that blocks the euphoric effects of heroin.

cytology The study of cells, usually in terms of shape and fine structure.

cytoplasm The cellular substances between the outer membrane and the intracellular membrane-bound structures. See also *nucleus.*

D

D and C Dilatation (enlargement) of the cervix and curettage (scraping) of the walls of the uterus.

DDT A water-insoluble insecticide used primarily against body lice, houseflies, mosquitos, and agricultural pests.

deciduous Destined to fall off and be replaced, as for example the primary, or "baby" teeth.

decongestants Drugs that act to clear mucous congestion from the nose, sinuses, or bronchial apparatus.

defense mechanism A reaction to frustration or conflict in which the individual deceives himself about his real motives and goals to avoid anxiety or loss of self-esteem. See also *compensation; displacement; projection; rationalization; reaction formation.*

delirium tremens (DTs) A symptom of alcohol withdrawal; it is characterized by a state of mental confusion and bodily trembling.

delusion A false belief, often a symptom of paranoid schizophrenia.

denial A form of defense mechanism in which a person refuses to acknowledge or identify a stressful situation.

dentin The material within a tooth that covers the pulp and lines the root canal.

deoxyribonucleic acid (DNA) The complex chains of nucleotides of which genes are composed.

depressants Drugs that slow or reduce the activity of bodily systems.

dermatitis Any inflammatory skin disorder.

dermatology The study and treatment of the diseases of the skin.

dermis The thick underlying layer of the skin that contains the sweat glands, sebaceous glands, and the hair follicles. See also *epidermis.*

diaphragm Anatomically, the domelike muscle that divides the chest or thoracic cavity from the abdominal cavity; contraction of this muscle forces the contents of the abdomen downward and expands the thoracic cavity, causing inhalation. Also, a term for a contraceptive device composed of a circular metal spring covered with rubber; it is inserted into the vagina and covers the opening to the cervix.

diastolic pressure Pressure of the blood within the arteries when the heart is resting between contractions. See also *systolic pressure.*

differentiation In embryology, the process by which cells of a developing fetus utilize select portions of the genetic information contained in their chromosomes and develop into different tissues and organs. Psychologically, the process by which forms of behavior become more complex and specialized.

digitalis A drug that stimulates a weak or failing heart.

disease Disability due to the incorrect functioning of an organ, part, structure, or system.

displacement The defense mechanism by which one transfers an emotional attachment from its proper object to a replacement.

disulfiram See *Antabuse.*

diuretic Any drug that removes body water through the production of urine.

DNA See *deoxyribonucleic acid.*

dominant gene A gene that will be phenotypically expressed whenever it is present. See also *codominance; recessive gene.*

douche Application of a stream of fluid, usually water, intended to flush out and clean the vagina.

Down's syndrome A genetic disease caused by the presence of an extra chromosome and characterized by mental retardation and several physical defects; also known as mongolism.

drug Any biologically active substance that is foreign to the body and is deliberately introduced to affect its functioning.

drug abuse The use of a drug to an extent that produces definite impairment of social, psychological, or physiological functioning.

DTs. See *delirium tremens.*

dysmenorrhea Menstrual pain or discomfort.

E

E. coli A bacterium endogenous to man that resides in the lower portion of the digestive tract.

eardrum See *tympanic membrane.*

eccrine glands The sweat glands covering most of the body that moisten the skin to prevent scaling of the horny layer and reduce body temperature by evaporation of fluid. See also *apocrine glands.*

ecology The study of the relationship between living things and their environment.

ecosystem A distinct physical space within which life forms exist and exchange materials with one another and with their environment.

eczema An inflammatory skin disorder of unknown cause characterized by redness, itching, blisters, and scaliness.

edema Swelling of the tissues due to the accumulation of excess fluids.

ejaculation The expulsion of seminal fluids.

electrocardiogram (ECG) A recording of the electrical activity and pattern of contraction of the heart.

electroencephalogram (EEG)   The electrical wave patterns recorded from the surface of the brain.

electroshock therapy   A form of therapy used chiefly with depressed patients in which high-voltage current is passed through the head, producing convulsions and unconsciousness.

embolus   A material, such as a blood clot fragment or an air bubble, that is carried in the bloodstream until it obstructs a small vessel.

embryo   The term used to refer to a developing human organism during the first three months of pregnancy. See also *fetus*.

emotion   Body changes (initiated in the CNS and mediated chiefly by the autonomic nervous system and the endocrine system) that result from the subjects' value response to a given stimulus; emotions are the physiological and psychological forms in which men experience their estimates of the harmful and helpful effects of stimuli.

enamel   A dense, hard substance that forms the crown of a tooth.

encounter group   An intensive group that meets for the purpose of developing and improving interpersonal communication.

endemic   Of normal occurrence in a specific population.

endocrine glands   Glands that secrete hormones directly into the bloodstream. See also *adrenal glands; gonads; pancreas; pituitary; thyroid*.

endodontics   Study and treatment of the interior tissues of the teeth.

endogenous   Developing or growing from within. See also *exogenous*.

endolymph   The fluid contained in the semicircular canals and in the scala media of the ear.

endometrium   The membrane lining of the inner walls of the uterus.

enzymes   Proteins that stimulate chemical changes through specific catalytic action. They are necessary for most chemical reactions that take place within the body.

epidemic   Referring to a disease that affects a larger number of people in an area than it normally would. See also *pandemic*.

epidemiology   The study of the frequency, distribution, causes, and control of diseases within a population.

epidermis   The upper layer of skin composed of four strata. See also *dermis*.

epididymis   The body of coiled tubes attached to each testis that collects and stores sperm cells.

epinephrine   See *adrenalin*.

episiotomy   Surgical incision in the vagina during childbirth to prevent tearing in the vaginal walls.

epithelium   The sheetlike tissues forming the surface of the skin and the lining of the respiratory, urinary, and digestive tracts.

Epstein-Barr virus   The organism that causes the most common form of infectious mononucleosis.

erection   The swollen and rigid state of an organ due to vasocongestion; usually refers to the male penis or female clitoris and nipples.

ergot   The fungus from which LSD is derived.

erogenous   Relating to the increase of sexual desire upon stimulation.

esophagus   The passage leading from the pharynx to the stomach.

essential hypertension   Persistent high blood pressure of unknown cause.

estrogen   A hormone produced by the ovaries that is responsible for the development of secondary female characteristics. See also *progesterone*.

ether   A central-nervous-system depressant occasionally used as a general anesthetic.

ethology   The study of animals in their natural habitat.

etiology   The study of the causes of disease.

eustacian tube   An air tube extending from the ear to the throat that maintains the pressure equilibrium on the eardrum and drains the middle ear.

excitatory   Relating to electrical nervous signals that trigger their target neurons into action. See also *inhibitory*.

existential therapy   A method of psychotherapy that attempts to restore in the patient the sense of freedom and responsibility for his own choices.

exocrine glands   Glands that secrete their products into ducts. See also *endocrine glands*.

exogenous   Produced from without. See also *endogenous*.

expectorants   Drugs that promote the spitting-up of mucus from the bronchi and throat.

exudate   Fluids that leak out of blood vessels into an inflamed area, causing swelling or edema.

F

Fallopian tubes   The two ducts that transport ova from the ovaries into the uterus; also called oviducts.

farsightedness   See *hyperopia*.

fatigue   A self-conscious state of discomfort or inability to perform physical or mental tasks. See also *mental fatigue; physical fatigue*.

fats   Highly caloric substances found in some form in most foods and composed of glycerol and fatty acids. See also *polyunsaturates; saturated fats; unsaturated fats*.

fear   A strong emotional response involving agitation and feelings of unpleasantness, coupled with a desire to flee.

fellatio   Oral stimulation of the penis. See also *cunnilingus*.

fertilization   The process that unites the sperm and the ovum.

fetishism   Sexual attraction to inanimate objects, such as female undergarments.

fetus   The term used to refer to the developing organism during the last six months of pregnancy. See also *embryo*.

fibrillation   Rapid ineffective non-rhythmic contractions of the heart.

fibrinogen   The protein that enables the blood to clot.

foreplay   Petting used as a preparation for coitus.

fossil fuels   Combustible fuels derived from organic fossil sources such as soft coal and oil.

fraternal twins   Twins that develop from separate zygotes. See also *identical twins*.

frigidity   The inability to experience sexual pleasure, or the lack of sexual desire in females.

fructose   A simple sugar predominantly found in fruits.

fungi   Parasitic plants that lack chlorophyll.

G

gall bladder   A pear-shaped sac containing bile and located on the underside of the liver.

gamete   A sex cell; an egg or a sperm.

gametic mutation   A mutation of a germ cell.

gamma globulins   The class of blood proteins to which antibodies belong.

ganglion cells   A layer of cells in the neural retina whose axons bundle together to form the optic nerve.

gastroenterology   The study and treatment of the disorders of the stomach and intestines.

gene recombination   See *crossing over*.

genes   The chromosomal units involved in the inheritance of a given genetic trait.

gentic code   The general term referring to the arrangement of codons within the genes to determine the ultimate instructions for protein synthesis.

genetic counseling   Advice to prospective parents based on identifying the various possibilities of their conceiving a genetically abnormal child.

genetic engineering   The attempt to treat genetically abnormal individuals by eliminating, replacing, or providing genes that are extra, defective, or missing, respectively.

genetic mutation   The alteration by chemicals or radiation of some portion of the DNA within the genes.

genetics   The science that studies the transmission of hereditary factors and the manner by which they express themselves during the development and life of an individual.

genitalia   The male or female external sex organs.

genotype   The genetic composition of an individual; the characteristics of an organism that are inherited and that can be transmitted to offspring. See also *phenotype*.

germ cell   See *gamete*.

gigantism   A condition characterized by excessive growth in childhood resulting from excessive production of growth-stimulating hormone (GSH).

gingivae   The mucous membranes that surround the teeth; also called *gums*.

gland   An organ made up of cells whose main function is to manufacture chemical products for secretion. See also *endocrine glands; exocrine glands*.

glands of Bartholin   Two small glands located on each side of the vaginal orifice that provide a lubricating fluid during sexual arousal.

glans   Head of the penis or clitoris.

glomeruli   The capillary tufts, each associated with one kidney tubule, from which blood waste products are filtered into the tubules. See also *nephron*.

glottis   The opening between the vocal cords.

glucose   The simple sugar used by the body: other sugars are usually converted into glucose by enzymes in the body before they can be used as energy sources.

glycerol   A thick syrupy liquid that is a component of fat.

glycogen   The form in which carbohydrates are stored in the liver.

goiter   An enlargement of the thyroid gland, causing a noticeable lump on the throat.

gonadotropins   Hormones secreted by the pituitary that stimulate the gonads.

gonads   The sex glands; testes in men and ovaries in women; they produce the sex cells (or gametes) and the main sex hormones.

gonococci   The bacteria that cause gonorrhea.

gout   A disease mainly affecting the joints and characterized by accumulation of a waste product called uric acid.

Graafian follicles   Small sacs inside the ovary in which ova mature.

granulocyte   A type of white blood cell produced in the bone marrow and involved in the destruction of foreign particles in the body.

growth-stimulating hormone (GSH)   A pituitary hormone necessary for proper growth. See also *acromegaly; gigantism; pituitary dwarf*.

guanine   An organic base that, with a sugar molecule and inorganic phosphate, forms a nucleotide, one of the building blocks of DNA.

gynecology   The study and treatment of diseases of the sexual-reproductive organs of women.

H

habituation   Behaviorally, the process of becoming accustomed to a particular set of circumstances or stimuli. In drug terminology, the state of psychological dependence on a drug. See also *addiction; tolerance*.

hair cells   The cells contained in the organ of Corti in the ear that transform fluid vibrations into electrical impulses.

hair cycle   The formation and growth of a hair followed by a resting period, loss of the hair, and the formation of a new hair in the same follicle.

hair follicle   A small cavity in the skin in which hair develops.

hallucination   Sensory experience for which there is no external stimulus.

hallucinogen   A drug that primarily produces hallucinations.

health   A sense of physical, mental, and social well-being; effective functioning, both within the individual and by the individual in his environment.

heart attack   Damage to the heart muscle resulting from the obstruction of a coronary artery by either an embolus or a thrombus.

heart block   Loss of the properties of conduction of nervous impulses that regulate the rhythmic contractions of the heart.

heart failure   A condition characterized by the inability of the heart to perform its proper pumping action.

hematology   The study and treatment of the diseases of the blood.

hemizygous   Referring to the alleles of the X chromosome in male cells.

hemodialysis   The process of filtering blood with an artificial kidney machine.

hemoglobin   The primary constituent of red blood cells and the protein responsible for the transport of oxygen and carbon dioxide.

hemophilia   A genetic disease characterized by excessive bleeding due to the deficiency of certain blood components necessary for rapid blood clotting.

hemorrhage   Bleeding.

heroin   A narcotic derived from morphine; known as "H" or "horse" by users.

heterosexuality   Sexual attraction to members of the opposite sex. See also *homosexuality*.

heterozygous   See *alleles*.

histamine   A chemical obtained from a modification of the amino acid histidine; it is released by body tissues in allergic reactions and causes the dilation of capillaries.

histology   The microscopic study of tissues.

hives   An allergic condition characterized by welting and itching of the skin.

homeostasis   The maintenance of stable, normal levels of body function.

homograft   The transplant of skin tissue from one individual to another of the same species. See also *autograft*.

homologues   The two chromosomes of a pair.

homosexuality   Sexual attraction to members of the same sex. See also *heterosexuality*.

homozygous   See *alleles*.

hormones   Chemicals secreted by endocrine glands or tissues and circulated through the bloodstream to act elsewhere in the body.

horny layer   See *stratum corneum*.

host   The recipient of extraneous materials, such as infectious agents or tissue transplants.

Huhner test   A female sterility test involving the microscopic examination of vaginal fluid shortly after intercourse to determine the presence of live sperm.

humoral antibodies   Antibodies that circulate in the bloodstream. See also *cellular antibodies*.

hydrocephalus   A congenital malformation characterized by the presence of water on the brain.

hydrochloric acid   An acid secreted by the walls of the stomach and aiding in the breakdown of food into its chemical constituents.

hymen   Circular fold of tissue usually present at the entrance of the vagina in virginal females.

hyperopia   A visual abnormality caused by a shortening of the diameter of the eye from front to back and characterized by the ability to see distant objects more clearly than near ones; also known as farsightedness. See also *myopia*.

hyperplasia   An abnormal increase in the number of cells in a given tissue; often associated with malignant tumors.

hypersensitivity   See *allergy*.

hypertension   Persistent high blood pressure.

hypnotic   Any drug that promotes sleep.

hypochondriasis Preoccupation with the body and with fear of diseases even though the body is in good health.

hypokinetic Relating to insufficient exercise.

hypophysis See *pituitary gland.*

hypothalamus A part of the brain that controls appetite, emotions, sexual reflexes, and visceral activities.

hysterectomy The surgical removal of the uterus.

hysterical neurosis, conversion type The conversion of mental conflict into extreme physical symptoms such as blindness, deafness, or paralysis.

hysterical personality A personality trait characterized by the attempt to control relations with others by simulation of sickness.

hysterotomy A miniature Caesarean operation done to abort a fetus after the twelfth week of pregnancy.

I

identical twins Twins that develop from the same zygote. See also *fraternal twins.*

immune mechanism The manufacture of antibodies in response to a foreign substance (or antigen), such as a disease-causing organism.

immunity The ability to resist infection or the development of a disease. See also *active immunity; passive immunity.*

immunology The study of immunity.

implantation The process by which the zygote burrows into the endometrium.

impotence The inability of a male to have or maintain an erection during intercourse.

imprint An irreversible behavior response learned early in life.

inborn errors of metabolism Gametic mutations causing certain enzymes or proteins to be defective.

incus A small bone of the middle ear that transmits vibrations from the tympanic membrane to the inner ear. See also *malleus; stapes.*

indole A compound to which serotonin, psilocybin, and other drugs are chemically related.

infarct An area of dead tissue resulting from the deprivation of blood; usually caused by an embolus.

infection The presence in the body of pathogenic organisms.

inflammation Redness, local warmth, swelling, and pain in body tissues resulting from intrusion of foreign matter.

inhibitory Relating to electrical nervous signals that prevent their target neurons from responding to an external stimulus. See also *excitatory.*

inlay A dental filling made outside the mouth and then cemented into place in the tooth.

inner ear See *labyrinth.*

insomnia The inability to sleep.

insulin A hormone produced by the islet cells of the pancreas that is necessary for sugar metabolism.

insulin shock therapy The inducement of a coma through large doses of insulin; used to relieve symptoms of extreme emotional disorders.

interferon A protein substance produced by the body that inhibits the growth of viruses.

internal medicine The study and treatment of the internal organs and systems of the body.

interneuron A nerve cell located along an electrical pathway between a sensory and motor neuron.

internist A physician specialized in the diseases of internal organs.

intrauterine device (IUD) Plastic or stainless-steel contraceptive device inserted into the uterus for the purpose of preventing conception.

ipecacuanha A root with the medicinal property of curing amoebic dysentery.

Iproniazid An early drug used to treat tuberculosis and later found to act as an antidepressant.

IQ (intelligence quotient) An index to the rate of mental growth obtained by dividing chronological age into mental-age score achieved on a test, then multiplied by 100.

iris The colored ring attached to the ciliary processes of the eye at the back of the anterior chamber; it is composed of circular and radial muscle fibers that control the size of the pupil and the amount of light admitted through it.

islet cells The cells of the pancreas that secrete insulin.

isoleucine One of the essential eight of twenty amino acids used in the human body.

Isoniazid A drug used to combat tuberculosis.

IUD See *intrauterine device.*

J

jaundice A symptom of several conditions leading to an excess of bile in the blood; it is characterized by yellowing of the skin and the whites of the eyes.

K

kidneys The two organs that filter impurities from the blood and produce urine.

Klinefelter's syndrome A genetic abnormality in which an extra X chromosome exists in a male's genetic make-up; it is characterized by abnormally small testicles and lack of mature sperm.

kwashiorkor A protein-deficiency disease of children characterized by weight loss, improper bone development, and possible mental retardation.

L

labia majora The outer folds of skin on either side of the vagina.

labia minora The inner flaps of soft skin on either side of the vagina.

labor pains Abdominal cramps resulting from contraction of the uterus during childbirth.

labyrinth (inner ear) A fluid-filled chamber containing the cochlea and the vestibular apparatus.

lacrimal gland The small gland located in the upper region of the eye orbit that secretes tears.

lacrimal sac A small cavity in the corner of the eye that collects tears.

lactose The form of sugar found in milk.

laparoscopy Sterilization achieved by electrically severing the Fallopian tubes through a small abdominal incision.

laryngology The study and treatment of the diseases of the throat.

larynx The voice-box.

laudanum A popular eighteenth-century cure-all consisting of opium dissolved in alcohol.

lead compounds Chemical air pollutants originating from the combustion of automobile fuels.

learning The acquisition of knowledge or skill through practice or experience.

lens The transparent fibrous structure of the eye located behind the pupil that focuses light on the retina.

lens ligament See *zonula.*

leucine One of the essential eight of twenty amino acids used in the human body.

leukemia Cancer of the white blood cells (leukocytes).

leukoplakia A whitish thickening in the mouth that is considered to be an early sign of cancer.

leukorrhea Vaginal discharge.

ligaments The fibrous connective tissues that hold bone joints together.

limbic system Structures in the upper portion of the brain that mediate the control of such emotive behavior as "rage."

linoleic acid An essential dietary fatty acid that helps prevent skin disorders in children.

lipids Organic chemicals made up of carbon, oxygen, and hydrogen; unlike carbohydrates, they are poorly soluble in water; also used for energy storage and fuel. Commonly referred to as fats.

lithium An element that is used in

drug form to treat persons diagnosed as being manic-depressive.

liver The largest organ of the body; a major function of the liver is the production of bile, but it also is a necessary organ for the metabolism of various nutrients.

lobotomy The surgical severing of the nerve tracts leading from the frontal association areas of the brain to the thalamus and hypothalamus; used to relieve symptoms of extreme psychosis.

lymph The fluid collected from tissue spaces once it has entered the lymph vessels.

lymph nodes Lumps of lymphoid tissue criss-crossed by distended lymph spaces.

lymphatic system An auxiliary circulatory system of vessels used to drain the body of fluids, to transport white blood cells, and to collect fatty nutrients from the intestinal villi.

lymphocyte A type of white blood cell produced from lymphoid tissue.

lymphoid tissue The tissue that comprises the lymph nodes and portions of the thymus and the spleen.

lymphoma A cancerous tumor derived from lymphoid tissue and localized to lymph nodes.

lymphosarcoma Cancers affecting both lymphoid and connective tissues.

lysine One of the essential eight of twenty amino acids used in the human body.

M

macrophages Large phagocytes usually found in the tissues rather than in the bloodstream.

malignant Dangerous to health or life; cancerous.

malleus A small bone of the middle ear resting on the tympanic membrane and transmitting vibrations to the inner ear. See also *incus; stapes.*

malnutrition The lack or insufficiency of certain dietary ingredients.

malocclusion Improper bite.

malpresentation A condition in which a fetus does not move through the birth canal in a normal manner; it requires a Caesarean operation to complete the delivery.

mammography An x-ray of the breast to determine the presence of a tumor; such an x-ray record is called a *mammogram.*

manic-depressive psychosis A psychotic reaction characterized by extreme variation in mood, ranging from a highly elated state to depression and back.

marasmus Severe malnutrition due primarily to calorie restriction or starvation.

marriage A coming together and union of two or more people for their common good and for the care of one another.

masochistic See *sado-masochism.*

masturbation Sexual self-stimulation.

materia alba A whitish food residue that adheres to the teeth near the gums.

mechanoreceptors The complex of nerve endings in the dermis that respond to such stimuli as touch, pressure, and tension.

medulla The center of a gland or organ.

meiosis The process of cell division in which the daughter cells receive half the normal number of chromosomes, thus becoming gametes. See also *mitosis.*

melanin The brown pigment that causes tanning and freckling and that colors the hair.

melanocytes The skin cells that produce the pigment melanin.

melanoma Cancer of the pigment-carrying cells of the skin.

membrane A thin layer of tissue, lining a body cavity; also, the "skin" of individual cells and the partitions within them.

menarche The onset of menstruation.

meninges The tissues covering the brain and spinal cord.

menopause The cessation of the menstrual cycle; also known as the climacteric.

menstruation A bloody discharge from the uterus at regular monthly intervals.

mental fatigue Fatigue resulting from mental exertion.

mental illness Impairment of psychological functioning due to neurosis, psychosis, or a personality disorder; deviance from social, psychological, ethical, or political norms.

metabolism The chemical processes of a cell, tissue, or organism by which food substances are transformed into chemical nutrients and energy.

metastases Sites of metastatic growth.

metastatic growth The transfer of cancer to other parts of the body through the lymphatic or circulatory system, producing secondary growths.

metazoa Multicellular animals, except sponges and wormlike mesozoa. Some, such as pinworms, tapeworms, and flukes, can be parasitic to man.

methadone A narcotic drug medicinally used as a substitute for heroin.

methionine One of the essential eight of twenty amino acids used in the human body.

microbe Any minute organism such as a bacterium or virus.

microelectrodes Tiny needles capable of carrying electrical current.

middle ear A small cavity in the ear containing the three ossicles that transmit vibrations from the tympanic membrane to the oval window.

midwife Any woman assisting a childbirth in the absence of a medical practitioner.

miscarriage Spontaneous abortion of an embryo or fetus.

mitochondria Sausage-shaped bodies, found in almost all cells, that use oxygen to process nutrients and produce the energy necessary for the cell to function.

mitosis A process of cell division involving the duplication of chromosomes and the production of two daughter cells identical to the original.

mongolism See *Down's syndrome.*

monoamine oxidase (MAO) inhibitor An antidepressant drug that elevates mood; used primarily in treating psychiatric patients.

monocyte A type of white blood cell produced in the bone marrow.

monogamy Marriage between two people. See also *polygamy.*

monosodium glutamate (MSG) A chemical used to enhance the flavor of foods.

morbidity Sickness or the presence of disease; the number of sick persons in a population, usually expressed in a ratio to the total population. See also *mortality.*

mortality Death; number of persons dying in a population, usually expressed as a ratio of the number of deaths per 100,000 persons. See also *morbidity.*

motivation A general term referring to factors within an organism that arouse and maintain behavior directed toward satisfying needs, drives, and values.

motor Referring to the branch of the nervous system that controls the various body activities. See also *autonomic nervous system; voluntary nervous system.*

motor-neural Relating to a motor nerve cell, its axon, and its target muscle cells.

MSG See *monosodium glutamate.*

mucosae The mucus-coated membranes that line the respiratory, digestive, and urogenital tracts.

multiphasic screening A type of health testing that combines a detailed computerized medical history and a series of diagnostic tests administered by paramedical personnel.

mutant Referring to a genotype that contains a mutation.

myocardial infarction The damaging or death of a portion of the heart muscle as a result of reduction of the blood supply to that area.

myoclonic jerk The spasm that sometimes occurs just as a person is falling asleep.

myopia A visual abnormality caused by a lengthening of the diameter of the eye from front to back and characterized by the ability to see near objects more clearly than distant ones; also known as nearsightedness. See also *hyperopia*.

myotonia Muscular tightness.

N

Naloxone A long-acting opiate antagonist that blocks the euphoric effects of heroin.

narcolepsy A mental disorder characterized by the constant desire to sleep.

narcotic Any of the opiate drugs.

naso-lacrimal duct A duct extending from the eye orbit to the nasal cavity that carries away excess lacrimal fluid, dust, or other foreign particles from the surface of the eye.

natural childbirth Childbirth without any form of anesthesia.

natural selection The relative reproductive success of those organisms best able to survive in a given environment.

naturopath A type of health practitioner who attributes disease to an imbalance of the natural forces within the body and treats disease by employing such natural forces as air, light, water, vibration, heat, electricity, dietetics, and massage.

nearsightedness See *myopia*.

neoplasm Tumor or new growth of tissue.

nephrons The small filtering units in the kidney that produce urine; a nephron is composed of a capillary tuft (glomerulus) and a kidney tubule.

nephrosis Noninflammatory kidney degeneration.

nerve A bundle of fibers from nerve cells, coursing together and carrying impulses between the neurons and their target tissues.

nerve fiber The portion of a neuron along which impulses travel.

neural retina The innermost layer of the posterior portion of the eye; it consists of photoreceptor cells, bipolar cells, and ganglion cells, among others.

neurasthenia An emotionally based fatigue in which an individual is unable to perform work.

neuritis A deficiency disease affecting peripheral nerves. It is caused by a lack of thiamin in the diet and characterized by constant burning sensations of the feet.

neurology The study and treatment of the diseases of the nervous system.

neuron A nerve cell, including all the long fibers extending from the cell.

neurosis A mental disorder that prevents the victim from dealing effectively with reality; it is characterized by anxiety and partial impairment of functioning, although the neurotic individual can still carry on in most areas of his life. See also *psychosis*.

neurotoxins Nervous-system poisons.

neurotransmitter A chemical released by one neuron across a synapse, triggering the next neuron into activity.

nicotine The most prevalent drug in tobacco; it affects the nervous system and produces both habituation and tolerance.

nitroglycerine A drug that dilates the arteries and is used to treat attacks of angina pectoris.

nocturnal emissions Ejaculations during sleep.

"no-lose" method A method of resolving parent-child conflict in which a solution acceptable to both the parent and child is reached through discussion.

nondisjunction The genetic phenomenon in which chromosome migration after replication is disturbed, resulting in an excess of chromosomes in one daughter cell and a deficiency in the other.

noradrenalin A hormone that maintains high blood pressure during periods of physical shock; also, the main chemical neurotransmitter utilized in the autonomic sympathetic nervous system. Also called norepinephrine.

norepinephrine See *noradrenalin*.

nucleotides The basic building blocks of a nucleic-acid (DNA or RNA) molecule; they are composed of sugars, inorganic phosphates, and bases.

nucleus The small spherical body within a cell that contains chromosomes and regulates the function of that cell.

nutrients The energy-yielding substances and building materials obtained from foods.

nutrition The science that relates the health and well-being of an organism to the food it consumes.

O

obsessive-compulsive behavior Behavior characterized by the persistent repetition of some thought or act.

obstetrics The medical specialty that deals with care of women during pregnancy, labor, and immediately after childbirth.

occipital lobe The back portion of the cerebral hemisphere, containing the visual sensory areas.

ocular muscles The six muscles attached to the outer surface of the eye that impart movement to it.

operant conditioning The form of conditioning in which the organism's response is instrumental in obtaining reinforcement. See also *classical conditioning*.

ophthalmology The study and treatment of the abnormalities and diseases of the eye.

opiate Any drug of the opium family; also known as opiate alkaloids.

optic nerve The nerve emerging from the back of the eye that transmits visual images to the brain.

optician A licensed technician who grinds and prepares eyeglass and contact lenses.

optometry The study of the optics and the visual problems of the eye and the prescription of corrective lenses.

oral contraceptives Drugs taken orally that prevent conception.

orbit The socket of bone in which the eyeball is encased.

organ A discrete combination of different tissues organized for a common specialized function.

organ of Corti A spiral-shaped organ within the cochlea containing the sensory nerve cells that transform sound vibrations into electrical nerve impulses.

orgasm The climax of sexual sensation.

orgasmic platform The vasocongested outer one-third of the vagina and the labia minora; together they form the anatomical basis for the physiological expression of orgasm.

orthodontics The study and correction of irregular dentition.

orthopedics The study and treatment of deformities and diseases of the bones, muscles, and joints.

ossicles The bones of the middle ear. See also *incus; malleus; stapes*.

osteopathy A branch of health care that attributed the causes of disease to irregularities in the skeletal structure; it is now almost identical to regular medicine.

otitis media A bacterial infection of the middle ear.

otology The study and treatment of the diseases of the ear.

oval window A membrane dividing the inner ear from the middle ear.

ovaries The sexual glands of the female that produce ova and the female hormones estrogen and progesterone.

oviduct See *Fallopian tubes*.

ovulation The process by which the ovum is ejected from the ovary.

ovum (plural ova) The reproductive cell of the female; the egg.

P

pacemaker An area of specialized heart tissue that rhythmically triggers contraction of the heart muscle even in the absence of autonomic neural signals.

pancreas A large abdominal gland that secretes enzymes into the intestine and insulin into the bloodstream.

pandemic The widespread distribution of a disease beyond its natural or characteristic boundaries. See also *epidemic.*

Pap smear See *Papanicolaou test.*

Papanicolaou test A diagnostic test to determine the presence of cancer of the cervix.

paranoia Psychotic behavior characterized by delusions of either grandeur or persecution.

parathormone A hormone secreted by the parathyroids.

parathyroids Four small glands in the neck that control the calcium and phosphate balances of the body.

parietal lobe The upper portion of the cerebral hemisphere between the occipital and frontal lobes.

passive immunity An immunity acquired through means other than the production of antibodies, usually through transfer of antibodies from an actively immune person. See also *active immunity; immunity.*

Pasturella pestis The bacterium that causes plague.

pathogen A disease-producing organism.

pathologist A physician who specializes in the diagnosis of disease through examination of tissue.

pathology The study of the nature and effects of disease.

patriarchy A form of family organization in which the father is the dominant authority.

pediatrics The medical specialty devoted to the study and treatment of children's diseases.

pedigree Genetic family history.

pedodontics The dentistry of children.

pedophilia Sexual attraction to children.

pellagra A disease caused by a lack of B vitamins, especially niacin, and characterized by mouth sores, bodily rash, and diarrhea; it is often associated with alcoholism.

penicillin An antibiotic drug derived from the mold *Penicillium glaucum.*

perception The active reception of stimuli in which the incoming message is interpreted in terms of the source or action that produced it and is expanded upon on the basis of the receiver's expectation. See also *sensation.*

perilymph The fluid contained in the scala vestibuli and the scala tympani of the ear.

periodontal ligament The ligament attaching each tooth to its socket in the jawbone.

periodontics The study and treatment of the diseases of the gums and underlying bones.

periodontium The area immediately around the teeth consisting of the gums, periodontal ligament, and the alveolar jawbone.

peripheral circulation The circulation of blood near the surface of the body.

peristalsis Wavelike muscular contractions forcing the contents of the intestinal tract onward.

peritoneum The abdominal lining enveloping the abdominal viscera.

pernicious anemia A disease caused by a deficiency of cyanocobalamin (vitamin B_{12}) in the diet or by the inability of the body to absorb the vitamin; it is characterized by a decrease in the number of red blood cells, irritability, drowsiness, and depression.

personality disorder Any deeply ingrained maladaptive pattern of behavior. See also *hysterical personality; sociopathic personality.*

petting Physical heterosexual stimulation not involving insertion of the penis into the vagina.

phagocyte A cell produced by the body that is able to engulf and digest invading pathogenic bacteria.

pharmacogenetics The scientific discipline that aims to identify genetic abnormalities that may cause a person to react adversely to certain drugs.

pharmacology The study of the effects and mechanisms of action of drugs on living systems.

pharynx The digestive passage leading from the mouth to the esophagus.

phenotype The observable characteristics of an individual; the outcome of the interaction between genotype instructions and internal and external environments. See also *genotype.*

phenylalanine hydroxylase An enzyme that converts the amino acid phenylalanine, a major component of any diet that becomes damaging in high concentrations, to the amino acid tyrosine.

phenylketonuria (PKU) A genetic disease caused by the absence of the enzyme phenylalanine hydroxylase and characterized by progressive mental retardation.

phenylthiocarbamide (PTC) A chemical that can be tasted by some people and not by others depending on a person's genotype.

phobia An irrational, strong fear.

phocomelia A condition characterized by congenitally stunted arms and legs.

photoreceptor cells The cells of the neural retina that respond to light. See also *cones; rods.*

physical dependence See *addiction.*

physical fatigue Fatigue resulting from physical exertion.

physiology The study of the functions of organs and systems of the body.

pigmented retina The inner layer of the eyeball covering the choroid.

pituitary The endocrine gland located at the base of the brain; it secretes numerous hormones that regulate other endocrine glands. Also known as hypophysis.

pituitary dwarfism A condition of stunted growth resulting from insufficient production of growth stimulating hormone (GSH) by the pituitary gland.

PKU See *phenylketonuria.*

placebo Any medication that has no active ingredient and is given to placate the patient.

placenta The organ that absorbs nutrients from the mother and distributes them to the developing child.

placenta previa A condition in which the placenta of an unborn child is situated over the cervix, making a normal birth impossible.

plaque The lipid deposits on the inside of an artery characteristic of atherosclerosis; also, a hardened composite of debris on the surface of a tooth, which is thought to play a role in tooth decay.

plasma The fluid portion of the blood.

plasma cell A bone-marrow-derived cell, present in lymphoid tissue and specialized in the production of antibodies.

plastic behavior A mode of behavior in which an action is dependent on the mood and history of an individual as well as on the stimulus that provokes the action. See also *stereotyped behavior.*

plastic surgery Surgical procedures used to reconstruct and reshape skin and bones; the repair of absent or defective tissue.

platelets A component of blood resembling colorless disks smaller than red blood cells and aiding in the formation of blood clots.

pneumococci A type of bacteria that can cause pneumonia.

podiatry The study and treatment of the diseases and conditions of the foot.

polygamy Marriage in which a person has more than one spouse at the same time. See also *monogamy.*

polygenic Referring to phenotypic qualities influenced by several genes.

polyunsaturates Fats that contain more than one pair of double-bonded carbon atoms and, therefore, fewer than the maximum number of hydrogen atoms in their chemical structure; usually they are vegetable fats rather than animal fats. See also *saturated fats; unsaturated fats.*

posterior chamber The fluid-filled space between the lens and the iris of the eye.

postsynaptic membrane A portion of nerve-cell membrane that receives messages across a synapse.

prepuce A flap of skin hooding the clitoris and penis.

presbycusis Progressive loss of hearing with age, characterized by the inability to hear high-pitched sounds.

presbyopia A visual abnormality characterized by the inability to clearly see near objects and generally associated with aging.

proctology The study and treatment of the diseases of the rectum and anus.

progesterone A hormone secreted by the ovaries that has an important role in embryonic development. See also *estrogen.*

progestin A synthetic hormone with properties similar to progesterone.

projection A form of defense mechanism in which one sees one's own traits and motives in others.

proof A measure of alcoholic content; the proof of a beverage is equal to twice the percentage of alcohol in that beverage.

prophylaxis Treatment for the prevention of a disease (adj. *prophylactic*).

prostaglandin A substance occurring naturally in most body tissues that also can be synthesized cheaply; it may have numerous medicinal properties including the ability to induce menstrual flow after intravaginal application.

prostate In males, a gland that surrounds the urethra where it joins the bladder and that secretes a fluid that forms a part of the semen.

prosthodontics The science of providing artificial replacements for missing teeth.

prostitute Any person who engages in sexual activity for pay.

proteins A category of vital organic chemicals that includes enzymes, hormones, and antibodies and constitutes one of the critical food substances.

protozoa Unicellular animals.

psychasthenia An emotionally based fatigue in which a person loses the ability to concentrate and is intellectually dull.

psyche The personal model of the world, including the self; the sum of all emotive and cognitive activities.

psychedelics Complex drugs that can produce excitement, agitation, hallucinations, depression, or other psychosislike changes in mood,

thinking, and behavior. Also called psychotogenics and psychotomimetics.

psychiatrist A medical doctor specializing in the study and treatment of mental and emotional disorders.

psychoactive Referring to any drug that produces a temporary change in a person's neurophysiological functions, affecting his mood, thoughts, feelings, or behavior; also called psychotropic.

psychoenergizers See *stimulants.*

psychogenic Referring to a functional disorder originating from the brain.

psychological dependence See *habituation.*

psychologist A specialist in the field of psychology, usually holding a master's degree or Ph.D. in psychology.

psychopharmacology The study of the effects and mechanisms of action of psychoactive drugs.

psychophysiological disorders The development of physical symptoms as a result of emotional imbalance; also known as psychosomatic disorders.

psychosis Severe mental disorder that prevents the individual from functioning in everyday life. See also *neurosis.*

psychosomatic See *psychophysiological disorders.*

psychotherapy The treatment of mental and emotional disorders by the application of psychological methods.

psychotic Referring to or associated with mental illness or psychosis.

psychotogenics See *psychedelics.*

psychotropic See *psychoactive.*

PTC See *phenylthiocarbamide.*

pubococcygeus muscles The muscles that surround the outer portion of the vagina.

pulmonary artery The artery extending from the right ventricle of the heart carrying venous blood to the lungs for aeration.

pulmonary stenosis A congenital heart defect characterized by obstruction or narrowing of the valve between the right ventricle and the pulmonary artery.

pulp The tissue within the tooth.

pulp canal See *root canal.*

pupil The aperture of the eye encircled by the iris.

pus The yellowish fluid that collects at a site of infection or inflammation.

Q

quackery The practice of health care by a medical charlatan.

quickening The mother's first sensations of the movements of her unborn child.

quinine A drug derived from the bark of the cinchona tree used to treat malaria.

R

radiology The branch of medicine that deals with x-rays and other radioactive substances in the diagnosis and treatment of disease; also called roentgenology.

rationalization A defense mechanism by which one justifies one's impulsive or irrational behavior by presenting false but acceptable reasons to oneself or to others.

rauwolfia The snake-root plant from which the drug reserpine is extracted.

reaction formation A defense mechanism involving the replacement in consciousness of an anxiety-producing impulse by its opposite.

reality therapy Psychological therapy aimed at confronting the patient with the reality of his situation and forcing him to accept the responsibilities for that situation.

receptor sites Special molecular groupings on cell membranes to which specific chemicals (for instance, neurotransmitters or drugs) or microorganisms can attach themselves prior to acting on the cell.

recessive gene A gene that will be phenotypically expressed only when it is homozygous. See also *codominant; dominant gene.*

rectum The last portion of the digestive tract, where feces are stored prior to voiding.

red blood cells The blood cells that transport oxygen and carbon dioxide between the lungs and the body tissues.

reflex arc The arrangement of sensory input pathway, control center, and motor output pathway that produces such reflex actions as the immediate removal of a hand from a hot surface before the brain can consider the action.

refractive Referring to the ability of the eye to focus light rays on the retina.

refractory Resistant to ordinary methods of treatment.

reinforcement The procedure of immediately following a response with a reward or punishment. See also *operant conditioning.*

Reissner membrane One of the two membranes that divides the cochlea into three chambers; also known as vestibular membrane. See also *basilar membrane.*

renal Referring to the kidneys.

replication The process by which DNA molecules and chromosomes reproduce themselves prior to cell division.

repression In psychoanalytic theory, the defense mechanism of unconsciously ejecting unpleasant memories or impulses from conscious awareness into the subconscious.

reserpine A tranquilizing drug often used to lower high blood pressure in hypertensive persons.

resistance The ability of the body to contact pathogenic organisms without being infected.

retina See *neural retina; pigmented retina.*

Rh factor An inherited component of blood-cell membranes present in some people but absent in others.

rhinology The study and treatment of the disease of the nose and nasal cavity.

rhodopsin The chemical substance found in the rod cells of the eye that is sensitive to low-intensity light; also called visual purple.

rhythm method A method of birth control based on determination of the time of ovulation and abstinence from coitus during this fertile period.

ribonucleic acid (RNA) Complex molecules that relay the genetic instructions of DNA to the protein-building machinery of the cell.

rickets A disease caused by the deficiency of vitamin D and characterized by softening of the bones, leading to bone deformities.

rickettsiae Bacterialike organisms responsible for typhus fever and other diseases.

RNA See *ribonucleic acid.*

rods The light-receptor cells of the retina that react to low-intensity light. See also *cones; rhodopsin.*

roentgenology See *radiology.*

root The portion of a tooth inside the bone beneath the gums.

root canal The cavity within a tooth that contains the pulp.

Rubin's test A female sterility test involving the injection of carbon dioxide gas into the Fallopian tubes to determine whether they are blocked.

S

saddle See *spinal block.*

sado-masochism Sexual pleasure obtained through giving or receiving pain or humiliation.

safety Cognizance of the possibility of accidents and action to reduce their probability and to minimize their consequences.

salpingitis Inflammation of the Fallopian tubes.

salting out A method of inducing abortion by injecting a salt solution into the uterus through the abdominal wall.

sarcoma Cancer arising in supportive tissue such as bones, cartilage, fat, or muscle.

saturated fats Fats that contain a maximum of hydrogen atoms in their chemical structure; they are usually animal fats. See also *polyunsaturates; unsaturated fats.*

schizophrenia A form of psychosis in which the patient becomes withdrawn and apathetic; hallucinations and delusions are common.

sclera The white outer layer of the eye.

scrotum The external pouch of skin that contains the testicles.

scurvy A disease caused by the deficiency of ascorbic acid (vitamin C) in the diet and characterized by anemia, swollen bleeding gums, and pain in the extremities.

sebaceous glands Skin glands that secrete a fatty substance called sebum.

sebum A fatty substance that emulsifies and retains water in the skin, thus preventing it from cracking and hardening.

secretin A digestive-tract hormone secreted by the cells of the small intestine that causes the pancreas to secrete digestive fluids into the small intestine.

sedative Any drug that produces relaxation.

sedative-hypnotics Drugs that promote relaxation in small doses and sleep in large doses by depressing the activity of the central nervous system. See also *barbiturates; depressants.*

self-actualization The process of developing one's own true nature and fulfilling one's potentialities.

self-esteem The amount and quality of the regard that a person has toward himself.

semen The fluid produced by the prostate and other glands of the male in which sperm cells are transported.

semicircular canals Three structures within the vestibular apparatus of the inner ear containing nerve fibers that transmit to the brain information regarding the orientation of the head in relation to the pull of gravity. See also *vestibular apparatus.*

seminal fluid See *semen.*

seminal vesicle A small gland located near each vas deferens that serves as a storage place for mature sperm and produces much of the fluid in which the sperm are suspended.

sensation The passive reception of stimuli through any receptor organ. See also *perception.*

sensitivity training The process of learning to be increasingly sensitive to a stimulus, often the emotions or feelings of other people.

sensorineural loss The loss of hearing due to interference with the reception of sound waves within the cochlea. See also *conduction loss.*

sensory Referring to the branch of the nervous system that gathers information and carries it to the central nervous system.

septum The muscular wall that separates the two halves of the heart. Septa also are present in the brain, nose, and elsewhere.

serotonin A brain amine thought to be important in emotional, perceptual, and cognitive functions.

serous Resembling blood serum.

serum The fluid that can be collected from blood after it has clotted.

sex chromosomes The chromosomes that determine the sex of an organism. See also *autosome.*

sex-flush A rash spreading from the chest over the lower abdomen and shoulders that occurs during sexual excitement.

sickle cell anemia A genetic disorder characterized by severe anemia and caused by defective hemoglobin in the red blood cells.

single-cell protein Protein produced by bacteria and rich in essential amino acids.

Skinner box A device developed by B. F. Skinner, a psychologist, to measure the reward value of a given signal. See also *operant conditioning.*

sociopathic personality A personality trait characterized by repeated conflict with society; in the extreme form the desire for self-gratification takes preference over all other values.

somatic mutation A genetic mutation of any cell other than a germ cell.

specificity The property of an antibody that enables it to recognize and combat only one type of foreign substance or organism.

sperm The reproductive cells (gametes) of the male.

spermatic cord The tube or canal that transports sperm from the testicles to the seminal vesicles.

spermatogenesis The process of sperm formation.

spermatogonia Cells that will develop into sperm.

spermatozoa See *sperm.*

sphincter A circular or ringlike muscle that regulates the opening and closing of a bodily opening or internal passageway.

sphingolipidoses Genetic diseases characterized by the accumulation of sphingolipids (fatty substances) in various parts of the body, including the brain.

spina bifida A congenital malformation of the spine characterized by a rupture of the spinal canal.

spinal block A common type of anesthesia administered during childbirth in which only the lower half of the body is anesthetized, leaving the woman conscious.

spinal column See *vertebral column.*

spinal cord   The lower portion of the central nervous system, located inside the vertebral canal.

spirochete   A corkscrewlike or spiral bacterium.

spleen   An abdominal organ that destroys old red blood cells and manufactures lymphoid cells.

sputum   Mucous fluid of the mouth.

squamous   Pertaining to a scaly surface.

stamina   The ability to mobilize energy to maintain movement over an extended period of time.

stapes   A small bone of the middle ear that transmits vibrations from the tympanic membrane to the inner ear. See also *incus; malleus.*

staphylococci   A type of bacteria responsible for several infectious diseases.

starch   A chainlike assembly of many carbohydrate molecules.

stereotyped behavior   Behavior in which a given stimulus always brings about a specific response. See also *plastic behavior.*

sternum (breastbone)   The midline bone of the chest.

stimulants   Drugs that elevate mood, increase alertness, and delay fatigue. See also *amphetamines; caffeine; nicotine.*

stratum corneum   The top layer of the epidermis composed of flattened dead cells; also called horny layer.

stratum germinativum   The deepest layer of the epidermis, it provides replacement cells for those lost from the stratum corneum; also called basal layer.

strength   The basic muscular force required for movement.

streptococci   A type of bacteria responsible for several infectious diseases.

stress   Some strain or bodily insult that disturbs a person's normal physical, mental, or emotional equilibrium.

stroke   A sudden brain injury usually caused by an embolus or rupture of a blood vessel.

succedaneous   Pertaining to a substitute or replacement, as in the case of the permanent teeth.

sucrose   The form of sugar that occurs in sugar cane and sugar beets and is commonly known as table sugar.

sulfa drugs   A family of antibacterial drugs.

sulfur dioxide   A noxious gas produced by the combustion of fossil fuels.

suppleness   The quality of muscles and joints that permits a full range of movement.

sweat glands   See *apocrine glands; eccrine glands.*

sympathetic system   A branch of the autonomic nervous system that carries signals to such internal organs as the heart, liver, smooth muscles, and lungs.

symptom   A well-defined sign of a disease. See also *syndrome.*

symptomatic treatment   Treatment designed to alleviate the overt manifestations of a person's illness without recognizing or dealing with the causes of that illness.

synapse   The point of close association between adjacent neurons where impulses leap from one nerve cell to the next, by use of neurotransmitters.

synaptic cleft   The space between neurons across which neural messages are transmitted.

synaptic vesicles   Small sacs that contain chemical neurotransmitters and are located within the neuron ending facing a synapse.

syndrome   A pattern of pathological symptoms occurring together but not yet assignable to a specific disease.

synesthesia   The blending of two sensory modalities or the transference of one sensation into another mode, such as "seeing" sounds.

systolic pressure   The maximum pressure of the blood under the force of the contracting heart. See also *diastolic pressure.*

T

Tay-Sachs disease   A genetic disease caused by the inability to metabolize certain fats and characterized by mental degradation, blindness, and death before the age of seven years.

tear gland   See *lacrimal gland.*

temporal lobe   The lower portion of each cerebral hemisphere in front of the occipital lobe.

tendon   The strong fibrous tissue connecting muscles to bones.

testes   The male sex glands. They produce sperm and the hormone testosterone, which is responsible for the development of male secondary sexual characteristics.

tetany   A condition of muscular spasms resulting from insufficient calcium in the blood.

tetraethyl lead   A lead compound contained in gasoline that forms an air pollutant on combustion.

tetralogy of Fallot   A congenital heart defect involving the pulmonary artery, the aorta, the septum, and the right ventricle.

T-group   An intensive group that emphasizes human-relations skills.

thalidomide   A sedative-hypnotic drug that can cause deformities to develop in the fetuses of pregnant women taking the drug.

thermograph   Any instrument that records changes in temperature.

thoracic cavity   The space above the diaphragm that is enclosed by the rib cage.

threonine   One of the essential eight of twenty amino acids used in the human body.

thrombus   A blood clot that forms inside the heart or blood vessels.

thymus   A thoracic gland largely made of lymphoid tissue that atrophies and becomes vestigial by the age of two.

thyroid gland   An endocrine gland in the neck. See also *thyroxin.*

thyroid stimulating hormone (TSH)   A hormone secreted by the anterior pituitary.

thyroxin   The hormone produced by the thyroid gland that regulates or influences body metabolism and growth.

tissue culture   The growth of cells in a laboratory environment outside the organism from which they were taken.

tolerance   The bodily adaptation to a particular drug that necessitates an increased dosage of that drug in order to produce the same effect.

tonometer   A small instrument used to measure the pressure within the antechamber of the eye.

toxin   A poison produced by pathogenic bacteria.

toxoid   A modified toxin used as a vaccine to induce antibody production.

trachea   The windpipe.

tranquilizer   A drug used to reduce anxiety and to induce relaxation. See also *reserpine.*

transcription   The process by which RNA molecules are made from DNA templates.

translation   The process by which amino-acid chains are made from RNA templates.

Treponema pallidum   The spirochete that causes syphilis.

triglycerides   Fatty organic chemicals composed of glycerol and fatty acids.

trisomic   Referring to the genetic abnormality in which three homologous chromosomes exist instead of the usual pair.

trophic levels   Nutritional levels based on their distance from the original source of energy, ranging from green plants (first level) to herbivores (second level) to carnivores (third level), and so on.

TSH   See *thyroid stimulating hormone.*

tubal ligation   Sterilization achieved by surgically interrupting the Fallopian tubes.

tubules   Small tubes within the kidney that surround capillary tufts, receive the filtrate from the blood, and carry that filtrate to the ureter.

tumescence Swelling, such as of the penis or clitoris.

tumor Abnormal mass of new tissue growing independent of its surrounding tissue structures.

Turner's syndrome A genetic abnormality in which a female genotype has only one X chromosome; it is characterized by the absence or vestigial presence of ovaries.

tympanic membrane (eardrum) A thin tissue membrane dividing the middle ear from the auditory canal.

tyrosine One of the twenty amino acids used in the human body.

U

umbilical cord The cord that attaches the embryo or fetus to the placenta.

unsaturated fats Fats that contain double-bonded carbon atoms and less than a full complement of hydrogen atoms in their chemical structure; usually they are vegetable fats rather than animal fats. See also *polyunsaturates; saturated fats.*

urea A white crystalline substance that is excreted by the body in the urine.

uremia A symptom caused by the inability of the kidneys to remove uric acid, urea, and other waste products from the blood.

ureter The tube that conveys urine from each kidney to the bladder.

urethra The duct that conveys urine from the bladder and semen from the vas deferens and accessory sex glands to the outside of the body.

urinalysis Examination of the urine to determine the presence of abnormal substances.

urine The liquid produced by the kidneys.

urology The study and treatment of diseases and abnormalities of the urogenital tract in men and the urinary tract in women.

uterus (the womb) A hollow muscular organ whose function is to hold and nourish the fetus.

utricle A small sac in the inner ear connecting the three semicircular canals.

V

vaccination The introduction into the body of a toxoid substance or live infectious agent to induce antibody production.

vagina The canal leading from the vulva to the cervix.

vagus nerve A nerve that regulates heartbeat and other visceral activities.

valine One of the essential eight of twenty amino acids used by the human body.

values The ideals of right or wrong, good or bad, that one holds.

vas deferens The duct leading from the epididymis to the urethra that carries sperm during ejaculation.

vascular Pertaining to blood vessels.

vasectomy A method of birth control for males in which the vas deferens is tied and severed, preventing sperm from leaving the testes.

vasocongestion The accumulation of blood in certain blood vessels.

vasodilation Dilation of the blood vessels resulting in increased blood flow.

vector Epidemiologically, an organism, food, or water supply from which man contracts an infectious disease.

veins Vessels carrying blood toward the heart.

venereal disease (VD) Any disease primarily transmitted through sexual intercourse and primarily affecting the genital organs or region.

ventricles The most muscular of the pumping chambers of the heart. See also *atria.*

venules The smallest vessels on the venous sides of capillary networks.

vertebrae The bones of the spine.

vertebral column The backbone or spine, made up of a stack of short bones, the hollow center of which forms the vertebral canal.

vestibular apparatus The structure of the inner ear that contains the semicircular canals and carries out the function of balance.

vestibular membrane See *Reissner membrane.*

villi Any small fingerlike projection of tissue, such as those in the lining of the small intestine.

virus A small disease agent or parasitic particle that is composed of a DNA core with a protein covering.

viscera A general term referring to the internal organs of the chest and abdomen.

visual purple See *rhodopsin.*

vitamins A group of organic chemicals essential in small amounts for normal metabolism.

vitreous humor The transparent fluid contained in the vitreous body of the eye.

voluntary nervous system The subsystem of the motor branch of the nervous system that can be consciously directed in its activity. See also *autonomic nervous system.*

vulva The external female genitalia.

W

wart A virus-induced skin lesion resulting in local overgrowth of cells; it has the potential to become cancerous.

Wassermann test A blood test used to confirm the presence of syphilis.

wet dreams See *nocturnal emissions.*

white blood cells Blood cells that destroy foreign substances or organisms. See also *granulocyte; lymphocyte; monocyte.*

withdrawal Psychologically, a form of defense mechanism in which a person retreats from reality in a stressful situation. In drug terminology, a temporary physical illness precipitated by the lack of a drug in the body of a person physically dependent on that drug.

X

x-rays Radiation that goes through the soft tissues of the body but not dense materials such as bone or abnormally packed masses of cells; it is used to examine the occurrence of abnormalities and for treatment of some types of cancer.

Z

zonula The circular ligament attached to the ciliary muscles and holding the eye lens in place.

zygote The fertilized egg cell.

A

abortion, 246, 260–262, *261*, 571
abscess, 431, 479
accidents, 507–525
  causes, 513–518
  home, 515
  motor-vehicle, 516
  occupational, 516
  prevention, 525
acetylcholine, 58, 70, 154, 173
acne, 398, 427
acromegaly, 481
action potential, 54, *54*, 61
acupuncture, *572*
addiction, drug, 124, *125*, 139–142
  alcohol, 165–169
  treatment, 195–199, *196–197*
Addison's disease, 483
adenine, 267
adenocarcinoma, 448
adenosinetriphosphate (ATP), 359
adrenal glands, 38, 368, 481–483
  see also adrenalin; noradrenalin
adrenalin, 38, 67, 71, 87, 279, 418, 474
aerobics, 359–360
affective appraisal, 78
affective psychosis, 106
Agnews State Hospital, 108
air pollution, 416, *490–491*, 498–500,
  499
Al-Anon, 169
Alateens, 169
alcohol, 153–169
  absorption of, 155–158
  blood levels of, 155–158
  historical perspective, 120
  laws governing, 162, 183
  physiological effects, 154–159
  psychological effects, 159–165
  sources and types of, 153
  youth and, 162
alcohol abuse, 153–169
  alcoholism, 123, 127, 165–169
  causes of, 165–168
  deaths due to, 157, 159, 165
  incidence, 162, 167–168
  tolerance, 161
  treatment, *168*, 169
  withdrawal illness, 126, 139, 154, 161
Alcoholics Anonymous, 169, 195
alcoholism. *See* alcohol abuse
alleles, 271

allergy, 367, 474
alveolar jawbone, 387
alveoli, 27, *28*, 477
  see also respiratory system
American Cancer Society, 454, 536
American College of Surgeons, 456
American Heart Association, 536
American Medical Association (AMA),
  124, 206, 410, 537, 550, 555
American Nurses Association, 537
American Pharmaceutical Society, 192
American Psychiatric Association, 103
American Public Health Association, 537
amino acids, 35, 37, 267–270, 279, 333
amniocentesis, 287, *287*
amnion, 241
amphetamines, 71, 143–145, 186, 189
amygdalae, *68*, 69
Amytal, 138
anaplastic cancer, 448
anatomy, human, 15–49, *passim*
  historical concepts, *6, 7, 9*
anemia, 244
  hemolytic, 475
  sickle cell, 278–279
angina pectoris, 466
Anichvok, N., 340
Antabuse, 169
antagonism (muscle), *20*, 21
antibiotics, 409–410, 419, 436, 440, 442,
  468, 543–544
  see also specific drugs
antibodies, 431–432, 473–475
antidepressants, 71, 110, 151, 521–522
antidiuretic hormone, 481
antihistamines, 474, 514
antisocial personalities, 109
anxiety, 101, 103
  drug-induced, 143
  neurosis, 365
apocrine glands, 399
appendicitis, 479
aqueous humor, 373
Ardrey, R., 79
Arnold, M., 76
arsenic, 500
arteries, *17*, 26–27, *460*
  see also circulatory system
arterioles, 26, 32, 38, 358
arthritis, rheumatoid, 475, *476*
artificial hearts, 470
artificial kidneys, 478–479
artificial resuscitation, 27

asbestos, 500
aspirin, 543
asthma, 368, 474, 500
astigmatism, 376
atherosclerosis, 340–342, 460, *460, 461*
ATP (adenosinetriphosphate), 359
atria, 26–27, 467
  see also heart
atrophy, 356
auditory nerve, 381
autograft, 401
autoimmune disease, 475
  and cancer, *452*, 453
autonomic control, 55–56
autonomic nervous system, 41
autosomes, 271
aversive conditioning, 111
axons, 38, 53
  see also neurons

B

Bachofen, J. J., 291
bacteria, 45, 415, *424*, 425–426, 427
  see also specific bacteria-caused diseases
Bandura, A., 86
barbiturates, 138–139, 156, 186
  deaths involving alcohol, 159
  poisoning, 139
  and suicide, 139, 186
Barr chromatin, 289
Bartholin, glands of, 45, 222
Beach, F., 297
Beck, J., 315
behavior
  abnormal, 93–115
  alcohol effects on, 159–165
  chemical basis of, 66–73
  drugs and, 71–73, 117–151
  emotional basis of, 75–91
  instinctive, 79–80
  nervous system and, 53–73
  plastic, *58, 59*, 67
  sexual, 213–231
  stereotyped, *58, 59, 68*
behaviorism, 84–88, 102
Benzedrine, 143, 186
benzopyrene, 173
beryllium, 500
bile, 32
biodegradation, 488
biological clocks, 367–368, 494
biomagnification, 492, *495*, 502

biopsy, 454
bipolar cells, 373
Birnback, B. S., 514
birth control, 252–263
  see also specific methods
birth defects, 285–287
birth process, 246–249, *246–247*
Blachly, P. H., 521
bladder, 35, 176
blind spot, *377*
blood
  alcohol level, 155–158
  cells, 24–26, *24*, 32, 272, *431*
  groups, 272–273
  rate of flow, 38
  see also circulatory system; hemoglobin
blood pressure, 462
Bloom, B. S., 314
Blue Cross–Blue Shield, 562
Blum, R. H., 542
Board Certified Specialists, 541
body, human, 15–49, *passim*
  autonomic control of, 55–56
  see also specific systems and tissues
body defenses, 429–431, *430*
Boisen, A., 107
bone marrow, 24, *431*
bones, 20–21
bootlegging, 189
botulism, 485, 502
brain, *40*, *42*, 61–73, *62, 63, 64, 65, 68*
  disorders, 94, 105, 484–485
  injury, 64, 94, 105
  see also central nervous system;
    nervous system
Branden, N., 91
Brave New World (Huxley), 117
breast, self-check for cancer, *455*
breathing
  controlled, 365
  mechanism of, 27–29, *29*
Brener, J., 56
bronchi, 27, 172, 175, 475–477, 500
  see also respiratory system
bronchitis, 172, 175, 475–477, 500
bubonic plague, 405
bulbourethral gland, 43, 234
Bunney, W., 368

C

Cade, J. F. J., 521
cadmium, 500

Caesarean section, 248
caffeine, 121, 142
California Rehabilitation Center (CRC),
  198
calories, 232
  expenditure of, 340
cancer, 445–457, *447*
  and biological clocks, 368
  causes, 450–453
  detection of, 454
  distribution of, 448, *449*
  immune theory of, *452*, 453
  prevention of, 453
  and smoking, 174–176, 450, 453
  treatment, 456
  types, 448
  virus theory of, 451, *451*
  see also carcinogens
cannabis, 120, 148–150, 190–191
capillaries, 23, *24*, 26, 32, 35, 38
  see also circulatory system
carbohydrates, 332
carbon monoxide, 175, 499
carcinogens, 173, 344, 349, 417, 450
carcinoma, 448
cardiac arrest, 466
cardiovascular disease, 340, 459–471
  see also specific diseases
CARE, 532
cataracts, 376
catecholamines. *See* adrenalin;
  noradrenalin
cells, 45–49, *46–47*
  bipolar, 373
  blood, 24–26, *24*, 32, 272, *431*
  division of, 47, 273–275
  ganglion, 373
  hair, 381, 398
  neurons, 38, *39, 52–53*, 54–73, *55*,
    381
  phagocytes, 429–432
  photoreceptor, 54, 373
  pigment, 400
  reproductive, 48, 233–234, 273–275
  uncontrolled growth in, 446
cementum, 387
central nervous system, 39, 58–73
  alcohol effects on, 154, 165
  disorders of, 484–485
  drug effects on, 138–151
  see also brain; nervous system
cerebral hemorrhage, 470, *470*
cervix, *44*, 222, 234–235, 253

chemotherapy, 419–421
  antibiotics, 419, 436, 440, 442, 468
  for cancer, 456
  sulfa drugs, 419
childbirth, 246–249
  rates, *310*
child-rearing. *See* parenthood
chiropractors, 545
chloral hydrate, 138–139
chlorine, 500
chlorpromazine, 108
cholesterol, 333, 462
cholera, 406, 416, 433
choroid, 373
Christian Science practitioners, 545
chromosomes, 45, 271–276, *271*
  abnormalities, 283–285, *283, 284, 287*
ciliary muscles, 373
circadian rhythms, 368
circulatory system, *17*, 23–27, *25*,
  459–461
  disorders of, 459–471
  voluntary control of, 55–56
  see also arteries; blood; heart; veins
circumcision, 229
cirrhosis of the liver, 155, *156*, 480
classical conditioning, 85
climacteric. *See* menopause
clitoris, 222–227
cocaine, 122, 145
cochlea, 380
codeine, 139
codon, 267
cognitive-developmental theory, 86
coitus, 43, 45, 217, 221–229, *226*,
  253–254
coitus interruptus, 255
colic, 479
colitis, 479, 505
color-blindness, 283, 377
Comer, J., 321–322
common cold, 434–435
communes, 300–304
communicable disease, 427
competence theory, 82
conditioning, 85, *85*, 111
condoms, 252, *257*
conflicts, emotional, 78, 95–103
congeners, 159
congenital defects, 285–287
conjunctiva, 373
consumer protection, 518–525
Consumers' Research, Inc., 523

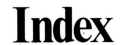

(Italic numbers refer to illustrations)

Consumers Union of U.S., Inc., 523
contact lenses, 377
contraception, 252–263, *256–257*
  see also specific methods
Coons, J., 344
Cooper, K. H., 359–360
cornea, 373
coronary thrombosis, 464, *465*
corpus luteum, 237
cost of health care, 10, 555–558
cough mechanism, *478*
Council on Environmental Quality, 501, 505
Cousins, N., 543
Crick, F., 267
cunnilingus, 216
Cushing's syndrome, 481
Cyclazocine, 199
cycles, biological, 367–368
cytoplasm, 47
cytosine, 267

D

Dabrowski, K., 107
Dann, J., 321
Davis, R. C., 57
day-care centers, 304–305, 322
Daytop, 195
DDT, 342, 487, 492
deciduous teeth, 386
defense mechanisms, 101
delirium tremens, 126, 154
Denfield, D., 299
dental caries, 389–390
dentin, 387
dentistry, 393–394, 546–547
deoxyribonucleic acid. *See* DNA
depressant drugs, 138–142
  see also specific drugs
depression, 104
dermatitis, 400
dermis, 397–400
Despert, J. L., 311
DET. *See* psychedelic drugs
Dexedrine, 143, 186
diabetes, 481, 483–484, *483*
diaphragm (contraceptive), 255, *256*
diaphragm (physiological), *17*, 29, *29*
diastolic pressure, 468
diet. *See* nutrition
dieting, 339–340
digestive system, *18*, 29–33, *30–31*
  diseases of, 479–481
diphtheria, 433
Directory of Medical Specialists, 541
disease, 405–505
  causes of, 413–419
  epidemiology, 406
  infectious, 415, 416, 423–443
  systemic, 472–485
  see also specific diseases
Ditran, 145, 148
divorce, 292, 295–296, *295*, 305
DMT. *See* psychedelic drugs
DNA, 266–270, *268–269*, 270, 413
  replication, 267, *268*
  transcription, *269*, *270*

Dodson, F., 316
Dole, V., 198–199
DOM. *See* psychedelic drugs
Doriden, 138
douching, 240, 254
Downing, J., 302
Down's syndrome, 284, *287*, 289
drug legislation
  Boggs Act (1951), 192
  Comprehensive Drug Abuse
    Prevention and Control Act (1970),
    193–194
  Drug Abuse Control Amendment
    (1965), 193
  Food and Drug Act of 1906, 192
  Harrison Narcotics Act (1914), 192
  Marijuana Act of 1937, 193
  Narcotic Drug Control Act of 1956,
    193
  Prohibition (1919–1933), 162, 183
drugs
  abuse, 122–131, 133–151, 183–201
  antipsychotic, 108, 110
  and biological clocks, 368
  chemotherapy, 419–421, 456
  generic, 409–410
  and neurotransmitters, 71
  perspective of, 203–209
  prescription, 409–410
  side effects, 110–145, 421
  traffic, 189–191, *190*
  see also specific drugs
Dubos, R., 493
Duchesne, E., 420
Duncan, W. R., 360
dwarfism, 481
Dwight, T., 295
dysmenorrhea, 239

E

ears, 378–383, *379*
  hearing aids, 383
  hearing losses, 381–383, *381*
  hearing tests, 383
  structure and function, 378–381
  vestibular apparatus, 380–381, *380*
ecological succession, 498
ecology, 489–498
ecosystems, 489, *496–497*
ectopic pregnancy, *248*
Edwards, C., 410
Ehrlich, P., 419
ejaculation, 228
electrocardiograph (ECG), 464, *465*
electroencephalograph (EEG), 366
electroshock therapy, 110
Ellis, A., 302
embolism, 470
embryo, 241, *242*, 267
  see also fetus; prenatal development
emotional disorders, 93–115
emotions, 75–91
emphysema, 175, 477, *477*
encephalitis, 484
endemic disease, 407
endocrine system, *18*, *36*, 37–38

disorders of, 481–484
  see also specific glands; hormones
endolymph, 380
endometrium, 235, 241
Engel, B., 58
enteritis, 479
environment
  and accidents, 517
  pollution, 382, 416–417, 487–505
  and psychological development,
    84–88
Environmental Protection Agency, 534
enzymes, 31–32, 479–481
epidemics, 407
epidemiology, 406–411, *408*
epidermis, 397
epididymis, 43, *44*, 234
epilepsy, 56, 63–64, 69, 105, 367, 410,
    485
epinephrine. *See* adrenalin
episiotomy, 249
Epstein-Barr virus, 437
Equanil, 138
Erikson, E., 82, *83*, 91
erogenous zones, 80
erythromycin, 421
esophagus, 31, 175–176
estrogen, 237
ethological theory, 79
eustachian tube, 378, 435
excretory system, *34*, 35–37
  disorders of, 477–479
  see also kidneys
exercise, 354–362
  aerobics, 359–360
  and heart disease, 359
  program for, 363
existential psychology, 102, 112
eyes, 371–378, *372*, *374*
  color-blindness, 283, 377
  contact lenses, 377
  function, 371–374
  muscles of, *22*, *23*
  nerve cells of, 62–64
  problems of, 376–379
  visual abstraction, 61
  visual fields, *65*
Eysenck, Hans, 112

F

Fabry's disease, 280
Fallopian tubes, 44, *44*, 234, 236, *237*,
    240, *241*, *248*, *250*
Fallot, tetralogy of, 467, *467*
family physician, 9, 530, 554
family therapy, 112
farsightedness, 375, *376*
fat cells, *339*
fatigue, 360, 362–366
fats, 333
FDA. See U.S. Food and Drug
    Administration
Federal Bureau of Narcotics and
    Dangerous Drugs, 199
Federal Communications Commission
    (FCC), 519
Federal Hazardous Substances Act, 520

Federal Trade Commission (FTC), 180, 519, 525
fellatio, 217
Fensterwald, B., 522
fertilizers, 343–344, 501
fetishism, 220
fetus, *240*, 241, *242*
  environmental factors affecting, 285–287, 344
Fetz, E., 56
fever, 430
fibrillation, 465
fight-flight response, 38, 66–68, *67*, 355–356
fish-protein concentrates, 334
fitness. *See* physical fitness
Fleming, A., 420
Fletcher, C. M., 181
Florey, H., 420
fluoridation of water, 395
food pollution, 416–422, 501–502
food web, 417, 489, *495*, 502
Ford, C., 297
Forster, F. M., 56
Fort, J., 117, 126
fossil fuels, 499
free clinics, 568
Freud, A., 82
Freud, S., 74, 81, *82*, 91, 425, *435*
  see also psychoanalytic theory
fructose, 333
fungi, 415, *424*, 427
Funk, C., 336
Furlong, W. B., 367

G

Gagnon, J., 300
gall bladder, 32
gamma globulin, 432
ganglion cells, 373
gastritis, 479–480
Gaucher's disease, 280
general practitioner, 9, 530, 554
genes, 266–280
genetic code, 267–271
genetic counseling, 287–289
genetics, 265–289, *273, 276, 288*
  see also heredity
genotype, 266
German measles. *See* rubella
Gestalt therapy, 112
Gibbon, E., 405
gigantism, 481
gingivae, 387
glaucoma, 373, 376
glomeruli, *34, 35*
  see also kidneys
glomerulonephritis, 478
glucose, 333
glycogen, 333, 483
Goldstein, M., 108
gonadotropins, 43
gonads, 43
  see also reproductive system
gonorrhea, 286, 416, *437, 438*, 440–443
Gordon, M., 299

government. *See* drug legislation; specific agencies
Graafian follicle, 236–237
granulocytes, 26, 32
Green Revolution, 345–349
Group Practice Prepayment Plan (GPPP), 561
group therapy, 112
growth-stimulating hormone (GSH), 481
guanine, 267
Guthrie, R., 280
Guttmacher, A., 262

H

habituation, drug, 124, *125*
Hahnemann, S., 543
hair, 398, *399*
Halberg, F., 368
hallucinogens. *See* psychedelic drugs
Hamburg, D., 494
Harlow, Harry, 80
Harrad Experiment, The (Rimmer), 301
Harvard University, 56
Haryou-Act Family Day Care, 322
hashish. *See* cannabis
Hauser, G., 343
hay fever, 474
Headstart, 322
health, *passim*
  basic concepts of, 571–573
  defined, 3, 11
  emotional, 91, 93–115
  exercise and, 354–362
  implementation, 6, 8, 572
  individual approach to, 11–13, 571–577
  means to, 6–9
  obstacles to, 9–11
health care, 529–551, 553–569
  community role, 566–569
  costs, 10, 555–558
  historical view, 529–531
  insurance, 555–556
  mental, 109–115
  organizations, 531–538
  practitioners, 9, 115, 538–547, 554–555, 574
  reforms, 558–566
health foods, 343–344
health organizations, 531–538
Health Rights Program, 567
health science, 3–9
hearing losses, 381–383, 502
heart, 458–459
  anatomy of, 26, *26, 28*
  artificial, 470–471
  diet effects, 462
  disease of, 459–471
  exercise effects, 357, 464
  muscles of, 23, *23, 27*
  transplants, 367, 470
  see also circulatory system
Heinlein, R., 301
hemoglobin, 24, 278, 333
hemolytic anemia, 475
hemophilia, 282, 287
hemorrhoids, 245

Henderson, L. J., 530
hepatitis, 142, 480
heredity, 78–84, 265–289
  see also genetics
heroin, 139–142, 184–186, 191
  compared to marijuana, 187–188
herpes simplex virus, 401
heterozygosity, 272
histamine, 474
Hodgkin's disease, 457
Holmes, O. W., 543
homograft, 401
homosexuality, 218, *218–219*, 302
homozygosity, 272
hormones, 37, 53, 481–484
  see also endocrine system; individual hormones
Horn, D., 181
hospitalization, 557
Houdini, H., 55
Hugo, V., 78
Huhner test, 250
humanistic theory, 88–91
Hunter's disease, *282–283*
Huxley, A., 117
hydrocephalus, 285
hydrochloric acid, 32, 479
hymen, 222
hyperplasia, 174–175, *175*
hypersensitivity, 474
hypertension, 358, 468, 500, 505
hypochondriasis, 104, 364
Hypokinetic Disease (Raab and Kraus), 355
hypokinetic disorders, 355–356
hysterectomy, 235, 544
hysterical neurosis, conversion type, 103
hysterical personality, 106
hysterotomy, 262

I

iatrogenic illness, 543–544
immunity, 431–434
  defective immune mechanism, 453
  disorders of immune system, 473, 475
immunization schedule, 433
imprinting, 79–80
Incaparina, 334
independent segregation, 275
infant mortality, 9, 413
infarct, 464
infectious diseases, 415–416, 423–443
  agents of, 424–427
  body defenses, 429
  common diseases, 434–442
  course of, 428
  immunity, 431
  prevention and treatment, 432
  spread of, 427
  venereal disease, 437–443
  see also specific diseases
infertility, 249–250, *250*
inflammation, 430
influenza, 433, 435
insomnia, 87, 104–105, 142, 369
insulin, 480–481, 483–484
insulin-shock therapy, 110
intelligence tests, 277

interferon, 431
International Rice Research Institute, 348
intestines, 32–33
  see also digestive system
intrauterine device (IUD), 256, 258
isometrics, 361
Iproniazid, 71
iris, 373
Isoniazid, 281

J

Jackson, J. H., 63
jaundice, 480
Jensen, A. R., 277
Johnson, V., 221–228
Judd, L., 108

K

Kaplan, J., 201
kidneys, 34, 35–36, 156, 176
  artificial, 478–479
  disorders of, 477–479
  transplants, 368, 479
  see also excretory system
Kinsey, A., 292
Kirkpatrick, C., 312
Klinefelter's syndrome, 284
Koch, R., 419
Kraus, H., 355
kwashiorkor, 334, 415

L

labia, 44, 45, 222, 224
lacrimal glands, 373
lactose, 333
Lang, P. J., 55–56
laparoscopy, 260
larynx, 175
laudanum, 121
laws. See drug legislation; sexuality
  and the law
L-dopa, 522
lead poisoning, 567
learning, 66
  conditioning, 85
  cognitive, 78
  parents' role in, 314–315
Leeuwenhoek, A. van, 423
Lemy, P. J., 409
lens (of the eye), 373
leukemia, 448
leukoplakia, 176
leukorrhea, 240
Levine, S., 88
Libman, E., 543
life expectancy, 9, 412–413, 415,
  420, 421
limbic system, 66–70, 68
linoleic acid, 333
lipids, 333
Lisina, M. I., 55
lithium salts, 151, 521–522
liver, 32, 155, 156, 165, 480
lobotomy, 113
Long, R., 410

Look Younger, Live Longer (Hauser), 343
Lorenz, K., 79
LSD. See psychedelic drugs
lungs, 17, 27–29, 174, 477, 478
  cancer of, 174, 450, 453
  and exercise, 358
  see also bronchitis; emphysema;
    respiratory system
Luria, A. R., 55
lymph nodes, 32, 33, 431
lymph system, 32, 33
lymphocytes, 26, 32, 431, 431
lymphoma, 448
lymphosarcoma, 448

M

macrophages, 430
Mafia, 191
malaria, 419, 492
malnutrition, 329–330, 334, 415
malocclusion, 387
maltose, 333
mammography, 454
manic-depressive psychosis, 106, 151
MAO inhibitors, 151
marasmus, 332
marijuana. See cannabis
Marijuana—The New Prohibition (Kaplan),
  201
marriage, 291–307
  effects of children on, 310
Maslow, A., 88–89, 90, 91
Masters, W., 221–228
masturbation, 187, 214
materia alba, 389
Mayer, J., 339
Mead, M., 300
mechanoreceptors, 400
Medicare and Medicaid, 535, 556–557
medicine
  in history, 6–12, 411
  recent advances in, 572–576
  see also chemotherapy; physicians
meiosis, 274, 275
melanin, 400
melanoma, 448
membrane
  basilar, 381
  cell, 45, 54–57
  postsynaptic, 57
memory, 66
menarche, 236
Mendel, G., 276
  see also genetics
meningitis, 484
Menninger, K., 107
menopause, 235, 237, 250–252, 251
menstruation, 45, 227, 239–240
mental illness, 93–115
  and biological clocks, 368
  institutionalization, 115
  role of stress in, 95–103
  therapy for, 109–115
meprobamate, 139
mercury contamination, 416, 502
mescaline, 73, 145, 155–156, 186
metabolism, 53
  and exercise, 358

inborn errors of, 278, 280–281
metastases, 446, 447
metazoa, 415, 424, 427
methadone maintenance, 198–199
Methedrine, 143
microelectrodes, 61, 68
midwives, 545, 547
Miltown, 138
Miner, J., 548
minerals, dietary, 336–337
  daily requirement, 337
  food sources, 337
  physiological role, 337
miscarriage, 246
mitochondria, 47
mitosis, 274, 275
mongolism. See Down's syndrome
monocytes, 26
mononucleosis, 437
monosodium glutamate, 349
Montagu, A., 300
morbidity rates, 407
morphine, 121, 139, 191
mortality rates, 344, 407, 413, 553
  accidental deaths, 508, 511
mother surrogates, 80
motivation, 61, 76
motives, 76
  hierarchy of, 89
motor-vehicle accidents, 512, 516
multiphasic screening, 563–565, 564
multiple sclerosis, 485
mumps, 433
muscles, 16, 20, 21–23, 21, 22
muscular system, 16, 21–23
  see also exercise
mutations, 270, 281
myocardial infarction, 465
myoclonic jerk, 366
myotonia, 222–228
myxedema, 483

N

Nader, R., 517
Naeye, R. L., 344
Naloxone, 199
narcotics. See heroin; opium
National Board of Medical Examiners,
  540
National Center for Health Statistics,
  173
National Health Service Corps, 534
National Institute of Mental Health,
  189, 368
National Institutes of Health, 534, 534
National Nutrition Survey, 414
National Research Council, 342
National Safety Council, 511–512
natural selection, 498, 505
naturopaths, 545
nearsightedness, 374–375, 376
Needham, A. E., 396–397
Nembutal, 138
nephritis, 478
nephrons, 34, 35
  see also excretory system; kidneys
nephrosis, 478
nerve fibers, 38, 39, 53, 400

nervous system, *19*, 38–43, 53–73
  autonomic control, 55–56
  and behavior, 53–73
  disorders of, 484–485
  and drugs, 71, 133–151
  nicotine effects on, 173
  sympathetic, 66
  see also brain; central nervous system
neurasthenia, 364
neuritis, 484
neurons, 38, *39, 52–53*, 54–73, *57*, 381
neurosis, 103–105
  see also mental illness
neurotransmitters, 38, 57
  acetylcholine, 58, 70, 154, 173
  drugs and, 71
  noradrenalin, 58, 70–73, 154, 279
  serotonin, 73, 154
New Left, 301
nicotine, 121, 173–175
Niemann-Pick disease, 280
Nisbett, R., 87
nitrates, 501
No-Doz, 142
noise pollution, 382, 502–505, *502*
noradrenalin, 56, 70–73, 154, 279
norepinephrine. *See* noradrenalin
nuclear weapons tests, 13
nucleotides, 267
nucleus, cell, 45
nursing, 9, 547
nutrition, 329–349
  components of, 330–336
  diet and heart disease, 340
  and fetus, 342
  Green Revolution, 345–349
  malnutrition, 329–330, 334, 415
  organic foods, 343–344, 346–347
  weight control, 338–339
  world food needs, 345
Nyswander, M., 198–199

O

obesity, 338, 414, 462
obsessive-compulsive behavior, 103
occipital cortex, 64
occlusion, 387, 390–391
oculist, 375
Oedipal conflict, 82
Oneida Community, 303
operant conditioning, 85
operant-feedback method, 55–56
ophthalmologist, 375
opium, 121, 139–142, 191
optician, 375
optometrist, 375, 545
oral contraceptives, *256*, 259
oral hygiene, 389–391, 395
organ of Corti, 381
orgasm, 43
  female, 223, 253–254
  male, 228, 254
orgasmic platform, 223
orthodontia, 387
Osler, W., 544
ossicles, 378
osteopathy, 539
otitis media, 380

otosclerosis, 382
ova, 43–44, 233–239
ovaries, 43–44, *44*, 233, 237–239, *237, 248*
overexertion, 361
overpopulation, 13, 303, 488
oviduct. *See* Fallopian tubes
ovulation, 236–237, *237*, 254

P

Pace, C. J., 187
pacemaker, *40*, 465
  artificial, *466*
pancreas, 32, 176
  islet cells of, 480, 483–484
pandemic disease, 407
Pap smear, 454
paraldehyde, 138
paranoia, 106
parenthood, 309–325
  discipline, 316–319
  effects on marriage, 310
  parent-child interaction, 315–319
  qualifications for, 309–310, 323–325
  social-class effects, 319, 321–322
  unwed mothers, 310
parietal cortex, 64
Partnership for Health Act, 566
Pasteur, L., 406, 419, 420, 493
pathogens, 423, *424*
  see also specific organisms
patriarchal monogamy, 292, 304–307
Patterns of Sexual Behavior (Ford and Beach), 297
pedophilia, 220
pellagra, 73
penicillin, 420–421, 440, 442, 468
  see also antibiotics
penis, 43, 227–228, 234
  see also reproductive system
peptic ulcer, 176, 479–480, *479*, 505
periodontal disease, 390
perilymph, 381
periodontium, 387
peripheral nervous system, 39
peristalsis, 31
peritonitis, 258, 479
personality disorders, 103, 106–109
personality theories, 78–84
petting, 214
peyote, 145, 148, 186
phagocytes, 429–430
pharmaceutical industry, 129, 189, 409–410, 521–522
pharmacogenetics, 281
pharmacology, 71
pharynx, 31
phenotype, 266
phenylketonuria (PKU), *266*, 279, *279*
phobias, 103
phocomelia, 286
physical fitness, 351–369
  exercise, 354–362
  and fatigue, 362–369
  and sleep, 366
physicians, 9, 115, 537–547
  education, 540
  and iatrogenic illness, 543–544

shortage of, 554–555
  specialization, 9, 540, 542, 554
  see also health care
Piaget, J., 86, 314
pigment, skin, 400
pituitary gland, 37, 43, 481
  see also endocrine system
placenta, *240*, 241
plague, *6*, 405
Planned Parenthood-World Population, 263
plasma, 24
plastic surgery, 401
platelets, 26
pneumonia, 436–437
podiatry, 545
polio, 432–433, 484
pollution, 13, 487–505, *490–491*
  air, 418, 498–500
  and ecology, 489–498
  food, 418–419, 501–502
  noise, 384, 502–505
  solutions, *503*
  water, 418, 500–502
population, 488–489
practical nurse, 547
pregnancy, 243–246, *244*
  dental care during, 389–390
  nutrition during, 342
  smoking and, 173
  see also prenatal development
prenatal development, *240*, 241–243, *242*
  see also embryo; fetus
presbycusis, 382
presbyopia, 375
progesterone, 237
Prontosil, 419
Proposition 31 (Rimmer), 301
prostaglandins, 262
prostate gland, 43, *44*, 228, 234
prosthetics, dental, 392
prostitution, 220, *221*
protein, 333
  see also amino acids
protozoa, 415, *424*, 427
psilocybin, 73, 145, 206
psychasthenia, 364
psyche, 76–91
psychedelic drugs, 73, 123, 126, 129 145, 149, 186, 189–190
  alcohol-LSD comparison, 155–156
  genetic effects, 205–206
  LSD effect, 146–148, *147*
  marijuana-heroin-LSD compared, 188
  schizophrenia-LSD compared, 108
Psychiatric Opinion, 522
psychiatry, 109–115
psychoactive drugs, 71–73, 110, 117–209
  causes of drug use, 126–131
  drug abuse, 122–131, 133–151, 183–201
  historical perspective, 120–122
  traffic in, 189–191, *190*
  see also drugs; specific drugs
psychoanalytic theory, 80, 101–102
  see also Freud, S.
psychological development, 75–91

cognitive-developmental theory, 86
competence theory, 82
ethological theory, 79
learning theory, 85
psychoanalytic theory, 80
psychosocial theory, 82
social learning theory, 86
psychologists, 115, 545
psychopharmacology, 71
psychophysiological disorders, 103, 109
psychosis, 103, 105–106
  see also mental illness
psychosocial theory, 82
psychosomatic disorders, 103, 109
psychotherapy, 109–115
  community psychiatry, 109
  family therapy, 112
  group therapy, 112
  psychoanalysis, 111
  symptomatic treatment, 110
  therapists, 115
psychotomimetic drugs, 73, 145
pubococcygeus muscles, 222
pulmonary stenosis, 467, *467*
pupil (of the eye), 373
pyelonephritis, 478

Q

quackery, 457, 548–551

R

Raab, W., 355
rabies, 433, 484
rapid eye movement (REM), 366
rauwolfia, 71
Rayner, R., 85
receptor sites, 57
rectum, 33
red blood cells, 24
Red Cross, 532
reflex arc, 41
Regional Medical Programs Act, 566
Reiss, I. L., 230
Reissner membranes, 381
renal disease, 477–479
repression, 78
reproductive system, *19*, 43–45, *44*,
  222–229, *224–226*, *228*, 233–239,
  253–254
reserpine, 71, 151
respiratory system, *17*, 27–29, *28*, *29*
  effects of smoking, 172, 174–175
  disorders of, 475–479
  see also lungs
retina, 61, 373
  abnormalities of, 377
"Revere, P.," 393
Rh factor, 244–245
rhesus monkeys, attachment in, 80–81,
  80
rheumatic heart disease, 468, 473
rheumatoid arthritis, as autoimmune
  response, 475, *476*
rhythm method of birth control, 255,
  257
ribonucleic acid. *See* RNA

rickettsiae, 415, *424*, 427
Rimmer, R., 301
RNA, 270
Robinson, D., 409
Rodale, R., 343
Rogers, C., 88–89, 91, 112
root-canal therapy, 391, *395*
Rorvick, D. M., 253
Rosebury, T., 425
rubella, 286, 416, 433
Rubin's test, 250

S

Sabin oral polio vaccine, 432
sado-masochism, 220
Sadove, M. S., 409
safety, 507–525
saliva, 31, 387, 389
Salk polio vaccine, 432
salpingitis, 236
sarcoma, 448
saturated fats, 333
Scarlet Letter, The (Hawthorne), 310
Schachter, S., 87
schizophrenia, 105, 107–108, 276
Schlemm, canal of, 373
sclera, 373
scrotum, 43, *44*, 227–228
sebaceous glands, 398
seconal, 138
secondary sex characteristics, 44–45
secretin, 37
sedative-hypnotic drugs, 138–142
  see also barbiturates
self-actualization, 89–91, 131
semen, 43, 228, 234
seminal vesicles, 43, *44*, 228, 234
septal heart defects, 467
Sernyl, 145, 148
serotonin, 73, 154
Seventh-Day Adventists, 172
sex-flush, 223–228
sexual intercourse, 43, 45, 217,
  221–231, *226*, 253–254
sexual reproduction, 233–263
  birth control, 252–263
  childbirth, 246–249
  infertility, 249–250
  pregnancy, 243–246
  prenatal development, 241–243
  see also reproductive system
sexuality, 213–231
  coitus, 43, 45, 217, 221–231,
    224–226, 253–254
  homosexuality, 218
  and the law, 217
  masturbation, 214
  petting, 214
  prostitution, 220
  psychosocial aspects, 213
  sex differences, 229
  sexual "revolution," 230–231
  sexual techniques, 229
Shearn, D., 55
Shettles, L. B., 253
shock therapy, 110
sickle cell anemia, 278–279, *278*

Silverman, J., 107
Singer, J., 87
sinusitis, 176
skeletal system, *16*, 20–21
skin, 396–401, *397*
  dermis, 397–400, *397*, *399*
  disorders, 400–401
  epidermis, 397, *397*, *399*
  nerve endings, 400
  pigment, 400
  plastic surgery, 401
Skinner box, 69
sleep, 366–369
smallpox, 433
smoking, 5, 110, 171–181
  advertising and, 176
  components of cigarette smoke, 173
  curtailment of, 180–181
  as disease agent, 174–176, 462
  historical perspective, 121, 176–177
  mortality rate, 172
  psychological dependence, 178
  see also nicotine
sociopathic personality, 106
spastic cerebral palsy, 286
specialization in medicine, 9, 542, 554
speech, 64–66
sperm, 43, 227, 234, 253–254
spermatogenesis, 234
sphincters, 22, 23, 32, 38, 43
sphingolipidoses, 280
spina bifida, 285
spinal column, 20–21
stamina training, 356–362, *357*
Stanford University, 494
starches, 333
sterilization, surgical, 259, *260*
Stern, B., 56
steroids, 333
Steward, W., 181
stimulants, 142–145
  amphetamines, 71, 143–145, 186, 189
  caffeine, 121, 142
  cocaine, 122, 145
stomach, 22, 32
  see also digestive system
Storms, M., 87
STP. *See* psychedelic drugs
Stranger in a Strange Land (Heinlein),
  301
streptomycin, 421
stress, emotional, 96–103, 417
  and fight-flight response, 66–68, *67*,
    355–356
Stroebel, C. F., 368
strokes, 469–470, *470*
succedaneous teeth, 386
succession, biological, 498, *498*
sucrose, 333
suicide, 104–105
  and barbiturates, 139
sulfa drugs, 419
sulfur dioxide, 499
Sullivan, H. S., 107
Surgeon General's Advisory Committee
  on Influenza, 436
sweat glands, 398, *399*
sympathetic nervous system, 66

Synanon, 195
synapse, 38, *39*, 53–57, *57*, 373
synesthesia, 146, 188
syphilis, 73, 286, 419, *437*, 438–440, *439*
systematic desensitization, 56
systemic diseases, 473–485
    cardiovascular system, 340, 459–471
    digestive tract, 479–481
    endocrine system, 481–484
    excretory system, 477–478
    immune system, 473–475
    nervous system, 484–485
    respiratory system, 475–477
    see also specific diseases
systolic pressure, 468
Szasz, T., 93–94

T

Tay-Sachs disease, 280
teeth, 385–396, *386, 387, 388, 389*
    care of, 395–396
    disease, 389–391
    prosthetics, 392–395, *392*
    restorative procedures, 391, *392, 395*
    structure, 386–389
tendons, 21
testes, 43, *44*, 227–228
tetanus, 433, 485
tetracycline, 421
T-groups, 113
thalidomide, 138, 205, 286, 521
thermal pollution, 501
Thorazine, 146, 151, 195
thrombosis, 464, 470
thymine, 267
thyroid gland, 37, 367, 483
thyroid-stimulating hormone (TSH), 37
thyroxin, 37, 279
Tinbergen, N., 79
toilet training, 84
tolerance, drug, 124, *125*, 139–146, 161
toxins, 424, 432
toxoids, 432
trachea, 27, 176
Trager, J., 343
tranquilizers, 71, 108, 110, 150, 189
triglycerides, 333
trophic levels, 492, *492*
trypanosomiasis, 419
tubal ligation, 260
tuberculosis, 412, 433, *436*
tumors, 446
Turner's syndrome, 284–285
twins
    in utero, 79

    studies of, 79, 276–277
typhoid, 433

U

ulcers, 176, 479–480, *479*
umbilical cord, 249
unconditional positive regard, 89–91
University of California, Los Angeles, 108
University of Oregon, 521
University of Pittsburgh, 55
University of Tennessee, 56
University of Washington, 56
University of Wisconsin, 55
unsaturated fats, 333
urea, 35
uremia, 478
ureter, 35
urethra, 43, 228, 234–235
U.S. Department of Agriculture, 414, 519, 525
U.S. Department of Commerce, 535
U.S. Department of Health, Education and Welfare (HEW), 178, 414, 534, 539
U.S. Department of Interior, 535
U.S. Food and Drug Administration (FDA), 199, 259, 349, 409, 519–523
U.S. Office of Economic Opportunity, 535, 567
U.S. Post Office Department, 519
U.S. Public Health Service (PHS), 195, 533
U.S. Veterans Administration, 409, 535
uterus, *44*, 44–45, 224, 234–235, *234, 240, 248, 250, 253*

V

vaccination, 432–434
vagina, *44*, 45, 222–226, 234–235, 253
Valins, S., 87
Vanderhost, L., 322
vas deferens, 43, *44*, 234
vasectomy, 260
veins, *17*, 26, *27*
    see also circulatory system
venereal disease, 412, 437–443, *437*
    gonorrhea, 286, 417, *437, 438*, 440–443
    syphilis, 73, 286, 419, *437*, 438–440, *439*
ventricles, 26
    see also heart
venules, 26, 32
vestibular apparatus, 380, *380*
villi, intestinal, 32, *33*

Vinci, L. da, *9, 72*
virus, 401, 415, *424*, 427, *427*, 434–436 451, *451*, 500
    see also specific virus-caused diseases
vision. *See* eyes
visual abstraction, 61
visual fields, *65*
vitamins, 334–336, 414
    daily requirement, 335–336
    deficiency syndromes, 335–336
    excess, results of, 336
    food source, 335–336
    physiological role, 335–336
vitreous humor, 373
vocational nurse, 547
voluntary nervous system, 41
vulva, 45

W

Walters, R., 86
warts, 401
Washington, G., 543
water pollution, 416, 500–502
Watson, J. 267
Watson, J. B., 85
weight control, 338
White, B., 88
white blood cells, 24–26
white noise, 369
White, R., 82, 86, 314
whooping cough, 433
withdrawal illness, 125
    alcohol, 139, 154, 161
    opiates, 140
    sedative-hypnotics, 139
women's liberation, 304–305
World Health Organization (WHO), 124, 181, 416, 529, 532

X

x-ray
    development of, 7
    radiation danger, 450, 453
    therapy, 456

Y

Yablonsky, L., 302
Yale University, 321
yellow fever, 406, 433
Yolles, S., 189

Z

zonula, 373
zygote, 234, 241, 267–273

Special thanks are extended to the following persons and sources for help in providing and developing graphics: San Diego Narcotics Bureau, San Diego Police Department; James H. Nelson, M.D.; Jack Baird, UCLA; Dr. Max Elliott, UCSD: Robert Dailey, County of Los Angeles Health Department, Alcoholism Rehabilitation Center; Captain Norvel Richardson, Dr. Don Schwerdtfeger, staff and patients at Vista Hill Hospital, Chula Vista, California; J. Robert Bobbitt Jr., D.D.S.   ¶ We also wish to extend special thanks for editorial contributions and help to: Silvio Varon, Ralph Grawunder, Sam Moffat, John Henahan, Nancy Marcus, and Sam Wilson; Albert Ax, Michigan Department of Mental Health; Leon Brody, New York University; Paul J. Fink, Hahnemann Medical College; Howard Leventhal, Harvard University; Smoking Research of San Diego.

Title page—Phil Kirkland

I FOUNDATIONS OF HEALTH SCIENCE

1 Introduction to Health Science

2—Diane McDermott; 4–5—Bill Mac-Donald/IBOL; 6—(*bottom left*) Museo Del Prado; (*bottom right*) Bettmann Archive, Inc.; (*top right*) Museum Yamato Bun-kakan; 7—(*top left and right, bottom left*) Bibliotheque Nationale, Paris; (*bottom right*) Musee Royal De L'Afrique Centrale; 8—Museo del Prado; 9—(*left*) Scala Fine Arts Publishers, Inc.; (*right*) Bettmann Archive, Inc.; 10—(*top*) Scala Fine Arts Publishers, Inc./Museo di Belle Arti, Ghent; (*bottom right*) Ciccione/Rapho-Guillumette Pictures; (*bottom left*) courtesy Harper & Row; 11—(*top*) Bettmann Archive, Inc.; (*bottom*) Scala Fine Arts Publishers, Inc.; 12—(*top left*) Philadelphia Museum of Art; (*bottom left*) courtesy of The Wellcome Trustees; (*top right*) photo by Byron, The Byron Collection, Museum of the City of New York; (*bottom right*) Public Health Service of the National Archives.

2 The Body in Action

14–15—John Dawson; 16–19—Millsap/Kinyon; 20—Patty Peck; 21—Felicia Fry; 22—(*top, center*) Gerry Efinger; (*bottom*) John Dawson; 23—Patty Peck; 24—Tom Lewis; 25—Tom Lewis; 26—John Dawson; 27—John Dawson, after Warren R. Guild, Robert E. Fuisz, and Samuel Bojar, *The Science of Health*, © 1969, p. 88; by permission of Prentice-Hall, Inc., Englewood Cliffs, N.J.; 28—John Dawson; 29—Tom Lewis; 30–31—Patty Peck; 33—(*left*) Tom Lewis; (*right*)

Patty Peck; 34—John Dawson; 36—Patty Peck; 39—(*left*) Millsap/Kinyon; (*top right*) COMPIX-UPI; (*bottom right*) Julius Weber; 40—(*top*) John Dawson, after Warren R. Guild, Robert E. Fuisz, and Samuel Bojar, *The Science of Health*, © 1969, p. 74; by permission of Prentice-Hall, Inc., Englewood Cliffs, N.J.; (*bottom*) John Dawson; 42—Tom Lewis; 44—John Dawson; 46—Tom Lewis; 47—Julius Weber; 48–49—Diane McDermott.

II MENTAL AND EMOTIONAL FUNCTIONING

3 Physiological Basis of Behavior

50—Diane McDermott; 52–53—Julius Weber; 54—A. L. Hodgkin; 57—Millsap/Kinyon; 58—Tom Lewis; 61—(*left*) Philip Daly; (*right*) Felicia Fry, after "The Visual Cortex of the Brain," by D. Hubel, *Scientific American*, November 1963, p. 57; 62—John Dawson; 63—Ron Estrine, after Penfield and Rasmussen, *The Cerebral Cortex of Man*, ©1950 The Macmillan Co.; reprinted with permission: 64—(*top*) Renald Von Muchow; (*center, bottom*) Philip Daly; 65—(*top*) Philip Daly; (*bottom*) Felicia Fry; 67—Ron Estrine; 68—John Dawson; 69—Dr. Jose Delgado; 70—(*top left, bottom left*) Dr. James Olds; (*right*) Steve McCarroll; 72—(*a*) Tom Suzuki; (*b*) University of Virginia Library; (*c*) Burndy Library, Norwalk, Conn.; (*d*) Philip Daly, courtesy National Educational Television; (*f, g*) Lawrence Parque.

4 The Healthy Personality

74–75—Terry Lamb; 77—Gary Van Der Steur; 79—Doug Armstrong; 80—

Regional Primate Research Center, University of Wisconsin; 83—Adapted from R. Bishof, *Interpreting Personality Theories*, Harper & Row, pp. 578–580; 84—Ken Heyman; 85—Felicia Fry; 87—Jason Lauré; 88–89—Dr. Burton L. White.

5 Mental Health and Mental Illness

92–93—Karl Nicholason; 94—Karl Nicholason; 96—(*top*) Leonard Freed/Magnum Photos, Inc.; (*bottom*) Dick Corten; 97—Howard Saunders; 98—(*top left, left center*) Burk Uzzle/Magnum Photos, Inc.; (*top right, bottom left*) Charles Harbutt/Magnum Photos, Inc.; (*bottom right*) Dan Morrill; 99—(*top*) Richard Balagur/Nancy Palmer Photo Agency; (*top center, bottom*) Charles Harbutt/Magnum Photos, Inc.; (*bottom center*) Allen Green/Nancy Palmer Photo Agency; 100—Bill MacDonald/IBOL; 102—Howard Saunders; 104—(*top left*) Warner Brothers Studios, courtesy Larry Edmunds Cinema Bookshop; (*center left*) Twentieth Century Fox, courtesy Museum of Modern Art/Stills Archive, New York; (*bottom left*) Walter Reade Organization, courtesy of the Museum of Modern Art/Stills Archive, New York; (*top right*) Paramont Pictures, courtesy of Museum of Modern Art/Stills Archive, New York; (*bottom right*) "Possessed" still #581 292, © 1931 Metro–Goldwyn–Mayer, Inc., courtesy of Larry Edmunds Cinema Bookshop; 110—National Association for Mental Health, Inc.; 111—John Oldenkamp/IBOL, taken at Vista Hill Hospital; 113—(*left, center right*) Arthur Schatz; (*top right*) J.M. Vincent/Camera 5; (*bottom right*) Ken Regan/Camera 5; 114—Karl Nicholason.

III CHEMICAL ALTERATION OF BEHAVIOR

6 The Role of Drugs in the Good Life

116 – Diane McDermott; 118 – 119 – Karl Nicholason; 121 – John Dawson; 122 – Patty Peck; 123 – Karl Nicholason; 125 – Susan Anson; 128 – Karl Nicholason.

7 Common Drugs of Misuse and Abuse

132 – 133 – Culver Pictures; 134 – 137 – (*bottom*) photos by Werner Kalber/PPS; 140 – Patty Peck; 141 – (*top, bottom right*) Ian Berry/Magnum Photos, Inc.; (*bottom left*) Archie Lieberman/Black Star; 144 – John Dawson; 147 – reproduced from *Triangle*, The Sandoz Journal of Medical Science, Vol. 2, No. 3, 1955, pp. 119 – 123; 149 – (*top, center*) Marilyn Silverstone/Magnum Photos, Inc.; (*bottom*) Charles Gatewood; 150 – Ronald Estrine.

8 Alcohol Abuse

152 – 153 – Paul Slick; 155 – Patty Peck; 156 – Dr. Max E. Elliott, University of California, San Diego; 157 – Shirley Dethloff; 160 – Karl Nicholason; 162 – Brown Brothers; 163 – Howard Saunders; 166 – Karl Nicholason; 168 – County of Los Angeles Health Department, Alcoholism Rehabilitation Center.

9 Smoking and Health

170 – 171 – Gerry Efinger; 172 – Doug Armstrong; statistics from U.S. Public Health Service; 174 – Dr. Max E. Elliott, University of California, San Diego; 175 – Tom Lewis; 177 – (*left*) John Dawson; (*right*) Dr. Max E. Elliott, University of California, San Diego; 179 – Karl Nicholason.

10 Controlling Drug Use and Abuse

182 – 183 – Karl Nicholason; 185 – Millsap/Kinyon; 190 – Tom Lewis, photo by Werner Kalber/PPS; 192 – National Audiovisual Center; 195 – (*top left, top right, bottom right*) COMPIX-UPI: (*bottom left*) Ken Regan/Camera 5; 196 – 197 – John Oldenkamp/IBOL, taken at Vista Hill Hospital; 200 – Phil Kirkland.

11 Drugs in Perspective

202 – Karl Nicholason; 208 – Shirley Dethloff.

IV FAMILY HEALTH

12 Human Sexuality

210 – Diane McDermott; 212 – 213 – Masami Teraoka; 215 – Howard Saunders; 216 – Howard Saunders; 218 – (*top*) Jack Brembeck – Director of Advertising and Public Relations, KABC-TV; Richter & Mracky-Bates, Inc. Advertising Agency for KABC-TV; Stanley Davis – Art Director, Richter & Mracky-Bates, Inc.; Carol Corbett – Copywriter, Richter & Mracky-Bates, Inc.; Robert M. Klosterman – Account Supervisor, Richter & Mracky-Bates, Inc.; (*bottom*) Richard Balagur/Nancy Palmer Photo Agency; 219 – Millsap/Kinyon; 220 – montage by Louis Neiheisel; 221 – (*top*) Troeller/Black Star; (*center*) Goksin Sipahioglu/Black Star; (*bottom*) Franklynn Peterson/Black Star; 224 – 225 – John Dawson; 226 – John Dawson; 227 – Doug Armstrong, after Masters and Johnson, *Human Sexual Response*, copyright © Little, Brown & Company, 1966; 228 – John Dawson; 230 – Diane McDermott.

13 Reproduction and Birth Control

232 – 233 – Elizabeth Wilcox; 234 – Tom Lewis; 235 – Tom Lewis; 236 – Doug Armstrong, after Tanner, 1962, *Growth and Adolescence*, Blackwell Scientific Publications, Ltd.; 237 – Tom Lewis; 238 – Tom Lewis; 239 – Tom Lewis; 240 – (*left*) Tom Lewis; (*right*) from Rugh and Shettles, *From Conception to Birth: The Drama of Life's Beginnings*, New York: Harper & Row, 1971; 242 – (*top left*) H. Nishimura; (*top right*) Rugh and Shettles; (*bottom*) Tom Lewis; 244 – John Dawson, after "Care During Pregnancy," *Story of Life*, 16, pp. 434 – 435; 245 – Tom Lewis; 246 – John Dawson; 247 – Elizabeth Wilcox; 248 – Tom Lewis; 250 – Tom Lewis; 251 – Adapted from B. Neugarten, "A New Look at Menopause," *Psychology Today*, December 1967, p. 44; 256 – 257 – drawings, Tom Lewis, photographs by Werner Kalber/PPS; chart after "To Be or Not To Be," *Story of Life*, 46, pp. 1274 – 1275; 260 – Tom Lewis; 261 – adapted from *Birth Control Handbook*, 7th ed., 1971.

14 Heredity and Health

264 – 265 – Culver Pictures; 266 – Felicia Fry; 268 – 269 – John Dawson; 270 – John Dawson; 271 – (*top*) William Laughman; (*bottom*) Patty Peck; 272 – (*top*) after Keeton, *Biological Science*, Norton, 1967, p. 539; (*bottom*) after H. Curtis, *Biology*, Worth Publishing, 1968, p. 378; 273 – Felicia Fry; 274 – Felicia Fry; 275 – Gerry Efinger, after H. Curtis, *Biology*, Worth Publishing, 1968, p. 365; 276 – Felicia Fry; 278 – Gabriele Wunderlich; 279 – Felicia Fry; 282 – 283 – Patty Peck; 283 – (*right*) Dr. O. W. Jones, University of California, San Diego; 284 – Tom Lewis; 285 – Tom Lewis, 286 – Courtesy Metropolitan Life Insurance Company; 287 – (*top*) John Dawson; (*center*) from Department of Neurosciences, University of California, San Diego; (*bottom*) Dr. O. W. Jones, University of California, San Diego; 288 – Doug Armstrong.

15 Marriage in American Society

Chapter adapted from "The Future of Marriage" by Morton Hunt; originally appeared in *Playboy* magazine, copyright © 1971 by Playboy; 290 – 291 – Larry Burchard, photo by Werner Kalber/PPS; 293 – (*top, bottom left*) Burt Glinn/Magnum Photos, Inc.; (*center*) Marilyn Silverstone/Magnum Photos, Inc.; (*bottom right*) Ted Schwartz, courtesy American Museum of Natural History; 294 – John Dawson; 295 – Felicia Fry; statistics from HEW, National Center for Health Statistics; 296 – Howard Saunders; 298 – Howard Saunders; 300 – (*left*) Sam Falk/Monkmeyer Press Photo Service; (*right*) montage by Louis Neiheisel; 306 – Phil Kirkland.

16 Parenthood

308 – 309 – Karl Nicholason; 310 – Doug Armstrong; 311 – Howard Saunders; 312 – Bill MacDonald/IBOL; 313 – Burk Uzzle/Magnum Photos, Inc.; 315 – Jason Lauré; 316 – Janet Colby; 317 – (*top*)

Credits and Acknowledgments

Lawrence Parque; (bottom) John Oldenkamp/IBOL; 318—Howard Saunders; 319—Ronald Estrine; 320—(top) Joan Sydlow/Monkmeyer Press Photo Service; (bottom) Fujihira/Monkmeyer Press Photo Service; 323—Susan Anson; 324—Terry Lamb.

V PERSONAL HEALTH CARE

17 Nutrition

326—Diane McDermott; 328–329—Ignacio Gomez; 330—Doug Armstrong; 331—Michelle Burchard; 332—Ronald Estrine; 333—Felicia Fry; 334—Roy Cummings; 339—Julius Weber; 340—Howard Saunders; 345—Tom Lewis; 348—Ignacio Gomez.

18 Physical Fitness

350–351—*Sports Illustrated;* 352—Young & Rubicam; 354—Bill MacDonald/IBOL; 355—Shirley Dethloff; 356—Leon Bolognese; 357—John Dawson; 358—Felicia Fry, after Astrand and Rodahl, *Textbook of Work Physiology,* McGraw-Hill, 1970, p. 131; 359—Doug Armstrong, after N. Shock, "The Physiology of Aging," *Scientific American,* January 1962, p. 110; 362—Bill MacDonald/IBOL; 363—adapted from "An Introduction to Physical Fitness," President's Council on Physical Fitness and Sports, 1970; 365—Paul Fusco, from *Sense Relaxation;* 366—after Naitoh & L. C. Johnson, "Sleep Patterns of Aquanauts During Tektite I," Navy Medical Neuropsychiatric Research Unit Report.

19 The Eyes and Ears

370–371—Paul Slick; 372—John Dawson; 374—(left) Tom Lewis; (right) Paul Slick; 376—Felicia Fry; 377—Felicia Fry; 378—Shirley Dethloff; 379—John Dawson; 380—John Dawson; 381—Tom Lewis; 382—Tom Lewis.

20 The Teeth, Skin, and Hair

384–385—painting on hand by Tom Lewis, photographed by Bill MacDonald/IBOL; 386—Shirley Dethloff; 387—photo by Werner Kalber/PPS; 388—John Dawson; 389—Joseph J. Schwarz, D.D.S., Chicago; 390—Tom Lewis; 391—Tom Lewis; 392—Shirley Dethloff; 395—Drs. Feldman, Solomon, Notaro & Moscowitz of Brooklyn, N.Y.; 396—Gerry Efinger; 397—John Dawson; 398—Gerry Efinger; 399—Luigi Giacometti.

VI HEALTH AND DISEASE

21 The Conquest of Disease

402—Diane McDermott; 404–405—Photographie Giraudon; 406—Tom Lewis; 408—Tom Lewis; 411—The Granger Collection; 412—Felicia Fry; statistics from HEW; 413—Felicia Fry; death rates from *World Health Organization Annual,* 1967; life expectancy figures from 1968 Data Sheet of the Population Reference Bureau; 414—Felicia Fry; 415—Felicia Fry; life expectancies from Public Health Service; infant mortality rates from *Statistical Yearbook,* 1968, Statistical Office of the United Nations, 1969; 415—Felicia Fry; 417—Michelle Burchard; 418—Karl Nicholason; 420—Ronald Estrine.

22 Infectious Diseases

422–423—Karl Nicholason; 424—Felicia Fry; 427—Tom Lewis; 428—Tom Lewis; 429—Ronald Estrine; 430—Karl Nicholason; 431—Tom Lewis; 432—Tom Lewis; 435—(left, center left, right) The Granger Collection; (center right) Bettmann Archive, Inc.; 436—Tom Lewis; 437—Doug Armstrong, after *PR Doctor,* © American Medical Association, January 1971; 438—Doug Armstrong; 439—Patty Peck; 422—Karl Nicholason.

23 Cancer

444–445—Julius Weber; 447—(top left) Max E. Elliott, University of California, San Diego; (top right) Patrick Thurston/Transworld Feature Syndicate, Inc.; (bottom) Tom Lewis; 449—Patty Peck; 451—Tom Lewis; 452—Ronald Estrine; 454—American Cancer Society, N.Y.; 455—Tom Lewis; 456—Ronald Estrine.

24 Cardiovascular Diseases

458–459—V-Dia/Scala Fine Arts Publishers; 460—Julius Weber; 461—Tom Lewis; 463—Karl Nicholason; 465—(top) Tom Lewis; (center, bottom) courtesy of Scripps Memorial Hospital; 466—Renald Von Muchow; 467—Tom Lewis; 469—Patty Peck; 470—Tom Lewis.

25 Systemic Diseases

472–473—Karl Nicholason; 474—Eli O. Meltzer, M.D.; 476—Tom Lewis; 477—Tom Lewis; 478—Tom Lewis; 479—Tom Lewis; 483—Patty Peck; 484—California Medical Publications.

26 Ecology and Pollution

486–487—Susan Anson, photo by Werner Kalber/PPS; 489—Diane McDermott; 490–491—illustrations © Mitchell Beazley, Ltd. 1971; 492—John Dawson; 495—John Dawson, after Woodwell, "Toxic Substances and Ecological Cycles," *Scientific American,* 1967; 496–497—John Dawson; 498—John Dawson, after Buchsbaum, *Basic Ecology,* Boxwood Press; 499—adapted from Warren R. Guild, Robert E. Feusz, and Samuel Bojar, *The Science of Health,* © 1969; reprinted by permission of Prentice-Hall, Inc., Englewood Cliffs, N.J.; 501—Susan Anson; 502—Shirley Dethloff, after Bernarde, *Our Precarious Habitat,* Norton, 1970; 504—Howard Saunders.

27 Accidents and Safety

506–507—Howard Saunders; 509—Howard Saunders; 510—Felicia Fry; 514—Gerry Efinger; 515—Ronald Estrine; 516—Howard Saunders; 517—Jack Baird, University of California, Los Angeles; 518–519—Ronald Estrine; 523—Department of Health, Education and Welfare; 524—Howard Saunders.

VII HEALTH CARE IN AMERICA

28 Health Providers

526—Diane McDermott; 528–529—Terry Lamb; 530—(top left) Culver Pictures; (top center) Elliott Erwitt/Magnum Photos, Inc.; (top right) Erich Hartmann/Magnum Photos, Inc.; (bottom) Photoworld-FPG; 531—Wide World Photos; 532—(top left) E. Schwab/World Health Organization; (top right) J. Mohr/World Health Organization; (bottom *left, bottom right)* P. Larsen/World Health Organization; 533—Millsap/Kinyon; 535—Felicia Fry; 536—National Tuberculosis and Respiratory Disease Association; 537—*(left)* National Counsel on Alcoholism; *(center)* American Cancer Society; *(right)* American Foundation for the Blind; 538—Millsap/Kinyon; 541—Susan Anson; 546—Doug Armstrong; statistics from HEW; 547—Doug Armstrong; statistics from HEW; 548—*(left)* John Oldenkamp/IBOL; *(right)* Doug Armstrong; statistics from HEW; 549—*(top right)* Karl Nicholason; *(bottom right)* John Oldenkamp/IBOL; 550—Howard Saunders.

29 Health Care Delivery
552–553—Renald Von Muchow; 554—Bruce Roberts/Rapho-Guillumette Pic-

tures; 555—Ted Spiegel/Rapho-Guillumette Pictures; 557—Doug Armstrong; data from U.S. Bureau of Labor Statistics; 559—Duke University Physicians Associate Program, Carolyn Vaughan, photographer; 561—Karl Nicholason; 564—*(left)* Jon Brenneis for *Scientific American*; *(right)* Permanente Medical Group; 565—Susan Anson, adapted from S. Garfield, "The Delivery of Medical Care," *Scientific American*, April 1970, p. 22; 567—Richard Balagur/Nancy Palmer Photo Agency; 568—*(top left, bottom left)* J. M. Vincent/Camera 5; *(top right, bottom right)* COMPIX-UPI.

30 Health and the Individual
570–571—Phil Kirkland; 572—*(top)* Paolo Koch/Photo Researchers, Inc.;

(bottom) Jerry Cooke/Photo Researchers, Inc.; 573—*(top)* Diane Rowson/Photo Researchers, Inc.; *(center)* Center for Disease Control, Atlanta; *(bottom)* Frederick Ayer/Photo Researchers, Inc.; 574—*(top)* Renald Von Muchow; *(bottom)* Carl Roodman/Photo Researchers, Inc.; 575—*(top)* Don Wong/Photo Researchers, Inc. *(center)* Alan Bernstein/Photo Researchers, Inc.; *(bottom)* Renald Von Muchow; 576—*(top left)* Carl Roodman/Photo Researchers, Inc.; *(top right)* Alan Bernstein/Photo Researchers, Inc.; *(center)* Renald Von Muchow; *(bottom)* Merck, Sharp & Dohme.

Cover design—Tom Lewis

Body painting—Karl Nicholason

Cover photograph—Werner Kalber/PPS

Film Supplement for
LIFE AND HEALTH Films

The Life and Health Film Series deals with two of the areas of health science that have the most serious implications to the majority of adult and adolescent Americans. The medium of film has been used to great advantage to document the rising incidence of heart disease and what can be done to combat it and to delve into the nature of and therapies for unhealthy human dependencies, treating drug abuse and alcoholism as cases in point. The following are synopses of the content of the four Life and Health Films.

The Heart: Attack

The films "Heart: Attack" and "Heart: Counterattack" are concerned primarily with the nature and prevention of heart disease. In focusing on this topic such areas of health as diet, genetics, exercise, smoking, stress, and the health-care delivery system are brought into perspective.

"Heart: Attack" presents the case of Joe Bowens, a fifty-one-year-old businessman who suffers a heart attack and is rushed to Long Beach Memorial Hospital for emergency treatment. His case is used as a jumping-off point for the examination of factors involved in the development of heart disease and for a presentation of methods of treatment.

Heart disease is the number one killer in America today—in fact, in all of the industrialized Western world. It is commonly thought to strike only during old age; however, the incidence of premature heart attack, and its extension into ever younger age groups, is mounting yearly. Today, one out of five American men will suffer a heart attack before he is sixty.

ATHEROSCLEROSIS

The heart pumps 4,000 gallons of blood through 60,000 miles of vessels each day. About one-twentieth of the blood is pumped to the heart itself, for its own nutrition. It receives this vital blood supply through a network of arteries about one-eighth of an inch in diameter. The most common and widespread form of heart disease involves these coronary vessels. It begins with *atherosclerosis*, a condition that is commonly termed "hardening of the arteries."

Atherosclerosis results when fatty materials, particularly cholesterol, begin to adhere to and occlude the inner lining of the artery walls. These deposits roughen the artery's normally smooth inner lining and narrow the channel for blood flow.

The heart begins to work harder to compensate. In the partially occluded artery, a spot, or *plaque*, appears. At first, it is only microscopic, but it grows as more fatty substances adhere and accumulate, further damming the channel, forcing the heart to work still harder. The gradual amassing of this "biological rust" eventually outstrips the ability of the artery cells to dispose of it.

Atherosclerosis—the narrowing, roughening, hardening, and eventual blocking of the arteries—can and, in the Western world often does, begin in youth, even in early childhood. By middle age, most Americans carry this pathological condition in some degree.

When an artery is wholly clogged, blood flow ceases. In peripheral areas of the cardiovascular system, ensuing circulatory disorders may take the form of painful ulcers in the legs, blindness, or, if the rupture damages the central nervous system, a paralyzing stroke. If a blood clot forms in either of the two main coronary arteries (those leading directly to the heart) the flow of blood and oxygen abruptly stops.

As pointed out in the film by Dr. Mervyn Ellestead, director of clinical physiology at Memorial Hospital, the blocking of a main coronary artery causes a condition termed *myocardial infarction*, or death of heart tissue. Myocardial infarction is one form of heart attack. When blood flow through an artery stops, the muscle normally nourished by it dies. In the mildest cases the condition may pass unnoticed. Perhaps 10 to 20 percent of all infarctions are "silent" in this manner. Myocardial infarctions may also be severe enough to cause cessation of heart function.

A second type of heart attack, *ventricular fibrillation*, often occurs after an infarction; it is caused by poor tissue oxygenation. Ventricular fibrillation affects the heart's pacemaker (an area of nervous tissue that controls the rate of heartbeat). When the function of the pacemaker is disrupted, heartbeat becomes erratic. If not treated immediately, the victim may die. The patient in the film, Joe Bowens, suffers from myocardial infarction and ventricular fibrillation. His heartbeat is restored to normal through emergency treatment with a machine called a defibrillator.

The symptom most commonly associated with coronary artery disease is *angina pectoris*, or chest pain. The pain is typically located under the sternum near the heart. It is often compared to the crushing pain of having someone step on one's chest. Characteristically the pain comes on with exertion and probably results from insufficient delivery of oxygen to the heart.

CHOLESTEROL

A principal agent implicated in atherosclerosis, and hence, heart disease, is the compound cholesterol. Cholesterol is a mushy, yellowish substance, smooth and oily to the touch. High magnification reveals a harsh, crystalline structure, with sharp, needlelike points. In atherosclerosis, these points embed in the artery walls, roughen and scar them, and trap other fatty materials from the passing bloodstream, ultimately creating a lethal impasse. Cholesterol is tough, hard, durable, and insoluble in water. It needs these attributes in order to perform its vital, normal functions, insulating the entire nervous system. The human body both manufactures cholesterol and takes it in through animal flesh and animal products in the diet—it does not occur in the plant kingdom.

As shown in the film, medical science has sought, for the better part of one hundred years, the reason why cholesterol appears to be involved in heart disease. Autopsies performed on large numbers of heart-attack victims almost invariably revealed high concentrations of waxy cholesterol blocking the stricken arteries. Presence did not prove causation, but it did increase suspicion that cholesterol played a role in heart disease.

Later experimenters tested the hypothesis that diet was the determinant in the accumulation of cholesterol in the blood and arteries. High-fat, high-cholesterol diets were fed to laboratory rats, rabbits, and monkeys. The invariable result was a marked degree of atherosclerosis, and, in the case of monkeys, occasional heart attacks with the same characteristics as those suffered by humans. When the same animals were allowed to resume their normal, largely vegetable diets, the incidence of atherosclerosis subsided.

Epidemiological studies of human populations around the world, past and present, have found little incidence of heart disease among peoples whose diets consist chiefly of foods low in calories, saturated fats, and cholesterol. Conversely, a high incidence of atherosclerosis always accompanies diets high in calories, saturated fats, and cholesterol.

THE FRAMINGHAM STUDY

"Heart: Attack" documents a study begun in 1948 to determine the cause or causes of heart diseases. In 1948, a group of heart specialists and medical technicians turned the town of Framingham, Massachusetts, into a "human laboratory" for the most extensive mass study of coronary heart disease ever undertaken. Five thousand townspeople, men and women with no apparent heart disease and no clinical signs of atherosclerosis at the outset, volunteered as subjects. For twelve years they continued in their normal, established ways of life, including dietary habits. Every four months, each volunteer underwent clinical tests for blood cholesterol level. Other parameters considered were blood pressure, weight loss and gain, lung capacity, and diabetes. In-depth medical interviews elicited extensive data on dietary habits, exercise and physical activity, smoking, tension and stress, and family history of heart disease. The resulting detailed medical profiles were cross-studied and statistically analyzed. A distinct and consistent pattern in the lives of heart victims became abundantly clear.

The Framingham study showed that men with a blood cholesterol level of 260 milligrams or higher suffered heart disease at *double* the rate of the general population, while those with a rate of only 200 had only *half* that of the general population. The risk of coronary disease steps up as cholesterol increases from low to high concentrations in the blood.

RISK FACTORS

High blood cholesterol was exposed as a chief conspirator in the epidemic of heart disease. It was not, however, the only one. In the great majority of heart-disease cases it worked in conjunction with one or more of eight other risk factors or was the result of them: high blood pressure, excess weight, overnutrition, diabetes, insufficient exercise, excessive smoking, extensive tension and stress, and heredity. Most of these factors are presented in detail in the second film, "Heart: Counterattack."

When there is reason to suspect hereditary heart disease, control of the other eight risk factors takes on greater importance. When hereditary tendency is certain, strict control becomes crucial. Interviewed in the film is Dr. Richard Casdorph, founder and director of the Casdorph Lipid Research Foundation, whose primary work is treating persons who suffer from a genetic blood fat abnormality called *hyperlipidemia*. This recently recognized inherited disease of the blood can cause premature atherosclerosis, heart attack, and death to thousands yearly and perhaps to many, many more. It is hoped that research into this and other areas of metabolic disorders may provide further understanding and control of heart disease.

The Heart: Counterattack

Every day, between 5,000 and 10,000 American men and women suffer heart attacks. More than 1,400 of these attacks are fatal. When the heart stops, the brain, deprived of blood flow, and therefore of oxygen, can survive for about four minutes. Unless circulation is restored in that time, the damage is irreparable, and death invariably results. About 40 percent of all first heart attacks are fatal, and 20 percent of the victims die within the first hour.

As both these films indicate, there are several factors that make people prone to heart attack. The ways of life in the industrialized nations of the Western world embody many social customs that lead to circulatory disorders. In nearly every case, a heart attack is the ultimate result of a combination of factors in the way the victim lives and has lived. Medical science has identified many of the causes of heart conditions. A potential victim, by fairly simple alterations in routine, can decrease the threat of heart disease.

The main areas in which people can act to reduce their risks of heart attack are related to diet, smoking, exercise, and stress.

DIET

In the film, noted heart specialist Jeremiah Stamler discusses the high-cholesterol, high-fat American diet. The foods most responsible for the build-up of atherosclerosis come from five main food groups:

high-fat meat products, high-fat dairy products, egg yolks, commercial baked goods excluding breads, and saturated fats (such as table spreads, shortening, and so on). Dr. Stamler recommends the deemphasizing of high-fat products in favor of those that are low in fat but nutritious: skim milk, cottage cheese, lean meat, substitution of egg whites for yolks, unsaturated oils.

Dr. Stamler suggests that the sources of the rising epidemic of heart disease lie in the enormous and widespread changes in the American way of life that have accompanied the spread of industrialization over the last several generations. Today's average American exercises little but still eats the heavy diet of his hard-working ancestors. Changes in life style also may have made heretofore latent hereditary weaknesses lethal and have brought new, damaging forms of tension and stress.

SMOKING

It can no longer be news to anyone that cigarette smoking imperils health. In addition to its association with lung cancer and emphysema, it gravely affects the entire cardiovascular system. It elevates serum cholesterol levels. Nicotine increases the work load of the heart. Carbon monoxide in inhaled tobacco smoke robs the heart of from 5 to 15 percent of its blood oxygen supply. These effects of smoking are immediate. Therefore, when one stops smoking, the benefits are immediate.

Because of such health concerns 10 million adults have quit smoking in the last four years, using a variety of methods. The film presents one such method, based on behavioral principles of positive reinforcement. It is based on the recognition that cigarette smoking is a *learned* habit. Therefore, cessation is a process of *re*-learning, whereby the patient teaches himself to be a nonsmoker. Therapy sessions utilizing this method are shown.

EXERCISE

One of the mixed blessings of the electronic age is that man's occupations and preoccupations become steadily more sedentary every year. Television creates not millions of weekend athletes, but millions of passive spectators. Other factors being equal, the sedentary man is twice as likely as the active man to develop heart disease. As is the case with high blood pressure, a sluggish circulation multiplies the chance for atherosclerotic occlusion of the arteries.

"Heart: Counterattack" shows executives of North American Rockwell participating in the heart fitness program established there ten years ago by Dr. Richard Morrison. Dr. Morrison explains the dynamics of exercise specifically designed for coronary needs and discusses jogging and bicycling, contrasting their effects on the cardiovascular system with those of weightlifting.

Dr. Morrison and other researchers into the physiology of exercise are interested in the possibility that exercise may open up certain tiny collateral vessels to the heart that, in the event of an attack, may provide enough oxygen to save the victim's life.

STRESS

The tension and stress of modern life are thought to have many adverse effects on the heart and cardiovascular system. Dr. Ray H. Rosenman, in an interview, explains that while the classical risk factors concerned with diet and nutrition, high blood pressure, inactivity, and smoking are associated with atherosclerosis, significant numbers of those with atherosclerosis never suffer heart attack. A ten-year study of 4,000 men in various professions confirms his hypothesis that heart attack is primarily emotional in origin.

Dr. Rosenman and his colleague, Dr. Meyer Friedman, in the course of their study have detected a behavior pattern in those predisposed to heart attack. He describes Type A, the prone type, and the psychological test-interview devised to distinguish Type A from Type B persons, who seem immune to heart attack even when high in the other risk factors. He produces and elucidates a graph showing correlated statistics on heart attack in terms of Type A and Type B.

Dr. Rosenman concludes that Type A people can modify their behavior to reduce the amount of stress in their lives, thus reducing their risks of sustaining a heart attack or other stress-induced disorders.

Dependence: A New Definition

Although the term *dependence* has often been used synonymously with addiction and habituation, this motion picture looks beyond constricting categories of "normal" and "abnormal" to seek an approach to the similarities of cause and effect that underlie all forms of dependence, healthy and unhealthy alike.

"Dependence" projects a view of all human beings as living in a fundamental state of dependence. The panorama of dependency thus extends over not only such abnormal patterns of behavior as alcoholism, drug addiction, compulsive eating, anxiety neurosis, and aggressive behavior, but over a variety of normal patterns of everyday living.

This film takes an unusual modular approach to natural dependence. With the assistance of feedback from the memory banks of a highly versatile computer, the film manages to transcend time and place and treat the subject matter as if it were a matrix of interrelated and mutually dependent points. The flexibility of this approach allows for coverage of a wider range of topics than one might expect.

BIOLOGICAL RHYTHMS

One area of normal living that suggests a dependency relationship is that of naturally occurring rhythms—the biological clock. The human body responds in countless ways to patterns in the environment. Solar periods can be traced in the operation of the liver, blood, urine, adrenal glands, and many diseases. Vulnerability to drugs, poisons, and pain are directly affected. Lunar and annual rhythms, too, hold sway over plants and animals.

Among other areas in which the film shows normal dependency relationships are gestation, birth, and postnatal development. Man's hereditary nature is the product of evolutionary processes reaching back perhaps 5 billion years. He has evolved with certain predetermined needs and phyllogenetic considerations that must be understood in a context of natural dependence. The film touches on considerations of maternal nutrition, birth trauma, intrauterine memory, parental vigilence, affectional response in primates, and that most amazing evolutionary gift, the human brain.

THE BRAIN

Perhaps man's ultimate dependence state is in relation to his brain: it has to carry and constantly recode an immense amount of complicated information. When this requirement of data storage is coupled with the requirement that the involved brain molecules replenish themselves every seven weeks, one can begin to see just how dependent man is upon the accurate and complete transfer of information to new molecules—repeatedly. This critical drama seems to take place during the REM phase of sleep (see text, Chapter 18). If the natural rhythms of sleep are disrupted, this all-important process of information rehearsal is endangered.

What does a human being depend upon for health during infancy and early childhood? To answer this complex question CRM's cameras turned to a conceptual model of infancy based upon Freud's theories of infantile sexuality. This basic approach to dependence helps spotlight crucial moments at which dependency needs go unfulfilled.

When people fail to satisfy their original needs and desires, primitive exaggerations of dependence often develop. If they cannot find ways to fulfill the powerful demands of their bodies and minds, they may sink into a state of pathological dependence that will rob them of the things they value most in life.

The film concludes that physical and psychological health arise only through the fulfillment of natural dependencies and the judicious substitution of healthy dependences for unhealthy ones.

Alcoholism: A Model of Drug Dependence

The concept of dependence as an omnipresent phenomenon fundamental to the human condition helps to explain why so many instances of pathological dependency occur. When natural dependency needs are not fulfilled, for whatever reason, they cause constant and intense suffering. If the need is physiological, the body will demand to be satisfied. Psychological unfulfillment will give rise to deep cravings and lusts that cannot be satiated because they are disguised, and their origins resist detection.

With a flair for joining the intimate loneliness of the dependency sufferer to the panoramic range of abuse in America, this cinematic essay focuses closely on the alcoholic as a paradigm of dependence pathology. Alcohol ranks as the fourth most serious health problem after heart disease, cancer, and mental illness. When one considers the devastation that alcohol helps to produce outside the body, as on the street and highway, he can begin to appreciate the wide range of lethal implications alcoholism has for user and nonuser alike.

DRUG ABUSE

Before taking up the particular problems of the alcoholic, the film surveys drug abuse as a general social phenomenon. Distinguishing between drug use and abuse, the film continues to explore the mechanisms of addiction and habituation, making clear comparisons and contrasts with the aid of a chemical analysis of euphoria, tolerance, and withdrawal.

A virtual epidemic of drug abuse is now occurring in America. In addition to abuse of narcotics, stimulants, amphetamines, and barbiturates, the devastations of smoking and obesity fall into this category of dependence pathology.

The film pays special attention to the effects of intoxication. Many factors influence the effects of alcohol upon the system: time and speed of ingestion, circadian rhythms, condition of the digestive track, and others. Consideration must be given to the role of carbon dioxide as a stimulus to faster diffusion of alcohol in the body and as a tranquilizer to the pyloric muscle controlling flow of alcoholic substances to the small intestine.

Recent biochemical research has brought forth substantial evidence that alcohol addiction is similar to, if not identical to, opiate addiction. Researchers studying metabolic changes in a biogenic amine called dopamine demonstrated that acetaldehyde, the primary metabolite of alcohol, inhibits an enzyme that governs the normal breakdown of dopamine; as a result of this inhibition, the metabolism of dopamine follows an alternate, rarely used metabolic pathway, resulting in the production of a substance also found as an intermediate step in the synthesis of morphine from opium. The film covers this exciting new research and visualizes the experiments that provide evidence that alcohol causes morphinelike and codeinelike substances to be produced in brain cells.

SLEEP

Only recently has it been possible to combine data about the biochemical mechanism of alcohol addiction with discoveries about the role of sleep in human physiology and psychology. Drug-withdrawal psychosis seems to be directly related to sleep deprivation. After a mere forty-eight hours of sleeplessness, the human body produces a stress-responsive chemical also found in the LSD family of drugs.

The film presents the results of current sleep

research: Stages of sleep as recorded on the electroencephalograph (EEG) give insight to delta sleep, rapid-eye-movement sleep, and the relationship between alpha waves and "microsleep."

All drugs disrupt the normal rhythmic patterns of dream activity, suggesting similar disruptions of sleep, upon which all people depend for mental and physical health. One exception, LSD, has been found to restore healthy sleep to those who have been deprived.

The film also presents part of the controversial history of LSD therapy with chronic alcoholics as conducted on government grant by psychiatrist Robert Lynch and his colleagues. No therapy has proven as effective as Alcoholics Anonymous, however. This amazing organization, since its beginnings in 1939, has helped thousands of chronic alcoholics to regain their self-respect and to begin to rehabilitate themselves through an ongoing commitment to the Twelve Steps of AA. Their goal is simple: sobriety; and nearly 50 percent of the people who have turned to AA have achieved their purpose through the effective substitution of healthy dependencies for unhealthy ones.